HANDBOOK OF

BIOGENERIC THERAPEUTIC PROTEINS

REGULATORY, MANUFACTURING, TESTING, AND PATENT ISSUES

HANDBOOK OF

BIOGENERIC THERAPEUTIC PROTEINS

REGULATORY, MANUFACTURING, TESTING, AND PATENT ISSUES

Sarfaraz K. Niazi, Ph.D.

CEO, Pharmaceutical Scientist, Inc.
Chicago, Illinois

Foreign Professor
HEJ Research Institute of Chemistry
Karachi University

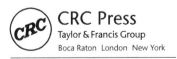

CRC Press
Taylor & Francis Group
Boca Raton London New York

CRC Press is an imprint of the
Taylor & Francis Group, an **informa** business

A TAYLOR & FRANCIS BOOK

First published 2006 by Taylor & Francis

Published 2019 by CRC Press
Taylor & Francis Group
6000 Broken Sound Parkway NW, Suite 300
Boca Raton, FL 33487-2742

© 2006 by Taylor & Francis Group, LLC
CRC Press is an imprint of Taylor & Francis Group, an Informa business

First issued in paperback 2019

No claim to original U.S. Government works

ISBN 13: 978-0-367-45481-4 (pbk)
ISBN 13: 978-0-8493-2991-3 (hbk)

Visit the Taylor & Francis Web site at
http://www.taylorandfrancis.com

and the CRC Press Web site at
http://www.crcpress.com

Library of Congress Cataloging-in-Publication Data

Niazi, Sarfaraz, 1949-
    Handbook of biogeneric therapeutic proteins : regulatory, manufacturing, testing, and patent issues / by Sarfaraz K. Niazi.
        p. ; cm.
    Includes bibliographical references and index.
    ISBN 0-8493-2991-4 (alk. paper)
    1. Protein drugs. 2. Generic drugs. 3. Recombinant proteins. 4. Pharmaceutical biotechnology industry.
I. Title.
    [DNLM: 1. Recombinant Proteins--therapeutic use. 2. Drug Industry. 3. Technology, Pharmaceutical.
QU 55 N577h 2005]

RS431.P75N53 2005
338.4'76153--dc22   2005040597

Library of Congress Card Number 2005040597

Dedicated to Gulzar Begum, whose teachings that nature does nothing in vain helped me appreciate the beauty in E. coli.

Foreword

When the International Center for Genetic Engineering and Biotechnology (ICGEB) was established in 1984 and later came under the auspices of the United Nations in 1987, the primary goals of the charter of the center were to assist developing countries in exploiting biotechnology to solve their indigenous problems and to foster international cooperation and research in the field of biotechnology. Today, with the membership of around 70 countries, the ICGEB is bringing remarkable benefits to the economies of the developing world by helping them in every area of the application of biotechnology and preparing them to comply with the standards of biosafety and responsible science. It is in this light of the charter of ICGEB that I view the book, *Handbook of Biogeneric Therapeutic Proteins: Regulatory, Manufacturing, Testing, and Patent Issues*, by Dr. Sarfaraz K. Niazi, a significant milestone in furthering the applications of biotechnology, in this case, the manufacturing of recombinant therapeutic proteins, throughout the world.

One of the greatest breakthroughs in the field of biotechnology came in the third quarter of the past century when scientists were able to clone the gene and combine it with host DNA to produce the desired target molecules; the recombinant technology was thus born and the first endogenous hormone that benefited millions of patients around the world was insulin. Indeed, today, the only major source of insulin is recombinant manufacturing in *E. coli*. However, the recombinant techniques became useful only after the U.S. Supreme Court ruling that a recombinant bacteria or a life form can be patented; since then, scores of endogenous molecules have been produced by recombinant techniques to bring relief to mankind for diseases that were once thought of as incurable. Indeed the mortality from the diseases related to deficiency of endogenous hormones and other proteins of patients has significantly decreased; yet, these drugs remain very expensive, due mainly to high investment required to manufacturing these drugs but also to patent protection given to these drugs, creating supply monopolies. All of this is about to change as the patents on many of these molecules are beginning to expire and an inevitable competition from the generic drug industry is about to become a reality. Nowhere would this impact be felt more palpably than in the developing world, where patients can ill afford these drugs because of a lack of organized health care systems in many developing countries. The teachings in the book you hold in your hand should go a long way in helping generic companies worldwide establish more efficient manufacturing systems while delivering a comparable quality product at a fraction of the price of the current innovator products. This should deliver a better quality of life and therefore an overall reduction in health care costs worldwide, one of the most serious concerns of global health care organizations such as the United Nations and the World Health Organization.

The *Handbook of Biogeneric Therapeutic Proteins* is the first comprehensive treatise on every aspect of manufacturing recombinant drugs; it is remarkable how such a large volume of information has been condensed in just a few hundred pages. Obviously, this is a handbook, not a textbook; therefore, the emphasis remains on practical applications rather than the theories behind the processes and methods. However, it is inevitable not to discuss some theory when describing these details. The book provides just the right balance between science and practical applications.

Chapter 1, "The Frontiers of Biotechnology," is a global view of the beginning or the roots of biotechnology leading to today's cloning techniques; while describing the new and novel applications, Dr. Niazi begins with a discussion of how biotechnology is interpreted worldwide, as a preamble to how "biogeneric" or "biosimilar" or "follow-on" products will be dealt with in the future. Given in this chapter are details of historic developments in the field of biotechnology that led to the deployment of various new modalities of therapy. At the end of the chapter there is an interesting timeline starting thousands of years B.C. all the way to 2004. It makes an interesting and rather amusing reading.

Chapter 2, "Marketing Opportunities," describes or rather lures generic companies into entering the market of biogeneric medicines; with a substantially higher growth in the market of biological products vis-à-vis chemically derived drugs, the financial rewards are indeed lucrative. A significant discussion in this chapter hovers around the politics, or more appropriately, the tussle, between the big pharmaceuticals and the generic counterpart in the industry. This is reminiscent of the fights that went on in the early 1980s prior to the establishment of Waxman-Hatch amendment in the U.S. that legalized generic drugs. Dr. Niazi predicts that should the regulatory authorities fail to develop guidelines to approve generic biological drugs in a timely basis, the governments will enforce this through legislative changes. The driving force behind this move is entirely the economics of health care. The arguments presented in the chapter include scientific rationale on proving similarity of products, the legal jurisdiction of regulatory authorities, and the case law that allows for approval of generic biological products. The marketing survey provided in this chapter also lists prominent patent expiries and literally lays out a business model for a potential generic manufacturer. An appendix to the book that is referred to in this chapter is an exhaustive information database on every approved therapeutic protein that is currently on the market. This encyclopedic information includes details on the formulation of products as well and should serve as a ready reference for all those involved in the manufacturing and marketing of therapeutic proteins.

Chapter 3, "Manufacturing Overview," is the largest chapter in the book and provides a broader view of the entire manufacturing process, from gene cloning to packaging of finished product in GMP environment; also included in this chapter are details regarding biosafety considerations. A prospective manufacturer should be able to get a fairly good idea of the scope of the entire technology, which is pivotal to manufacturing recombinant drugs. An important aspect of this general chapter on manufacturing is the practical advice interspersed throughout, amid regulatory guidelines. Establishing recombinant drug manufacturing can be a daunting task, as it requires much greater understanding of science, establishing higher standards of environmental controls, requiring more intense training of personnel, and a need to continuously improve and monitor the processes, than what is generally required in traditional chemical-based pharmaceutical manufacturing. The amount of science needed to manufacture therapeutic proteins is generally not available at traditional generic pharmaceutical manufacturers, and the biotechnology companies more used to gene cloning exercises may not have strong enough regulatory compliance attitudes; as a result, many mergers between pharmaceutical and biotech companies have not fared well. The chapter on the general aspects of manufacturing of therapeutic proteins should be read by the top management just as intensely as it deserves to be read by the scientists and technicians working on the floor if the divide between the need for science and the need for compliance is to be met effectively.

Chapter 4, "Genetically Modified Cells," deals with methods on creating generically modified cells, bacteria, yeast, mammalian cells, insect cells, and transgenic animals. This chapter makes certain basic assumptions that the reader is well aware of, such as, the basic technology of gene cloning, the use of vectors, and selection of host systems; however, when I examined the extensive glossary of terms included as an appendix to the book, it became clear to me that even novices in the field should be able to understand the science described in the chapter with the help of this voluminous, encyclopedic appendix. Therefore, this chapter should prove useful for both the experienced scientists and the novice technicians. In this chapter, the emphasis is placed on a comparative evaluation of the various expression systems available; this chapter, however, should not be viewed as a complete guide to creating genetically modified cells, despite the support information, particularly the availability of canned systems by commercial suppliers, provided. In all likelihood, a generic pharmaceutical manufacturer is less likely to work on this phase of development in-house; the expertise required for this purpose is generally not available to traditional generic manufacturers. At ICGEB we deal with these issues on a daily basis and find that creation of genetically modified cells remains somewhat of an art despite the remarkable advances made in the science and the availability of newer tools. Unless a manufacturer is willing to make a substantial investment, the construction of GMCs is best left to well-equipped biotechnology companies or institutions. This is also the advice given by Dr. Niazi in this book. Additionally, we now face another problem — of biosafety standard compliance. Whereas, any material that comes in contact with a genetically modified cell should be properly decontaminated, the issues in the creation of GMCs can be difficult to address and accidents have happened in the past where modified cells with random gene insertions have been released into the environment at great potential for peril to the public. It should be remembered that the science of GMC creation is fast changing with the availability of newer techniques, and the need to induct safer organisms, such as the use of yeast, is becoming more popular though *E. coli*, which with all of its disadvantages, remains the workhorse of the industry. This is because of a thorough understanding of the genetic structure of the organism, its robustness, and ease of handling. The use of mammalian cells, though essential for some molecules requiring posttranslational modification, is severely disadvantaged because of the issue of viral contamination. Whereas the current ICH guidelines on characterization of cell lines are extensive, a clean cell line does not necessarily allow reducing the steps related virus clearance and decontamination. We have worked for years on solving these problems and find that the process development should be more intensely studied and validated. The more recent recommendations of the U.S. FDA and EMEA in statistical testing of critical parameters can be very expensive to implement, yet, when it comes to handling GMCs, it is advisable that the manufacturers make this investment in time and money upfront to allow them to streamline and optimize the processes in later manufacturing stages. Each of the type of cell lines has its own disadvantage, from endotoxins to contamination with prions, and handing these problems at the very initial steps is highly recommended. Another aspect related to creation of GMCs is their robustness over a period of time. It often takes several hundred passes before we know how stable a cell line we have in our possession, and that requires time and extensive studies supporting the thesis to outsource the job of construction of GMCs where possible to induct a time-tested cell line instead of creating a new one.

Chapter 5, "Upstream Processing," deals with unit operations that start the manufacturing process. This chapter is an overview of these manufacturing systems with a follow up on specific systems in the next chapter. The basics of bacterial fermentation types, mammalian cell secretion systems, yeast systems, insect cells, and transgenic animals are described in sufficient detail to give the reader a good understanding of the difficulties incumbent in each process. With a broader choice of upstream systems available today, from roller bottles to wave reactors to cell cubes, and the fact that GMCs can be modified to provide optimal performance in any of these systems, the selection process has become more difficult. The bigeneric manufacturer, however, faces a different type of dilemma than that faced by the innovator companies; the regulatory risk of modifying an approved system is too large for the generic manufacturers, even though it may compromise the cost of production. A case in point, as described by Dr. Niazi, is the manufacturing of erythropoietin; originally approved for manufacturing in roller bottles, a process that continues to be used by the innovators, the generic manufacturer may not have the liberty of switching to perhaps more efficient systems since this will require a validation exercise that the biogeneric manufacturer may not be able to make.

Chapter 6, "Manufacturing Systems," deals with each of the most popular systems, from bacterial to transgenic animals, in sufficient details. For each of the system, this chapter describes the method of creating the genetically modified cells and offers extensive reference to commercial sources of products available for the purpose. I agree with Dr. Niazi that where proprietary and intellectual property considerations do not hinder, one should consider use of these commercial systems as they have been thoroughly tested and tried in a variety of circumstances and applications; in addition, the supplier of these systems often have a large database to assist the developer in many phases of development. Obviously, the choice of expression system chosen will depend to a great deal on the system that was originally chosen by the innovator. Over a period of decades the technology has evolved and the expression systems have become more efficient, for example, the use of fusion systems has remarkably changed the final yield and cost of production; these systems may not have been available to the innovators when they created their GMC and patented it. The question arises whether the generic manufacturer should choose an archaic system or risk the cost of additional validation by choosing a smarter systems; I will prefer to use a more efficient system, as the overall cost of production may actually be lower even if it requires higher investment in the beginning. This chapter uses a similar format for each expression system, wherein both upstream and downstream processing are described, including efforts to optimize the systems with appropriate in-process controls; monoclonal antibodies are discussed in the mammalian cell section. Extensive treatment of viral clearance and decontamination is included in the chapter as well. Whereas the world is yet to see a useful products made from insect cells and transgenic animals, a broad discussion of these two types is included here, perhaps projecting that these systems will offer considerable commercial advantages in the future.

Chapter 7, "Downstream Processing," is an extension of the previous chapter, wherein the steps in downstream processing for each of the expression systems are dealt with in greater detail. Extensive discussion of the chromatographic techniques used and the selection of buffers and processing conditions are discussed with respect to different types of proteins to establish a rationale between the type of protein and the selection of downstream processing steps. Whereas most downstream purification steps will make use of at least three unit operations, their choice will determine whether a product is cost-effective to produce; minimizing the number of steps is the key to not only optimizing the cost but also to the quality of product and the yield obtained; each step strains the protein and reduces yield. Given the fact that two-third of the cost of production goes into downstream processing, this chapter is of greatest significance to the generic manufacturers; comparative analysis, extensive tabulation, and broad choice offered in this chapter should be carefully read and evaluated. Of interest is the discussion about the expanded bed technology that can combine several steps in the purification process and the use of chromatographic techniques to reduce the viral burden.

Chapter 8, "Purification Techniques," is a detailed review of the unit operations used in downstream processing; a lot of practical details, identification of specific equipment, media, and supplies, make this chapter indeed very practical and a useful read for all those who want to develop a new process or to improve on an existing method.

Chapter 9, "Quality Assurance Systems," is a large and intensive chapter description of the evolving philosophy in ensuring quality of biological products; the current theme that the quality must be built into and not just tested in the products is explained in greater detail, including statistical models used to validate the choice and the range of critical parameters. Whereas quality assurance is the key element of all GMP regulations, when it comes to biological products, the importance of a good question-answer system is decidedly more critical mainly because we still do not fully understand the complex interplay between the large number of parameters that govern the manufacturing process of biological products; take, for example, the process of bacterial fermentation vis-à-vis chemical synthesis of a complex molecule. The number of parameters involved in a biological process is by far more and their interactivity is determined only by empirical methods; in a chemical synthesis the rules are clearly laid out. This chapter, therefore, presents a much desired reading into developing quality systems for biological manufacturing; this should be of equal importance to pharmaceutical manufacturers entering biological manufacturing and biotechnology companies or institutions planning a GMP-based manufacturing process.

Chapter 10, "Quality Control Systems," is a classic section on testing of biological products; some of the purification techniques described under manufacturing are also used on a different scale and with different perspective in the testing of products. The aim of testing products is to control the quality since obviously not all units produced will be tested; therefore, the methods should be statistically validated and established for robustness. This chapter describes in detail the testing of products in accordance with the pharmacopoeia requirements. More attention is given in this chapter to such complex issues as identifying the various physical forms and chemical degradants of proteins as well as testing for viral and adventitious agent contamination. Again, pharmaceutical manufacturers used to testing sterile products may find several new elements of caution here as they handle proteins. For example, studies have shown that if erythropoietin solution is shaken, it may result in a change in its structure to a point where it can become more immunogenic; such is not the case for many chemical-based testing procedures.

Chapter 11, "Regulatory Affairs," is where this book provides a unique insight not just for the biogeneric companies but also for the regulatory authorities. The regulatory issues related to therapeutic proteins are complex, and most of the confusion is caused by the difficulties in defining what a biogeneric product is. A lot of politics and business pressures have further confounded the issue. The only question that is raised by the regulatory authorities today is whether it is possible to manufacture an exact copy of an innovator product without having to go through detailed evaluation. Two observations must be made: first, the innovator product is indeed a copy of a natural product and the generic product is a copy of the copy. (If a generic manufacturer tries to copy the original, this will not qualify for a generic application.) Obviously, by approving the first copy the agencies have admitted that it is possible to make an exact copy of the endogenous protein. Now after years of use, wherein, I am sure not all batches produced by the innovators were exactly the same, though they certainly fell within the range of parameters determined by the manufacturer. If a generic manufacturer is allowed to stay within that range of parameters, would this not be similar to what the innovator does? However, the argument is not played out so simply. The in-process control parameters that the innovator follows are either known to the manufacturer or to the regulatory authorities; they consider it proprietary information. Though there are no patents involved, this does fall under the rubric of intellectual property, nevertheless. However, how much the regulatory authorities should rely on their knowledge of the system when reviewing a generic application remains to be determined. The innovators claim that the process makes the product and the generic manufacturer claims that the product is well defined and the process is not critical; a support to the argument comes from the example of growth hormone that is produced by all different methods yet ending up with the exact same product. Europe is moving fast with establishing guidelines for biogeneric filings and has allowed its first such filing in October 2004 for interferon alpha; the U.S. FDA will soon follow the lead and once guidelines have been put in place, the race to biogeneric manufacturing will heat up. It is at this juncture that I believe this book will prove handy in resolving many logistics and technical issues.

Chapter 12, "Intellectual Property Issues," is a long chapter on patenting, particularly pharmaceutical products and pointedly biological products; Dr. Niazi being a patent agent with the U.S. Patent and Trademark office, brings a rare insight for scientists; he insists that scientists should educate themselves on the technical aspects of patenting to give themselves a better vision of what has been invented and more so on how to go around inventing — a most critical step for biogeneric manufacturers. However, I believe the depth and breadth of this chapter should be of equally great value to innovator scientists as well. It is fascinating how the difference in the patent laws between the U.S. and the rest of the world make it so difficult to properly evaluate if a product is out of patent or not. For a generic manufacturer, it is not just the molecule but the various steps involved in the upstream and downstream processing that must be individually evaluated to ensure that no patents are infringed, because there are just so many patents out there.

The appendices to this book make this book an encyclopedia; an exhaustive glossary of terms, a detail on each and every therapeutic protein currently used in humans and a long bibliography referring to each chapter consolidates the robustness of this treatise. Whereas it is not possible to acknowledge every source of information and to properly quote in a book of this size, Dr. Niazi has chosen to list the references for each of the chapters separately. I am very pleased to see a book on a very complex and difficult issue condensing most useful practical advice into just a few hundreds pages. Those who are interested in exploring further would find the bibliography very useful and the other appendices should serve as a daily reference for scientists as well as marketing personnel.

It was a pleasure to review this book by Dr. Niazi, who has an eloquent style of expression and ability to condense a large volume of data into a lucid format; I hope that more people will benefit from this emerging field of biotechnology through this book and from the experience of Dr. Niazi in the field. I am particularly hopeful that those in the developing world, which is our major focus at ICGEB, will benefit from the timely, up-to-date information provided in this book to develop products that are now off patent and make these products available to the public at a price they can afford while maintaining the quality standards. I hope that prospective manufacturers will gain much from the discussion of quality systems in the book and accordingly build facilities that are of the highest standards; this is the only way to ensure the safety of biological products.

Professor Francisco Baralle
Trieste, Italy

Professor Francisco Baralle is the second director general of the International Center for Genetic Engineering and Biotechnology (ICGEB) in Trieste, Italy, since the inception of the institute under a charter of the United Nations in 1984. Professor Baralle heads hundreds of scientists worldwide in developing applications of biotechnology to resolve endogenous problems of the developing countries. He has made substantial contributions to the science of molecular biology, proteomics, and recombinant techniques. A former professor of pathology at the University of Oxford, member of Magdalen College, elected member of the Molecular European Biology Organization, Professor Baralle has pioneered cloning techniques and developed several new biological drugs. The ICGEB also provides extensive training in the field of constructing genetically modified cells and offers assistance in the field of recombinant therapeutic protein manufacturing.

Preface

Therapeutic proteins are essential indigenous molecules, which are administered as supplements to individuals who have developed deficiencies of these proteins. Historically, these proteins were extracted from biological fluids at a very large cost and it was impossible to supply them in sufficient quantity. Now, as a result of the development of recombinant DNA techniques, therapeutic proteins are widely used, savings millions of lives. With the first recombinant DNA product, insulin, the doors opened wide for a new class of drugs to emerge about 25 years ago. With the U.S. Supreme Court ruling that life forms can be patented, drug companies rushed to create hosts that will produce a variety of therapeutic proteins. The intellectual property protection on the techniques of recombinant manufacturing also created one of the largest monopolies in the history of drug therapy — a $10 billion molecule, erythropoietin, owned by one company. Such monopolies created over the past two decades are fast crumbling as the patents have begun expiring on some of the most widely sold therapeutic proteins.

Generally, the biotechnology companies have fared well, achieving sales of over half a million dollars per employee, compared to about one-half that in traditional pharmaceutical companies. The recombinant therapeutic protein market is projected to be a $60 billion industry from the current $40 billion market share; this has stirred great interest in manufacturing therapeutic proteins by pharmaceutical companies. Through buyouts of biotechnology companies, pharmaceutical companies are fast securing their presence in this dramatic market expansion, though not all mergers have been successful. It is also anticipated that generic biological products will soon become reality, stiff opposition by the big pharmaceutical companies and their political lobbying organizations notwithstanding. However, the regulatory authorities are cautious in approving generic versions of these drugs.

Most recently, in October 2004, a Swiss biopharmaceuticals company BioPartners filed its first application in Europe for a generic version of interferon alpha, a biological drug. If approved, the "biosimilar" could be on the market as early as next year. This development comes shortly after the U.S. government turned down an application to market Omnitrope (somatropin), a generic version of recombinant human growth hormone developed by Sandoz, citing problems in establishing an appropriate regulatory route for biogeneric products. Last year, the European Parliament approved new pharmaceutical legislation that, among other things, set out a legal framework for the registration of so-called biosimilars, biological therapies that are therapeutically the same as existing, approved biological products. Sandoz had also filed for approval with the European Medicines Evaluation Agency (EMEA) for Omnitrope, but was unable to process the application.

Some of the largest-selling biological drugs developed during the first phase of the biotechnology revolution in the 1980s, including hGH, interferon alpha, and insulin, have patent protection opening opportunities for generic companies to compete, but only if a regulatory route to market can be worked out. To date, the development of the market for biosimilar drugs outside regions with less stringent intellectual property protection such as Asia has been patchy, to say the least. Last year, SICOR (now part of Teva) gained approval in Lithuania for a generic version of granulocyte colony stimulating factor (G-CSF), the active principle in Genentech's Neupogen (filgrastim) drug for treating neutropenia in patients undergoing cytotoxic cancer chemotherapy. Meanwhile, other companies, for example Wockhardt (with erythropoietin) and GeneMedix (with granulocyte macrophage colony stimulating factor or GM-CSF), have concentrated on Asian markets until such time as a route to market for these drugs in the U.S. and Europe opens up. China and Korea are widely distributing therapeutic protein products to unregulated markets.

The U.S. FDA (Food and Drug Administration) and European Medicines Evaluation Agency (EMEA) are in the process of establishing guidelines to approve biological drugs, particularly therapeutic proteins. The European guidelines are likely to be released sooner than the FDA guidelines. In September 2004, the FDA called its first public hearing session to establish certain ground rules, including how these drugs should be addressed, for example, as biogenerics or follow-on biologicals. While there is fierce opposition to generic biologicals by the brand name leaders as represented by the Biotechnology Industry Organization (BIO) group (http://bio.org), the U.S. Congress is reviewing the laws to amend them to allow generic entry for generic biological products. This unique situation arises because biological products are not included in the Waxman-Hatch amendment that created the category of bioequivalent generic pharmaceutical products. Back in the mid-1980s, therapeutic proteins were too new to be considered serious drugs, and few understood the nature of these molecules, let alone could draw guidelines on proving their bioequivalence. Therapeutic proteins are approved under a Biological License Application (BLA) in the U.S., while only approvals under Section 505 are subject to generic evaluation despite the fact that therapeutic proteins are now under the purview of the Center for Drug Evaluation and Research (CDER, which handles Section 505 filings) and not under the Center for Biologics Evaluation and Research (CBER, where BLAs were handled) and despite the fact that some biologicals were approved as drugs and not as biologicals; all of this has created an extremely confusing scenario, legally, logistically, and above all, morally.

The innovators are insisting that when it comes to biological products, process defines the product, and since they have exclusive knowledge of the process (as perfected over years), there can be no generic equivalent for these drugs. Some enthusiastic orators representing big pharmaceuticals have declared biogeneric as an oxymoron. The generic manufacturers on the other hand cite an example of a human growth hormone that had been approved from several host sources (not as generic) for years, but which resulted in an identical product. The FDA claims that it does not have the tools to evaluate generic equivalence, while, at the same time, it allows the innovator to change the entire process, every step of it, including the host system, and still requires any additional clinical data to approve these changes under the Comparability Protocol (most appropriately, paradox). Since a lot of planning by generic companies hinges on how this Protocol is interpreted, this issue will be discussed throughout the book, to provide tools to the industry to make a successful generic filing. An opinion written by the author on the issue of biosimilar drug approvals is available through the US FDA dockets at: www.fda.gov/ohrms/dockets/dockets/04n0355/04N-0355-EC-9-Attach-1.pdf.

Given the strong political impetus behind the fact that the technology is well caught up with the needs to develop tools to answer the questions the regulatory authorities may raise, it is inevitable that the FDA and EMEA will soon allow biogeneric products, though the entry would most likely be first for those products that have been on the market the longest and wherein sufficient data exist that safety is not a major issue; this will comprise simpler nonglycosylated products, readily expressed and purified. My guess is that the first biogeneric approved by the FDA would be insulin and growth hormone, followed by interferons and filgrastim and finally those products that require translational modification such as epoetin.

In approving biogeneric products, the primary safety concern that the regulatory authorities will have is the immunogenicity of the product; since the purpose of generic approval is to reduce the cost of development by not requiring extensive clinical trials, the issue of immunogenicity evaluation has taken roots in the minds of regulatory authorities as an irresolvable issue. The irony is that even when full-blown clinical trials are conducted, such as in the approval of a new BLA or an NDA, the number of subjects tested is not enough to detect the potential for immunogenicity; in other words, even if the second entry sponsor were required to submit a new NDA or BLA, the issue of immunogenicity will still not be resolved. In fact, in every approval granted for a new BLA or NDA, it has always been the postmarketing studies that have identified immunogenicity. However, this argument does not fair well with innovators who continue to insist that they have a better knowledge of the in-process controls that are essential to guarantee safety of products. There is indeed a certain merit to this argument, but only to the point where we can accept that the in-process controls and other proprietary techniques developed represent just *one* of the many ways to control process, not *the* only way. To lend more support to this thesis, it is often necessary to examine how fast the technology for upstream and downstream processing has advanced and how the newer methods of testing, not available at the time when the innovator products were approved two decade ago, can add significantly to safety evaluation of biogeneric products. For example, the following techniques were generally not available two decades ago:

- Deletion of protease genes or engineering for overexpression of rare-codon tRNAs, foldases, or chaperones.
- Gene multimerization as beneficial in improving production yields.
- Affinity fusions used to streamline purification process (fusion proteins).
- Modified isoelectric point (pI) and hydrophobic properties for improved downstream processing.
- Combinatorial protein engineering to generate tailor-made product-specific affinity ligands that will additionally allow less immunogenic yields. This strategy, which allows efficient recovery of a recombinant protein in its native form, is likely to be increasingly used in industrial-scale bioprocesses, since novel protein ligands have been described that can be sanitized using common industrial cleaning-in-place (CIP) procedures.
- Technical developments in the scaling of fermentation cycles using hollow membrane fibers, expanded bed systems; product-specific chromatographic media, and newer analytical testing procedures such as 2- and 3-D NMR (nuclear magnetic resonance), CD (circular dichroism), thermodynamic evaluation of 3- and 4-D presentation of molecules, etc., making it easier to manufacture and validate a safer product.

The most relevant inquiry today is whether an *in vitro* test can be constructed that would adequately predict immunogenicity. I believe a battery of tests that dwell on three-dimensional characterizations should be sufficient to eliminate any gross risks. In a recent approval by the FDA for darbepoietin alfa, the FDA was provided data wherein only one out of around 1600 patients showed significant antibody formation; the FDA was more interested in Amgen developing sensitive testing for levels of antibodies; however, the application was approved in the interim, but the levels reported into nanogram levels were found to be not low enough. This indicates the thinking of regulatory authorities wherein picogram level tests for antibodies would be required; given the available testing technologies, it is quiet possible to achieve these targets. What this example teaches us is that the regulatory authorities are willing to accept the risk posed by drugs like darbepoietin, which is a modified form of erythropoietin, and thus has a much larger risk factor, than to allow drugs that have been used in millions of patients with good safety record, only because there is no legal structure to allow this. In my opinion, this is a question of semantics, not science. As a result, I pontificate that biogeneric product will soon be a reality.

The *Handbook of Biogeneric Therapeutic Proteins* that you hold in your hand is the first comprehensive treatise written to review and analyze the status of technology, regulatory environment, and intellectual property issues — in brief, all that a manufacturer would need to plan development of biogeneric products and complete the process of regulatory filing. The book addresses the four major issues — manufacturing, regulatory, testing, and intellectual property — associated with the development of therapeutic protein drugs. As a comprehensive treatise, the book offers a complete description (as of the time of going to press) of every approved therapeutic protein, and it includes an extensive glossary of terms to assist researchers, product developers, regulatory personnel and authorities, intellectual property practitioners, and generic manufacturers in general to establish a firm understanding of these issues and prepare detailed plans and policies on developing generic versions of therapeutic proteins. The book is, however, not exhaustive, as this not possible given the complexities involved in establishing manufacturing of therapeutic proteins.

Hopefully this book proves useful in preparing regulatory applications for biogeneric products; however, companies need to evaluate their strengths and weaknesses when diversifying into the biotechnology arena if they are already not involved in it. Historically, mergers between pharmaceutical and biopharmaceutical companies have not fared well. Where the surviving company is the pharmaceutical company, it creates difficulty in understanding the elaborate scientific nature of production techniques; where the biopharmaceutical company survives the merger, the problems have been visualizing beyond the research horizon and translating the bioprocess into a commercially feasible, validated process. In my opinion, the best solutions are offered through outsourcing, as the technical requirements are highly specific and elaborate to manufacture these products in-house on a piece meal basis. Creation of gene construct and the genetically modified cell (or animal) is a different science than the science of fermentation and the science of downstream purification, and certainly it is quite different from routine pharmaceutical manufacturing of chemical-based drugs. Even the process of finishing the product, formulating the purified protein in a vial or ampule, requires a different understanding in controlling the process. For example, excessive stress to a protein solution can result in loss of structure or cause aggregation, both resulting in increased immunogenicity of the product; such awareness is not part of routine chemical drug manufacturing process.

It is difficult, if not impossible, for the generic company to carry the burden of all the diverse disciplines of manufacturing and finishing biological drugs under one roof. Limited financial resources, compressed timelines, and new regulatory constraints faced by the generic companies suggest that most companies would do well in outsourcing all phases of an active pharmaceutical ingredient (API) manufacturing and only keep the final filling operation in-house. My estimation shows that the cost per gram of therapeutic protein produced by a contractor may not be significantly higher than if produced in-house; this is a result of a rather large carrying cost of infrastructure, both in the manufacturing and testing phases, which is necessary to carry out the production. In a typical pharmaceutical manufacturing setup, any existing facilities and personnel are least likely to fit the new mold. Obviously, at some point when the sales justify, the entire process can be brought in-house; this is particularly important since there is no clear indication as to when the FDA would release its definitive guidelines. Waiting for these guidelines is a mistake, as the race after the guidelines will leave many companies way behind in the game. It is recommended that the companies start developing and characterizing their genetically modified cells now and complete initial guanosine monophosphate (GMP) production runs through a contract research organization (CRO) to get ready for the newer testing requirements that the FDA might impose. I have included in this book a list of possible CROs; the list is continuously growing and the companies are advised to make a thorough search to find the best fit. The purpose of listing CROs and also the suppliers of various instruments and supplies is to provide a quick reference and not necessarily an endorsement of any individual or a company.

In writing this practical book, I have sought and received help from many individuals and institutions; I would be remiss if I did not acknowledge them fully and completely. However, it would be impossible for me to acknowledge and recognize all. First and foremost, I am indebted to the International Center for Genetic Engineering and Biotechnology (ICGEB), a United Nation's organization located in Trieste, Italy, for providing ongoing interaction and knowledge about technology development and technology transfer. Professor Francisco Baralle, the director general of ICGEB, has been a good friend and mentor to me in this field. His kindness in writing a Foreword to this book is deeply appreciated. ICGEB is a premier institution that assists the developing world with solutions to indigenous problems using biotechnology and has pioneered recombinant engineering that is now widely and successfully used around the world. Dr. Sergio Tsiziminsky of the ICGEB is the chief architect of many genetically modified cells now widely used throughout the world; I had the distinct pleasure and honor of knowing him and working jointly to transfer the technology worldwide. Dr. Mojtaba Tabatabae is a great scientist, a good friend, and above all an expert who knows how to make cells express whenever he demands. I have learned a lot from him; Dr. Mohsen Nayebpour knows more about putting together a business plan for manufacturing therapeutic protein than most, and the remarkable success he has acquired in a very short time speaks largely about his understanding of science and art involved in the business of therapeutic protein manufacturing. Sam Trippie and Joe Ioppilleto know pharmaceutical manufacturing well, and it was a pleasure working with them in assisting them in their diversity of manufacturing interests. Jeff Yordon has been a long-time visionary friend who believes, with me, that biogenerics are just down the horizon; he has been a great motivator to me in the writing of this book. Jabbar Saya is a close friend who always appreciated my efforts and kept me motivated to finish the work. Abdul Razzaq Yousef is a renaissance man, one who scales mountains with ease. Dr. Riazuddin Shaikh of CEMB in Pakistan has been a good supporter of my efforts and I am highly thankful to him, just as I am indebted to Dr. Mojtaba Naqvi and Dr. Qasim Mehdi. Dr. Amy Rosenberg at the FDA is responsible for developing protocols to test immunogenicity of therapeutic proteins; her work will literally carve how the business of biogenerics explodes in U.S. and worldwide. I have met her several times and attended many of her detailed and lucid presentations on the subject; her talks have helped determine the focus of this book. When it comes to scientific leadership and innovation in education, Professor Attaur Rahman, a long-time friend and colleague, has been a role model for me. His recognition of my humble efforts and his encouragement, including appointing me to the Foreign Professorship at his prestigious research institute, is highly appreciated; Professor Iqbal Choudhary is a well-known and recognized scientist and visionary; his assistance to me has been exemplary.

The manufacturing of therapeutic proteins is made to look easy by scores of professional companies who have developed products, processes, and equipment that make it possible for novices like myself to practice this trade. Whereas I have benefited broadly from the information provided by these companies, this work would not have been possible without the consistent and out-of-the-way support granted to me by one of the clear leaders in the industry, Amersham (now GE Life Sciences). It is difficult for anyone to not come in contact with Amersham if they are in the business of therapeutic protein manufacturing; from the prepacked columns to expanded bed to gene construction, there is everything available in the famous Amersham catalog. The folks at Amersham who helped me beyond the call of duty were Frances Bach, Gregg Krueger, Linda Henry (Linda.henry@amersham.com), Hillevi Jansony (hillevi.janson@amersham.com), both associated with Amersham's Proteins Separations group. Hillevi and Linda coordinated support in allowing me to review their remarkable website at BioProcess (http://www.bioprocess.com), which is clearly the most important practical source for any manufacturer intending to enter biogeneric market. In this regard, my longtime friend Thomas Flynn III was always available to coordinate my access to useful data, processes, and material for my book, besides loading me up with tons of motivation to complete the manuscript as he kept telling me to put into practice what I was teaching others. Irwin Morris, when not riding his Harley, in his own friendly way gave me enough challenge and admiration to ride the difficult task of collecting and writing (and rewriting several times) the information contained in this book.

A book of this size could not be produced without the recognition and arduous support of the publisher. Stephen Zollo, senior editor at CRC Press, knows how to motivate authors, and I am indebted to him as well as others at CRC Press for taking on this task; thanks are also due to production editors at CRC Press, particularly Gail Renard, and others, without whose untiring effort this book could not have been completed and delivered on time. The editorial staff of CRC, with whom I have worked for years, has always been kind to me, perhaps realizing my shortcomings, and always demonstrated patience of remarkable proportion, for which I cannot be thankful enough.

Last, but not the least, I am thankful to scores of scientific and professional colleagues and particularly those whom I came to know through the landmark literature in the field but have never met. I may have quoted their work thinking subconsciously that the information was all in public domain; I hope they would excuse me for taking this liberty, as it would be impossible to recognize them adequately. An elaborate bibliography, as provided here, does not necessarily replace this obligation. Even though I have extensively benefited from published works, the errors, whatsoever remaining, and I am sure there will be many, are altogether mine. I would appreciate readers bringing these to my attention so that I may correct them in the future editions of the book. An e-mail in this regard to niazi@niazi.com will be highly appreciated.

I would be remiss if I did not acknowledge the continuous support, loyalty, and love of my wife, Anjum, who never complained of being ignored while I worked on this and several other books that took an inordinate amount of my time away from family. She is that part of genetic code that makes me write. The recombinant association — matrimony of more than 30 years ago — has been good to me.

Sarfaraz K. Niazi, Ph.D.
Deerfield, Illinois

About the Author

Professor Sarfaraz K. Niazi is the chief executive officer of Pharmaceutical Scientist Inc., a consulting company for the pharmaceutical and biotechnology industry (http://www.pharmsci.com). He is also Foreign Professor at the HEJ Research Institute of Chemistry at Karachi University in Pakistan. Professor Niazi has been involved in the licensing, technology transfer, process development, and turnkey pharmaceutical and therapeutic protein manufacturing operations worldwide. Professor Niazi is also licensed to practice patent law before the U.S. Patent and Trademark office and an inventor with scores of patents on new drugs and drug delivery systems. Professor Niazi has been teaching and conducting research for over 35 years and has authored over 100 research articles and written scores of books in the field of pharmaceutical and biotechnology manufacturing, pharmacokinetics, literature, and poetry. His most recent book, *Handbook of Pharmaceutical Manufacturing Formulations*, is a six-volume work, the largest of its kind ever published. Professor Niazi lives in Deerfield, Illinois, and Karachi, Pakistan.

Author's Comments

While I have made every effort to acknowledge contributions of others in writing this book, it is inevitable to have omitted many, particularly where general principles and guidance are discussed; I have benefited enormously from the literature and guidance provided by one of the most prominent leaders in the industry, Amersham Biosciences; without this support, this book could not have been made so comprehensive and useful to the industry and academia. Tables 3.2, 3.4, 3.5, 3.6, 4.1, 4.2, 4.6, 4.7, 4.8, 5.1, 6.1, 6.2, 6.3, 7.1, 7.3, 7.4, 7.5, 7.6, 7.9, 7.10, 8.2, 10.2, 10.3, 10.4, 10.5, 10.6, 10.7, 10.8, 10.9, 10.10, 10.11 and Figures 7.1, 8.1, 8.2, 9.2, and 9.3 are reproduced here courtesy of Amersham as they contain the data provided by Amersham. Amersham provides an extensive development tool at http://www.bioprocessguide.com, which is available on a licensing basis only from Amersham. The information contained in this source is updated every three months and represents an excellent means of evaluating the current state of the art in every aspect of manufacturing of therapeutic proteins and other biological products.

Similarly, I have benefited from the information provided by various equipment and supply vendors, particularly, Amersham, Pall, Sartorius, New Brunswick, Novogen, and many others. The guidance provided by BioMetics, a premier engineering firm in the field of biological manufacturing is highly appreciated. A large number of vendors are specifically mentioned in the book and their specific products recommended — this is always done as an example and not necessarily to endorse these specific products. The author has no vested interest in making any recommendation in this book.

List of Figures

List of Tables

Contents

1 The Frontiers of Biotechnology

INTRODUCTION

Man has done well utilizing other life forms to his own advantage. From the taming of the cattle to making recombinant therapeutic proteins using yeast, the history of man interacting with nature is full of great and exciting surprises, genius exploitation, and pursuit of solutions to problems of mankind in nature. The first wave of this interaction began very early when man fermented food articles to make bread, wine, cheese, and yogurt long before he had any knowledge of the invisible, microbial world. The thesis that technology does not necessarily depend on science is well proven here. The next wave arrived when man learned the scientific basis of the biological world and began manufacturing drugs and other essential components from biological tissues; the discovery of penicillin opened the way for this research. Antibiotics were then routinely manufactured by the process of fermentation. The third wave of technologic and scientific breakthrough came in the late 1970s and 1980s when the new technology related to cell culture, fusion, bioprocessing, and genetic engineering took roots in the industry. Today, prokaryotes, eukaryotes algae, glycophytes, and halophytes are all likely to contribute to products of the future. The techniques of DNA manipulation, monoclonal antibody preparation, tissue culture, protoplast fusion, protein engineering, immobilized enzymes, cell catalysis, antisense DNA, and so forth are the leading technology helping mankind find solutions to his problems, what began with a glass of brewed grape juice that made man feel good.

Biotechnology is the application of biological systems and organisms to technical and industrial processes. In its broadest definition, biotechnology refers to the use of living organisms, including isolated mammalian cells, in the production of products having beneficial use. This places alcohol brewing, antibiotic production, and dairy processing, for example, within the scope of biotechnology. The use of yeast to ferment grain into alcohol has been ongoing for centuries. Likewise, farmers and breeders use a form of "genetic engineering" to produce improved crops and stock by selecting for desirable characteristics in plants and animals. Only recently have "new" biotechnology techniques enabled scientists to modify an organism's genetic material at the cellular or molecular level. These methods are more precise, but the results are similar to those produced with classical genetic techniques involving whole organisms. Biotechnologically derived products are those derived from the new biotechnology techniques. The development of these products offers many challenges, integration of many sciences, and an almost art-like implementation of technology to achieve consistent results.

However, the current interest in biotechnology is a result primarily of two major advances:

1. The development of recombinant DNA (rDNA) technology, which allowed the genes of one species to be transplanted into another species (gene coding). Thus, gene coding for the expression (production) of a desired protein (usually human) could be inserted into a host prokaryotic (e.g., bacteria) or eukaryotic (e.g., mammalian) cell in such a manner that the host cell would then express (yield) usable (commercially) quantities of the desired protein.
2. The development of techniques for producing large quantities of monoclonal antibodies (i.e., antibodies arising from a single lymphocyte).

TABLE 1.1
Global Definitions of Biotechnology

Country/Region (Source)	Definition	Analysis
British (British Biotechnologist)	Application of biological organisms, systems, or processes to manufacturing and service industries.	Broad, noncommittal, technology driven, bureaucratic differentiating manufacturing and services industries.
European (European Federation of Biotechnology)	The integrated use of biochemistry, microbiology, and engineering sciences in order to achieve technological (industrial) applications of the capabilities of microorganisms, cultured tissue cells, and parts thereof.	Legal deconstruction of the term defining components and targets and beginning with "integrated," to reflect the union.
Japan (Japanese Biotechnologists)	A technology using biological phenomena for copying and manufacturing various kinds of useful substances.	Pure technologic exploitation; the use of "copying" and "various kinds" is significant as it is leading to "useful" substances.
USA (National Science Foundation)	The controlled use of biological agents, such as microorganisms or cellular components, for beneficial use.	Control, concern about its unlawful exploitation, and deleterious effects using microorganisms is obvious.

The definition of "biotechnology" is relatively new and how it is accepted worldwide is worth examining as it reflects how the regulatory controls of biotechnology derived products would be evaluated. Table 1.1 lists the definitions of the world's major regulatory regions. Later, we will analyze how different regulatory agencies label "biogeneric," from what it should be to all types of variations like, "follow-on," "biosimilar," or "generic biologicals," all reflecting a bias, a disbelief (or perhaps amazement) at how fast the age of biogenerics products has arrived.

As we get closer to regulatory approvals of the first biological products in their "generic" forms, the above differences in how different countries view biotechnology are beginning to become obvious. For example, Europeans would prefer to call the products marketed by competitors after the expiry of patents as "follow-on biologicals," "similar biologicals," whereas the push in the U.S. is to call it "biogeneric," as it *is* a generic product. Billions of dollars are riding on the hair splitting differences between these interpretations. Lobby groups like Biotechnology Industry Organization (BIO) in the U.S. are supported by the big pharmaceutical companies and they work incessantly to block the introduction of biogeneric products, whereas the legislature, the generic companies, and government-supported Medicare are insisting on cheaper biological products — the biogenerics. These differences will be further discussed in Chapter 11.

BIOTECHNOLOGY FRONTIERS

"Biotechnology, the combination of biology and technology, includes biologic applications, diagnostic tools and businesses that improve everyday life by providing solutions to some of life's most vexing problems," describes the BIO. Since 1982, hundreds of millions of people have been helped by about 200 biotechnology drugs and vaccines, with many more in the pipeline treating diseases that were just a couple of decades ago were considered untreatable, from AIDS to Alzheimer's disease to stroke prevention. Prevention of diseases like cancer appears possible within a short time. Many enzymes used to make food products are likely to be produced by recombinant techniques, as are the ingredients in most processed foods. A newer generation of oils without trans fats and cholesterol are now available that reduce the incidence of heart disease; "golden rice" fortified with vitamins and allergen-free foods is now common as are safer meats.

Today, over 2500 biologicals are used to fight nearly 200 different animal diseases. To make animal products safe, products are made to keep animals free of infectious bacteria (e.g., *E. coli* O157:H7) and to identify animals with DNA tagging to trace outbreaks of disease; bovine spongiform encephalopathy (BSE)–resistant bovine species are also being cloned. New plastics made with corn and other plants, not petroleum, serve ecology, as are the plants that consume carbon dioxide rather than exude it to control environment warming. New fuels for automobiles would come from soybeans and other crops, as would biodegradable grease and industrial lubricants. Bacteria are used to clean up oil spills and other contaminants. Energy consumption in production is reduced drastically, and crop yields are enhanced and made resistant to disease (e.g., virus-resistant cotton plants).

Today, farmers in 18 countries are growing more than 167 million acres of crops improved through biotechnology, helping feed the world population at a lower cost than ever before. Fiber made from goat's milk is used as body armor and mustard plant is modified to serve as "sentinel plants," to warn against chemical or biological warfare agents. DNA typing and testing is now routinely settling the criminal investigation and paternity suits. Other advances are limited only by our imagination — such is the power of biotechnology.

What we need to understand today is the projected impact of biotechnology in the future in light of fast changing sciences that are bound to impinge on this technology. An excellent projection of this scenario is made in a recent report by the Rand Corporation, funded by the National Security Administration of the U.S. government. According to this report, life in 2015 will be revolutionized by the growing effect of multidisciplinary technologies across all dimensions of life: social, economic, political, and personal. The report identifies biotechnology, nanotechnology, and materials technology as the technologies that will make the most impact.

Biotechnology, in the near future, will enable us to identify, understand, manipulate, improve, and control living organisms, which obviously includes human beings as well. Smart materials, agile manufacturing, and nanotechnology will change the way we produce devices while expanding their capabilities. These technologies may also be joined by what is called long-shot or "wild cards," such as novel nanoscale computers, molecular manufacturing, and self assembly in 2015 if barriers to their development are resolved in time. Biotechnology will begin to revolutionize life most significantly by 2015. Disease, malnutrition, food production, pollution, life expectancy, quality of life, crime, and security will be significantly addressed, improved, or augmented. Some advances could be viewed as accelerations of human-engineered evolution of plants, animals, and in some ways even humans with accompanying changes in the ecosystem. Research is also under way to create new, free-living organisms. Given below is a bird's eye view of how these technologies will revolutionize our lives.

ENHANCED QUANTITY AND QUALITY OF HUMAN LIFE

A marked acceleration is likely by 2015 in the expansion of human life spans along with significant improvements in the quality of human life. Better disease control, custom drugs, gene therapy, age mitigation and reversal, memory drugs, prosthetics, bionic implants, animal transplants, and many other advances may continue to increase human life span and improve the quality of life. Some of these advances may even improve human performance beyond current levels (e.g., through artificial sensors).

EUGENICS AND CLONING

By 2015 we may have the capability to use genetic engineering techniques to "improve" the human species and clone humans. These will be very controversial developments — among the most controversial in the entire history of mankind. It is uncertain whether cloning of humans will be technically feasible by 2015; however, some serious attempts such as gene therapy for genetic diseases and cloning by rogue experimenters will be inevitable. The revolution of biology will not come without issue and unforeseen radicalism. Significant ethical, moral, religious, privacy, and environmental debates and protests are already being raised in such areas as genetically modified foods, cloning, and genomic profiling. There is much more to come. The evolution of biology would rely not just on technological trends but also on microelectromechanical systems, materials, imaging, sensor, and information technology. The fast pace of technological development and breakthroughs makes foresight difficult, but advances in genomic profiling, cloning, genetic modification, biomedical engineering, disease therapy, and drug developments are accelerating and should continue at a rapid pace.

Despite these potentials, the controversy continues over such issues as:

- Eugenics;
- Cloning of humans, including concerns over morality, errors, induced medical problems, gene ownership, and human breeding;
- Gene patents and the potential for either excessive ownership rights of sequences or insufficient intellectual property protections to encourage investments;
- The safety and ethics of genetically modified organisms;
- The use of stem cells (whose current principal source is human embryos) for tissue engineering; this issue was boldly played out in the recent U.S. presidential race, with George W. Bush taking a cautious step and John Kerry trying to cash in on the lack of general awareness about the issue; Kerry lost. However, California voted in research on stem cells, which makes it look like the gold rush has begun again;
- Concerns over animal rights brought about by transplantation from animals as well as the risk of trans-species disease;
- Privacy of genetic profiles (e.g., nationwide police databases of DNA profiles, denial of employment or insurance based on genetic predispositions);
- The danger of environmental havoc from genetically modified organisms (perhaps balanced by increased knowledge and control of modification functions compared to more traditional manipulation mechanisms);
- An increased risk of engineered biological weapons (perhaps balanced by an increased ability to engineer countermeasures and protections). The use of synthetic oligonucleotides to make viruses as recently reported in 2003 has substantially raised the risk of biological weapons coming into hands of rogue elements. Nevertheless, biomedical advances (combined with other health improvements) will continue to increase human life span and productivity.

TECHNOLOGY TRENDS: GENOMICS

Biotechnology will continue to improve and apply its ability to profile, copy, and manipulate the genetic basis of both plants and animal organisms, opening wide opportunities and implications for understanding existing organisms and engineering organisms with new properties. Research is even under way to create new free-living organisms, initially microbes with a minimal genome. One of the most dramatic findings was reported in 2003 when Smith et al. of the Institute of Biological Energy Alternatives (Rockville, MD) reported "Generating a synthetic genomy by whole genome assembly: X174 bacteriophage from synthetic nucleotides." This was dubbed as the first successful experiment to create a virus totally *in situ*. Whether a virus can be labeled as a living organism or not is a different issue, but the technology of Smith et al. dramatically shortened the time required for accurate assembly of 5-6-kb segments of DNA from synthetic nucleotides and to test it; assembly of the complete infectious genome of bacteriophage from a single pool of chemically synthesized oligonucleotides has raised many questions as it has razed many barriers in man's ability to conquer life, and if the dogmatic purveyors of religion will allow me, to create life. We are indeed living in very exciting times wherein man's effort can shatter many core belief systems and scientific paradigms.

GENETIC PROFILING AND DNA ANALYSIS

DNA analysis machines and chip-based systems will accelerate the proliferation of genetic analysis capabilities, improve drug searches, and enable development of biological sensors. The genomes of plants (ranging from important food crops such as rice and corn to production plants such as pulp trees) and animals (ranging from bacteria such as *E. coli,* through insects and mammals) will continue to be decoded and profiled. To the extent that genes dictate function and behavior, such extensive genetic profiling would provide an ability to better diagnose human health problems, design drugs tailored for individual problems and system reactions, better predict disease predispositions, and track disease movement and development across global populations, ethnic groups, and other genetic pools. Note that a link between genes and function is generally accepted, but other factors such as the environment and phenotype play important modifying roles. Gene therapies will continue to be developed, although they may not mature by 2015. Genetic profiling could also have a significant effect on security, policing, and law. DNA identification may complement existing biometric technologies (e.g., retina and fingerprint identification) for granting access to secure systems (e.g., computers, secured areas, or weapons), identifying criminals through DNA left at crime scenes and authenticating items such as fine art. Genetic identification will likely become a more commonplace tool in prosecuting kidnapping, paternity, and fraud cases.

Biosensors (some genetically engineered) may also aid in detecting biological warfare threats, improving food and water quality testing, continuous health monitoring, and medical laboratory analyses. Such capabilities could fundamentally change the way health services are rendered by greatly improving disease diagnosis, understanding predispositions, and improving monitoring capabilities. Such profiling may be limited by technical difficulties in decoding some genomic segments and in understanding the implications of the genetic code. Our current technology has decoded nearly all of the human gene sequence. More important, although there is a strong connection between an organism's function and its genotype, we still have large gaps in understanding the intermediate steps in copying, transduction, isomer modulation, activation, and immediate function and its effect on larger systems in the organism.

PROTEOMICS

Proteomics (the study of protein function and genes) is the next big technological push after genomic decoding. Progress may rely on advances in bioinformatics, genetic code combination and sequencing (akin to hierarchical programming in computer languages), and other related information technologies. Despite current optimism, a number of technical issues and hurdles could moderate genomics progress by 2015. Incomplete understanding of sequence coding, transduction, isomer modulation, activation, and resulting functions could form technological barriers to wide engineering successes. Extensive rights to own genetic codes may slow research and ultimately the benefits of the decoding. At the other extreme, the inability to secure patents from sequencing efforts may reduce commercial funding and thus slow research and resulting benefits. In addition, investments in biotechnology have been cyclic in the past. As a result, advances in research and development (R&D) may come in surges, especially in areas where the time to market (and thus time to return on investment) is long.

CLONING

Artificially producing genetically identical organisms through cloning will be significant for engineered crops, livestock, and research animals. Cloning may become the dominant mechanism for rapidly bringing engineered traits to market, for continued maintenance of these traits, and for producing identical organisms for research and production. Research will continue on human cloning in unregulated parts of the world with possible success by 2015, but ethical and health concerns will limit wide-scale cloning of humans in regulated parts of the world. Individuals or even some states may also engage in human or animal cloning, but it is unclear what they may gain through such efforts. The Human Genome Project and Celera Genomics have released drafts of the human genome. The drafts are undergoing additional validation, verification, and updates to weed out errors, sequence interruptions, and gaps. Additional technical difficulties in genomic sequencing include short, repetitive sequences that jam current DNA processing techniques as well as possible limitations of bacteria to accurately copy certain DNA fragments. Cloning, especially human cloning, has already generated significant controversy across the globe. Concerns include moral issues, the potential for errors and medical deficiencies of clones, questions of the ownership of good genes and genomes, and eugenics. Although some attempts at human cloning are possible by 2015, legal restrictions and public opinion may limit their extent. Fringe groups, however, may attempt human cloning in advance of legislative restrictions or may attempt cloning in unregulated countries. (See, for example, the human cloning program announced by Clonaid.) Although expert opinions vary regarding the current feasibility of human cloning, at least some technical hurdles for human cloning will need to be addressed for safe, wide-scale use. "Attempts to clone mammals from single somatic cells are plagued by high frequencies of developmental abnormalities and lethality," says Dr. Pennisi. Even cloned plant populations exhibit "substantial developmental and morphological irregularities," according to Dr. Matzke. Research will need to address these abnormalities or at the very least mitigate their repercussions. Some believe, however, that human cloning may be accomplished soon if the research organization accepts the high lethality rate for the embryo and the potential generation of developmental abnormalities.

One of the hottest debated issues on cloning were related to stem cells; in November 2004, California offered its Proposition 71 to raise a few billion dollars to support research on stem cells; the proposition was approved 59.1% (6.6 million) saying yes to 40.9% (4.6 million) saying no. Never in history has science been at the forefront of political debate as it is today where stem cell research was one of the key issues in presidential debates.

GENETICALLY MODIFIED CELLS

Beyond profiling genetic codes and cloning exact copies of organisms and microorganisms, biotechnologists can also manipulate the genetic code of plants and animals and will continue efforts to engineer certain properties into life forms for various reasons. Traditional techniques for genetic manipulation (such as cross-pollination, selective breeding, and irradiation) will continue to be extended by direct insertion, deletion, and modification of genes through laboratory techniques. Targets include food crops, production plants, insects, and animals. Desirable properties could be genetically imparted to genetically engineered foods, potentially producing: improved taste; ultra-lean meats with reduced "bad" fats, salts, and chemicals; disease resistance; and artificially introduced nutrients (so-called nutraceuticals).

Genetically modified cells (GMCs) can potentially be engineered to improve their physical robustness, extend field and shelf life (e.g., the Flavr-Savr™ tomato), tolerate herbicides, grow faster, or grow in previously unproductive environments (e.g., in high-salinity soils, with less water, or in colder climates). Beyond systemic disease resistance, *in vivo* pesticide production has already been demonstrated (e.g., in corn) and could have a significant effect on pesticide production, application, regulation, and control with targeted release. Likewise, organisms could be engineered to produce or deliver drugs for human disease control. Cow mammary glands might be engineered to produce pharmaceuticals and therapeutic organic compounds; other organisms could be engineered to produce or deliver therapeutics (e.g., the so-called prescription banana). If accepted by the population, such improved production and delivery mechanisms could extend the global production and availability of these therapeutics while providing easy oral delivery.

In addition to food production, plants may be engineered to improve growth, change their constitution, or artificially produce new products. Trees, for example, will be engineered to optimize their growth and tailor their structure for particular applications such as lumber, wood pulp for paper, fruiting, or carbon sequestering (to reduce global warming) while reducing waste by-products. Plants might be engineered to produce biopolymers (plastics) for engineering applications with lower pollution and without using oil reserves. Biofuel plants could be tailored to minimize polluting components while producing additives needed by the consuming equipment.

Genetic engineering of microorganisms has long been accepted and used. For example, *E. coli* has been used for mass production of insulin. Engineering of bacterial properties into plants and animals for disease resistance will occur. Other animal manipulations could include modification of insects to impart desired behaviors, providing tagging (including GMC tagging), or preventing physical uptake properties to control pests in specific environments to improve agriculture and disease control. Research on modifying human genes has already begun and will continue in a search for solutions to genetically based diseases.

Although slowed by recent difficulties, gene therapy research will continue its search for useful mechanisms to address genetic deficiencies or for modulating physical processes such as beneficial protein production or control mechanisms for cancer. Advances in genetic profiling may improve our understanding and selection of therapy techniques and provide breakthroughs with significant health benefits. Some cloning of humans will be possible by 2015, but legal restrictions and public opinion may limit its actual extent. Controls are also likely for human modifications (e.g., clone-based eugenic modifications) for nondisease purposes. It is possible, however, that technology will enable genetic modifications for hereditary conditions (i.e., sickle cell anemia) through *in vitro* techniques or other mechanisms. GMCs are also having a large effect on the scientific community as an enabling technology. Not only do "knock-out" animals (animals with selected DNA sequences removed from their genome) give scientists another tool to study the effect of the removed sequence on the animal, they also enable subsequent analysis of the interaction of those functions or components with the animal's entire system. Although knock-outs are not always complete, they provide another important tool to confirm or refute hypotheses regarding complex organisms.

BROADER ISSUES AND IMPLICATIONS

Extant capabilities in genomics have already created opportunities yet they have also generated a number of issues. As more organisms are decoded and the functional implications of genes are discovered, concerns about property and privacy rights for the sequencing will continue. The ability to profile an individual's DNA is already raising concerns about privacy and excessive monitoring. Examples include databases of DNA signatures for use in criminal investigations, and the potential use of genetically based health predispositions by insurance companies or employers to deny coverage or to discriminate. The latter may raise policy issues regarding acceptable and unacceptable profiling for insurance or employment. This issue is further worrisome because the exact code-to-function mechanisms that trigger many disease predispositions are not well understood. Issues may also arise if a strong genetic basis of human physical or cognitive ability is discovered. On the positive side, understanding a person's predisposition for certain abilities (or limitations) could enable custom educational or remediation programs that will help to compensate for genetic inclinations, especially in early years when their effect can be optimized. On the negative side, groups may use such analyses in arguments to discriminate against target populations (despite, for example, the fact that ethnic distribution variances of cognitive ability are currently believed to be wider than ethnic mean differences), aggravating social and international conflicts.

Although the genetic profiles of plants have been modified for centuries using traditional techniques, questions regarding the safety of genetically modified foods have sparked international concerns in the United Kingdom and Europe, forcing a campaign by biotechnology companies to argue the safety of the technology and its applications. Some have argued that genetic engineering is actually as safe or safer than traditional combinatorial techniques such as irradiated seeds, since there often is strong supporting information concerning the function of the inserted sequences. Governments have been forced into the issue, resulting in education efforts, food labeling proposals, and heated international trade discussions between the United States and Europe on the importation of GMCs and their seedlings.

As genetic modification becomes more common, it may become more difficult to label and separate GMCs, resulting in a forcing function to resolve the issue of how far the technology should be applied and whether separate markets can be maintained in a global economy. This debate is starting to have global effects as populations in other countries begin to notice the impassioned debates in the United Kingdom and Europe. Some have likened the antibiotechnology movement to the antinuclear-power movement in scope and tactics, although the low cost and wide availability of basic genomic equipment and know-how will allow practically any country, small business, or even individual to participate in genetic engineering. Such wide technology availability and low entry costs could make it impossible for any movement or government to control the spread and use of genomic technology. At an extreme, successful protest pressures on big biotechnology companies, together with wide technology availability, could ultimately drive genomic engineering "underground" to groups outside such pressures and outside regulatory controls that the global technology revolution helps ensure safe and ethical uses. This could ironically facilitate the very problems that the antibiotechnology movement is hoping to prevent. Cloning and genetic modification also raise biodiversity concerns. Standardization of crops and livestock has already increased food supply vulnerabilities to diseases that can wipe out larger areas of production.

Genetic modification may increase our ability to engineer responses to these threats, but the losses may still be felt in the production year unless broad-spectrum defenses are developed. In addition to food safety, the ability to modify biological organisms holds the possibility of engineered biological weapons that circumvent current or planned countermeasures. On the other hand, genomics could aid in biological warfare defense (e.g., through improved understanding and control of biological function both in and between pathogens and target hosts as well as improved capability for engineered biosensors). Advances in genomics, therefore, could advance a race between threat engineering and countermeasures. Thus, although genetic manipulation is likely to result in medical advances, it is unclear whether we will be in a safer position in the future.

The rate at which GMC benefits are felt in poorer countries may depend on the costs of using patented organisms, marketing demands and approaches, and the rate at which crops become ubiquitous and inseparable from unmodified strains. Consider, for example, current issues related to human immunodeficiency virus (HIV) drug development and dissemination in poorer countries. Patentability has fueled research investments, but many poorer countries with dire needs cannot afford the latest drugs and must wait for handouts or patent expiration. Globalization, however, may fuel dissemination as multinational companies invest in food production across the globe. Also, the rewards from opening previously unproductive land for production may provide the financial incentive to pay the premium for GMCs. Furthermore, widely available genomic technology could allow academics, nonprofit small businesses, and developing countries to develop GMCs to alleviate problems in poorer regions; larger biotechnology companies will focus on markets requiring capital-intensive R&D. Finally, moral issues may play a large role in modulating the global effect of genomics trends. Some people simply believe it is improper to engineer or modify biological organisms using the new techniques. Unplanned side effects (e.g., the imposition of arthritis in current genetically modified pigs) will support such opposition. Others are concerned with the real danger of eugenics programs or of the engineering of dangerous biological organisms.

THERAPIES AND DRUG DEVELOPMENT

TECHNOLOGY

Beyond genetics, biotechnology will continue to improve therapies for preventing and treating disease and infection. New approaches might block a pathogen's ability to enter or travel in the body, leverage pathogen vulnerabilities, develop new countermeasure delivery mechanisms, or modulate or augment the immune response to recognizing new pathogens. These therapies may counter the current trend of increasing resistance to extant antibiotics, reshaping the war on infections. In addition to addressing traditional viral and bacterial problems, therapies are being developed for chemical imbalances and modulation of chemical stasis. For example, antibodies are being developed that attack cocaine in the body and may be used to control addiction. Such approaches could have a significant effect on modifying the economics of the global illegal drug trade while improving conditions for users.

Drug development will be aided by various technology trends and enablers. Computer simulations combined with proliferating trends for molecular imaging technologies (e.g., atomic-force microscopes, mass spectroscopy, and scanning probe microscopes) may continue to improve our ability to design molecules with desired functional properties that target specific receptors, binding sites, or markers, complementing combinatorial drug search with rational drug design. Simulations of drug interactions with target biological systems could become increasing useful in understanding drug efficacy and safety. For example, Dennis Noble's complex virtual heart simulation has already contributed to U.S. Food and Drug Administration (FDA) approval of a cardiac drug by helping to explain the mechanisms and significance of an effect noticed in the clinical trial. For some better understood systems such as the heart, this approach may become a dominant complement to clinical drug trials by 2015, whereas other more complex systems (e.g., the brain) will require more research on the system function and biology.

SURGICAL AND DIAGNOSTIC BIOTECHNOLOGY

Biotechnology and materials advances are likely to continue producing revolutionary surgical procedures and systems that will significantly reduce hospital stays and cost and increase effectiveness. New surgical tools and techniques and new materials and designs for vesicle and tissue support will continue to reduce surgical invasiveness and offer new solutions to medical problems. Techniques such as angioplasty may continue to eliminate whole classes of surgeries; others such as laser perforations of heart tissue could promote regeneration and healing. Advances in laser surgery could refine techniques and improve human capability (e.g., LASIK® eye surgery to replace glasses), especially as costs are reduced and experience spreads.

Hybrid imaging techniques will improve diagnosis, guide human and robotic surgery, and aid in basic understanding of body and brain function. Finally, collaborative information technology (e.g., telemedicine) will extend specialized medical care to remote areas and aid in the global dissemination of medical quality and new advances.

BROADER ISSUES AND IMPLICATIONS

The research and development costs for drug development are currently extremely high and may even be unsustainable, with averages of approximately $800 million per drug brought to market. These costs may drive the pharmaceutical industry to invest heavily in technology advances with the goal of long-term viability of the industry. Combined with genetic profiling, drug development tailored to genotypes, chemical simulation and engineering programs, and drug testing simulations may begin to change pharmaceutical development from a broad application trial-and-error approach to custom drug development, testing, and prescription based on a deeper understanding of subpopulation response to drugs. This understanding may also rescue drugs previously rejected because of adverse reactions in small populations of clinical trials. Along with the potential for improving success rates, reducing trial costs, and opening new markets for narrowly targeted drugs, tailoring drugs to subpopulations will also have the opposite effect of reducing the size of the market for each drug. Thus, the economics of the pharmaceutical and health industries will change significantly if these trends come to fruition. Note that patent protection is not uniformly enforced across the globe for the pharmaceutical industry. As a result, certain regions (e.g., Asia) may continue to focus on production of nonlegacy (generic) drugs, and other regions (e.g., the U.S., United Kingdom, and Europe) will continue to pursue new drugs in addition to such low-margin pharmaceuticals.

RECOMBINANT PRODUCTION SYSTEMS

The choice of an expression system for the high-level production of recombinant proteins depends on many factors. These include cell growth characteristics, expression levels, intracellular and extracellular expression, posttranslational modifications, and biological activity of the protein of interest, as well as regulatory issues in the production of therapeutic proteins. In addition, the selection of a particular expression system requires a cost breakdown in terms of process, design, and other economic considerations. The relative merits of bacterial, yeast, insect, and mammalian expression systems have been examined in detail, and later chapters in this book will dwell on these topics in detail.

An efficient prokaryotic expression vector should contain a strong and tightly regulated promoter, an SD (Shine-Dalgarno) site that is positioned approximately 9 bp 5 to the translation initiation codon and is complementary to the 3 end of 16S rRNA, and an efficient transcription terminator positioned 3 to the gene coding sequence. In addition, the vectors require an origin of replication, a selection marker, and a gene that facilitates the stringent regulation of promoter activity. This regulatory element may be integrated either in the vector itself or in the host chromosome. Other elements that may be beneficial include transcriptional and translational "enhancers," as well as "minicistrons" in translationally coupled systems. These may be gene specific; therefore, their utility must be tested case by case. The translational initiation region of a gene must be free of secondary structures that may occlude the initiation codon or block ribosome binding. UAAU is the most efficient translation termination sequence in *E. coli*.

There are many different prokaryotic vectors that allow the tight regulation of gene expression. The experimental approaches to achieve tight regulation of promoter activity range from the simple repositioning of the operator in *lac*-based systems to the construction of elaborate "cross-regulation" systems. These vectors are efficient, and each system has its own niche in prokaryotic gene expression. The demonstrated effectiveness of a thermosensitive *lac* repressor now allows the thermal regulation of *lac*-based promoters in lieu of using IPTG (isopropyl-β-D-thiogalactopyranoside). To date, there is no generally applicable strategy to prevent the degradation of a wide variety of mRNA species in *E. coli*.

Although certain 5- and 3-stem-loop structures have been shown to block mRNA degradation, these seem to stabilize only specific mRNAs, under restricted conditions. One exception appears to be the 5 UTR of the *E. coli ompA* transcript, which prolongs the half-life of a number of heterologous mRNAs in *E. coli*. The use of strains deficient in specific RNAs has been ineffective for enhanced gene expression.

Each of the four "compartments" for targeted protein production (i.e., the cytoplasm, periplasm, inner and outer membranes, and growth medium) offers advantages and disadvantages for gene expression, depending on the experimental objectives. The formation of inclusion bodies can be minimized by a variety of techniques, but it remains a significant barrier to high-level protein production in the cytoplasm. To date, the effectiveness of molecular chaperones has been protein-specific. It is possible that this is due to conditions that prevent the formation of a thermodynamically stable end product, such as the production of severely truncated proteins or single domains from multisubunit protein complexes, lack of formation of disulfide bonds, suboptimal growth conditions, absence of posttranslational modifications, and the normally concerted action of multiple types of chaperones *in vivo*. Nevertheless, molecular chaperones have been used very successfully for the enhanced production of specific proteins.

The wide variety of existing fusion partners have utility in the production, detection, and purification of recombinant proteins. Specific fusion moieties can increase the folding, solubility, resistance to proteolysis, and secretion of recombinant proteins into the growth medium.

Protein misfolding, attributed to the intracellular concentration of aggregation-prone intermediates, may be minimized by a combination of experimental approaches: replacement of amino acid residues that cause aggregation, coexpression of molecular chaperones and foldases, reduction of the rate of protein synthesis, the use of solubilizing fusion partners, and the careful optimization of growth conditions.

Codon usage can have adverse effects on the synthesis and yield of recombinant proteins. However, the mere presence of "rare" codons in a gene does not necessarily dictate poor translation of that gene. Currently, we do not know all the rules that link codon usage and translation of a transcript. The lack of consistent results in the published literature on codon usage may be due to several variables, such as positional effects, the clustering or interspersion of the rare codons, secondary structure of the mRNA, and other effects. Positional effects appear to play an important role in protein synthesis. Thus, the presence of rare codons near the 5 end of a transcript probably affects translational efficiency. This problem may be rectified by the alteration of the culprit codons or the coexpression of the cognate tRNA genes.

Much progress has been made in the elucidation of specific determinants of protein degradation in *E. coli*. Effective approaches for minimization of proteolysis in *E. coli* include the targeting of protein to the periplasm or the culture medium, the use of protease-deficient host strains, the construction of fusion proteins, the coexpression of molecular chaperones, the coexpression of the T4 *pin* gene, the elimination of protease cleavage sites through genetic engineering, and the optimization of fermentation conditions. Host strains that are deficient in the *rpoH* (*htpR*) locus are among the best, particularly for thermally induced expression systems.

Future challenges in the use of *E. coli* for gene expression will involve the following factors. First is the achievement of enhanced yields of correctly folded proteins by manipulating the molecular chaperone machinery of the cell. Perhaps this might be done by the coexpression of multiple chaperone-encoding genes or by methods that activate a large battery of chaperone molecules in the cell. Second is the realization of a "true" and robust secretion mechanism for the efficient release of protein into the culture medium. There are several available systems that facilitate secretion of recombinant proteins into the culture medium. Some of these are based on the use of signal peptides, fusion partners, and permeabilizing agents that cause disruption and limited leakage of the outer membrane. Other efforts are directed at pirating existing secretion pathways that promise greater specificity of secretion. Work in this area will necessitate an improved understanding of the various secretion pathways in *E. coli*. Third is the endowment of the prokaryotic cell with the ability to perform some of the posttranslational modifications found in eukaryotic proteins, such as glycosylation. This might be done by engineering eukaryotic glycosylating enzymes into the *E. coli* chromosome.

DRUG DELIVERY SYSTEMS

Recently, the more patient-friendly modes of drug delivery have drawn a lot of attention. Oral, nasal, transdermal, and even buccal and rectal routes are being investigated as potentially feasible routes to administer protein drugs. With the alternative methods of drug delivery there are two major problems. One is that the site, or route, of administration of the drug is frequently hostile to polypeptides (e.g., orally delivered proteins are subjected to harsh conditions prior to absorption through the gastrointestinal tract, or during absorption through the nasal mucosa considerable metabolism may occur). Second, the absorption of sufficient amounts of drug through the respective barrier layers after administration may be a significant factor in achieving a pharmacological response. Strategies to improve absorption of usually hydrophilic (hence poorly absorbed) compounds include encapsulation into hydrophobic carriers, combination with penetration enhancers, active electrical transport, or chemical modification to increase hydrophobicity.

ENCAPSULATION TECHNOLOGIES

Encapsulation involves the entrapment of the polypeptide drug within a polymeric, phospholipid, or carbohydrate particulate delivery system such as microspheres, liposomes, and nanoparticles. Encapsulation can confer several beneficial effects to a polypeptide drug, including slow or controlled release of the drug, improvement of drug stability, promotion of cutaneous delivery, or bioadhesion to tissue surfaces.

TRANSDERMAL APPLICATIONS

Although numerous cytokines have been genetically cloned and expressed, only a few are being used clinically, mainly due to their relatively short half-lives and rapid clearance (e.g., IFN has a half-life of approximately 10 min in serum). Many cytokines have received attention as potential topically applicable proteins. For example, applying human epidermal growth factor in liposomes, a 200% increase in wound tensile strength could be achieved, whereas epidermal growth factor in saline had no wound-healing effect. Niosomes (liposomes made of nonionic surfactants) may also be useful for peptide drug delivery through the pilosebaceous route in the skin. Vesicles composed of glyceryl dilaurate cholesterol and polyoxyethylene-10-stearyl ether enhance the absorption of interferon alpha and cyclosporine. Another type of liposome preparation, transfersomes (a phosphatidylcholine/sodium cholate mixture), can be used to deliver insulin through topical application *in vivo*. One of the functions of the stratum corneum is to act as a "protective barrier" against exogenous factors that may invade the body. Consequently, it is not unexpected that the transdermal delivery of proteins and peptides is limited by the very low permeability of the skin due to properties such as hydrophilicity and high molecular mass. The various approaches to delivering peptides through the skin have so far utilized methods that temporarily compromise the integrity or physicochemical characteristics of the skin, including the use of penetration enhancers such as *N*-alkylazacycloheptanones (Azone) for desglycinamide arginine vasopressin. The nonionic surfactant n-decylmethyl sulfoxide enhances the penetration of Leu-enkephalin through hairless mouse skin *in vitro* and a urea/ethanol/menthol/camphor/methyl salicylate hydroxypropylcellulose gel enhanced absorption of the nonapeptide leuprolide (a luteinizing-hormone-releasing hormone analogue) through a hydration and keratolytic effect.

Iontophoresis, a method based on electrical stimulation of skin permeability for mostly ionized molecules, has been employed by a number of researchers in the past few years for the enhancement of delivery of short peptides (model tripeptides, vasopressin), growth-hormone-releasing factor (amino acids 1–44), insulin and luteinizing-hormone-releasing hormone. Ultrasonic vibration was tried for delivery *in vivo* of insulin, with some success. The latest approach in the transdermal delivery of proteins and peptides is electroporation. Electroporation uses ultra-short pulses, lasting a few msec, with an intensity of a few hundred volts to induce changes in the skin and enable hydrophilic compounds to pass.

CHEMICAL MODIFICATION

Hydrophobic peptides such as cyclosporin appear to penetrate the intestinal barrier to a greater degree than hydrophilic peptides. Based on this and other similar observations, lipophilic derivatives of insulin and thyrothropin-releasing hormone by fatty acylation with palmitic or lauric acid have been tested for improving permeability across intestinal and rectal barriers. The modified drug molecules can spontaneously form vesicle-like structures (Prosome®, Pharmacosome®), which apparently greatly increases the bioavailability and circulation time of the drug in patients.

PULMONARY DELIVERY

Pulmonary drug delivery offers the potential for noninvasive administration of a wide variety of macromolecules. Nearly every biotherapeutic product that treats chronic or long-term illness would benefit from noninvasive delivery by providing a competitive advantage with current therapeutics. This advantage could expand the market for each product or enable new indications to be considered. Inhalation delivery of macromolecules can extend the life of a drug, increase patient compliance because of prompt effectiveness, and reduce the total costs of long-term health care. The future of drug administration by inhalation will expand vastly. The development of new macromolecule drugs that can treat diseases that previously were either not treatable or only partially treatable has led to renewed interest in noninvasive drug delivery technology. Many new agents are now under investigation for pulmonary delivery: interleukin-1 receptor (asthma therapy), heparin (blood clotting), human insulin (diabetes), α-1 antitrypsin (emphysema and cystic fibrosis), interferons (multiple sclerosis and hepatitis B and C), and calcitonin and other peptides (osteoporosis). Inhalation delivery methods may apply gene therapy via tissue targeting and organ targeting. Inhale's novel dry powder formulation, processing, and filling, combined with aerosol device technology, will provide many patients who previously received injections with the ability to independently and painlessly inhale medicine into the deep lung, where it will be absorbed into the bloodstream naturally and efficiently.

A TIME LINE OF BIOTECHNOLOGY DEVELOPMENT

8000 B.C.

- Humans domesticate crops and livestock.
- Potatoes first cultivated for food.

4000–2000 B.C.

- Biotechnology first used to leaven bread and ferment beer, using yeast (Egypt).
- Production of cheese and fermentation of wine (Sumeria, China, and Egypt).
- Babylonians control date palm breeding by selectively pollinating female trees with pollen from certain male trees.

1750 B.C.

- The Sumerians brew beer.

500 B.C.

- The Chinese use moldy soybean curds as an antibiotic to treat boils.

100 A.D.

- First insecticide: powdered chrysanthemums (China).

1322

- An Arab chieftain first uses artificial insemination to produce superior horses.

1590

- Zacharias Janssen invents the compound microscope.

1665

- Robert Hooke discovers existence of the cell.

1675

- Antonin van Leeuwenhoek discovers bacteria.

1761

- Josef Gottlieb Koelreuter reports successful crossbreeding of crop plants in different species.

1796

- Edward Jenner inoculates a child with a viral vaccine to protect him from smallpox.

1830

- Proteins discovered.

1833

- First enzyme discovered and isolated.

1835–1855

- Mathias Schleiden and Theodor Schwann propose that all organisms are composed of cells, and Rudolf Virchow declares, "Every cell arises from a cell."

1857

- Louis Pasteur proposes microbes cause fermentation.

1859

- Charles Darwin publishes the theory of evolution by natural selection. The concept of carefully selecting parents and culling the variable progeny greatly influences plant and animal breeders in the late 1800s despite their ignorance of genetics.

1865

- Science of genetics begins: Austrian monk Gregor Mendel studies garden peas and discovers that genetic traits are passed from parents to offspring in a predictable way — the laws of heredity.

1870–1890

- Using Darwin's theory, plant breeders crossbreed cotton, developing hundreds of varieties with superior qualities.
- Farmers first inoculate fields with nitrogen-fixing bacteria to improve yields.
- William James Beal produces first experimental corn hybrid in the laboratory.

1877

- A technique for staining and identifying bacteria is developed by Robert Koch.

1878

- The first centrifuge is developed by Carl Gustaf Patrik de Laval.

1879

- Walther Fleming discovers chromatin, the rod-like structures inside the cell nucleus that later came to be called chromosomes.

1900

- *Drosophila* (fruit flies) used in early studies of genes.

1902

- The term *immunology* first appears.

1906

- The term *genetics* is introduced.

1911

- The first cancer-causing virus is discovered by Francis Payton Rous.

1914

- Bacteria are used to treat sewage for the first time in Manchester, England.

1915

- Phages, or bacterial viruses, are discovered.

1919

- First use of the word *biotechnology* in print, by a Hungarian engineer.

1920

- The human growth hormone is discovered by Herbert McLean Evans.

1928

- Penicillin discovered as an antibiotic by Alexander Fleming.
- A small-scale test of formulated *Bacillus thuringiensis* (Bt) for corn borer control begins in Europe. Commercial production of this biopesticide begins in France in 1938.
- Georgi Karpechenko crosses radishes and cabbages, creating fertile offspring between plants in different genera.
- Alexander Fleming Laibach first uses embryo rescue to obtain hybrids from wide crosses in crop plants — known today as hybridization.

1930

- U.S. Congress passes the Plant Patent Act, enabling the products of plant breeding to be patented.

1933

- Hybrid corn, developed by Henry Wallace in the 1920s, is commercialized. Growing hybrid corn eliminates the option of saving seeds. The remarkable yields outweigh the increased costs of annual seed purchases, and by 1945, hybrid corn accounts for 78% of U.S.-grown corn.

1938

- The term *molecular biology* is coined.

1940

- American Oswald Avery demonstrates that DNA is the "transforming factor" and is the material of genes.

1941

- The term *genetic engineering* is first used, by Danish microbiologist A. Jost in a lecture on reproduction in yeast at the technical institute in Lwow, Poland.

1942

- The electron microscope is used to identify and characterize a bacteriophage — a virus that infects bacteria.
- Penicillin mass-produced in microbes.

1943

- Selman Abraham Waksman isolates streptomycin, an effective antibiotic for tuberculosis.

1944

- DNA is proven to carry genetic information by Oswald T. Avery.

1946

- Discovery that genetic material from different viruses can be combined to form a new type of virus, an example of genetic recombination.
- Recognizing the threat posed by loss of genetic diversity, the U.S. Congress provides funds for systematic and extensive plant collection, preservation, and introduction.

1949

- Linus Pauling shows that sickle cell anemia is a "molecular disease" resulting from a mutation in the protein molecule hemoglobin.

1950

- Artificial insemination of livestock using frozen semen (a longtime dream of farmers) is successfully accomplished.

1951

- Barbara McClintock discovers transposable elements, or "jumping genes," in corn.

1953

- The scientific journal *Nature* publishes James Watson and Francis Crick's manuscript describing the double helical structure of DNA, which marks the beginning of the modern era of genetics.

1955

- An enzyme involved in the synthesis of a nucleic acid is isolated for the first time.

1956

- Arthur Kornberg discovers the enzyme DNA polymerase I, leading to an understanding of how DNA is replicated. The fermentation process is perfected in Japan.

1958

- Sickle cell anemia is shown to occur due to a change of a single amino acid.
- DNA is made in a test tube for the first time.

1959

- Systemic fungicides are developed. The steps in protein biosynthesis are delineated.

ALSO IN THE 1950s

- Discovery of interferons.
- First synthetic antibiotic.

1960

- Exploiting base pairing, hybrid DNA-RNA molecules are created.
- Messenger RNA is discovered.

1961

- USDA registers first biopesticide: *Bacillus thuringiensis,* or Bt.

1963

- New wheat varieties developed by Norman Borlaug increase yields by 70%.

1964

- The International Rice Research Institute in the Philippines starts the Green Revolution with new strains of rice that double the yield of previous strains if given sufficient fertilizer.

1965

- R.A. Harris and L.J. Watkins successfully fuse mouse and human cells.

1966

- The genetic code is cracked, demonstrating that a sequence of three nucleotide bases (a codon) determines each of 20 amino acids. (Two more amino acids have since been discovered.)

1967

- The first automatic protein sequencer is perfected.

1969

- An enzyme is synthesized *in vitro* for the first time.

1970

- Norman Borlaug receives the Nobel Peace Prize (see 1963).
- Discovery of restriction enzymes that cut and splice genetic material, opening the way for gene cloning.

1971

- First complete synthesis of a gene.

1972

- The DNA composition of humans is discovered to be 99% similar to that of chimpanzees and gorillas.
- Initial work with embryo transfer.

1973

- Stanley Cohen and Herbert Boyer perfect techniques to cut and paste DNA (using restriction enzymes and ligases) and reproduce the new DNA in bacteria.

1974

- The National Institutes of Health forms a Recombinant DNA Advisory Committee to oversee recombinant genetic research.

1975

- Government first urged to develop guidelines for regulating experiments in recombinant DNA: Asilomar Conference, California.
- The first monoclonal antibodies are produced.

1976

- The tools of recombinant DNA are first applied to a human inherited disorder.
- Molecular hybridization is used for the prenatal diagnosis of alpha thalassemia.
- Yeast genes are expressed in *E. coli* bacteria.
- The sequence of base pairs for a specific gene is determined (A, C, T, G).
- First guidelines for recombinant DNA experiments released: National Institutes of Health–Recombinant DNA Advisory Committee.

1977

- First expression of human gene in bacteria.
- Procedures developed for rapidly sequencing long sections of DNA using electrophoresis.

1978

- High-level structure of virus first identified.
- Recombinant human insulin first produced.
- North Carolina scientists show it is possible to introduce specific mutations at specific sites in a DNA molecule.
- Thirumalachar issued patent for a process for the production of insulin by genetically transformed fungal cells.

1979

- Human growth hormone first synthesized.

ALSO IN THE 1970s

- First commercial company founded to develop genetically engineered products.
- Discovery of polymerases.
- Techniques for rapid sequencing of nucleotides perfected.
- Gene targeting.
- RNA splicing.

1980

- The U.S. Supreme Court, in the landmark case *Diamond v. Chakrabarty,* approves the principle of patenting recombinant life forms, which allows the Exxon oil company to patent an oil-eating microorganism.
- The U.S. patent for gene cloning is awarded to Stanley Cohen and Herbert Boyer.
- The first gene-synthesizing machines are developed.
- Researchers successfully introduce a human gene — one that codes for the protein interferon — into a bacterium.
- Stanley Cohen gets a patent for a process for producing biologically functional chimeras.
- Nobel Prize in Chemistry awarded for creation of the first recombinant molecule: Paul Berg, Walter Gilbert, Frederick Sanger.

1981

- Scientists at Ohio University produce the first transgenic animals by transferring genes from other animals into mice.
- Chinese scientist becomes the first to clone a fish — a golden carp.

1982

- Applied Biosystems, Inc., introduces the first commercial gas phase protein sequencer, dramatically reducing the amount of protein sample needed for sequencing.

- First recombinant DNA vaccine for livestock developed.
- First biotech drug approved by FDA: human insulin produced in genetically modified bacteria.
- First genetic transformation of a plant cell: petunia.

1983

- The polymerase chain reaction (PCR) technique is conceived. PCR, which uses heat and enzymes to make unlimited copies of genes and gene fragments, later becomes a major tool in biotech research and product development worldwide.
- The first genetic transformation of plant cells by TI plasmids is performed.
- The first artificial chromosome is synthesized.
- The first genetic markers for specific inherited diseases are found.
- First whole plant grown from biotechnology: petunia.
- First proof that modified plants pass their new traits to offspring: petunia.
- Richard Axel gets a patent for a process of inserting DNA into eukaryotic cells and for producing proteinaceous materials.

1984

- The DNA fingerprinting technique is developed.
- The first genetically engineered vaccine is developed.
- The entire genome of the human immunodeficiency virus is cloned and sequenced.

1985

- Genetic markers found for kidney disease and cystic fibrosis.
- Genetic fingerprinting entered as evidence in a courtroom.
- Transgenic plants resistant to insects, viruses and bacteria are field-tested for the first time.
- The NIH approves guidelines for performing gene-therapy experiments in humans. Protropin® is approved for the treatment of growth hormone deficiency in children.

1986

- First recombinant vaccine for humans: hepatitis B.
- First anticancer drug produced through biotech: interferon.
- The U.S. government publishes the *Coordinated Framework for Regulation of Biotechnology*, establishing more stringent regulations for rDNA organisms than for those produced with traditional genetic modification techniques.
- A. Tramontano describes how to combine antibodies and enzymes (abzymes) to create pharmaceuticals.
- The first field tests of transgenic plants (tobacco) are conducted.
- The Environmental Protection Agency approves the release of the first transgenic crop — gene-altered tobacco plants.
- The Organization of Economic Cooperation and Development (OECD) Group of National Experts on Safety in Biotechnology states: "Genetic changes from rDNA techniques will often have inherently greater predictability compared to traditional techniques" and "risks associated with rDNA organisms may be assessed in generally the same way as those associated with non-rDNA organisms."
- Albutein® is approved for treatment of hypovolemic shock.

- Intron A® is approved for treatment of hairy cell leukemia. Orthoclone OKT3® is approved for the reversal of acute kidney transplant rejection.
- Recombinate® rAHF, a blood-clotting factor VIII for the treatment of hemophilia A, is approved.

1987

- First approval for field test of modified food plants: virus-resistant tomatoes.
- Frostban, a genetically altered bacterium that inhibits frost formation on crop plants, is field-tested on strawberry and potato plants in California, the first authorized outdoor tests of a recombinant bacterium.
- Activase® is approved for treatment of heart attacks.
- Infergen® is approved for treatment of hepatitis C.
- Recombivax-HB®, a hepatitis B vaccine for adolescents and high-risk infants, is approved.

1988

- Harvard molecular geneticists are awarded the first U.S. patent for a genetically altered animal — a transgenic mouse.
- A patent for a process to make bleach-resistant protease enzymes to use in detergents is awarded.
- Congress funds the Human Genome Project, a massive effort to map and sequence the human genetic code as well as the genomes of other species.

1989

- First approval for field test of modified cotton: insect-protected (Bt) cotton.
- Plant Genome Project begins.
- Epogen® is approved for the treatment of renal disease anemia.
- The gene responsible for cystic fibrosis is discovered.
- Alferon N® is approved for treatment of genital warts.
- Kogenate®, which replaces blood-clotting factor VIII for the treatment of hemophilia A, is approved.

Also in the 1980s

- Studies of DNA used to determine evolutionary history.
- Recombinant DNA animal vaccine approved for use in Europe.
- Use of microbes in oil spill cleanup: bioremediation technology.
- Ribozymes and retinoblastomas identified.

1990

- Chy-Max™, an artificially produced form of the chymosin enzyme for cheese-making, is introduced. It is the first product of recombinant DNA technology in the U.S. food supply.
- The Human Genome Project — an international effort to map all the genes in the human body — is launched.

- The first experimental gene therapy treatment is performed successfully on a 4-year-old girl suffering from an immune disorder.
- The first transgenic dairy cow — used to produce human milk proteins for infant formula — is created.
- First insect-protected corn: Bt corn.
- First food product of biotechnology approved in U.K.: modified yeast.
- First field test of a genetically modified vertebrate: trout.
- Actimmune® is approved for treatment of chronic granulomatous disease.
- Adagen® is approved for treatment of severe combined immunodeficiency disease (SCID).
- CytoGam® is approved for the prevention of cytomegalovirus (CMV) in kidney transplant patients.
- Procrit® is approved for the treatment of anemia in AZT-treated HIV-infected patients.

1991

- Neupogen® is approved for the treatment of low white blood cells in chemotherapy patients.
- Leukine®, used to replenish white blood cell counts after bone marrow transplants, is approved.
- Ceredase® is approved for the treatment of type 1 Gaucher's disease.

1992

- American and British scientists unveil a technique for testing embryos *in vitro* for genetic abnormalities such as cystic fibrosis and hemophilia.
- The FDA declares that transgenic foods are "not inherently dangerous" and do not require special regulation.
- Proleukin® is approved for the treatment of renal cell cancer.
- American and British scientists unveil a technique for testing embryos *in vitro* for genetic abnormalities such as cystic fibrosis and hemophilia.

1993

- Merging two smaller trade associations creates the Biotechnology Industry Organization (BIO).
- FDA approves bovine somatotropin (BST) for increased milk production in dairy cows. Betaseron® is approved as the first treatment for multiple sclerosis in 20 years. Pulmozyme® is approved for mild to moderate cystic fibrosis.

1994

- First FDA approval for a whole food produced through biotechnology: FLAVRSAVR™ tomato.
- The first breast cancer gene is discovered.
- Approval of recombinant version of human DNase, which breaks down protein accumulation in the lungs of CF patients.
- BST commercialized as POSILAC bovine somatotropin. The FLAVRSAVR™ tomato — the first genetically engineered whole food approved by the FDA — is on the market.

- The first breast cancer gene is discovered.
- Approval of genetically engineered version of human DNase, which breaks down protein accumulation in the lungs of CF patients.
- Oncaspar® is approved for treatment of acute lymphoblastic leukemia. ReoPro™ is approved to reduce acute blood-clot-related complications for high-risk angioplasty patients

1995

- The first baboon-to-human bone marrow transplant is performed on an AIDS patient.
- The first full gene sequence of a living organism other than a virus is completed, for the bacterium *Hemophilus influenzae.*
- Gene therapy, immune system modulation and recombinantly produced antibodies enter the clinic in the war against cancer.
- Abelcet® is approved for treatment of invasive fungal infections in patients who are refractory to or intolerant of conventional amphotericin B.
- Doxil® is approved as a second-line therapy for Kaposi's sarcoma in AIDS patients.
- Photofrin® is approved for palliative treatment of totally and partially obstructing cancers of the esophagus.
- Venoglobulin®-S is approved for the treatment of primary immunodeficiencies.
- WinRho SDF® is approved for the prevention of Rh isoimmunization in pregnant women and for the treatment of thrombocytopenic purpura (TP).

1996

- The discovery of a gene associated with Parkinson's disease provides an important new avenue of research into the cause and potential treatment of the debilitating neurological ailment.
- AlphaNine® SD it approved to prevent and control bleeding in patients with factor IX deficiency due to hemophilia B.
- AMPHOTEC® is approved as a second-line treatment of invasive aspergillosis infections.
- DaunoXome® is approved as a first-line treatment for HIV-related Kaposi's sarcoma.
- Fertinex™ is approved for treatment of female infertility to stimulate ovulation disorders and in women undergoing assisted reproductive technologies treatment.
- Retavase™ is approved for the management of acute myocardial infarction in adults.
- RespiGam® is approved for the prevention of respiratory syncytial virus in children under 2 with bronchopulmonary dysplasia or history of prematurity.
- Serostim® is approved for cachexia (AIDS-wasting).
- Tripedia® is approved as a vaccine for infants 2, 4, and 6 months of age and first booster at 15–18 months.
- TriHIBit™ is approved for childhood immunization between 15 and 8 months for acellular pertussis, diphtheria, tetanus, and HIB infection.
- VISTIDE® is approved for the treatment of cytomegalovirus (CMV) retinitis in AIDS patients.

1997

- First animal cloned from an adult cell: a sheep named Dolly in Scotland.
- First weed- and insect-resistant biotech crops commercialized: Roundup Ready® soybeans and Bollgard® insect protected cotton.

- Biotech crops grown commercially on nearly 5 million acres worldwide: Argentina, Australia, Canada, China, Mexico, and the U.S.
- A group of Oregon researchers claims to have cloned two Rhesus monkeys.
- A new DNA technique combines PCR, DNA chips and a computer program providing a new tool in the search for disease-causing genes.
- Abbott HTLV-1/HTLV-II EIA is approved for the detection of HTLV-I/HTLV-II antibodies in serum or plasma.
- AmBisome® is approved for primary treatment of presumed fungal infections in patients with depressed immune function and fevers of unknown origin (FUO).
- Carticel™ is approved for treatment of knee cartilage damage.
- Follistim™ is approved as a recombinant follicle-stimulating hormone for treatment of infertility.
- Gonal-F is approved for functional infertility not due to primary ovarian failure.
- Neumega® is approved for the prevention of severe chemotherapy-induced thrombocytopenia in cancer patients.
- Prandin is approved as an anti-diabetic agent for treatment of type 2 diabetes.
- Regranex® Gel is approved as a platelet-derived growth factor treatment of diabetic foot ulcers.
- Rituxan™ is approved for treatment of relapsed or refractory low-grade or follicular, CD20-positive B-cell non-Hodgkin's lymphoma.

1998

- University of Hawaii scientists clone three generations of mice from nuclei of adult ovarian cumulus cells.
- Human embryonic stem cell lines are established.
- Scientists at Japan's Kinki University clone eight identical calves using cells taken from a single adult cow.
- The first complete animal genome, for the *C. elegans* worm, is sequenced.
- A rough draft of the human genome map is produced, showing the locations of more than 30,000 genes.
- Five Southeast Asian countries form a consortium to develop disease-resistant papayas.
- Apligraf® is approved for treatment of venous leg ulcers.
- Enbrel® is approved for treatment of rheumatoid arthritis.
- Herceptin® is approved for treatment of patients with metastatic breast cancer.
- LYMErix™ is approved for the prevention of Lyme disease.
- PROVIGIL® is approved to improve wakefulness in patients with excessive daytime sleepiness (EDS) associated with narcolepsy.
- Rebetron® is approved as a combination therapy for treatment of chronic hepatitis C in patients with compensated liver disease who have relapsed following alpha interferon treatment.
- Refludan® is approved for treatment of anticoagulation in patients with heparin-induced thrombocytopenia and associated thromboembolic disease in order to prevent further thromboembolic complications.
- Remicade® is approved for short-term management of moderately to severely active Crohn's disease including those patients with fistula.
- Renagel® capsules are approved for the reduction of serum phosphorus in patients with end-stage renal disease.
- SYNAGIS™ is approved for prevention of serious lower respiratory tract disease caused by respiratory syncytial virus (RSV) in pediatric patients at high risk of RSV disease.

- Thyrogen® is approved as an adjunctive diagnostic tool for serum thyroglobulin (Tg) testing with or without radioiodine imaging in the follow-up of patients with thyroid cancer.
- Vitravene™ is approved for the treatment of cytomegalovirus (CMV) retinitis in patients with AIDS.
- Integrilin™ is approved for treatment of patients with acute coronary syndrome and angioplasty.

ALSO IN THE 1990S

- First conviction using genetic fingerprinting in the U.K.
- Discovery that hereditary colon cancer is caused by defective DNA repair gene.
- Recombinant rabies vaccine tested in raccoons.
- Biotechnology based biopesticide approved for sale in the U.S.
- Patents issued for mice with specific transplanted genes.
- First European patent on a transgenic animal issued for transgenic mouse sensitive to carcinogens.
- Isolation of gene that clearly participates in the normal process of regulating weight.
- Breast cancer susceptibility genes cloned.
- Biotechnology Industry Organization is established.

2000

- First complete map of a plant genome developed: *Arabidopsis thaliana.*
- Biotech crops grown on 108.9 million acres in 13 countries.
- "Golden rice" announcement allows the technology to be available to developing countries in hopes of improving the health of undernourished people and preventing some forms of blindness.
- First biotech crop field-tested in Kenya: virus-resistant sweet potato.
- Rough draft of the human genome sequence is announced.
- First complete map of the genome of a food plant completed: rice.
- Chinese National Hybrid researchers report developing a "super rice" that could produce double the yield of normal rice.
- Complete DNA sequencing of the agriculturally important bacteria, *Sinorhizobium meliloti,* a nitrogen-fixing species, and *Agrobacterium tumefaciens,* a plant pest.
- A single gene from *Arabidopsis* inserted into tomato plants to create the first crop able to grow in salty water and soil.

2001

- Aranesp™ (darbepoetin alfa).
- Campath® (alemtuzumab) Kineret™ (anakinra).
- Natrecor® (nesiritide) NovoLog® (insulin aspart).
- PEG-Intron™ (pegylated version of interferon alfa-2b).

2002

- The first draft of a functional map of the yeast proteome, an entire network of protein complexes and their interactions, is completed. A map of the yeast genome was published in 1996.

- International consortia sequence the genomes of the parasite that causes malaria and the species of mosquito that transmits the parasite.
- The draft version of the complete map of the human genome is published, and the first part of the Human Genome Project comes to an end ahead of schedule and under budget.
- Scientists make great progress in elucidating the factors that control the differentiation of stem cells, identifying over 200 genes that are involved in the process.
- Biotech crops grown on 145 million acres in 16 countries, a 12% increase in acreage grown in 2001. More than one-quarter (27%) of the global acreage was grown in nine developing countries.
- Researchers announce successful results for a vaccine against cervical cancer, the first demonstration of a preventative vaccine for a type of cancer.
- Scientists complete the draft sequence of the most important pathogen of rice, a fungus that destroys enough rice to feed 60 million people annually. By combining an understanding of the genomes of the fungus and rice, scientists will elucidate the molecular basis of the interactions between the plant and pathogen.
- Scientists are forced to rethink their view of RNA when they discover how important small pieces of RNA are in controlling many cell functions.
- Aranesp™ (darbepoetin alfa).
- Elitek® (rasburicase).
- Follistim™ (follitropin beta).
- FORTEO® (teriparatide).
- HUMIRA™ (adalimumab).
- INFUSE™ Bone Graft/LT-CAGE™ (device utilizing recombinant human bone morphogenetic protein [rhBMP-2-]).
- Neulasta™ (pegfilgrastim).
- Pegasys® (peginterferon alfa-2a).
- Rebif® (interferon beta 1-a).
- Zevalin™ (ibritumomab tiuxetan).

2003

- First synthetic bacteriophage. Hamilton Smith et al. of the Institute of Biological Energy Alternatives, in Rockville, MD, publish their paper on the creation of first bacteriophage from synthetic oligonucleotides. This research will revolutionize the field of biotechnology, raising serious concerns about biological warfare hazards.
- FDA reorganized its biological division taking all recombinant drugs from Center for Biologicals Evaluation and Research (CBER) to Center for Drug Evaluation and Research (CDER); FDA also issues guidelines on comparability protocols for biologicals starting a system that will eventually result in the approval of biogeneric products in the U.S.
- Zorbtive™ (Serostim®) (somatotropin).
- Xolair® (omalizumab; recombinant DNA-derived humanized monoclonal antibody targeting immunoglobulin-E [subcutaneous]).
- Synagis™ (palivizumab; recombinantly produced, humanized monoclonal antibody).
- SOMAVERT® (pegvisomant; pegylated version of a recombinant human growth hormone analog structurally altered to act as a GH receptor antagonist).
- REMICADE® (infliximab; recombinantly produced, chimeric monoclonal antibody).
- RAPTIVA™ (efalizumab; selective, reversible T-cell blocker [subcutaneous injection; self-administered]) Humatrope® (somatotropin).
- ENBREL® (etanercept; recombinant product; dimeric fusion protein consisting of tumor necrosis factor receptor linked to the Fc portion of human IgG1).

- BEXXAR® (tositumomab and I-131 tositumomab; monoclonal antibody targeting the CD20 antigen and radiolabeled version of the antibody).
- Betaseron® (interferon beta-1b).
- Avonex® (interferon beta-1a; recombinant).
- Amevive® (alefacept; recombinant, dimeric fusion protein; targets CD45RO+ T-cells).
- Advate (recombinant antihemophilic factor produced without any added human or animal plasma proteins and albumin).

2004

- FDA refuses to accept biogeneric application for somatropin by Sandoz.
- FDA holds its first public hearing and opens forum for discussion of "follow-on" biologic products.
- BioPartners files biogeneric application for interferon in Europe; it is accepted for review as "biosimilar" product.
- Aventis receives approval for recombinant insulin glulisine (Apidra).
- California approves Proposition 71 to allow and fund research on stem cell cloning.

2 Marketing Opportunities

INTRODUCTION

The therapeutic protein market grew by 20% between 2002 and 2003, faster than the pharmaceutical industry as a whole, and is forecast to achieve sales of over $60 billion by 2010 with key market growth in the following order: erythropoietins, insulins, monoclonal antibodies (cancer), interferon alfa, blood clotting factor, colony stimulating factors, interferon beta, monoclonal (others), growth hormone, therapeutic vaccine, plasminogen activator, growth factor, interleukin, and so forth. Detailed information on each of the categories with market segmentation is available from Datamonitor; market statistics are available free from several investment bankers, particularly, ABN Amro, PriceWaterhouse, and so forth. This growth has been led by the continued expansion of the erythropoietin and insulin classes, which accounted for 26% and 15% of the total market, respectively. Monoclonal antibodies represent a newer, emerging class of therapeutic proteins.

Therapeutic compounds are divided into two broad categories: small molecules, which comprise most of the traditional drugs, and biologics. Biologics includes medically important substances like erythropoietin (Epogen®) for treating anemia, Humulin® (recombinant insulin) for diabetics, and Interleukins for treating Parkinson's disease. Small molecules, which include chemical substances like aspirin, and psychotropic drugs like Prozac®, are typically chemical compounds that are synthesized in the laboratory in a precisely controlled way by a defined sequence of chemical reactions. The nature of these molecules is such that once they are made their exact structure and composition can be determined by sophisticated laboratory tests, ensuring that if a manufacturer sets out to make a precise molecular copy of fluoxetene (Prozac®) it can know with certainly whether or not it has succeeded. Biological drugs on the other hand cannot be made in this way.

In most cases, manufacture of biologics relies on engineering live cells grown in a laboratory to produce the material of interest and then purifying and characterizing that material. There are an increasing number of sophisticated assays and tests that can be done to characterize the structure, composition, and activity of a manufactured biological drug. But, unlike with small molecules, these tests by themselves do not guarantee the clinical effectiveness or safety of a biologic. The reason is that while the synthesis of small molecules can be completely controlled to yield a precisely defined entity, the cell-based synthesis of biological drugs is much more difficult to control. Subtle alterations in cell growth conditions, nutrient supply, and host cell origin can make a significant impact on the composition of the end product.

Luckily, the fact that such subtle alterations cannot be easily detected is not typically a problem for biologic manufacturers. This is because manufacturers go to great lengths to ensure that every batch of biologic made is manufactured in precisely the same way, and in the same place, as the last batch. Indeed, review and approval of the manufacturing process and facility as well as the controls used to ensure consistency are integral parts of getting a biologic approved by the Food and Drug Administration (FDA). Thus, one might say that for biological drugs to adhere to strict manufacturing protocols becomes a substitute for the rigorous determination of structure and composition that is possible for small molecules. This argument augments well if you are the inventor of the manufacturing process and you know the details and subtleties of your specific biologic. The FDA requires you to have already manufactured a substantial supply of your biologic before you test it in humans, and that you have the facility and the process of manufacture approved.

Moreover, they will have to approve the battery of tests to be done to prove that each batch of biologic you make is as much like the last as possible. The principle is that if you have a defined process, and you use the material from that process in a clinical trial and it works, then the process and the output of that process and the manner of testing of that output are deemed acceptable.

The stakes in biogeneric drugs are high; judging by the innovator's sales of small molecules, we can easily predict huge profits for the generic companies entering the field of biological products; for example, when Lilly's blockbuster drug Prozac® came off patent, its sales fell more than 70% in 2002 due to the introduction of generic substitutes. The biotechnology industry has good reason to worry about the scenario of a generic manufacturer producing a duplicate biological molecule, using sophisticated tests to show that it is the same as the original, and then referencing the original manufacturers clinical tests to demonstrate efficacy. Still, the cost of developing biogeneric drugs is going to be higher than what the pharmaceutical industry is used to, in the development of small molecule generic versions; this is likely to reduce the price to the public but not to the same extent as experienced with small molecules.

It is at this juncture that multiple interest groups are converging to do battle. The FDA has issued statements suggesting that it may be amenable to some form of abbreviated approval process for generic biological drugs, following the principles of the abbreviated new drug application (ANDA) process currently used for small molecule drugs that go off patent. The FDA has also indicated that this new process may take advantage of section 505(b)(2) of the Federal Food Drug and Cosmetic Act (FDCA) which allows FDA applications to reference data and material to which they do not necessarily have access. Such material could include for example the safety and efficacy data filed by the original manufacturer of the biologic. The implication is that if a new manufacturer can prove that it can manufacture the same entity as the original manufacturer, it could simply reference the safety and efficacy data of that manufacturer for the original material which is in the hands of the FDA and seek approval without having to conduct lengthy and expensive clinical trials. Despite lengthy legal and logistics issues, the move to approve biogeneric products is getting stronger and with the recent filing and acceptance of a "biosimilar" interferon alfa application in Europe in October 2004, the footprint is just about complete.

Understandably, this is a scenario that has set the biotechnology industry and, in particular, the Biotechnology Industry Association (BIO) to work hard to discredit biogeneric products. Pioneer manufacturers of biological drugs would face the same threat to their monopolies and economic well-being that manufacturers of small molecule drugs now face. BIO submitted a 67-page petition to the FDA (BIO Citizen Petition [21CFR 10.30] Follow-on therapeutic proteins) objecting to the statements made by the FDA about generic biological drugs and requesting public hearings to review the process by which follow-on or generic biological drugs must be approved. The public hearing held by the FDA in September 2004 on the issue of "follow-on" biological drugs brought a strong representation from the big pharmaceuticals demonstrating why the "product is process" reality cannot be overlooked and that the FDA should not and cannot use the proprietary data submitted to support their original applications. These data include mostly the proprietary in-process controls, parameter tolerance intervals, and other such elements that define the process. If the FDA knows and is convinced what it takes to make a safe and efficacious product, should the FDA rely on this information in evaluating a biogeneric application? These are the kinds of questions currently being debated, rather hotly, in the scientific and lay press.

The arguments presented in the BIO petition are many and complex but center on one important element. They challenges the application of section 505(b)(2) to biological drugs by stating that for biological drugs specifically the agency lacks the authority to rely on one sponsor's data in support of another's application. The reason for this is that section 505 (b)(2) requires that new therapeutic molecules first be shown to be identical to the pioneer molecules that they mimic. BIO's petition makes the statement "Because of the scientific complexities of therapeutic protein products it is virtually impossible to isolate much less compare, the active ingredients of two of these products." This is a statement that might well cause considerable anxiety in patients who rely on these products for their survival, particularly in light of the Comparability Protocol that allows innovators to change the entire process including the genetically modified cells (GMCs), yet not be required to conduct any expensive clinical trials to support the safety and efficacy issues.

How much truth is there in this statement? If assays that are good enough to document batch-to-batch identity to the FDA's satisfaction exist, why can those same assays not be used to certify identity of a new version of the biologic from a different manufacturer in a different manufacturing facility? The FDA has already answered this in principle in approving Avonex® manufactured in the U.S.

The problem is that biological drugs are in fact complicated to make, and no one really believes that all the assays used to prove batch-to-batch comparability guarantee molecular identity. Indeed, as noted in the BIO petitions "Scientifically, one never demonstrates sameness, rather ... the absence of differences according to a set of tests and criteria." Turn the process over to a new group of people in a different plant and even though they may be following the same manufacturing process as the original manufacturer and using the same characterization and release assays, there is no guarantee they are making the same thing. Even worse, have the new group make the biologic by a process different from the original and the concerns become even more acute. The complexity of biological drugs requires a degree of caution beyond that applied to chemicals.

Everyone agrees that the prevailing attitude must be one of caution. However, when caution has a major economic impact on the affordability of health care, the degree of caution must be evaluated, and creative solutions must be sought.

As noted above the FDA has shown that it can accommodate complex medical and economic realities. In approving U.S. manufactured Avonex®, the FDA showed considerable flexibility on one cautionary principle, that of associating manufacturing details with approval, while retaining another, that of manufacturing know-how. It is unreasonable to ask that if the FDA approved transfer of manufacture to a different site and a new cell line operated by certified manufacturers, it might also allow transfer of those manufacturing skills from one group to another.

In fact, why not require that the original manufacturer of a biologic whose patent has expired make all the details of the manufacturing process available to those who wish to manufacture generic versions of the compound? And why not compensate such companies for their effort by extending their patent protection by 1 year, using the same principle that was applied in the orphan drug act to encourage manufacturers to work for the public good?

All of this assumes that the manufacture of generic biological drugs could be done at significant cost savings and that there is manufacturing capacity available, both questionable tenets. However, these are economic factors and not legal or regulatory ones. Whether it is practical and economically beneficial to produce generic biological drugs should have no bearing on the decision to make it legally possible to do so in a manner that can best benefit health care consumers and manufacturers alike.

What is the path forward for such approval? Some have suggested that biological drugs can be grouped into classes, each requiring different levels of comparability data depending on the expected consequences of subtle alterations in protein structure or modification. The simplest class would be those proteins for which such alterations have been shown to have little or no effect on activity, as in the case of glycosylation of human growth hormone. For this class of biological drugs only animal studies and human pharmacokinetic data might be sufficient to demonstrate comparability. More complex cases in which minor alterations or differences in composition may compromise activity or induce severe immunogenicity would likely need to be treated as a new chemical entity. Intermediate classes of biological drugs with correspondingly intermediate levels of comparability data can also be defined. It is just this kind of detailed ranking of potential generic biological drugs that the pharmaceutical and biotechnology industries need to get involved in as soon as possible.

Who besides the consumer will benefit from such a process? Clearly manufacturers of generics will benefit provided they can acquire or contract for the facilities needed to manufacture biological drugs. Given that current estimates indicate that biologic manufacturing capabilities are operating at maximum capacity, this suggests that new facilities may need to be built and that companies that do so proactively may be in a position to benefit from a biogeneric policy once it is approved.

SALES, PATENTS, AND APPROVALS

The biopharmaceutical market has come a long way since 1982 when the first biopharmaceutical product, recombinant human insulin, was launched. Over 120 such products are currently being marketed around the world including nine blockbuster drugs. The global markets for biopharmaceuticals, which was valued in 2003 at US$41 billion, has been growing at an impressive compound annual growth rate of 21% over the previous 5 years. With over one third of all pipeline products in active development being biopharmaceuticals, this segment is set to continue outperforming the total pharmaceutical market and could easily reach US$100 billion by the end of the decade. Erythropoietins, with a market size of around US$10 billion and rising, monoclonal antibodies, with a market size approaching US$7 billion and a stratospheric growth rate, human insulins, interferons, and colony stimulating factors are some of the main biopharmaceutical classes. Table 2.1 lists the top ten market leaders, their current products, and prospective market leads.

More than 20 years ago, the first biopharmaceutical products were patented in the U.S. Over the next 5 years, more than $15 billion worth of products will be coming off patent (Table 2.2). Recognizing an untapped opportunity, the pharmaceutical and biotechnology companies worldwide are focusing on the development and commercialization of generic biopharmaceutical products. Although no regulatory infrastructure presently exists in the U.S. for such an undertaking, the regulatory systems are fast responding to this need, in response to intense political pressure and the strong stance taken by the generic pharmaceutical industry in the U.S. It is likely that such filings will first take place in foreign countries, where the regulatory authorities are better prepared to accept such submissions.

The key therapeutic proteins that will fully play the market in the next few years include (some under development):

- Erythropoietins: Procrit/Eprex (epoietin alfa), Epogen (epoietin alfa) and Aranesp (darbepoietin alfa), NeoRecormon/Epogin (epoietin beta).
- Interferons Intron family, Intron A (interferon alfa-2b), PEG Intron (peg interferon alfa-2b), Rebetol (ribavirin), Rebetron (interferon alfa-2b + ribavirin), Roferon-A (interferon alfa-2a) and Pegasys (pegylated interferon alfa-2a), Avonex (interferon beta-1a), Rebif (interferon beta). Insulins: Novolin (insulin), Humulin (insulin), Humalog (insulin lispro), Lantus (glargine insulin), NN304 (insulin Detemir), AERx iDMS, Exubera (inhaled insulin).
- Monoclonal antibodies: Mabthera/Rituxan (rituximab), Remicade (infliximab), Herceptin (trastuzumab), Humira (adalimumab), Xolair (omalizumab), Bexxar (tositumomab), Raptiva (efalizumab), Erbitux/IMC-C225 (cetuximab).
- Blood factors: Activase/TNKase (alteplase/tenecteplase), NovoSeven (rh factor VIIa).
- Colony stimulating factors: Neupogen (filgrastim), Neulasta (pegfilgrastim).
- Growth hormones: Genotropin (somatropin), Nutropin/Protropin, somatropin/somatrem), Norditropin/Norditropin SimpleX (r-Somatropin), Saizen (somatropin), Serostim (somatropin).
- Interleukins: Proleukin (interleukin-2).
- Growth factors: Regranex (beclapermin), Fiblast (trafermin), Stemgen (ancetism), Keratinocyte growth factor.
- Therapeutic vaccines: Melacine (theraccine), M-Vax, OncoVax.
- Other therapeutic proteins: Enbrel (etanercept), Cerezyme (imiglucerase), Xigris (drotrecogin alfa).

TABLE 2.1
Top 10 Biopharma Companies and Their Products

Company (2003 Revenue, $ millions)	Recently Approved	Pending	Phase IIIB and Beyond	Early Research	Top Sellers
Amgen ($7868)	Enbrel (psoriasis) Neulasta (moderate risk febrile neutropenia) Aranesp (chronic kidney disease) Sensipar (secondary hyperparathyroidism in kidney disease)	Palifermin (toxicity from chemotherapy/ radiation therapy)	Panitumumab (colorectal carcinoma) AMG 714 (rheumatoid arthritis) Alfimeprase (peripheral arterial occlusion) AMG 531 (immune thrombocytopenic purpura) GDNF (Parkinson's disease) AMG 162 (osteoporosis) 11B – HSD1 (metabolic disease, type II diabetes)	Aranesp (congestive heart failure) AMG 162 (metastatic bone disease) AMG 706 (cancer)	Epogen (anemia) Aranesp (chemotherapy-induced neutropenia) Neupogen (chemotherapy) Neulasta (chemotherapy-induced neutropenia) Enbrel (rheumatoid arthritis, psoriatic arthritis)
Genentech ($2621)	Rituxan (rheumatoid arthritis) Raptiva (chronic plaque psoriasis) Avastin (metastatic colorectal cancer)	Nutropin & Nutropin AQ (idiopathic short stature)	Herceptin (adjuvant breast cancer) Lucentis (age-related macular degeneration) Nutropin Depot (adult growth hormone deficiency) Rituxan (aggressive frontline) Hematology/ Oncology (non-Hodgkin's lymphoma Rituxan (ANCA-associated vasculitis, lupus, refractory) Immunology (rheumatoid arthritis) Tarceva (lung cancer, pancreatic cancer) Xolair (pediatric asthma) Veletri (acute heart failure)	Omnitarg (breast cancer, lung cancer, ovarian cancer, prostate cancer) Raptiva (psoriatic arthritis) Immunology (multiple sclerosis) Tarceva (glioblastoma multiforme) Xolair (peanut allergy) G –024856 (basal cell carcinoma) PRO1762 (APO2L/TRAIL) (cancer therapy) PRO70769 Anti-CD20) (rheumatoid arthritis) PRO128115 (VEGF) (wound healing)	Rituxan (non-Hodgkin's lymphoma) Herceptin (breast cancer) Nutropin/Protropin (growth hormone)

Continued.

TABLE 2.1 (Continued)
Top 10 Biopharma Companies and Their Products

Company (2003 Revenue, $ millions)	Recently Approved	Pending	Phase IIIB and Beyond	Early Research	Top Sellers
Serono ($1858)	Zorbtive (short bowel syndrome)	Luveris (female infertility) Gonal – F (dosage form) Prefilled pen Raptiva (psoriasis) Saizen (small gestational age babies)	Microencapsulated (female infertility) R- FSH Anastrozole (ovulation induction, improved follicular development) Emfilermin (R-LIF) (embryo implantation enhancement) Atexakin-A (R-IL-6) (peripheral neuropathy) Serostim (HARS/lipodystrophy) R – interferon BETA (chronic hepatitis C in Asian patients) Tadekinig –A (IL –18 BP) (psoriasis) Onercept (R- TBP –1) (psoriasis)	FSH – Chimera (female infertility) Prostanoid FP (pre-term labor) Receptor antagonist oxytocin (pre-term labor) Receptor antagonist MMP- 12 (multiple sclerosis) Chemokine inhibitor (multiple sclerosis) JNK inhibitor (multiple sclerosis) Oral cladribine (multiple sclerosis) PTP1B inhibitor (diabetes, obesity) TACI- 1G (lupus, rheumatoid arthritis) Tadekinig –A- 1 –18 BP (rheumatoid arthritis)	Gonal – F (infertility) Rebif (multiple sclerosis) Saizen (growth retardation) Serostim (wasting)
Biogen Idec ($1852)	Rituxan (replaced indolent B –cell non-Hodgkin's lymphoma) Zevalin (certain B-cell non-Hodgkin's lymphoma) Avonex (multiple sclerosis – relapsing forms, monosymptomatic)	Antegren (multiple sclerosis)	Rituxan (replaced chronic lymphocytic leukemia, newly diagnosed aggressive & indolent non-Hodgkin's lymphoma, rheumatoid arthritis) Antegren (Crohn's disease, rheumatoid arthritis) Anti-CD80 MAB (non-Hodgkin's lymphoma) Avonex (chronic inflammatory demyelinating) Amevive (psoriatic arthritis) BG – 12/ (psoriasis) Oral fumarate	Kappaproct (ulcerative colitis) Anti – CD 23 MAB (chronic lymphocytic leukemia, allergic asthma & rhinitis) Interferon beta cancer Gene delivery BG-12 (multiple sclerosis) Oral fumarate (replasing forms) Adentri (congestive heart failure)	Avonex (multiple sclerosis) Rituxan (lymphoma)

Genezyme General ($1141)	Aldurazyme (mucopolysaccharidosis I) Fabryzme (Fabry disease) Cerezyme (Gaucher disease) Renagel (renal disease) Synvisc (osteoarthritis)	Myozyme (infantile Prompe disease) Tolevamer (C. *difficile* colitis) Synvisc (hip – U.S.) Synvisc (for other joints, Europe — ankle, shoulder).	Genz – 112638 (lysosomal storage disorders) Acid sphingomyelinase (type B Niemann Pick disease) Anti-TGF beta (renal and other diseases) Second Generation (chronic kidney disease) Sevelamer Thyrogen (ablation of thyroid cancer) Iron chelator (iron overload diseases) DX – 88 (hereditary angioedema) RDP-58 (ulcerative colitis and Crohn's disease) Anti-TGF Beta (diffuse scleroderma) Thymoglobulin (bone marrow transplant, liver transplant) Genz–29155 (multiple sclerosis) Anti-TGF beta (pulmonary fibrosis)	Cerezyme (Gaucher disease) Rena gel (hemodialysis)
Chiron ($1117)	Betaseron SC Injection (multiple sclerosis)		Tifacogin (community-acquired pneumonia) Daptomycin (gram-positive bacteria) Cyclosporin (acute lung transplant rejection) Menjugate (meningococcal C disease) HCV vaccine (HCV) HIV vaccine (HIV)	Proleukin (non-Hodgkin's lymphoma) CHIR258 (cancer) TOBI (dry powder for pseudomonal infection) TOBI (bronchiectasis)	Fluvirin (flu vaccine) TOBI (cystic fibrosis) Betaseron (multiple sclerosis) Proleukin (cancer)
Medimmune ($993)	Flumist (influenza) Cytogam (cytomegalovirus) Respigam (respiratory syncytial virus) Neutrexin (moderate-to-severe *Pneumocystis carinii* pneumonia)		CAIV-T (dosage form) Flumist liquid HPV vaccine (cervical cancer) Ethyol (mucositis in non-small cell lung cancer)	Epstein – BARR Vaccine (Epstein – Barr virus) Vitaxin (rheumatoid arthritis, psoriasis, cancer) Ethyol (acute myelogenous leukemia) Cytomegalovirus vaccine (cytomegalovirus) Numax (respiratory syncytial virus RSV) IL-9 antagonists (asthma, other respiratory disease)	Synagis (RSV) Ethyol (renal toxicity from chemotherapy)

Continued.

TABLE 2.1 (Continued)
Top 10 Biopharma Companies and Their Products

Company (2003 Revenue, $ millions)	Recently Approved	Pending	Phase IIIB and Beyond	Early Research	Top Sellers
Gilead Sciences ($836)	Viread (HIV /AIDS) Ambisome (severe fungal infections) Hepsera (hepatitis B) Emtriva (HIV/AIDS) Vistide (CMV retinitis) Tamflu (influenza A/ B)	Coformulation (HIV/AIDS)	Emtricitabine (hepatitis B)	GS 7340 (HIV/AIDS) GS 9005 (HIV/AIDS)	Viread (HIV) Ambisome (fungal infection)
Millennium Pharm. ($244)	Integrilin (prevents occlusion of the arteries, used in balloon angioplasty) Velcade (multiple myeloma)		Integrilin (ACS) (ST – segment elevation myocardial infarction, coronary artery bypass graft surgery) Velcade (colorectal, lung cancer, other solid tumors, non- Hodgkin's lymphoma) MLN02 (Crohn's disease, ulcerative colitis) MLN1202 (rheumatoid arthritis)	MLN519 (anti- inflammatory) MLN 2222 (reperfusion injury resulting from coronary artery bypass grafting) MLN591RL (prostate cancer) MLN518 (brain tumors) MLN2704 (metastatic prostate cancer) MLN576 (solid tumors) MLN944 (advanced solid cancers) MLN273 (proteasome inhibitor)	Integrilin (cardiovascular disease) Velcade (multiple myeloma)
Intermune ($154)	Actimune (chronic granulomatous disease, severe malignant osteoporosis) Amphotec (Aspergillosis) Inferagen (hepatitis C)		Interferon Gamma (idiopathic pulmonary fibrosis, ovarian cancer) Oritavancin (complicated skin and skin structure infection) PEG –Alfacon –1 (hepatitis C) Pirfenidone (idiopathic pulmonary fibrosis)		Actimmune (chronic granulomatous disease, malignant osteoporosis)

TABLE 2.2
Biotechnology Drugs Coming Off Patent in Recent Years

Brand Name (Generic Name)	Marketing Company	Indication	2002 Sales ($, millions)	US Patent Expiry
Robetron™ Combination Therapy (Ribavirin and Interferon alfa-2b)	Schering-Plough	Chronic hepatitis C	1361	2001
Ceredase® (aglucerase)	Cenzyme	Gaucher disease	537	2001
Cerezyme® (imiglucerase)	Cenzyme	Gaucher disease	537	2001
Humulin® (human insulin)	Novo Nordisk	Diabetes	500	2002
Intron® A (interferon alfa-2b)	Schering Plough	Leukemia; hepatitis B and C, melanoma; lymphoma	2700	2002
Avonex® (interferon beta-1a)	Biogen	Multiple sclerosis	1034	2003
Humatrope® (somatropin)	Eli Lilly & Co	Growth hormone deficiency	329	2003
Nutropin®/Nutropin AQ® (somatropin)	Genentech	Growth hormone deficiency	226	2003
Epogen® (epoietin alfa)	Amgen	Anemia	2300	2004
Procrit® (epoietin alfa)	Johnson & Johnson	Anemia	4283	2004
Geref® (sermorelin)	Serana Laboratories	Growth hormone deficiency	0.07	2004
Synagis® (palivizumab)	Abbott	Respiratory syncytial viral	480	2005
Activase® (alteplase)	Genentech	Myocardial infarction, stroke, pulmonary embolism	180	2005
Protropin® (somatrem)	Genentech	Growth hormone deficiency	2100	2005
Neupogen® (filgrastim)	Amgen	Neutropenia	1400	2005
Albutein® (human albumin)	Enzon	Shock and hemodialysis	4509	2006

The FDA has approved a large number of recombinant DNA and monoclonal antibodies recently (see Appendix I). The biotechnology derived product market is growing much faster than small-molecule therapeutic drugs, and this adds to the financial benefits in developing biogeneric products (Table 2.3). However, because of the intrinsic differences from conventional pharmaceuticals, as well as differences in the oversight and manner in which they are regulated, generic biopharmaceutical products face a number of unresolved issues inhibiting progress toward establishing rules for the approval and marketing of such compounds. Nonetheless, significant changes are under way to create biogeneric products. The research-based pharmaceutical industry is fighting hard to keep biogenerics off the market, claiming that products manufactured from different cell lines cannot be rendered equivalent.

BIOGENERIC PRODUCTS PATHWAY

Whereas there is much politics involved, there have been several events in the past that point clearly to emergence of law that will allow biogeneric biotechnology products, the foremost being the filing of the first "biosimilar" product, an alfa interferon in Europe in October 2004. At the same time Sandoz is involved in litigation in Europe over its somatropin product, which was also filed but refused by the FDA. The FDA is likely to take a cautious path wherein some, but not all, products may be candidates for biogenerics. The first candidates are likely to be simple proteins to be followed by therapeutic proteins with complex glycosylation and monoclonal antibodies. The early drugs will likely be nonglycosylated proteins with known tertiary structure and known mechanism of action and where analytical comparisons with original product are possible. The product would have to demonstrate an acceptable safety profile and meet both a validated clinical surrogate for efficacy as well as a short-term objective clinical endpoint. The FDA is likely to be stricter on the control of the Master Cell Bank than it would concern itself with differences in

TABLE 2.3
Historical Worldwide Sales of Recombinant Drugs

Product	Protein	Effects/Therapeutic Use	Marketed By	Worldwide Sales ($, millions)						
				1997	1998	1999	2000	2001	2002	2003
Epogen	Erythropoietin	Stimulation of the production of erythrocytes	Amgen	1161	1380	1760	1960	2200	2300	2400
Procrit/ Eprex	Erythropoietin alfa	Stimulation of the production of erythrocytes	J&J/ Ortho Biotech	1000	1460	1505	2709	3430	4283	3984
NeoRecormon	Erythropoietin beta	Stimulation of the production of erythrocytes	Roche	—	—	—	—	443	1192	998
Aranesp	Darbepoietin alfa	Stimulation of the production of erythrocytes	Amgen	—	—	—	—	42	400	1500
Intron (incl. PEGylated alfa-interferon/ Ribavirin)	Alfa-interferon (+ PEGylated alfa-interferon)	Antitumor (anti-HCV)	Schering-Plough	598	—	650	1361	1447	2700	1851
Avonex	Interferon beta-1a	Multiple sclerosis	Biogen	240	394.9	621	761	972	1034	1168
Rebif	Interferon-beta-1a	Multiple sclerosis	Ares Serono	19	44	143	254	379.6	548.8	630.8
Betaseron/ Betaferon	Interferon beta-1b	Multiple sclerosis	Schering AG	297	321	395	546	592	830	770
Neupogen	G-CSF	Stimulation of the production of granulocytes	Amgen	1056	1120	1260	1220	1300	1400	1300
Neulasta	G-CSF PEG conjugate	Stimulation of the production of granulocytes	Amgen	—	—	—	—	—	—	1300
Leukine	GM-CSF	Stimulation of leukocytes	Immunex/ Schering AG	53	63.8	69.1	88.3	108.4	n.a. (04/03)	n.a. (02/04)
Humulin	Insulin	Diabetes	Eli Lilly	936	959.2	1087.5	1114.5	1060.6	1004	1060
Humalog	Insulin	Diabetes	Eli Lilly	—	—	—	350.2	627.8	1004	1021
Rituxan (in EU: Mabthera)	Rituximab (humanized antibody)	Leukemia and lymphomas	Genentech/ Roche	—	162.6	279.4	444.1	818.7	1163	2220
Herceptin	Trastuzumab (anti-HER-2 antibody)	Breast cancer	Genentech/ Roche	—	30.5	188.4	275.9	346.6	385	942

Product	Substance/Type	Indication	Company							
Enbrel	Etanercept (fusion protein of antibody-Fc and p75-TNF receptor protein)	Rheumatoid arthritis	Immunex/Amgen	1300	802	761.9	652.4	366.9	—	—
Remicade	Infliximab (chimeric antibody)	Rheumatoid arthritis, morbus Crohn	Schering-Plough	n.a. (02/04)	337	166	57	—	—	—
Humatrope	Human growth hormone (HGH) Somatotropin	Dwarfism	Eli Lilly	n.a. (02/04)	329	312.7	301	300	268	260
Protropin/Nutropin	Human growth hormone (HGH) Somatotropin	Dwarfism	Genentech	297	250	226.6	221.2	214	224	—
Serostim	Human growth hormone (HGH)	Dwarfism	Ares Serono	88.8	95.1	125.3	137.1	137.4	88.2	38.8
Saizen	Human growth hormone (HGH)	Dwarfism	Ares Serono	151.5	124	107.3	90.0	—	—	—
Cerezyme/Ceredase	Glucocerebrosidase	Gaucher's disease	Genzyme	n.a. (02/04)	619	570	537	479	411	333
Synagis	Humanized mAb	Respiratory syncytial virus prevention	Abbott/Medimmune	n.a. (02/04)	668	516	427	293	110	—
Gonal F	Follitropin alfa	Stimulation of ovulation	Ares Serono	526.1	450.4	410.5	365.9	348.7	243.8	116
Activase	Tissue plasminogen activator	Coronary infarct	Genentech	n.a. (02/04)	180	197	206	236	213	—
ReoPro	GBIIb/IIIa-antibody	Inhibition of thrombosis	Eli Lilly/Centocor	n.a. (02/04)	384	431.4	418.1	447.3	365.4	254
Kogenate	Factor VIII	Hemophilia	Bayer	n.a. (02/04)	424	—	427	327	335	262
Engerix-B	Envelope protein of the hepatitis B virus	Vaccine	SmithKline Beecham	n.a. (02/04)	n.a. (04/03)	—	—	540	574	584
Pulmozyme	Human DNAse	Mucoviscidosis	Genentech	n.a. (02/04)	138	123	121.8	111.4	93.8	92
Proleukin	Interleukin	Cancer	Chiron	n.a. (02/04)	114	93	113	112	93	71

down-stream processing, which has improved substantially in recent years. The clinical studies required will likely not be the full clinical package but it will not be limited to PK (as allowed in ANDA), and some small clinical studies will be required.

CASE LAW

The case of *Serono v. Shalala* established that the power to determine "sameness" lay with FDA and that a therapeutically equivalent biologic can be achieved. FDA's determination of what is required to establish "sameness" was upheld in an appeals court decision. Essentially, FDA is entitled to a "high level of deference" for "evaluations of scientific data within its area of expertise." The significance of this ruling is that it established the authority for the determination of "sameness" solely with FDA — a point that the FDA advocated and the courts upheld. In addition, FDA exemplified that a generic or therapeutically equivalent biologic can be achieved.

In *Amgen Inc. v. Hoechst Marion Roussel, Inc. and Transkaryotic Therapies, Inc.*, it was disclosed in district court proceedings that Transkaryotic Therapies' product is not significantly different from Amgen's product. At the same time, TKTX's product was reported to FDA as equivalent in therapeutic properties to Amgen's product. This suggests that simple amino acid changes in a biologic do not result in a different product, unless the changes result in functional differences. As such, a generic manufacturer may engineer a biologic, which would be considered the "same" as the originator's one.

According to the FDA, there are multiple approval processes for interchangeable drugs, but there are legal issues surrounding biological drugs. Interchangeable products will require evidence to demonstrate therapeutic equivalence, which is scientifically based, technology driven, and product dependent. The biotechnology derived drugs can be divided into two groups — macromolecules and small molecules. Macromolecules comprise proteins, genes, and mononuclear antibody-drug conjugates. Small molecules cover antibiotics, amino acids, vitamins, and other cell metabolites. Current policy on biotechnology derived products comes from the Federal Registrar (51 FR 23309) dated June 26, 1986. Points to consider in the production testing of new drugs and biologicals produced by recombinant DNA technology were issued on April 10, 1986. An Investigational New Drug (IND) and full New Drug Application (NDA) (505 (b)(1)) are required, and a Chemistry, Manufacturing, and Control (CMC) supplement is not acceptable. FDA released its first Comparability for Protein Drugs guidance in 1994. Within the same manufacturer's product before and after manufacturing changes, clinical studies may be waived. This is separate from equivalents (21 CFR 320.1 (c) and (e)), which are between products manufactured by different manufacturers. The Pharmaceutical Research and Manufacturers of America (PhRMA) and BIO are sensitive to this issue because FDA has stated: "We are postulating a path for the recombinant molecule that gets an AB rating in the Orange Book, that does not come in under the [ANDA] route, it comes in under the (b)(2) route." The FDA has proposed a potential pathway for generic biologic approval using an established procedure. This is demonstrated by several major initiatives by the FDA.

- Approval of Biogen's Avonex® by the FDA for multiple sclerosis showed that the product produced from a different cell line than the one used to produce the current marketed product can be same. The Avonex® case illustrates that after extensive characterization and analysis that two different cell lines can be proven comparable. It demonstrates that biological drugs can be quantified, that different cell lines and manufacturing processes can be utilized to produce the same clinically efficacious compound, and that issues of safety and immunogenicity are manageable. This directly refutes BIO's claim that products produced by different cell lines cannot be equivalent.
- Transfer of therapeutic proteins and some other drugs from FDA's Center for Biologics Evaluation and Research (CBER) to the Center for Drug Evaluation and Research (CDER) where possibility of filing generic applications exists.

- Issuance of a number of guidelines such as the comparability protocols for biotechnology drugs, evaluation of immunogenicity of products, prevention of viral contamination, characterization of cell lines, and so forth, discussed in greater details elsewhere in this book.
- The FDA released on May 7, 2003, a new guidance document: *FDA's Guidance for Industry: Independent Consultants for Biotechnology Clinical Protocols* (Docket No. 03D-0112, Federal Register May 7, 2003, Pages 24486-24487), which allows use of outside consultants to review clinical testing protocols. This guidance document announcement of a new procedure by which the biotechnology product sponsors can request the FDA to appoint an expert consultant to receive their input during the review of proposed clinical trials. This is a result of understanding that biotechnology products are often novel and complex, requiring a study design with a high level of expertise to build and justify. More specifically, this includes a 60-day extension for the scheduling of a meeting that is subject to this guidance; this is to allow FDA time to consider and screen potential consultants and allows the consultant time to review the scientific issues. The guidance states that the FDA may decide not to select a consultant from the list suggested by the sponsor and does not specify how the consultant's input will be shared with the sponsor or how there would be dispute resolution if the sponsor does not agree with the rationale for denial.
- FDA has been accepting proposals for a regulatory pathway. At this point, CDER has decided that the traditional ANDA route does not allow for sufficient evidence to approve a generic biopharmaceutical. This is partly because CDER cannot ask for additional preclinical or clinical testing under an ANDA. FDA has sought a compromise application, which offers data from the innovator product and the potential for additional information. In following this approval process, a recombinant protein would technically not be filed under an ANDA, as generic drugs are, rather it would be filed under section 505(b)(2) of the Food Drug and Cosmetic Act, not 505(j), making it a "me too" product with "AB" substitution. A 505(b)(2) application is a new drug application where the sponsor relies on data it does not own. It may be considered a hybrid between the regular NDA with full, independent data or data for which the applicant has the rights, called a 505(b)(1), and the 505(j), which is a generic drug application (ANDA). An approved 505(b)(2) receives NDA patent protection. The sponsor, therefore, creates a branded generic.

PHARMACOPOEIA EFFORTS

The U.S. Pharmacopoeia (USP) establishes and disseminates officially recognized standards of quality and authoritative information for the use of medicines and other health care technologies. USP has suggested use of the term "pharmaceutical equivalence" when comparing moieties of biotech products to which changes have been made, and potentially for comparing products developed by different manufacturers. USP believes that the way to determine the critical differences in a highly complex molecular structure is to perform replicative crossover studies. Crossover studies would show proof of concept by following patients who have been switched from the original product to the generic and vice versa. These would typically be designed as small Phase III trials. However, it is anticipated that the FDA will primarily be interested in safety studies, relying on other information, such as bioequivalence, for approval. The Health Care Financing Administration (HCFA) policy brings a controversy. Section 1861(f)(1) of the Social Security Act of 1965 states that in order to obtain Medicare reimbursements, drugs and biological drugs must be either included or approved for inclusion in a select number of compendia such as the USP-NF. BIO is resisting such a policy shift due to the implications of monographs for biological drugs, which raises the issue of intellectual property. Industry is under the impression that biologic monographs will provide a "how to" on the manufacture of biological drugs.

Monographs are an important step in the standardization of biological drugs even if the HCFA may reverse its policy under political pressure. The USP is likely to follow the BP and EP and start including monographs for biotechnology products soon. The USP has begun setting up standards for the characterization of generic biological drugs, providing a highly respected, independent voice in favor of the concept. In addition to developing guidance documents such as for submission of scientific and technical documentation for approval of somatotropin (hGH) and human insulin drug products under section 505(b)(2, the USP 27 (2004) includes several guidance documents of relevance to biotechnology products:

- <1045> Biotechnology-Derived Articles
- <1047> Biotechnology-Derived Articles Tests
- <1048> Quality of Biotechnological Products: Analysis of the Expression Construct in Cells Used for Production of r-DNA Derived Protein Products
- <1049> Quality of Biotechnological Products: Stability Testing of Biotechnological/Biological Products
- <1050> Viral Safety Evaluation of Biotechnology Products Derived from Cell Lines of Human or Animal Origin
- <1078> Good Manufacturing Practices for Bulk Pharmaceutical Excipients
- <1086> Impurities in Official Articles

LEGISLATIVE ACTION

There is growing interest within the legislature toward establishing new regulations for the approval of generic biological drugs as part of a comprehensive reform of the overall Waxman-Hatch framework.

The Medicare Bill is a landmark legislation that ensures that the patients who need biotechnology medicines the most will have access to them. It also removes a major layer of uncertainty for the companies and investors developing those medicines. The bill stabilizes and protects federal reimbursement of biotechnology products and other drugs for some 40 million Medicare beneficiaries. Although the new program is slated to take effect in 2006, many of the legislation's provisions will have a near-term impact. Three months after enactment, the Medicare program will launch a $500 million demonstration project covering oral cancer drugs and self-injectable biotech products for rheumatoid arthritis and multiple sclerosis. Until now, Medicare did not cover these medicines. The legislation also will reverse the deep Medicare cuts (instituted in 2002) to biotech products used in the hospital outpatient setting, and it prohibits future application of the concept of functional equivalence, a controversial mechanism by which a new drug could be deemed "functionally equivalent" to an older one and reimbursed at the same rate. For the biotechnology industry, this legislation is a major milestone.

TECHNOLOGY ADVANCES

Technologic advances have made downstream processing much more consistent and less likely to a source of concern to regulatory authorities. Some examples include: MALDI-TOF Spectroscopy, Reflectometric Interference Spectroscopy, Capillary electrochromatography, Signal Transduction Fingerprinting, Bioinformatics, including Microarray Technology and Pharmacogenomics. The crux of the other reservations, besides the issue of immunogenicity, generally revolves around science's ability to manufacture and measure such products. Since those early reservations, there has been a combination of technological advances, which are fulfilling the necessary requirements for such an undertaking. This is particularly true for improved production and assay techniques (e.g., *in vitro*/biochemical and analytical assays).

TABLE 2.4
Some Contemporary Issues in Regulatory Approvals of Biogeneric Products and Their Solutions

Problems	Potential Solutions
Complex chemical structure closely associated with biological activity, clinical safety, and efficacy	Physiochemical testing
Physiochemical tests with limitation	Biological testing
Biological activity assays imprecise, unable to detect small chemical changes	Clinical relevance
Same solution formulation containing the same protein, with different PK/PD profiles when produced by different manufacturers or different processes	Standard requirements
Isoforms with different PK/PD profiles	PK/PD testing
Assays for PK are problematic	Clinical efficacy (in the absence of meaningful bioassays and/or *in vivo* biomarkers)
Inherent microgenicity	Preclinical safety (e.g., impurity qualification) and clinical safety (e.g., immunogenicity)
Determining critical differences in a product	Crossover studies

Source: After ABN "AMRO Special Report: Generic Biologics — The Next Frontier, 2001."

SCIENTIFIC RATIONALE

It is generally accepted that any generic biologic would have to be considered on a case-by-case basis. There is a sound scientific rationale to resolving the problems currently facing the evaluation of biogeneric products (Table 2.4).

3 Manufacturing Overview

INTRODUCTION

Macromolecular (large molecules) substances (e.g., therapeutic proteins) are manufactured by a number of methods, including extraction from natural sources (as done in the past to extract erythropoietin from urine), modification of naturally occurring protein, mammalian cell culture *in vitro*, mammalian cell culture *in vivo*, production by microorganisms, and chemical syntheses. The overall regulatory scheme for biotechnology derived products is the same as for products in the same category produced by traditional manufacturing methods, with the addition of specific requirements suited to the biotechnology derived product. As an example, somatropin (human growth hormone) was approved by the FDA on July 30, 1976, derived from natural sources (Asellarcin® of Serono) and in April 1979 (Crescormon® of Genentech); both of these products have since been discontinued and replaced with recombinantly produced somatropin in 1993. The entire technical package relating to purity and characterization of somatropin remains the same for the product except there are new steps of production added.

Generally, manufacturing recombinant therapeutic proteins involves:

- Cloning of a specific gene in the laboratory, or the construction of a synthetic gene;
- Insertion into a host cell and subcloning in a microorganism or cell culture;
- Process development on a pilot scale to optimize yield and quality;
- Large-scale fermentation or cell culture processes;
- Purification of the macromolecular proteins;
- Animal testing, clinical testing, regulatory approval, and marketing.

This applies to both recombinant deoxyribonucleic acid (rDNA)-derived products as well as monoclonal antibody products. Biotechnology derived products are therefore readily differentiated from proteins or peptides that have been obtained by isolation from natural source materials such as plasma, serum, or tissue, or by chemical synthesis even though the nature of the product is the same and even labeled as such, for example, hEPO (human erythropoietin) or hIFN (human interferon); except for the undesirable changes that may arise as a result of processing, these products are indeed an exact replica of what the body produces.

MANUFACTURING PROCESS

The manufacturing processes follow similar basic requirements for process validation, environmental control, aseptic manufacturing, and quality control/quality assurance systems as required for pharmaceutical products, though with a great deal more complexity, as the processes of cell propagation, purification methods, and analytical controls are significantly different and more detailed. Most pharmaceutical companies are not likely to have in-house expertise to handle this new requirement slanted toward biological rather than chemical aspects. It is always inevitable not to recruit specialized manpower for the manufacturing of biological products. This applies not just to the recombinant phase of manufacturing but also the formulation aspects that offer unique handling and therefore validation problems.

Overall, the process of manufacturing is comprised of *upstream, downstream,* and *formulation* processing. Upstream refers to cell culture, leading to fermentation. The downstream segment of process begins with the harvest step where the cells are separated, the target proteins are separated from host and process-related impurities, an intermediate purification step (or further separation from host), followed by a polishing step to separate target protein from impurities. The yield at this point is called drug substance. The formulation step involves preparing a dosage form ready for administration to humans by converting drug substance into drug product. This is an equally important step as studies show that protein structures can be significantly altered depending on how the batch is handled. For example, a recent change in the label for erythropoietin indicates that the vial should *not* be shaken prior to administration to protect the protein structure. In upstream the major strategic issue is whether the cell culture should be run in the batch, fed-batch, or in continuous mode, the latter being very attractive at low expression levels because of higher yields in continuous processing. Whereas the recombinant process outline is to some extent determined by the expression system used, most recombinant processes follow identical patterns. The target protein is expressed in cellular systems (bacteria, mammalian cells, and insect cells), transgenic animals, or plants (upstream part). The harvest is purified by means of several purification unit operations divided into capture, intermediary purification, and polishing (downstream), resulting in the purified bulk material (drug substance). Finally, the drug substance is transformed into a product acceptable for use in humans (drug product). Upstream refers to protein expression and harvest; downstream refers to capture, intermediate purification, and polishing, and formulation refers to conversion of the drug substance to drug product.

The entire manufacturing process must be tightly connected at each unit of operation of upstream and downstream processing. Yield variation, impurity diversity, and potency achieved are the factors that can significantly affect all steps. As a result, the manufacturing process is carefully laid out in a lengthy exercise of process definition and development, a flow chart that identifies slacks as well as sizing issues. These charts are presented elsewhere in the book.

CELL CULTURE EXPRESSION SYSTEMS

The starting material for manufacturing therapeutic proteins are the bacterial, yeast, insect, or mammalian cell culture that expresses the protein product or monoclonal antibody of interest. To ensure identity and purity of the starting raw material, manufacturers use the cell seed lot system. A cell seed lot consists of aliquots of a single culture. The master cell bank (MCB) is derived from a single colony (bacteria, yeast) or a single eukaryotic cell, stored cryogenically to ensure genetic stability, and composed of sufficient ampoules of culture to provide source material for the working cell bank (WCB). The WCB is defined as a quantity of cells derived from one or more ampoules of the MCB, stored cryogenically and used to initiate the production batch.

The most common cellular expression systems used to manufacture therapeutic proteins include bacteria (*E. coli, Bacillus subtilis, Lactococcus lactis*), yeast (*Saccharomyces cerevisiae, Pichia pastoris*), mammalian cells (Chinese hamster ovary, baby hamster kidney), and insect cells where the baculovirus expression system is used to some extent and may prove itself as a future biopharmaceutical expression system; currently, there are no products approved using insect cell lines or transgenic animals, though several are under development (Table 3.1).

The choice of expression system depends on factors such as type of target protein, posttranslational modifications, expression level, intellectual property rights, and economy of manufacture. The *E. coli* expression system offers rapid and cheap expression, but cannot express complex proteins, and it includes *in vitro* folding and tag removal into the downstream process. Yeast generally expresses the target protein in its native form to the medium, but expression levels are very low. Insect cells provide many advantages of the mammalian cell characteristics. Table 3.2 lists the advantages and disadvantages of each of these systems.

Table 3.1
Cell Lines Used for Commercially Produced Recombinant Products as Approved by the FDA

Type of Cell	rDNA Product (Brand)
African monkey kidney cells (COS-1)	Antihemophilic factor (Advate®)
Baby hamster kidney cells	Antihemophilic factor (Helixate® and Kogenate®FS)
Chinese hamster ovary cell	Adalimumab (Humira®)
	Alefacept (Amevive®)
	Alemtuzumab (Campath®)
	Algasidase beta (Fabrazume®)
	Alteplase (Activase®, Cathflo®)
	Antihemophilic factor (Bioclate®, Recombinate® Rahf®, ReFacto®)
	Choriogonadotropin alfa (Ovidrel®)
	Coagulation factor IX (BeneFix®)
	Darbepoetin alfa (Aranesp®)
	Dornase alfa (Pulmozyme®)
	Drotrecogin alfa (Xigris®)
	Efalizumab (Raptiva®)
	Epoietin alfa (Epogen®, Procrit®)
	Etanercept (Enbrel®)
	Follitropin alfa (Gonal-F®)
	Follitropin beta (Follistim®)
	Ibritumomab tiuxetan (Zevalin®)
	Imiglucerase (Cerezyme®)
	Interferon beta 1-alfa (Avonex®)
	Laronidase (Aldurazyme®)
	Omalizumab (Xolair®)
	Rituximab (Rituxan®)
	Tenecteplase (TNKase®)
	Thyrotropin alfa (Thyrogen®)
	Trastuzumab (Herceptin®)
E. coli	Aldesleukin Proleukin, IL-2®
	Alfa interferon+ribavarin Reberon®
	Alfa-interferon (Intron A®)
	Anakinra (Kineret®)
	Bone morphogenetic protein [rhBMP-2-] device (Infuse® Bone Graft/LT-CAGE®)
	Coagulation factor VIIa (NovoSeven®)
	Denileukin difitox (Ontak®)
	Filgrastim (Neupogen®)
	Growth Hormone (BioTropin®)
	Insulin (Humalog,® Humulin®, Velosulin®, BR Novolin®, Novolin L®, Novloin R®, Novolin® 70/30,Novloin N®)
	Insulin aspart (Novolog®)
	Insulin glargine (Lantus®)
	Insulin glulisine (Apidra®)
	Interferon alfa-2a (Roferon-A®)
	Interferon alfacon-1 (Infergen®)
	Interferon beta 1-a (Rebif®)
	Interferon beta 1-B (Betaseron®)
	Interferon gamma-1b (Actimmune®)
	Nesiritide (Natrecor®)
	Oprelvekin (Neumega®)
	Pegfilgrastim (Neulasta®)
	Peginterferon alfa-2z (Pegasys®)

Table 3.1 (Continued)
Cell Lines Used for Commercially Produced Recombinant Products as Approved by the FDA

Type of Cell	rDNA Product (Brand)
E. coli (Continued)	Pegvisomant (Somavert®)
	Pegylated interferon alfa-2b (PEG-Intron®)
	Reteplase (Retavase®)
	Somatotropin (Humatrope®)
	Somatrem (Protropin®)
	Somatropin (Norditropin®, Nutropin® / Nutropin AQ®) Nutropin Depot®
	GenoTropin® Geref®)
	Teriparatide (Forteo®)
Lymphocyte activated	Daclizumab (Zenapax®)
Mouse C 127	Growth hormone (Saizen®, Serostim®)
Mouse myeloma	Basiliximab (Simulect®)
Myeloma NSO	Gemtuzumab ozogamicin (Mylotarg®)
Mammalian	Tositumomab with I-131(Bexxar®)
	Abciximab (ReoPro®)
Prostate epithelium cell	Capromab pendetide with In-111 (ProstaScint®)
Saccharomyces cerevisiae	Becaplermin gel (Regranex® Gel)
	Glucagon (GlucaGen®)
	Granulocyte macrophage colony-stimulating factor (Leukine®)
	Haemophilus B conjugate (Comvax®)
	Hepatitis A inactivated and hepatitis B vaccine (Twinrix®)
	Hepatitis B and inactivated polio-virus vaccine (Pediarix®)
	Hepatitis B vaccine (Engerix-B®, Recombivax-HB®)
	Lepirudin (Refludan®)
	OspA lipoprotein (LYMErix®)
	Rasburicase (Elitek®)

TABLE 3.2
Comparison of Various Expression Systems, Advantages, and Disadvantages

Qualifier	Bacteria	Yeast	Insect Cells	Mammalian Cells	Transgenic Animals
Example	E. coli	*Saccharomyces cerevisiae, Pichia pastoris*	*Lepidopteran*	Chinese hamster ovary cell	Cattle
Level of expression	High	Medium	Medium	Medium	Very high
Time to produce expression system	Fast	Fast	Medium	Slow	Very slow
	5 days	14 days	4 weeks	4–8 weeks	6–33 months
Cost	Low	Low	High	High	Medium
Extracellular expression	No	Yes	Yes	Yes	Yes
Met-Protein expression	Yes	No	No	No	No
Posttranslation modifications	No	No	Yes	Yes	Yes
Major impurities	Endotoxins	Glycosylated products	Viruses	Viruses	Viruses and prions
In vitro protein refolding	Yes	No	No	No	No
Unintended glycosylation	No	Possible	Possible	Possible	Possible
Host cell protein expression	No	No	No	No	Yes
Regulatory track record	Good	Good	N/A	Good	n/a

BACTERIA

The common bacterial expression systems make use of gram negative (e.g., *E. coli*), and gram positive host cells (*Bacillus* and *Lactococcus*) allow both intracellular and extracellular expression of target protein, however, without posttranslational modifications. It takes about 5 days from introduced gene to protein production at acceptable levels of a few hundred mg/L to g/L. Bacterial systems are easy to scale up from culture flask to fermenters with capacity into thousands of liters because of their simpler nutrition and aeration requirements and their ability to withstand shear force. Several types of culture processes are used such as batch and fed-batch, making this system highly flexible. The major adventitious agents are host cell proteins and endotoxins from *E. coli*; viruses are of little concern, except what may be required to control general exposure during processing. Critical steps including control of impurities arising out of released proteolytic enzymes and endotoxins, besides the handling of inclusion bodies, *in vitro* folding and cleavage of the N-terminal extension introduced to overcome the problem with expression of Met-protein. As a result, the downstream processing is often complicated, which can limit the choice of this expression system. However, the regulatory record is impressive (Table 3.2); at this stage only gram-negative organisms have been approved.

YEAST

The yeast species *Saccharomyces cerevisiae* and *Pichia pastoris* are also used, with their use quickly growing (Table 3.1 and Table 3.2) as these systems offer high efficiency (short doubling times, high cell densities, high yields from better mass transfer of nutrients in unicellular growth morphology) and low fermentation costs. The media cost and scale-up considerations are similar to those encountered in bacterial systems; however, the development time frame is a bit longer, about 14 days from gene construct to production. Both batch and fed-batch culture methods are used. The target protein is usually expressed directly to the medium in its native form, although some proteins tend to undergo degradation upon expression (e.g., proinsulin). A low redox potential of the medium/harvest is sometimes observed, resulting in cleavage of disulfide bonds. Yeast has GRAS (generally regarded as safe) FDA status, and host-related impurities are very low since the organism has a rigid cell wall and the expressed protein is secreted to the medium. Like the bacterial cultures, viruses are of little significance as contaminants. The purification process is usually simpler compared to the bacterial system (since the product is secreted in yeast), and no extra host-cell-related operations are required. However, the disadvantages include lack of posttranslational modifications and unexpected formation of mono- and diglycosylated forms of the target proteins that may be difficult to remove.

INSECT CELLS

Insect cells constitute a promising, yet unproven, alternative to bacterial and yeast expression systems for a wide range of target proteins requiring proper posttranslational modifications. The difficulties in scale-up arise because of difficulties in aeration and type of infection needed for high-level expression. The use of baculovirus system is very quickly becoming accepted; it has been used to transform *lepidopteran* insect cells into high-level expression systems in the range of 1 to 600 mg/L. Preparation and purification of the recombinant virus is faster than the process in mammalian cells and can be completed in about 4 weeks. In the fermentation cycle, the insect cells grow 50-fold in about a week but only in single batches or in semicontinuous batches because of the sensitivity of the cells to shear force. The costs for culture media are moderate (serum free media) to expensive compared to bacteria and yeast media. The system is suited for expression of cell toxic products since the cells can be grown in a healthy state before infection. Insect cells lack the ability to properly process proteins that are initially synthesized as larger inactive precursor proteins (e.g., peptide hormones, neuropeptides, growth factors, matrix metalloproteases). Baculoviruses are not infectious to vertebrates and therefore do not pose a health threat, though the risk of adventitious viruses is still not settled, requiring virus inactivation and active filtration. Also, the cyclic killing and lysis of the host cell releases intracellular proteins and nucleic acids into the medium, severely straining the downstream purification steps (like in the case of bacterial cells with inclusion bodies). The regulatory record of insect cells remains poor as no products have been approved by the FDA yet.

Mammalian Cells

Mammalian cells like Chinese hamster ovary (CHO), human cervix (HeLa), African green monkey kidney (COS), baby hamster kidney (BHK) cells and hybridomas are widely used for the production of monoclonal antibodies and complex posttranslational eukaryotic proteins. The target protein is generally expressed directly to the medium in its native form. The development timeline from gene construct to production is 4 to 5 months and the yields obtained range from a few mg/L to g/L. Since the protein is expressed to the low viscosity medium and the content of host cell proteins is usually low, the purification processes are relative simple; however, these processes must remove components like peptone, antifoam reagents, growth factors, and so forth when used as well as the released host cell proteins and nucleic acids due to apoptosis and cell sensitivity to shear forces. Mammalian cells are difficult and slow to grow and are more fragile than microbial cells, making them very sensitive to shear forces; batch or fed-batch cultures are often used for antibody production, while other recombinant protein also may be produced in continuous cultures over 4 to 8 weeks. Culture media are expensive relative to those used for microbial and yeast protein expression. Since viral contamination is a real risk, inactivation and removal must be designed into the downstream process and extensive control procedures established (e.g., end of production testing, virus validation). The relative low expression levels combined with high prices on culture media and expensive quality control programs make it generally more expensive to produce recombinant proteins in animal cells than in microbial systems. However, complex proteins cannot be expressed in microbial systems, leaving transgenic animals or plants as the only alternative. The regulatory record of the use of mammalian cells is very good (Table 3.2).

Transgenic Animals

Transgenic animals have the most promising recombinant protein expression systems in the biopharmaceutical industry. The first product, an antibody expressed in goats, is about to be approved by the FDA. In this system, even complex posttranslational modified proteins are successfully expressed in their native biologically active form, thus making it possible to produce plasma proteins, human antibodies, and other proteins not easily derived from other sources at industrial scale. It takes 6 to 33 months (depending on host organism) from gene construct to product expression, usually in the mammary gland, often at high protein concentrations (50 mg/ml), resulting in up to a yearly production of 10 to 100 kg per animal (cows). Transgenic animals coexpress species-specific target protein, which can be difficult to separate from the recombinant target protein. Virus inactivation and removal procedures must be included. Even though rarely recorded, prions as well as the most likely viruses undergo virus inactivation and removal and with extensive control procedures must be established (e.g., end of production test, virus validation). The skim milk fraction is an excellent starting material after capture of fat and casein. For large-scale production (> 100 kg/yr), the costs of raw products are one tenth for transgenic animals compared to mammalian cell cultures, mainly because of reduction in capital investment. The regulatory record in the use of transgenic animals is poor (Table 3.2).

CELL LINES AND CHARACTERIZATION

Since the genetic stability of the cell bank during storage and propagation is a major concern, it is important to know the origin and history (number of passages) of both the MCB and WCB. An MCB ampoule is kept frozen or lyophilized and only used once. Occasionally, a new MCB may be generated from a WCB. The new MCB should be tested and properly characterized in accordance with the prescribed ICH protocol. For biological products, a product license application or amendment must be submitted and approved before a new MCB can be generated from a WCB. Information about the construction of the expression vector, the fragment containing the genetic material that encodes the desired product, and the relevant genotype and phenotype of the host cell(s) are submitted as part of a product application. The major concerns of biological systems are genetic stability of cell banks during production and storage, contaminating microorganisms, and the presence of endogenous viruses in some mammalian cell lines. As part of the application document, manufacturers are required to submit a description of all tests performed to characterize and qualify a cell bank.

It must be emphasized that the tests required to characterize a cell bank will depend on the intended use of the final product, the host/expression system, and the method of production including the techniques employed for purification of the product. In addition, the types of tests may change as technology advances. The MCB is rigorously tested using the following tests, though the testing may not be limited to these tests:

- Genotypic characterization by DNA fingerprinting;
- Phenotypic characterization by nutrient requirements, isoenzyme analysis, growth, and morphological characteristics;
- Reproducible production of desired product;
- Molecular characterization of vector/cloned fragment by restriction enzyme mapping, sequence analysis;
- Assays to detect viral contamination;
- Reverse transcriptase assay to detect retroviruses;
- Sterility test and mycoplasma test to detect other microbial contaminants.

It is not necessary to test the WCB as extensively as the MCB; however, limited characterization of a WCB is necessary. The following tests are generally performed on the WCB, but this list is not inclusive:

- Phenotypic characterization;
- Restriction enzyme mapping;
- Sterility and mycoplasma testing;
- Testing the reproducible production of desired product.

The MCB and WCB must be stored in conditions that ensure genetic stability. Generally, cells stored in liquid nitrogen (or its vapor phase) are stable longer than cells stored at 70˚C. In addition, it is recommended that the MCB and WCB be stored in more than one location in the event that a freezer malfunctions.

MEDIA

Media must be carefully selected to provide the proper rate of growth and the essential nutrients for the organisms, thus producing the desired product. Raw materials should not contain any undesirable and toxic components that may be carried through the cell culture, fermentation, and the purification process to the finished product. Water is an important component of the media and the quality of the water will depend on the recombinant system used, the phase of manufacture, and the intended use of the product. Raw materials considered to be similar when supplied by a different vendor should meet acceptance criteria before use. In addition, a small-scale pilot run followed by a full-scale production run is recommended when raw materials from a different vendor are used to ensure that growth parameters, yield, and final product purification remain the same.

Most mammalian cell cultures require serum for growth. Frequently, serum is a source of contamination by adventitious organisms, especially mycoplasma, and firms must take precautions to ensure sterility of the serum. There is an additional concern that bovine serum may be contaminated with bovine spongiform encephalopathy (BSE) agent. Because there is no sensitive *in vitro* assay to detect the presence of this agent, it is essential that the manufacturers know the source of the serum and request certification that the serum does not come from areas where BSE is endemic. Other potential sources of BSE may be proteases and other enzymes derived from bovine sources. Biological product manufacturers have been requested to determine the origin of these materials used in manufacturing.

The media used must be sterilized generally by sterilizing in place (SIP) or by using a continuous sterilizing system (CSS) process. Any nutrients or chemicals added beyond this point must be sterile. Air lines must have sterile filters. The following checklist, though not inclusive, should be used frequently:

• Confirm the compliance of the source of serum.
• Confirm that the sterilization cycle has been properly validated to ensure that the media will be sterile.
• Verify that all raw materials have been tested by quality control. Determine the origin of all bovine material.
• Document instances where the media failed to meet all specifications.
• Verify that expired raw materials have not been used in manufacture.
• Check that media and other additives have been properly stored.

CULTURE GROWTH

Cell cultures are run in batch, fed-batch, or continuous mode depending on expression system used. Continuous systems may take weeks to complete and may result in several harvest pools, making it necessary to define clearly the batch strategy. Bioreactor inoculation, transfer, and harvesting operations must be done using validated aseptic techniques. Additions or withdrawals from industrial bioreactors are generally done through steam sterilized lines and steam-lock assemblies. Steam may be left on in situations for which the heating of the line or bioreactor vessel wall would not be harmful to the culture.

It is important for a bioreactor system to be closely monitored and tightly controlled to achieve the proper and efficient expression of the desired product. The parameters for the fermentation process must be specified and monitored. These may include: growth rate, pH, waste by-product level, viscosity, addition of chemicals, density, mixing, aeration, and foaming. Other factors that can affect the finished product include shear forces, process-generated heat, and effectiveness of seals and gaskets.

Many growth parameters can influence protein production. Some of these factors affect deamidation, isopeptide formation, or host cell proteolytic processing. Although nutrient-deficient media are used as a selection mechanism in certain cases, media deficient in certain amino acids may cause substitutions. For example, when *E. coli* is starved of methionine or leucine while growing, the organism will synthesize norleucine and incorporate it in a position normally occupied by methionine, yielding an analogue of the wild-type protein. The presence of these closely related products will be difficult to separate chromatographically; this may have implications both for the application of release specifications and for the effectiveness of the product purification process.

Computer programs used to control the course of fermentation, data logging, and data reduction and analysis should be validated in accordance with 21 CFR 11.

Bioreactor systems designed for recombinant microorganisms require not only that a pure culture is maintained, but also that the culture be contained within the systems. The containment can be achieved by the proper choice of a host-vector system that is less capable of surviving outside a laboratory environment and by physical means, when this is considered necessary. The *National Institutes of Health* (NIH) *Guidelines* are described under the "Environment Control" section below.

EXTRACTION, ISOLATION, AND PURIFICATION

Several techniques have been used to condition the sample for the first chromatographic capture step: centrifugation, filtration, and microfiltration. In some cases, the harvest and capture steps have been united by means of expanded bed technology. Due to the large volumes handled, major changes in ionic strength or pH are not recommended. Instead, a purification principle matching the characteristics of the application sample should be selected. The recovery process begins with isolation of the desired protein from the fermentation or cell culture medium, often in a very impure form. The advantage of cell culture and yeast-derived products is that many of these proteins are secreted directly into the medium, thus requiring only cell separation to obtain a significant purification. For *E. coli*-derived products, lysis of the bacteria is often necessary to recover the desired protein. It is important in each case to achieve rapid purification of the desired protein because proteases released by the lysed organisms may cleave to the desired product. Such trace proteases are a major concern in the purification of biotechnology derived products because they can be very difficult to remove, may complicate the recovery process, and can significantly affect final product stability. The recovery process is usually designed to purify the final product to a high level. The purity requirement for a product depends on many factors, although chronic use products may be required to have much higher purity than those intended for single-use purposes. Biotechnology products contain certain impurities that the recovery processes are specifically designed to eliminate or minimize. These impurities include trace amounts of DNA, growth factors, residual host proteins, endotoxins, and residual cellular proteins from the medium.

CAPTURE

Once the fermentation process is completed, the desired product is separated, and if necessary, refolded to restore configuration integrity, and purified. The first part of the downstream process, capture separates the expressed protein from major impurities (water, cell debris, lipoproteins, lipids, carbohydrates, proteases, glycosidases, colored compounds, adventitious agents, fermentation additives, fermentation by-products) and conditions the sample for further intermediary purification steps.

The target protein should be concentrated and transferred to an environment, which will conserve the biological activity. The main purpose of the capture step is to get rid of water, host, and process-related impurities. Due to the large volumes handled and the nature of the application sample, the first chromatographic purification step is built on the on/off principle aiming for selective binding of the protein to the matrix. Large particle sizes are used to avoid clotting of the column and low resolution should be expected. One of the fundamental principles for capture operations is to focus on the target protein properties to achieve effective binding and pay less attention to contaminants, since purity is not the issue at this stage. The high selectivity of affinity chromatography is an attractive approach for capture provided that the affinity ligand stability does not put severe restrictions on the use of efficient cleaning and sterilization regimes. The most frequent purification principles used are packed bed or expanded bed affinity and ion exchange chromatography. In expanded bed technology, direct application of the cell culture, is possible, thereby reducing the number of unit operations. Capture operations should make use of simple technologies, broad parameter intervals, high flow rates, cheap chromatographic media, and large particle sizes to ensure process robustness, consistency, and economy. The outcome of the capture operation is a severe reduction in sample volume, reduction of the amount of impurities, and a sample, which is conditioned for the next step.

For recovery of intracellular proteins, cells must be disrupted after fermentation. This is done by chemical, enzymatic, or physical methods. Following disruption, cellular debris can be removed by centrifugation or filtration. For recovery of extracellular protein, the primary separation of product from producing organisms is accomplished by centrifugation or membrane filtration. Initial separation methods, such as ammonium sulfate precipitation and aqueous two-phase separation, can be employed following centrifugation to concentrate the products. Further purification steps primarily involve chromatographic methods to remove impurities and bring the product closer to final specifications. Extraction and isolation requires either filtration or centrifugation:

- Ultrafiltration is commonly used to remove the desired product from the cell debris. The porosity of the membrane filter is calibrated to a specific molecular weight, allowing molecules below that weight to pass through while retaining molecules above that weight. Filtration is an integrated part of every downstream process in order to condition the sample for chromatographic purification and to perform sterile filtrations. The filtration techniques comprise conventional filtration, microfiltration, ultrafiltration, and the use of specific filters for removal of defined impurities such as endotoxins, viruses, or prions. In-depth filtration consists of separation of particles from the solute using large pore size filters. Most samples are filtered before entering the chromatographic column to prevent increase in back pressure. Microfiltration consists of separation of particles from the solute using specifically designed tangential flow-over membranes with pore sizes ranging from 0.1 to 0.3 pm. Shear forces may destabilize the protein. Ultrafiltration separates the protein from low molecular solvent molecules using specifically designed tangential flow-over membranes with a cut-off range from 1 to 100000 kDa. Filters with specific ligands are used and specific filters for virus and prion removal are entering the market. They may be used in future processes to increase product safety. Filtration is used throughout for sample conditioning. Microfiltration is used for clarification of the harvest. Ultrafiltration is used for buffer exchange or sample concentration. It is not recommended to use the technique as the final step in the downstream process, as the shear forces may affect protein stability.
- Precipitation is rarely used as a purification technique, but rather as an intermediary step between two chromatographic unit operations. The trend is to avoid precipitation for reasons of economy, time, compliance issues, and convenience. However, it may be useful to precipitate the protein for the purpose of storage. Precipitation is rarely used in capture due to the large volumes handled.
- Centrifugation can be open or closed. The environment where centrifugation is performed must be controlled. Centrifugation is commonly applied to remove cells, cell debris, and precipitates from the harvest. The technique is labor demanding and may soon be replaced with microfiltration techniques or expanded bed technology.
- Crystallization is protein specific. It offers both purification and the ability to store the protein in a convenient way. Crystallization may be used for some intermediary products.
- Virus inactivation or active filtration is added as an extra unit operation when using mammalian cells or transgenic animals as the expression system.

PURIFICATION

The intermediate purification steps include removing the majority of the key impurities, cellular proteins, culture media components, DNA, viruses, endotoxins, and so forth. It is the first stage of the purification process. Medium-size particles are used in a variety of chromatographic techniques, and for chemical or enzymatic modifications of the protein. Higher resolution between related compounds is accomplished by applying more selective desorption principles such as multistep or continuous gradient elution procedures, and more specific chromatographic matrices, using smaller particles (offering better resolution) and technically more advanced solutions (gradients); made possible by higher purity and generally lower viscosity of the samples applied. It is ideal for packed bed technology.

POLISHING

The polishing steps include: high-resolution chromatographic methods to separate even closely related compounds (des-amido forms, oxidized forms, etc.). Polishing requires expensive, small uniform media particles with reversed phase and ion exchange chromatography as the dominant chromatographic principles. It involves recommended size exclusion chromatographic (SEC) or desalting operation as the final polishing step. Use of SEC as the final step may serve a number of purposes:

- Removal of di- and polymers;
- Possible buffer exchange to any buffer requested for formulation of drug substance bulk;
- Increase of protein stability;
- Uniform composition of the bulk material.

The eluant from the polishing operation should be a stable well-defined bulk material (drug substance) meeting specifications and with a composition acceptable for further formulation.

Chromatography in at least three distinct steps carefully adjusted to the capture, intermediary, and polishing principle offers the ideal solution to purification. The selection of chromatographic medium depends on the composition of the sample. Cosolvents generally do not affect the binding of the protein to the column. For every chromatographic technique used, there is a balance between resolution, speed, capacity, and recovery. The procedures given below can handle large volumes except SEC; they also require low protein concentration except in the case of SEC.

AC (affinity chromatography) works on the basis of structural epitome recognition and works at any pH that applies provided there is low to medium ionic strength. AC is a selective technique wherein the on/off principle fits very well into the capture mode, where large amounts of impurities are removed. Proteins normally elute from the column at low pH; a common practice is to apply the sample at neutral to slightly alkaline pH.

AEC (anion exchange chromatography) works on the principle of electrostatic interactions. It works best in pH > pI and low ionic strength; ethanol, urea, and nonionic detergents are tolerated. AEC is the most common chromatographic technique in use. It suits capture, intermediate purification, and polishing, making use of the highly specific media developed with defined particle sizes, spacers, and ligands. HIC offers, generally, less resolution than ion exclusion chromatography (IEC), but selectivity can be high when the proper ligand has been defined.

CEC (cation exchange chromatography) is used at pH < pI; low ionic strength; ethanol, urea, and nonionic detergents are tolerated.

HAC (hydroxyapatite chromatography) matrix does not tolerate acidic pH; it works best at low to high ionic strength; ethanol is tolerated. HAC often provides excellent solutions to purification challenges. The high resolution RPC technique is primarily used for proteins of molecular weight

TABLE 3.3
Relative Importance of Various Chromatographic
Methods in Various Downstream Processes

Principle	Capture	Intermediary Purification	Polishing
Affinity	+++	+	+
Crystallization	+	++	+++
Filtration	+++	+++	+++
HAC	+	+++	+
HIC	++	+++	+
IEC	+++	+++	+++
IMAC	+++	++	+
Microfiltration	+++	+	+
Precipitation	+	+++	+++
RPC	+	+	+++
SEC	+	+	+++
Ultrafiltration	+++	+++	+++

lower than 25 kDa, as the binding constant for higher molecular weight proteins is too high. Elution in organic solvents is common and protein stability in these buffers is a major issue.

HIC (hydrophobic interaction chromatography) works at any pH that applies; it has medium to high ionic strength. HIC is often used in combination with ion exchange, making use of the binding of proteins at high salt concentrations and elution at low salt concentrations. The presence of hydrophobic antifoam agents in fermentation broth and cell cultures may lower the binding capacity if HIC is used in the capture step. It may also be a less attractive capture technique if the feed volume is large and addition of salt is needed in order to increase the ionic strength of the solution. Thus, the large salt quantities needed add to the manufacture costs and cause a waste disposal problem.

IMAC (immobilized metal affinity chromatography) works on complex binding between metal-ligand and proteins. It works best at neutral pH; it has high ionic strength and denaturants, detergents, and ethanol are tolerated. IMAC is rarely exploited in industrial downstream processing. It is a powerful capture technique for a number of proteins and a unique tool for histidine tagged proteins. It is also a salt-tolerant technique, a useful feature considering typical ionic strength in biological starting materials. Selectivity can be very high and depends on the combined efforts of primary, secondary, and tertiary structure of proteins.

RPC (reversed phase chromatography) has hydrophobic interaction; its silica-based matrices do not tolerate alkaline pH, but organic solvents can be used.

SEC (size exclusion chromatography) has steric exclusion from the intraparticle volume; the sample volume is restricted to a maximum 5% of the column volume. It works at any pH and ionic strength or with any solvent. SEC is recommended as the final purification step. Although the sample volume rarely exceeds 5% v/v of the column volume, the technique offers removal of di- and polymeric compounds, transfer to a well-defined buffer, and, in many cases, enhanced protein stability.

Relative importance of each of the unit operations is given in Table 3.3.

IMPURITY REMOVAL

A variety of impurities that these chromatographic techniques are expected to remove and the testing methods used to ascertain this removal include:

- Aggregated proteins: SDS-PAGE, HPSEC
- Amino acid substitutions: amino acid analysis, peptide mapping, MS, Edman degradation analysis
- Deamidation: IEF, HPLC, MS, Edman degradation analysis
- DNA: DNA hybridization, UV spectrophotometry, protein binding
- Endotoxin: Bacterial Endotoxins Test (Pyrogen Test)
- Formyl methionine: Peptide mapping, HPLC, MS
- Host cell proteins: SDS-PAGE, immunoassays
- Microbial (bacteria, yeast, fungi): Microbial limit tests, sterility tests, microbiological testing
- Monoclonal antibodies: SDS-PAGE, immunoassays
- Mycoplasma: Modified 21 CFR method, DNAF
- Other protein impurities (media): SDS-PAGE, HPLCb, immunoassays
- Oxidized methionines: Peptide mapping, amino acid analysis, HPLC, Edman degradation analysis, MS
- Protein mutants: Peptide mapping, HPLC, IEF, MS
- Proteolytic Cleavage: IEF, SDS-PAGE (reduced), HPLC, Edman degradation analysis, MSS
- Viruses (endogenous and adventitious): CPE and HAd (exogenous virus only), reverse transcriptase activity, MAP

FORMULATION

The formulation of the drug product is a crucial step; most therapeutic proteins are either packaged in liquid form or in lyophilized form, both requiring a certain minimum final liquid volume of the concentrate obtained to contain the final drug product volume. As a result, it may be necessary to include a size-exclusion or desalting step to reduce the volume. Whereas much attention has been paid to the upstream and downstream step determining the final characterization of the product, the formulation step can significantly affect the safety and efficacy of the product. In the case of a lyophilized product, there are likely to be no added ingredients, but in a liquid formulation, there could be several common ingredients. Examples include albumin, sucrose, polysorbates, buffer salts, etc. The composition of a few such examples is give below.

Oprelvekin Injection (Interleukin IL-11)

Bill of Materials (Batch Size 1 L)					
Scale/mL		Item	Material	Quantity	UOM
1.00	mg	1	Oprelvekin (Interleukin IL-11)	1.00	g
4.60	mg	2	Glycine	4.60	g
0.32	mg	3	Dibasic sodium phosphate heptahydrate	0.32	g
0.11	mg	4	Monobasic sodium phosphate monohydrate	0.11	g
qs	mL	5	Water for injection, qs to	1.00	L

Interleukin Injection (IL-2)

Bill of Materials (Batch Size 1 L)					
Scale/mL		Item	Material	Quantity	UOM
0.25	mg	1	IL-2	0.25	g
0.70	mg	2	Sodium laurate	0.70	g
10.00	mM	3	Disodium hydrogen phosphate	10.00	M
50.00	mg	4	Mannitol	50.00	g

Bill of Materials (Batch Size 1 L) (Continued)					
Scale/mL		Item	Material	Quantity	UOM
Qs	mL	5	Hydrochloric acid for pH adjustment 1 M	qs	
qs	mL	6	Water for injection, qs to	1.00	L

Interferon Alfa-2a Injection

Bill of Materials (Batch Size 1 L)					
Scale/mL		Item	Material	Quantity	UOM
3 million	IU	1	Interferon alfa-2a	3B	IU
7.21	mg	2	Sodium chloride	7.21	g
0.20	mg	3	Polysorbate 80	0.20	g
10.00	mg	4	Benzyl alcohol	10.00	g
0.77	mg	5	Ammonium acetate	0.77	g
qs	mL	6	Water for injection, qs to	1.00	L

Interferon Beta-1b

Bill of Materials (Batch Size 1 L)					
Scale/mL		Item	Material	Quantity	UOM
0.30	mg	1	Interferon beta-1b	0.30	g
15.00	mg	2	Albumin human	15.00	g
15.00	mg	3	Dextrose	15.00	g
5.40	mg	4*	Sodium chloride	5.40	g
qs	mL	5	Water for injection, qs to	1.00	L

Note: This item is packaged separately as 0.54% solution (2 mL diluent for lyophilized product)

Interferon Beta-1a Injection

Bill of Materials (Batch Size 1 L)					
Scale/mL		Item	Material	Quantity	UOM
33.00	mcg	1	Interferon beta-1a	33.00	mg
15.00	mg	2	Albumin (human)	15.00	g
5.80	mg	3	Sodium chloride	5.80	g
5.70	mg	4	Dibasic sodium phosphate	5.70	g
1.20	mg	5	Monobasic sodium phosphate	1.20	g
qs	mL	6	Water for injection, qs to	1.00	L

Interferon Alfa-n3 Injection

Bill of Materials (Batch Size 1 L)					
Scale/mL		Item	Material	Quantity	UOM
5 million	U	1	Interferon alfa-n3	5B	U
3.30	mg	2	Liquefied phenol	3.30	g
1.00	mg	3	Albumin (human)	1.00	g
8.00	mg	4	Sodium chloride	8.00	g
1.74	mg	5	Sodium phosphate dibasic	1.74	g
0.20	mg	6	Potassium phosphate monobasic	0.20	g
0.20	mg	7	Potassium chloride	0.20	g
qs	mL	8	Water for injection, qs to	1.00	L

Interferon Alfacon-1 Injection

Bill of Materials (Batch Size 1 L)					
Scale/mL		Item	Material	Quantity	UOM
0.03	mg	1	Interferon alfacon-1	0.03	g
5.90	mg	2	Sodium chloride	5.90	g
3.80	mg	3	Sodium phosphate	3.80	g
qs	mL	4	Water for injection, qs to	1.00	L

Interferon Gamma-1b Injection

Bill of Materials (Batch Size 1 L)					
Scale/mL		Item	Material	Quantity	UOM
200.00	mcg	1	Interferon gamma-1b	200.00	mg
40.00	mg	2	Mannitol	40.00	g
0.72	mg	3	Sodium succinate	0.72	g
0.10	mg	4	Polysorbate 20	0.10	g
qs	mL	5	Water for injection, qs to	1.00	L

Infliximab for Injection

Bill of Materials (Batch Size 1 L)					
Scale/mL		Item	Material	Quantity	UOM
10.00	mg	1	Infliximab	10.00	g
50.00	mg	2	Sucrose	50.00	g
0.05	mg	3	Polysorbate 80	0.05	g
0.22	mg	4	Monobasic sodium phosphate monohydrate	0.22	g
0.61	mg	5	Dibasic sodium phosphate dihydrate		
qs	mL	6	Water for injection, qs to	1.00	L

Daclizumab for Injection

Bill of Materials (Batch Size 1 L)					
Scale/mL		Item	Material	Quantity	UOM
5.00	mg	1	Daclizumab	5.00	g
3.60	mg	2	Sodium phosphate monobasic monohydrate	3.60	g
11.00	mg	3	Sodium phosphate dibasic heptahydrate	11.00	g
4.60	mg	4	Sodium chloride	4.60	g
0.20	mg	5	Polysorbate 80 (Tween®)	0.20	G
qs	mL	6	Water for injection, qs to	1.00	L
qs	mL	7	Sodium hydroxide for pH adjustment	qs	
qs	mL	8	Hydrochloric acid for pH adjustment	qs	
qs	cuft	9	Nitrogen gas	qs	

Coagulation Factor VIIa (Recombinant) Injection

Bill of Materials (Batch Size 1000 vials)					
Scale/vial		Item	Material	Quantity	UOM
1.20	mg	1	rFVIIa	1.20	g
5.84	mg	2	Sodium chloride	5.84	g
2.94	mg	3	Calcium chloride dihydrate	2.94	g
2.64	mg	4	Glycine	2.64	g

Bill of Materials (Batch Size 1000 vials) (Continued)					
Scale/vial		Item	Material	Quantity	UOM
0.14	mg	5	Polysorbate 80	0.14	g
60.00	mg	6	Mannitol	60.00	g

Reteplase Recombinant for Injection

Bill of Materials (Batch Size 1000 vials)					
Scale/vial		Item	Material	Quantity	UOM
18.10	mg	1	Reteplase	18.10	g
8.32	mg	2	Tranexamic acid	8.32	g
136.24	mg	3	Dipotassium hydrogen phosphate	136.24	g
51.27	mg	4	Phosphoric acid	51.27	g
364.00	mg	5	Sucrose	364.00	g
5.20	mg	6	Polysorbate 80	5.20	g

Alteplase Recombinant Injection

Bill of Materials (Batch Size 1000 vials)					
Scale/vial		Item	Material	Quantity	UOM
58 million	IU	1	Alteplase	100.00	g
3.50	g	2	L-Arginine	3.50	kg
1.00	g	3	Phosphoric acid	1.00	kg
11.00	mg	4	Polysorbate 80	11.00	g
qs	mL	5	Water for injection, qs to	1.00	L

Several formulations require added components for stabilization of proteins; albumin is one of the most commonly used stabilizer, e.g., in the case of darbepoietin alfa, interferon beta 1a and 1b, interferon alfa 2b, antihemophilic factor, epoietin alfa (also available without albumin), recombinant factor VIII (also available without albumin), and laronidase. Extra care is needed as albumin is a known carrier of viruses; validated sources must be used to supply human albumin.

VALIDATION

Chemicals used in chromatography methods, either in the stationary (bonded) phase or in the mobile phase, may become impurities in the final product and the burden of validation (i.e., demonstrating removal of potentially harmful chemicals) lies on the manufacturer. A column material supplier certification regarding leaching of chemicals is not sufficient since the contamination is process and product dependent. Validation is necessary when isolating end-product monoclonal antibodies or using a technique that contains a monoclonal antibody purification step. The process must demonstrate removal of leaching antibody or antibody fragments. It is also required to ensure the absence of adventitious agents such as viruses and mycoplasmas in the cell line that is the source of the monoclonal antibodies. The main concern is the possibility of contamination of the product with an antigenic substance whose administration could be detrimental to patients. Continuous monitoring of the process is necessary to avoid or limit such contamination. The problem of antigenicity related to the active as well as host proteins is one that is unique to biotechnology derived products in contrast to traditional pharmaceuticals. Manufacturing methods that use certain solvents should be monitored if these solvents are able to cause chemical rearrangements that could alter the antigenic profile of the drug substance. The manufacturer is also obligated to produce evidence regarding performance consistency of novel chromatographic columns. Considerations for single-use products such as vaccines may differ because they are not administered continuously and, in this case, antigenicity is desirable. On the other hand, validating the removal of ligand or extraneous protein contamination is necessary. Unlike drugs derived from natural sources, manufacturers of biotechnology derived products have been required to provide validation of the removal of nucleic acids during purification. Vaccines may again be different in this regard because of the accumulated clinical history on these products.

PROCESS OVERVIEW

Table 3.4 gives an overview of the unit operations for different expression systems.

PROCESS MATURITY

Manufacturing of therapeutic proteins is a complex process that goes through well-defined development stages; however, in situations where a company is used to developing small molecules and not appreciative of the difficulties, it may choose to use a less than mature process to manufacture clinical test samples. This can create a serious regulatory problem where a major process change, either for economic or safety reasons, will significantly delay the launch of the product. As a result, there is a need to define the process maturity level a priori. Ideally, criteria listed in Table 3.5 should be accomplished before technology transfer, but the real world is not perfect and certain tasks may remain unfinished at scale up with the risk of major adjustments and perhaps process redesign at a later stage. Some companies plan with a process redesign between Phase II and Phase III as a compromise between time to market and extra development costs. Maturity criteria for technology transfer and scale up are described in Table 3.5.

SCALE UP

The downstream process is designed in a linear manner such that most parameters are fixed and only column diameter in chromatographic unit operations, and the membrane area in filtration operations change. The perpetual conflict between the pilot scale mentality and the commercial sale requirements continues to be the greatest impediment — the human factor. The FDA's Process and Analytical Technology (PAT) Initiative (http://www.fda.gov/cder/OPS/PAT.htm) offers an ideal solution adopting the concept of "design in," where issues related to process safety, robustness, cGMP compliance, facility constraints, economy, and time to market are build into the process at small-scale development. The process is tested in small scale before transfer against predefined process maturity factors, such as parameter intervals, in-process control points, critical parameters and their interactions, robustness, yield, documentation level, raw material qualification, and maturity of analytical procedures. This concept challenges the classic stepwise scale up (a short-cut approach to accommodate unrealistic timelines), where cell culture and initial purification steps (e.g., capture) are scaled up before the process is developed in small scale. The stepwise scale up procedure creates much confusion, is time consuming, and invites redesign to late process. It is also common to outsource this stage of work, particularly if the company plans to outsource manufacturing as well. Transferring an immature process into the pilot environment may result in delayed Phase I and Phase II clinical material manufacture as process changes may raise doubts of the stability, virus validation, and preclinical data. Immature process indicators include:

- Yields are low or vary from batch to batch
- Target protein instability
- Changing impurity profiles
- UV-diagrams are not super imposable
- Too many batches are discarded or do not meet specifications
- Manufacture is terminated during processing

Table 3.4
Process Overview of Unit Operations for Different Expression Systems

System	Unit Operation	Comment
General	Cell culture	Batch, fed batch or perfusion; 3 to 40 days.
	Harvest	Centrifugation/filtration; omit if using expanded bed.
	Capture	Chromatographic unit operation is typically based on affinity or IEC. Remove major host and process related impurities and water.
	Variable Unit operation	The unit operation may be refolding (if *E. coli* is used) or virus inactivation if insect cells, mammalian cells, or transgenic animals are used.
	Intermediate purification	Chromatographic unit operation typically based on HIC, IEC, or HAC stepwise gradient technology used to remove host and process related impurities.
	Variable Unit operation	This unit operation may include tag removal (if *E. coli* is used) or virus removal by filtration if insect cells, mammalian cells, or transgenic animals are used.
	Polishing	Chromatographic unit operation typically based on HP-IEDC or HP-RPC stepwise/linear gradient technology used to remove product related impurities.
	Variable Unit operation	SEC or ultra-filtration to ensure proper drug substance formulation.
	Drug substance	The conversion of the drug substance to drug product typically includes change of buffer, precipitation, or crystallization.
	Formulation	Batch manufacturing often including stabilizers such as albumin.
	Finished Drug product	Filling in appropriate containers such as vials or prefilled syringes.
E. coli (Gram negative)	Fermentation	Expression of N-terminally extended target protein to overcome formation of Met-protein.
	Harvest	Harvest of cells by centrifugation prior to cell disruption.
	Cell Disruption	Disruption with French press or like; wash out inclusion bodies.
	Extraction	Extraction under reducing and denaturing conditions (e.g., 0.1 M cysteine, 7 M urea pH 8.5).
	Capture	Purification under reducing and denaturing conditions (e.g., IEC or IMAC if protein is His-tagged).
	Renaturation	Controlled folding of the target protein using hollow fiber, SEC, dilution, or buffer exchange.
	Intermediate Purification	Purification of the folded target protein (e.g., IEC, HIC, HAC).
	Enzyme cleavage	Cleavage of the N-terminal extension with exo- or endo- proteases.
	Polishing 1	Purification of the target protein (e.g. HP-IEC, HP-RPC)
	Polishing 2	Purification of the target protein by SEC (not always included).
	Drug substance	The purified bulk product.
	Formulation	Re-formulation of the drug substance preparing for administration to humans.
	Drug product	The final product.
Gram Positive Bacteria	Fermentation	Expression the target protein to the periplasmatic room or medium.
	Harvest	Harvest of cells by centrifugation prior to cell disruption. This step may be bypassed by means of expanded bed technology.
	Capture	Purification of the target protein from the supernatant.
	Intermediate purification	Purification of the target protein (e.g., IEC, HIC, HAC).
	Polishing 1	Purification of the target protein (e.g., HP-IEC, HP-RPC).
	Polishing 2	Purification of the target protein by SEC (not always included).
	Drug substance	The purified bulk product.
	Formulation	Reformulation of the drug substance preparing for administration to humans.
	Drug substance	The final product.

Table 3.4 (Continued)
Process Overview of Unit Operations for Different Expression Systems

System	Unit Operation	Comment
Yeast	Fermentation	Expression the target protein to the medium.
	Harvest	Harvest of cells by centrifugation prior to cell disruption. This step may be bypassed by means of expanded bed technology.
	Capture	Purification of the target protein from the supernatant or by expanded bed technology.
	Intermediate purification	Purification of the target protein (e.g., IEC, HIC, HAC).
	Polishing 1	Purification of the target protein (e.g., HP-IEC, HP-RPC).
	Polishing 2	Purification of the target protein by SEC (not always included).
	Drug substance	The purified bulk product.
	Formulation	Reformulation of the drug substance preparing for administration to humans.
	Drug product	The final product.
Insect Cells	Cell culture	Expression the target protein to the medium.
	Harvest	Harvest of cells by centrifugation prior to cell disruption. This step may be bypassed by means of expanded bed technology.
	Capture	Purification of the target protein from the supernatant or by expanded bed technology.
	Virus inactivation	Inactivation by means of low pH, high temperature, detergents, etc.
	Intermediate purification	Purification of the target protein (e.g., IEC, HIC, HAC).
	Virus filtration	Nano-filtration.
	Polishing	Purification of the target protein (e.g., HP-IEC, HP-RPC, SEC).
	Drug substance	The purified bulk product.
	Formulation	Reformulation of the drug substance preparing for administration to humans.
	Drug product	The final product.
Mammalian Cells	Cell culture	Expression the target protein to the medium.
	Harvest	Harvest of cells by centrifugation prior to cell disruption. This step may be bypassed by means of expanded bed technology.
	Capture	Purification of the target protein from the supernatant or by expanded bed technology.
	Virus inactivation	Inactivation by means of low pH, high temperature, detergents, etc.
	Intermediate purification	Purification of the target protein (e.g., IEC, HIC, HAC).
	Virus filtration	Nano-filtration.
	Polishing	Purification of the target protein (e.g., HP-IEC, HP-RPC, SEC).
	Drug substance	The purified bulk product.
	Formulation	Reformulation of the drug substance preparing for administration to humans.
	Drug product	The final product.
Transgenic Animals	Raw milk	Milking of animals according to Good Agricultural Practices.
	Skim milk	Centrifuged raw milk with low fat content.
	Capture	Purification of the target protein from the skim milk.
	Virus inactivation	Inactivation by means of low pH, high temperature, detergents, etc.
	Intermediary Purification	Purification of the target protein (e.g., IEC, HIC, HAC).
	Virus filtration	Nano-filtration.
	Polishing	Purification of the target protein (e.g., HP-IEC, HP-RPC, SEC).
	Drug substance	The purified bulk product.
	Formulation	Reformulation of the drug substance preparing for administration to humans.
	Drug product	The final product.

TABLE 3.5
Indicators of Maturity of Unit Processes in Deciding Technology Transfer

Maturity Criteria	Comments
Cell line	QA release of the MCB required prior to transferring cells into the cGMP facility.
Process design	Design should be robust with provisions for removal of host-, process-, and product-related impurities. Where refolding is involved, include a well-defined renaturation step; where virus contamination can be an issue, integrate virus removal and inactivation steps with due consideration for denaturation of protein.
Raw materials	A list of raw materials should be provided; do not use materials not qualified to be used in cGMP manufacturing.
Intermediary compounds	Data from three small-scale batches should be provided; critical parameters and their interaction should be defined. Holding times of relevance to large-scale operations should be provided.
Drug substance	Short-term stability of the intermediary compounds is to be documented.
Drug product	Formulation to be flexible enough to change composition of the bulk; short-term stability documented.
In-process control	Parameters stated in intervals (validated and proven acceptable ranges) and monitored; analytical method description plus data for in-process analyses to be provided.
Specifications	Acceptance criteria for drug substance and drug product provided where possible.
Quality control	Drug substance and product to have a well-defined quality control plan and analytical method described along with representative data.

- Reworking of unit operations is necessary
- The process is frequently being redesigned.

TECHNOLOGY TRANSFER

The key to an effective technology transfer lies in good communication between the development laboratory and the pilot scale production staff; both of which have somewhat different goals. One intends to provide an elegant process design, the other is interested in practical solutions; often these goals do not meet. The information contained in a technology transfer package varies with the type of product, but it should generally include the following:

- Overview: Process rationale and brief strategy of production.
- Molecule: Physical and chemical properties of target protein.
- Cell line: History of cell line; MCB vials, WCB vials, WCB release documentation; safety profile; reworking and propagation documentation.
- Process: List of raw materials and equipment; hazardous element identification; development history documentation; description of unit operations; manufacturing process protocol; small batch data; critical parameters; related impurities description: host, process, and product-related; process flow sheet; major impurity removal steps; batch production plan.
- Fill and finish: Master production document; batch record; formulation deviation parameters; development history document; compliance record.
- Storage: Conditions for all in-process materials, drug substance, and drug product.
- Shipping: Conditions and instructions, packaging specifications for both drug substance and drug product.
- In-process controls: Required tests and when needed; parameter intervals (tolerance and specifications) for pH, conductivity, redox potential, protein concentration, temperature, holding time, load, transmembrane pressure, linear flow, etc.

- Specifications: Acceptance criteria for appearance, identity, biological activity, purity, and quantity; pharmacopoeial specifications where applicable.
- Analytical methods: Description, typical data, method qualification level, methods transfer protocols, and reference material.
- Stability: Real-time data and extrapolated data on both drug substance and drug product.
- Virus validation: Documentation and protocol; compliance report.
- Master validation plan: Update.
- Training: Employee training protocol, end of training objectives and on-going support.

This phase of communication is important particularly if the company is planning to outsource any portion of the manufacturing operations; in such instances, a master plan should be devised on formal communication lines between the sponsor and the Contract Manufacturing Organization (CMO).

PROCESS OPTIMIZATION AND COST REDUCTION

The most important factor that determines the choice of process optimization and scale up is the cost of the product; a good understanding of the cost components is needed by both the development as well as pilot and full-scale commercial production teams. Recombinant manufacturing involves processes that may be not be scaled up linearly, requiring in-depth studies of commercial production requirements and availability of process techniques that might be complementary to each other. Table 3.6 lists the factors that go into calculation of the finished product cost; other factors may be included, particularly those related to environment controls such as disposal of waste, etc. The relative contribution of each of the steps or components should be the first criterion of selection on which step to rework to reduce costs. However, relative costs should be considered in terms of long-term impact. For example, a 1% recurring cost can add a substantial savings if reduced.

Once the process is scaled up the process design is finalized, it is time to optimize the process within the established and proven acceptable ranges of parameter intervals. The optimization exercise should result in improved yields, economy, robustness, enhanced column lives, labor savings, and other such regulatory considerations that may impinge on the documentation and filing to regulatory authorities.

The economy of the manufacturing process (facility depreciation, raw material costs, quality control, and quality assurance) must match the expected results. As a rule of thumb, the expenses on manufacture should not exceed 15% of the price per dose (vial). Some of the factors influencing the process economy are labor, chromatographic media, filters and membranes, buffers, other raw materials, number and type of in-process control analyses, and the overall yield obtained. Additional cost comes from complying with environmental requirements. Where organic solvents are used, their disposal is further costly. Waste disposal, particularly the requirement that all material in contact with the genetically modified cells must be properly sterilized and disposed, adds considerable overhead to the overall production costs.

Typically, manufacturers develop purification processes on a small scale and determine the effectiveness of the particular processing step. When scale up is performed, allowances must be made for several differences when compared with the laboratory-scale operation. Longer processing times can affect product quality adversely, since the product is exposed to conditions of buffer and temperature for longer periods. Product stability, under purification conditions, must be carefully defined. It is important to define the limitations and effectiveness of the particular step. Process validation on the production size batch should then compare the effect of scale up. Whereas the data on the small scale can help in the validation, it is important that validation be performed on the production size batches. There are specific situations such as where columns are regenerated to allow repeated use; this requires proper validation procedures performed and the process periodically monitored for chemical and microbial contamination.

TABLE 3.6
Cost Calculation for Therapeutic Protein Manufacturing

Category	Issue	Index	Comments
General	Expression level	A1	Amount in g/L expressed
	Number of batches	A2	
	Process yield	A3	% of purified protein (drug product)
	Dose	A4	Mg/dose
	Pack size	A5	Mg/vial
	Vials needed	A6	Number of vials/dose
Upstream	Facility	B1	Yearly cost ($) of using upstream component of cGMP facility (including maintenance and manpower)
	Utilization	B2	Number of months the upstream component is used for given project
	Culture volume	B3	Volume in liters in a given batch
	Media cost	B4	Price in $/L of culture media
	Utensils	B5	Price in $ for utensils used (e.g., filters, bags, etc.)
Downstream	Facility	C1	Yearly cost ($) for using downstream component of the cGMP facility (including maintenance and manpower)
	Utilization	C2	Number of months the downstream component is used for a given project
	Chromatography steps	C3	Number of chromatography steps
	Binding capacity	C4	Average binding capacity in mg/mL
	Media cost	C5	Chromatography media cost in $/L
	Buffer volume	C7	Total consumption in L (on an average 15 column volumes are used/step)
	Buffer cost	C8	$/L
	Utensils	C9	Cost in $ for components used (filters, membranes, bags, etc.)
	Raw materials	C10	Cost in $ for expensive reagents, enzymes, etc.
	Formulation	C11	Cost in $ for formulation of drug substance
Fill and pack	Number of vials	D1	Vials/batch
	Price	D2	Price/vial
	Shipping cost	D3	
In-process control	Number of analyses	E1	Total number per batch
	Cost of analysis	E2	Average in $/IPC analysis
DS quality control	Number of analyses	F1	Total number of drugs substance quality analysis per batch
	Cost	F2	$/analysis
DP quality control	Number of analyses	G1	Total number per batch of drug product
	Cost	G2	$/analysis
QA release	Cost	H1	$/batch

Upstream cost = (B1*B2)/12 + B3 * B4 + B5 (asterisk is used for multiplier). Downstream = (C1*C2)/12 = (B3 * A1 * C5 * C3)/(C4 * C6 * 1000) + (C7 * C8) + C9 + C10 C11. Fill and pack = D1 * D2 * + D3. Total cost/batch = Upstream + Downstream + Fill and pack + E1 * E2 + F1 * F2 + G1 * G2 + H1. Yield/batch = (B3 * A1 * A3)/100,000. Cost/G = Total cost/yield (per batch). Cost per vial = Cost per batch/D1. Cost per dose = (Cost per batch/D1) * A6

Where batches are rejected, it is important to identify the specific manufacturing and control systems that resulted in the failure and thus appropriate an action plan to prevent reoccurrence of the mistake.

Process design should be distinguished from process optimization, where factors such as labor, automation, lean management, column life-time, reuse of utensils, and batch planning affect the process economy. The latter issues are dealt with at a later development stage, typically when the process design has been locked.

- Expression system selection, and eventually cell line, takes place early in the process and is the most important decision. The choice depends on the nature of the target protein (glycosylation, phosphorylation, acylation, size, etc.), expected expression levels, expression system development time, risk of batch failure, safety considerations, amount needed, and regulatory record.
  - The target proteins without posttranslational modifications can be expressed in all expression systems (bacteria, yeast, insect cells, mammalian cells, transgenic animals, or transgenic plants); the bacterial system is historically preferred for cost considerations but better expression yields have been obtained with yeast, mammalian cell cultures, and the introduction of transgenic animals and plants over the past 10 years challenge the bacterial systems, where intracellular expression of Met-protein and *in vitro* folding increases the complexity of the downstream process. Posttranslational modified proteins or more complex proteins are expressed in insect cells, mammalian cells, transgenic animals, or plants. Microbial systems cannot be used.
  - Expression level varies with the host organism used and the nature of the target protein. Typical expression levels vary widely. In most hosts these range at less than 1 g/L; *E. coli* generally gives a better yield of 1 to 4 g/L while mammalian cells when used for antibodies generally produce much higher levels; transgenic animals provide the highest yield of 5 to 40 g/L; the yield in transgenic plants is uncertain and not widely available for evaluation. The nature and quality of the expressed protein influences the purification yield. Although expression levels of *E. coli* usually are high, expression of N-terminal extended target protein and the need for *in vitro* refolding significantly influence the overall process yield. Further, stressed cells tend to express less stable protein, resulting in great losses during purification or production of drug substance/product with shortened lifetime.
  - Expression system development time varies widely between various expression systems. However, for most hosts, 4 to 6 months are required to develop the system. Once developed, the time to target protein expression depends on the bioreactor system deployed but generally ranges from a few days e.g., 5 days for *E. coli* and other bacteria, 2 weeks for yeast, 4 weeks for insect cells, and 2 to 16 weeks for mammalian cells. The longer development time for transgenic goats and cows (18 to 24 months) is partly compensated for by the relative high expression levels and the fast access to target protein, once the system has been developed.
  - Risk of batch failure is mainly due to infections; large-scale mammalian cell cultures, having long cell expansion times including several bioreactors and running over long time intervals, are associated with higher risk factors than other expression systems. Due to the high cell culture media cost, the economic loss can be substantial.
  - Safety considerations add to the cost significantly. Insect cells, mammalian cells, and transgenic animals can be infected with viruses. Costly virus testing, virus reduction unit operations, and validation programs are needed to ensure product safety. The potential prior infection risk of sheep, goats, and cows is being debated, emphasizing the need for controlled herds.
  - The amount needed can vary. A 1000 L bioreactor with an expression level of 1 g/L produces 1 kg of target protein per reactor volume. A batch or fed-batch culture typically runs for 7 days, offering a productivity of 100 g/day. A 1000 L perfusion bioreactor with a 2 × flow per 24 hours and with an expression level of 1 g/L produces 200 g/day. A transgenic cow expressing 20 g/L milk produces 400 g/day, assuming a volume of 20 L milk per day. In terms of output, the transgenic cow is a far more efficient expression system than the cell culture-based systems and probably less risky. Animal-based expression systems should therefore seriously be considered for large-scale operations.

- Regulatory records of insect cells, transgenic animals, and plants are poor. This is an important consideration when selecting a system to ensure that favorable regulatory review is forthcoming.
- Raw materials are very different in price between culture media used for microbial, insect, and mammalian cell cultures and commercial scale fermenter media, the former being the most expensive per liter. Unfortunately, mammalian cell cultures usually offer relatively low expression levels compared to microbial systems, making expenses to culture media a major cost contributor. An expression system yielding 1000 g/L with 40% yield, the contribution of the cost of media is about $25/g of protein; when the expression level drops to 10 g/L, the cost contribution of media rises to $2500/g of protein. Obviously, low mammalian cell expression levels adversely affect the process economy.
- Cell growth is normally achieved in batch, fed-batch, or continuous mode, the latter mainly being used for mammalian cell bioreactors up to a volume of maximum 300 liters, at present. A bioreactor run in the batch mode has a fixed working volume and the cell culture is grown to a defined cell density before harvest. The harvest volume defines the batch and the yield is the expression level × harvest volume. For example, a bioreactor of 100 L working volume with an expression level 300 mg/L results in a batch yield of 30 g. The productivity is thus 30 g/week or 0.3 g/L culture medium assuming it takes 1 week to complete the batch. A bioreactor run in fed-batch mode may result in a final volume of 130 L equivalent to a productivity of 39 g/week or 0.3 g/L culture medium, assuming identical culture time and expression level. A 100 L working volume bioreactor run in continuous mode at a flow of 2 reactor volumes per day and an expression level of 100 mg/L produces $100 \times 2 \times 7 \times 100 = 140$ g per week or 140/1400 = 0.1 g/L culture medium or one third of the batch culture. The increased overall productivity may compensate for the decreased productivity per L culture medium. Cell cultures offer the most opportunities and the most problems in scale up. For example, large-scale animal cell cultures are fundamentally different from conventional microbial fermentation due to the fragility of mammalian cells. The cells are easily damaged by mechanical stress, making it impossible to use conditions of high aeration and agitation; this includes the use of the newly introduced Wave bioreactors. Fortunately, animal cells grow slowly and at less cell densities and therefore do not require the high oxygen inputs typical of microbial cultures. Cell culture scale up often results in changes in the cell culture supernatant composition, which may affect the downstream process. However, except for reactor volume, other parameters like culture medium, pH, temperature, redox potential, osmolality, agitation rate, flow rate, ammonia, glucose, glutamine, lactate concentrations, pCO_2, etc., remain constant within the prescribed interval limits.
- In-process control is less expensive for batch and fed-batch systems compared to continuous cultures, but the overall cost may not be too different and is worth considering in light of the PAT Initiative of the FDA. Milking procedures may result in production of small volume bags, increasing the cost for analytical control programs. The insect and mammalian cell end-of-production test comprising sterility, fungi, mycoplasma, and virus testing should be included in the cost calculations.
- Yield is the composite of each purification step's output. A downstream process comprising 10 unit operations with an average recovery of 95% will result in an overall yield of 57%, which is acceptable. However, an average recovery of 80% will result in a total yield of 11%, which in most circumstances is not acceptable. In several cases more than 10 unit operations are needed to guarantee a safe product, making it fair to conclude that one should aim for more than 95% recovery in most if not all unit operations. Some of the most recent trends to alter the molecular structure, e.g., pegylation, has met with lower yields. Because of the mathematical nature of proportional reduction, small changes in step yields result in dramatic changes in the total yield. For example, a step yield of 95% where 15 steps are

involved gives 46% total yield; the same 15 steps in 75% step yield would give only 1% of the total yield. In most instances 5 to 10 steps are minimally involved; at 10 steps, therefore, the total yield ranges from 60% to 6% in 95% to 75% step yield transition. The cost is inversely proportional to quantity produced, ranging from about $85/mg for insulin to $1000+/mg for some cytokines. For expensive products, it may be worthwhile not to look at production cost optimization, as timely entry may be more relevant.

- Batch size is decided on a variety of consideration, not all of them have economic optimization. Large batches require automated facilities, but results in a relative small number of samples to analyze. Batch is defined as the *batch* or fed-batch cell culture volume processed in downstream as a combined amount of material resulting in the drug substance. In continuous cell cultures or by transgenic animal technology, the harvest or milk may be pooled in subfractions, making it more difficult to define the batch, and the batch scheme must provide information about the flow, the harvest procedures, pools, analytical in-process control programs, and intermediary compounds. Also included here are details if several columns are used or where parallel processing or splitting of processing is envisioned. Because inclusion bodies can be combined from several fermentation batches and then processed together, clear identification of starting subbatches is required.
- Chromatographic media costs are a minor fraction of the entire manufacturing cost, and it may be wise to select media from other criteria than price per liter. Service, trouble-shooting, linking media, column, and equipment to the same supplier, and regulatory support files may be far more important aspects as the number of failed batches can be reduced by such actions. Suppliers like Amersham or others with a wide range of offering and validation should be the first choice as media vendors. The major factors influencing the economy of chromatographic unit operations are media cost, binding capacity, recovery, column lifetime, linear flow, and shelf life.
- Utensils are bags, filters, or any other equipment exchanged at regular intervals. It has become common practice to use bags, filters, tubes, etc. only once in order to reduce cost and time to cleaning in place procedures.
- The number of steps in a process directly affects cost and yield; however, reducing the number of steps in a process can affect robustness and safety and even later costs in additional testing as may be required by the regulatory authorities. For example, a choice may have to be made whether to add an additional adventitious agent removal process of validate the system.
- Formulation, fill, and pack operations of the active pharmaceutical ingredient (API) can also be subject to cost reduction depending on the formulation. Obviously, a lyophilized product will cost more and if a ready to inject formula can be developed, that should be a better choice. The components such as syringes, pen systems, etc. added at this stage add substantially to the cost of the product.
- In-process control testing should be minimal and this is only possible with a well-defined system, which may incur higher costs initially. The trend is to reduce the number of in-process analytical methods and to expand on monitoring of parameters and responses, thereby keeping strict control of the process in real time. The number of samples to analyze is inversely related to the batch size; large batches reduce the cost for in-process control. Another way to reduce costs is to use the Process Analytical Technology (PAT) approach recently suggested by the FDA (http://www.fda.gov/cder/guidance/5815dft. htm). PAT is considered to be a system for designing, analyzing, and controlling manufacturing through time measurements of critical quality and performance attributes of raw and in process materials and processes with the goal of ensuring final product quality. The goal of PAT is to understand and control the manufacturing process as quality cannot be tested into products, but should be build-in. This approach can be taken during the development phase extending the in-process control program to not only include tradi-

tional analytical testing, but also real-time monitoring of the process parameters and responses. A desired goal of the PAT framework is to design and develop processes that can consistently ensure a predefined quality at the end of the manufacturing process. Such procedures would be consistent with the basic tenet of quality by design and could reduce the risks to quality and regulatory concerns while improving efficiency. A third way to reduce costs is to lower the price per sample by ensuring a continuous flow of samples, thereby reducing time spent on method set up and calibration.

- Quality control testing is performed on both the drug substance (DS) and the drug product (DP) (see BP/EP/USP). The testing typically comprises from 10 to 15 different analytical methods with an average price between $500 to $3000/sample. If outside laboratories are inducted to provide additional testing, the cost can skyrocket. For example, the National Institute for Biological Standards and Control (NIBSC) would typically charge about $20,000 to test one sample; animal assays and viral assays can be extremely expensive when outsourced; yet, outsourcing is still the preferred way of doing these assays to obviate the large cost of maintaining animal houses or viral containment systems and validating the methods.
- Quality assurance systems should ensure that the process scale up does not alter process safety, robustness, or compliance with regulatory demands. If the process is redesigned during scale up, the validity of preclinical data should be considered. Robust systems introduce strict control of unit operation parameters and define parameters in intervals rather than set points. The parameter intervals are tested and justified in small scale (proven acceptable range), making room to adjust the intervals according to large-scale needs. In the linear scale concept these parameter intervals are kept constant upon scale up. Other factors, such as reactor volumes, sample loads, and column diameters, are increased — all in a linear fashion.
- Batch variations document specifies variability and lack of reproducibility; this may be due to scale up procedure because of formation of concentration gradients in large reactors or containers.
- Buffer preparation at large scale that cannot be handled requires automation and robotics management to create an entirely different set of validation requirements and tools including computer validation (see section 211.68 (a, b) of FDA cGMP for validation of automated systems, mechanized racks, and computers).
- Column life, when prolonged, reduces cost significantly; remember that almost 70% of total production cost goes into downstream processing, mainly in the cost of chromatographic media. Measures taken to prolong column life include longer usage, recharging, etc., and they must be properly validated and documented.
- Environmental issues relate to disposal of large waste; for example, use of ammonium sulfate will severely affect the environment in large-scale operations.
- Equipment interaction can determine the choice of chemicals used; sodium chloride is a corrosive agent to stainless steel; whereas sodium acetate is not. These issues should be addressed as early as possible in process development.
- Facility costs can be very high because of specialize area requirements, specialized manpower required, environment controls and waste disposal needs, etc. A prospective biogeneric marketer would be wise to look into outsourcing manufacturing especially if several products are involved that may require separate processing suites. One of the control areas often not given full budgeting is the monitoring of the environment; a 5000 ft^2 facility may cost upward of $2 million per year only to comply with the monitoring standards. As the regulatory environment is still evolving, the area requirements are likely to change, which may cost substantial redesigning, another reason to outsource manufacturing until such time that the market is firmly established. The price per gram of drug substance is significantly reduced by linking process design, scale-up factor, and batch logistics to the facility design and thereby reduces the occupancy time. This requires

several levels of set up, one for transfer of technology to pilot scale, from pilot scale to first-stage manufacturing, and from first-stage manufacturing to full-scale manufacturing.

- Validation of biological processes is an expensive exercise that continues throughout commercial manufacturing operations. Typically, validation steps are initiated when all separation and purification steps are described in detail and presented with flow charts. Adequate descriptions and specifications should be provided for all equipment, columns, reagents, buffers, and expected yields. The FDA defines process validation in the May 1987 "Guideline on General Principles of Process Validation" as: "validation — establishing documented evidence which provides a high degree of assurance that a specific process will consistently produce a product meeting its pre-determined specifications and quality attributes." As a result, there is a need to establish comprehensive documentary proof to justify the process and demonstrate that the process works consistently. Validation reports for the various key processes would be dependent on the process involved; for example, if an ion-exchange column is used to remove endotoxins, there should be data documenting that this process is consistently effective as done by determining endotoxin levels before and after processing. It is important to monitor the process before, during, and after to determine the efficiency of each key purification step. One method commonly used to demonstrate validation is to "spike" the preparation with a known amount of a contaminant and then demonstrate its absence.
- Harvesting can be programmed to store inclusion bodies for a longer time (even two years), and most large-scale operations should validate this storage step.
- Holding times can be long and add cost in commercial production; these are often not considered in developing processes; it is advisable that in the initial phases, realistic times should be validated. This aspect is related more to logistics than to science. It takes much longer to empty a 4000 L tank than it does to dump a 2 L flask. Often the practical consideration of shift-change (if the process requires more than 8 hours) is necessary in designing the process.
- Cleaning, sanitizing, and storing columns, equipment, and utensils are integrated parts of the manufacturing program. Whereas liberties are routinely taken in small-scale production, these issues can add substantial costs in a poorly designed process and facility but also raise contamination risks that may not be acceptable by the regulatory authorities.
- Precipitation step scale up involves only a change in the amount of sample and the volume of reagent as all other parameters like sample pH, conductivity, temperature, concentration, redox potential, holding time, reagent concentration, and precipitation time remain constant within interval limits. The procedure of precipitation also remains identical.
- Chromatography scale up produces more problems than any other operation in the process. Larger equipment may cause extra-column zone broadening due to different lengths and diameters of outlet pipes, valves, monitor cells, etc. An increase in column diameter may result in decreased flow rate due to a reduction in supportive wall forces (at constant pressure drop). For example, a decrease in flow of 30% to 45% is observed for a column packed with Sepharose 6 FF when the diameter is increased from 2.6 to 10 cm. Prolonged sample holding times on column may result in precipitation of material, resulting in clotting of pipes, valves, or chromatographic columns. Parameters that are changed proportionally (linear scale up) include sample volume, sample load, column diameter, column area and column volume, and flow rate; residence time remains constant (an alternate method would keep residence time constant, allowing for variations in both column area and height. Parameters that remain constant within the interval limits include: sample pH, conductivity, temperature, concentration, redox potential, holding time, bed height, residence time, linear flow rate, binding capacity, back pressure, buffers, equilibration procedure, wash procedure, elution procedure, and cleaning-in- place (CIP) procedure. Gradients should not be changed linearly but step-wise.

- Filtration step scale up does not change the interval limits for pH, redox potential, temperature, concentration, conductivity, holding time, membrane type, transmembrane pressure, retentate pressure, feed pressure, cross-flow velocity, filtrate velocity, Cwall, flux, or CIP procedures. Parameters that are increased linearly include sample volume and membrane area.
- Equipment change is the most significant aspect of scale up from laboratory scale to production scale. Not all equipment is available in scalable type. This consideration should be the prime deciding factor in laboratory scale development. Manufacturers like New Brunswick, Amersham, Pall, etc., offer a broad line of products in terms of capacity and are always preferred to single source suppliers, even if the initial cost is higher to use this equipment. Large-scale hardware often has a different design (e.g., pump design may change from high precision piston or displacement pumps to rotary, diaphragm, or peristaltic pumps). Similarly, low volume multiport valves are replaced by simple one-way valves, which combined with large-scale tubing, may expand volumes of equipment accessories substantially and lead to extra dispersion of the target protein molecules. Large-scale equipment is often constructed from stainless steel and does not withstand high concentrations of sodium chloride. The scale-up issues to consider in relation to large-scale equipment include differences in chromatographic column physics of movement, the choice and placement of tubing, valve, and reservoir, chemical resistance of construction material, the choice of CIP and SIP, etc.

PROCESS MATERIALS

The quality of water should depend on the intended use of the finished product. For example, FDA's Center for Biologics Evaluation and Research (CBER) requires water for injection (WFI) quality for process water. On the other hand, for *in vitro* diagnostics, purified water may suffice. For drugs, the quality of water required depends on the process. Also, because processing usually occurs cold or at room temperature, the self-sanitization of a hot WFI system at 75°C to 80°C is lost.

For economic reasons, many of the biotech companies manufacture WFI by reverse osmosis rather than by distillation, which may result in contaminated systems because of the nature of processing equipment that is often difficult to sanitize. Any threads or drops in a cold system provide an area where microorganisms can lodge and multiply. Some of the systems employ a terminal sterilizing filter. However, the primary concern is endotoxins, and the terminal filter may merely serve to mask the true quality of the WFI used. The limitations of relying on a 0.1 ml sample of WFI for endotoxins from a system should also be recognized. The system should be designed to deliver high purity water, with the sample merely serving to ensure that it is operating adequately. As with other WFI systems, if cold WFI is needed, point-of-use heat exchangers can be used.

Buffers can be manufactured as sterile, nonpyrogenic solutions and stored in sterile containers. Some of the smaller facilities have purchased commercial sterile, nonpyrogenic buffer solutions. The production or storage of nonsterile water that may be of reagent grade or used as a buffer should be evaluated from both a stability and microbiological aspect.

WFI systems for biological manufacturing are the same as WFI systems for other regulated products. As with other heat sensitive products, cold WFI is used for formulation. Cold systems are prone to contamination. The cold WFI should be monitored both for endotoxins and microorganisms.

ENVIRONMENT CONTROL

Microbiological quality of the environment during various stages of processing is very important, particularly as the process continues downstream, more intensive control and monitoring is recommended. The environment and areas used for the isolation of the biologically derived product (BDP) should also be controlled to minimize microbiological and other foreign contaminants. The typical isolation of BDP should be of the same control as the environment used for the formulation of the solution prior to sterilization and filling.

NIH GUIDELINES FOR HANDLING DNA MATERIAL

Recombinant technology is associated with a number of safety issues related to the expression system used, cell banking, fermentation and cell cultures, raw materials used, downstream processing, and unintended introduction of adventitious agents (bacteria, viruses, mycoplasma, prions). One of the major purposes of the purification process is to provide a rational design ensuring the removal of said adventitious agents and other harmful impurities. A rule of thumb says that at least three different chromatographic principles should be used in a biopharmaceutical downstream process. If insect cells, mammalian cells, or transgenic animals have been used, a virus inactivation step and an active virus filtration step should be considered. The adventitious agents and their relation to the expression system used are simply understood as endotoxins, nucleic acids, bioburden, viruses, and prions and can be an issue in all systems of expression except that viruses and prions are not an issue in microbial systems; prions are also not an issue in other systems except in transgenic animals. The use of raw materials should be carefully investigated. Only raw materials suited for biopharmaceutical processing should be accepted, based on solid documentation on safety and quality.

The purpose of the *NIH Guidelines* is to specify practices for constructing and handling: (1) rDNA molecules, and (2) organisms and viruses containing rDNA molecules. Any rDNA experiment, which according to the *NIH Guidelines* requires approval by NIH, must be submitted to NIH or to another federal agency that has jurisdiction for review and approval. Once approval, or other applicable clearance, has been obtained from a federal agency other than NIH (whether the experiment is referred to that agency by NIH or sent directly there by the submitter), the experiment may proceed without the necessity for NIH review or approval. For experiments involving the deliberate transfer of rDNA, or DNA or RNA, derived from rDNA, into human research participants (human gene transfer), no research participant shall be enrolled until the risk assessment certificate (RAC) review process has been completed.

In the context of the *NIH Guidelines*, rDNA molecules are defined as either: (1) molecules that are constructed outside living cells by joining natural or synthetic DNA segments to DNA molecules that can replicate in a living cell, or (2) molecules that result from the replication of those described in (1) above. Synthetic DNA segments that are likely to yield a potentially harmful polynucleotide or polypeptide (e.g., a toxin or a pharmacologically active agent) are considered as equivalent to their natural DNA counterpart. If the synthetic DNA segment is not expressed *in vivo* as a biologically active polynucleotide or polypeptide product, it is exempt from the *NIH Guidelines*.

Genomic DNA of plants and bacteria that have acquired a transposable element, even if the latter was donated from a recombinant vector that is no longer present, are not subject to the *NIH Guidelines* unless the transposon itself contains rDNA.

Risk assessment is ultimately a subjective process. The investigator must make an initial risk assessment based on the risk group (RG) of an agent. Agents are classified into four risk groups according to their relative pathogenicity for healthy adult humans by the following criteria: (1) Risk Group 1 (RG1) agents are not associated with disease in healthy adult humans; (2) Risk Group 2 (RG2) agents are associated with human disease that is rarely serious and for which preventive or therapeutic interventions are *often* available; (3) Risk Group 3 (RG3) agents are associated with serious or lethal human disease for which preventive or therapeutic interventions *may be* available; (4) Risk Group 4 (RG4) agents are likely to cause serious or lethal human disease for which preventive or therapeutic interventions are *not usually* available.

Considerable information already exists about the design of physical containment facilities and selection of laboratory procedures applicable to organisms carrying rDNA. The existing programs rely upon mechanisms that can be divided into two categories: (1) a set of standard practices that are generally used in microbiological laboratories; and (2) special procedures, equipment, and laboratory installations that provide physical barriers that are applied in varying degrees according to the estimated biohazard.

There are six categories of experiments defined in the *NIH Guidelines* involving rDNA that require:

1. Institutional Biosafety Committee (IBC) approval, RAC review, and NIH Director approval before initiation. Experiments considered as *Major Actions:* The deliberate transfer of a drug resistance trait to microorganisms that are not known to acquire the trait naturally, if such acquisition could compromise the use of the drug to control disease agents in humans, veterinary medicine, or agriculture, will be reviewed by RAC.
2. NIH/OBA and Institutional Biosafety Committee approval before initiation. Experiments Involving the Cloning of Toxin Molecules with LD_{50} of Less than 100 Nanograms per Kilogram Body Weight. Deliberate formation of recombinant DNA containing genes for the biosynthesis of toxin molecules lethal for vertebrates at an LD_{50} of less than 100 nanograms per kilogram body weight (e.g., microbial toxins such as the botulinum toxins, tetanus toxin, diphtheria toxin, and *Shigella dysenteriae* neurotoxin). Specific approval has been given for the cloning in *Escherichia coli* K-12 of DNA containing genes coding for the biosynthesis of toxic molecules which are lethal to vertebrates at 100 nanograms to 100 micrograms per kilogram body weight.
3. Institutional Biosafety Committee and Institutional Review Board approvals and RAC review before research participant enrollment. Experiments Involving the Deliberate Transfer of Recombinant DNA, or DNA or RNA Derived from Recombinant DNA, into One or More Human Research Participants. For an experiment involving the deliberate transfer of recombinant DNA, or DNA or RNA derived from recombinant DNA, into human research participants (human gene transfer), no research participant shall be enrolled until the RAC review process has been completed. In its evaluation of human gene transfer proposals, the RAC will consider whether a proposed human gene transfer experiment presents characteristics that warrant public RAC review and discussion. The process of public RAC review and discussion is intended to foster the safe and ethical conduct of human gene transfer experiments. Public review and discussion of a human gene transfer experiment (and access to relevant information) also serves to inform the public about the technical aspects of the proposal, meaning and significance of the research, and any significant safety, social, and ethical implications of the research.
4. Institutional Biosafety Committee approval before initiation. Prior to the initiation of an experiment that falls into this category, the Principal Investigator must submit a registration document to the Institutional Biosafety Committee which contains the following information: (i) the source(s) of DNA; (ii) the nature of the inserted DNA sequences; (iii) the host(s) and vector(s) to be used; (iv) if an attempt will be made to obtain expression of a foreign gene, and if so, indicate the protein that will be produced; and (v) the containment conditions that will be implemented as specified in the *NIH Guidelines*.
   a. Experiments Using Risk Group 2, Risk Group 3, Risk Group 4, or Restricted Agents as Host-Vector Systems. Experiments involving the introduction of recombinant DNA into Risk Group 2 agents will usually be conducted at Biosafety Level (BL) 2 containment. Experiments with such agents will usually be conducted with whole animals at BL2 or BL2-N (Animals) containment.
   b. Experiments Involving the Use of Infectious DNA or RNA Viruses or Defective DNA or RNA Viruses in the Presence of Helper Virus in Tissue Culture Systems Caution: Special care should be used in the evaluation of containment levels for experiments which are likely to either enhance the pathogenicity (e.g., insertion of a host oncogene)

or to extend the host range (e.g., introduction of novel control elements) of viral vectors under conditions that permit a productive infection. In such cases, serious consideration should be given to increasing physical containment by at least one level.

c. Experiments Involving Whole Animals. This section covers experiments involving whole animals in which the animal's genome has been altered by stable introduction of recombinant DNA, or DNA derived therefrom, into the germ-line (transgenic animals) and experiments involving viable recombinant DNA-modified microorganisms tested on whole animals. For the latter, other than viruses which are only vertically transmitted, the experiments may *not* be conducted at BL1-N containment. A minimum containment of BL2 or BL2-N is required.

d. Experiments Involving Whole Plants. Experiments to genetically engineer plants by recombinant DNA methods, to use such plants for other experimental purposes (e.g., response to stress), to propagate such plants, or to use plants together with microorganisms or insects containing recombinant DNA.

e. Experiments Involving More than 10 Liters of Culture. The appropriate containment will be decided by the Institutional Biosafety Committee. Where appropriate, Appendix K, *Physical Containment for Large Scale Uses of Organisms Containing Recombinant DNA Molecules*, shall be used. Appendix K describes containment conditions Good Large Scale Practice through BL3-Large Scale.

5. Institutional Biosafety Committee notification simultaneous with initiation. Examples include experiments in which all components derived from non-pathogenic prokaryotes and non-pathogenic lower eukaryotes and may be conducted at BL1 containment.

a. Experiments Involving the Formation of Recombinant DNA Molecules Containing No More than Two-Thirds of the Genome of any Eukaryotic Virus. Recombinant DNA molecules containing no more than two-thirds of the genome of any eukaryotic virus (all viruses from a single Family being considered identical may be propagated and maintained in cells in tissue culture using BL1 containment. For such experiments, it must be demonstrated that the cells lack helper virus for the specific Families of defective viruses being used. The DNA may contain fragments of the genome of viruses from more than one Family but each fragment shall be less than two-thirds of a genome.

b. Experiments Involving Whole Plants

Experiments Involving Transgenic Rodents

6. Are exempt from the *NIH Guidelines*. The following recombinant DNA molecules are exempt from the *NIH Guidelines* and registration with the Institutional Biosafety Committee is not required:

a. Those that are not in organisms or viruses.

b. Those that consist entirely of DNA segments from a single nonchromosomal or viral DNA source, though one or more of the segments may be a synthetic equivalent.

c. Those that consist entirely of DNA from a prokaryotic host including its indigenous plasmids or viruses when propagated only in that host (or a closely related strain of the same species), or when transferred to another host by well established physiological means.

d. Those that consist entirely of DNA from an eukaryotic host including its chloroplasts, mitochondria, or plasmids (but excluding viruses) when propagated only in that host (or a closely related strain of the same species).

e. Those that consist entirely of DNA segments from different species that exchange DNA by known physiological processes, though one or more of the segments may be a synthetic equivalent. A list of such exchangers will be prepared and periodically revised by the NIH Director with advice of the RAC after appropriate notice and opportunity for public comment.

    f. Those that do not present a significant risk to health or the environment as determined by the NIH Director, with the advice of the RAC, and following appropriate notice and opportunity for public comment.

BIOSAFETY LEVELS

There are four biosafety levels. These biosafety levels consist of combinations of laboratory practices and techniques, safety equipment, and laboratory facilities appropriate for the operations performed and are based on the potential hazards imposed by the agents used and for the laboratory function and activity. Biosafety Level 4 provides the most stringent containment conditions, Biosafety Level 1 the least stringent. Experiments involving rDNA lend themselves to a third containment mechanism, namely, the application of highly specific biological barriers. Natural barriers exist that limit either: (1) the infectivity of a vector or vehicle (plasmid or virus) for specific hosts, or (2) its dissemination and survival in the environment. Vectors, which provide the means for rDNA or host cell replication, can be genetically designed to decrease, by many orders of magnitude, the probability of dissemination of rDNA outside the laboratory.

Since these three means of containment are complementary, different levels of containment can be established that apply various combinations of the physical and biological barriers along with a constant use of standard practices. Categories of containment are considered separately in order that such combinations can be conveniently expressed in the *NIH Guidelines*.

Physical containment conditions within laboratories may not always be appropriate for all organisms because of their physical size, the number of organisms needed for an experiment, or the particular growth requirements of the organism. Likewise, biological containment for microorganisms may not be appropriate for all organisms, particularly higher eukaryotic organisms. However, significant information exists about the design of research facilities and experimental procedures that are applicable to organisms containing rDNA that is either integrated into the genome or into microorganisms associated with the higher organism as a symbiont, pathogen, or other relationship. This information describes facilities for physical containment of organisms used in nontraditional laboratory settings and special practices for limiting or excluding the unwanted establishment, transfer of genetic information, and dissemination of organisms beyond the intended location, based on both physical and biological containment principles. Research conducted in accordance with these conditions effectively confines the organism.

Revision of Appendix K of the *NIH Guidelines* in April 2002 (http://www4.od.nih.gov/oba/rac/guidelines/guidelines.html) reflects a formalization of suitable containment practices and facilities for the conduct of large-scale experiments involving rDNA-derived industrial microorganisms. Appendix K replaces portions of Appendix G when quantities in excess of 10 L of culture are involved in research or production. For large-scale research or production, four physical containment levels are established: GLSP, BL1-LS, BL2-LS, and BL3-LS.

- GLSP: (Good Large-Scale Practice) level of physical containment is recommended for large-scale research of production involving viable, nonpathogenic, and nontoxigenic recombinant strains derived from host organisms that have an extended history or safe large-scale use. The GLSP level of physical containment is recommended for organisms such as those that have built-in environmental limitations that permit optimum growth in the large-scale setting but limited survival without adverse consequences in the environment.
- BL1-LS: (Biosafety Level 1-Large Scale) level of physical containment is recommended for large-scale research or production of viable organisms containing rDNA molecules that require BL1 containment at the laboratory scale.

- BL2-LS: Level of physical containment is required for large-scale research or production of viable organisms containing recombinant DNA molecules that require BL2 containment at the laboratory scale.
- BL3-LS: Level of physical containment is required for large-scale research or production of viable organisms containing rDNA molecules that require BL3 containment at the laboratory scale.
- BL4-LS: No provisions are made at this time for large-scale research or production of viable organisms containing rDNA molecules that require BL4 containment at the laboratory scale.

There should be no adventitious organisms in the system during cell growth. Contaminating organisms in the bioreactor may adversely affect both the product yield and the ability of the downstream process to correctly separate and purify the desired protein. The presence or effects of contaminating organisms in the bioreactor can be detected in a number of ways — growth rate, culture purity, bacteriophage assay, and fatty acid profile.

To ensure compliance with the *NIH Guidelines*:

- Verify that there are written procedures to ensure absence of adventitious agents and criteria established to reject contaminated runs.
- Maintain cell growth records and verify that the production run parameters are consistent with the established pattern.
- Establish written procedures to determine what investigations and corrective actions will be performed in the event that growth parameters exceed established limits.
- Ensure proper aseptic techniques during cell culture techniques and appropriate in-process controls in their processing.

The FDA is responsible under the National Environmental Policy Act (NEPA) for ascertaining the environmental impact that may occur due to the manufacture, use, and disposal of FDA-regulated products. The FDA makes sure that the product sponsor is conducting investigations safely. Typically, a product sponsor describes environmental control measures in environmental assessments (EAs) that are part of the product application. When the product is approved, the EA is released to the public. Of particular importance are the *NIH Guidelines for Recombinant DNA Research* and particularly Appendix K (2002), regarding the establishment of guidelines for the level of containment appropriate to "Good Industrial Large Scale Practices." It must be ensured that the equipment and controls described in the EA as part of the biocontainment and waste processing systems are validated to operate to the standards and that the equipment is in place, is operating, and is properly maintained. Such equipment may include, for example, HEPA filters, spill collection tanks with heat or hypochlorite treatment, and diking around bioreactors and associated drains. Standard operating procedures (SOPs) should be established for the cleanup of spills, for actions to be taken in the case of accidental exposure of personnel, for opening and closing of vessels, for sampling and sample handling, and for other procedures that involve breaching containment or where exposure to living cells may occur.

GOOD MANUFACTURING CONTROLS OF ACTIVE PHARMACEUTICAL INGREDIENTS

The "Good Manufacturing Practices" prescribed for the active pharmaceutical ingredient (API) depend to a great degree on the type of API manufactured; for example, Table 3.7 shows the increasing compliance requirement in various API manufacturing types.

TABLE 3.7
Application of the cGMP Guidance in Drug Substance Manufacturing

Type of Manufacturing		Application of cGMP to Steps (shown in italic)			
Chemical manufacturing	Production of the API starting material	*Introduction of the API starting material into process*	*Production of intermediate(s)*	*Isolation and purification*	*Physical processing, and packaging*
API derived from animal sources	Collection of organ, fluid, or tissue	Cutting, mixing, or initial processing	*Introduction of the API starting material into process*	*Isolation and purification*	*Physical processing, and packaging*
API extracted from plant sources	Collection of plant	Cutting and initial extraction(s)	*Introduction of the API starting material into process*	*Isolation and purification*	*Physical processing, and packaging*
Herbal extracts used as API	Collection of plants	Cutting and initial extraction		*Further extraction*	*Physical processing, and packaging*
API consisting of comminuted or powdered herbs	Collection of plants and/or cultivation and harvesting	Cutting/comminuting			*Physical processing, and packaging*
Biotechnology: fermentation/ cell culture	Establishment of master cell bank and working cell bank	*Maintenance of working cell bank*	*Cell culture or fermentation*	*Isolation and purification*	*Physical processing, and packaging*
"Classical" fermentation to produce an API	Establishment of cell bank	Maintenance of the cell bank	*Introduction of the cells into fermentation*	*Isolation and purification*	*Physical processing, and packaging*

MANUFACTURING SYSTEMS AND LAYOUT

Each unit operation will require careful adjustment of the sample parameters (pH, conductivity, protein concentration, redox potential, load). In some cases, desalting, ultrafiltration, or addition of cosolvents is needed in order to ensure proper conditions. One should be aware that ion exchange generally requires samples of low ionic strength, while hydrophobic interaction chromatography is generally used for samples of high ionic strength. Such observations can be used in the design of the process, thus reducing the number of unit operations. The particle size of the media will decrease from capture to polishing to accommodate the need for resolution by decreasing zone spreading on the column. The manufacturing layout will depend on the unit operations' manufacturing system.

A biopharmaceutical manufacturing process must fulfill the criteria of consistency and robustness, meaning that the outcome of each of the unit operations and the entire process shall be the same from lot to lot. Not only shall the acceptance criteria of the drug substance specification program be met, but also in-process acceptance criteria must be specified and met. Each parameter of each of the unit operations should be defined as a proven acceptable range within which the operation has to take place. It is today common practice to qualify and validate the downstream process unit operations by means of statistical factorial design analysis. Small variations in handling procedures or in parameter set points must not influence the outcome of the manufacturing process.

Most proteins are unstable in aqueous solutions and the demand for robustness is not easily obtained. Procedures that are easy to carry out in a laboratory scale (pH adjustment, chromatographic gradients, fraction collection) are technically complicated in large scale. Much can be gained if the process designers think ahead by, for instance, defining broad parameter intervals.

Where multiple products manufacturing is envisioned, the manufacturer is faced with the dilemma of design parameters that would comply with the regulatory requirements internationally. Given the cost of establishing such facilities, global compliance, rather than a regional approval, is recommended. It is well established that whereas the FDA follows certain strict requirements, the European Union (EU) requirements of cGMP compliance often exceed the FDA requirements. Whereas the FDA has moved therapeutic proteins from the CBER to the Center for Drug Evaluation and Research (CDER), these remain pretty much covered under the same regulations as are the biological products, including the timely visits and approvals by the agency, of the manufacturing facility. BLA 357 provides details of this inspection schedule. The fundamental question whether a facility can be used to manufacture a multitude of molecules needs examination. If we broadly classify the processes involved based on the type of fermenter required, the decision can be relatively straightforward. Bacterial and yeast fermentation requires a faster agitating fermenter, requiring at least two sets of line production, one for mammalian cells (which require slow and more gentle stirring) and one for other types that require relatively more agile stirring. Many newer systems now offer an opportunity for a closed system of transfer of culture to the larger fermenting vessels, reducing the environment definition, say from 100,000 area classification to pharmaceutical grade (unclassified) conditions. With computerized CIP and SIP available on most equipment, such systems are highly recommended. However, where closed systems are not utilized, the rooms where fermentation is installed should be at least of 100,000 class. In all areas where the product is exposed such as in the cell culture transfer and downstream processing purification, the rooms must be class 10,000 with separation equipment placed under class 1000 laminar flow curtains. Most regulatory authorities will not allow GMCs (genetically modified cells) to be let out in the environment. This requires an elaborate setup to sterilize the media prior to its discharge. A word of caution applies here where bacterial inclusion bodies are involved. Whereas most of the cells are ground up, some remain, requiring an equally intensive treatment of media.

Figure 3.1 shows a typical layout for a biotechnology manufacturing unit. The manufacturing layout of biological products is determined by two major factors: the size of production and the type of production; in most cases the conditions of containment described above and the need to process products under clean room conditions are similar to the processing of sterile products otherwise. As a rule of thumb, the environment should be comparable to preparation room environment for sterile products. There are four major types of work performed in a biological product manufacturing, and the requirements for each of these phases are:

1. Master Cell Bank and Working Cell Bank. A dedicated room is to be made available for each GMC; this room includes a cold storage system (often a liquid nitrogen system) and a cold (−70°C) cabinet. The cells in the MCB are used to create WCB and both of these are kept under high security. It is recommended that this be a vaulted area with class 100,000 environment; generally a 100 to 200 ft^2 area would suffice for this purpose. Some manufacturers divide the room, one section for MCB and one for WCB with restricted entrance to each. In some designs a direct transfer from WCB to the inoculum/culture room (see below) is allowed through a transfer window under negative pressure. However, this practice is questioned on the basis of need to maintain a certain area classification; as a result, the MCB/WCB is to be considered as the supply center at the time of use, processed through materials dispensing. In all instances a duplicate MCB shall be maintained off site from the immediate manufacturing area. These rooms should have a backup supply of electricity to ensure no power breakdown losses along with alarms to record temperature variations in the cabinets storing the GMCs; an

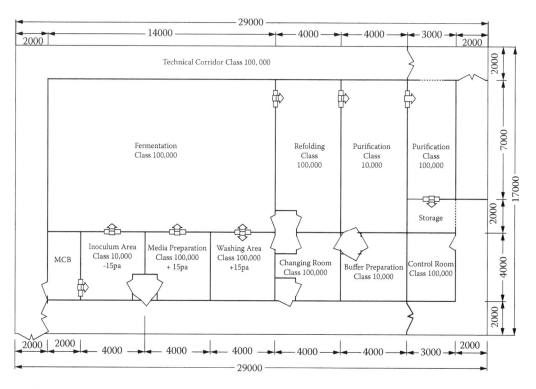

FIGURE 3.1 A typical layout of manufacturing of therapeutic proteins.

electronic recording device that would transmit the temperature at which the GMCs are stored should be installed. The room should also be equipped with an automated system of pressure differential; the room to be maintained negative as opposed to the corridor. This room is dedicated to each GMC; the reason being to avoid mixing cultures, access restrictions to different personnel, and the storage requirements.

2. Inoculum Room. This is first room where the culture tubes are opened for the purpose of making WCB, or for making the inoculum for fermentation and it should be a class 10,000 room. If the fermentation system used is a closed inline system then this room will also have a 4 to 8 L fermenter to make the starter culture; the culture will then be directly transferred to larger size fermenters. Where roller bottles are used, this room will serve as the staging room to prepare the culture for inoculation into the bottles, which would be done in another room because of the size of operation involved. The culture is handled under a biosafety laminar flow hood (the biosafety hoods prevent exposure of operator). The room should have a 10,000 classification with class 100 under the laminar flow hood. Generally, this room will be connected to the fermentation area, the recovery area, and the roller bottle preparation area, preferably through a negative pressure passing carousel. The room should be the smallest size possible (100 to 200 ft²).

3. Fermentation Room. This is generally the largest room of the facility or may comprise a series of rooms depending on the size of production. Where larger fermenters such as 25,000 L sizes are involved, this may take a three-stage fermenting. A facility of this size would likely be a 20,000+ ft² facility that may comprise several floors to accommodate large fermenters. However, for many therapeutic proteins of low dosing, fermenters of 500 L should be sufficient and these can be accommodated on a single floor basis.

The area classification for this room is 100,000 unless a complete closed system is use (which is recommended) wherein general pharmaceutical grade classification (unclassified) may be used.

4. Roller Bottle Room. Where mammalian cell cultures are used in roller bottles, the fermentation room (above) is replaced with two rooms, one for staging the roller bottles and the other a 37°C room to roll the bottles. The classification of both rooms is 100,000 with bottles being opened under a class 100 biosafety laminar flow hood. There are several issues involved in using roller bottles, the most important being the cost and time constraints in processing large number of bottles. Newer systems offer robotic controls and also recently, a multiple bottle automated continuously flowing system; these will be discussed later in the manufacturing details. Where large quantities are involved, manufacturers will be advised to develop a fermentation-based system; much progress has been made in this area and it would be discussed later as well. The size of roller bottle room will depend on the number of rolling racks involved and the size of staging room will depend on the type of process involved (robotics, manual, continuous flow, etc.). For a medium-scale operation, the 37°C room is about 150 ft^2 and the staging area about 400 ft^2.

5. Recovery Room. The product of fermentation (either from fermenters or from roller bottles) is brought to this room for the first stage of processing. Where inclusion bodies are involved (such as in the use of bacterial cultures) this room will be cold centrifuge and cell disrupters; for the mammalian culture systems where the protein is secreted, this will the first stage of reduction of volume through filtration. This room is also used to store the product where refolding is involved at 2 to 8°C environment generally (provided by walk in refrigerators). This area classification of this room remains 100,000. A room of about 500 ft^2 is required for this purpose.

6. Downstream Processing Room. This is the second 10,000 classification room with large square footage under laminar flow hoods for the purification process. It is noteworthy that dedicated contact equipment (columns, vessels, etc.) is required for each product. A room of about 500 ft^2 is required as a minimum; the size of room will depend on the volume of production and the steps involved; in some instances this may take more than 5000 ft^2 where large-scale filtration equipment is involved and may comprise several floors. Some manufacturers do their downstream processing in different facilities; in such instances, there should be proper SOPs describing the packaging and transportation of the fermentation product.

7. Media and Buffer Preparation Rooms. Each process requires a specific buffer and media; depending on the size of operation, the quantity of these liquids can be substantial. For example, when using large fermenters (1000 L or up), it may be advisable to switch to closed systems of media preparation and transfer to fermenters; however, for most medium- and small-scale operations, a large media preparation room is required (500 ft^2) with 10,000 classification and work under class 100 hood; the media prepared is then transferred to a storage area and issued a specification code; the same applies to buffers used in downstream processing. Buffers should be prepared in a separate room and transported in closed containers to the storage area prior to dispensing.

8. Storage Rooms. Incoming material is stored in special environment controlled areas; a large refrigerated space is required for many components including media and buffer. This room is also a 100,000 classification room of about 1000 ft^2. A part of the room is dedicated to staging of supplies at the time of batch issue for production wherein material will be gathered from the WCB, media, and buffer rooms.

9. Finished Product Storage Room. This is a relatively small room, about 100 ft^2, where concentrate is stored at refrigerated temperature. The classification remains 100,000.

CLEANING PROCEDURES

Validation of the cleaning procedures for the processing of equipment, including columns, should be carried out. This is especially critical for a multiproduct facility. The manufacturer should have determined the degree of effectiveness of the cleaning procedure for each BDP or intermediate used in that particular piece of equipment. Validation data should verify that the cleaning process will reduce the specific residues to an acceptable level. However, it may not be possible to remove absolutely every trace of material, even with a reasonable number of cleaning cycles. The permissible residue level, generally expressed in parts per million (ppm), should be justified by the manufacturer. Cleaning should remove endotoxins, bacteria, toxic elements, and contaminating proteins, while not adversely affecting the performance of the column. There should be established a written equipment cleaning procedure that provides details of what should be done and the materials to be utilized. Some manufacturers list the specific solvent for each BDP and intermediate. For stationary vessels, CIP is often used and in these instances necessary diagrams should be drawn to identify specific parts (e.g., valves, etc.) that are part of the cleaning protocol.

After cleaning, there should be some routine testing to ensure that the surface has been cleaned to the validated level. One common method is the analysis of the final rinse water or solvent for the presence of the cleaning agents last used in that piece of equipment. There should always be direct determination of the residual substance.

The efficiency of the cleaning system would depend to a large degree on the robustness of the analytical system used to characterize the cleaning end points. The sensitivity of modern analytical apparatus has lowered some detection thresholds below ppm, even down to parts per billion (ppb). The residue limits established for each piece of apparatus should be practical, achievable, and verifiable. There should be a rationale for establishing certain levels that must be documented to prove their scientific merit. Another factor to consider is the possible nonuniform distribution of the residue on a piece of equipment. The actual average residue concentration may be more than the level detected.

PROCESSING AND FILLING

The products of biotechnology are proteins and peptides that are relatively unstable molecules compared to most organic pharmaceuticals. Most biotechnology processes involve the transfer of proteins from one stabilizing or solubilizing buffer to another during the purification process. Ultimately, the protein is exchanged into its final solution dosage from where long-term stability is achieved. In addition, these products often require lyophilization to achieve long-term stability because of the potential for degradation by a variety of mechanisms, including deamidation, aggregation, oxidation, and possible proteolysis by trace levels of host cell proteases. The final dosage form of the protein usually contains stabilizing compounds that result in the optimal pH and solution conditions necessary for long-term product stability or the desired properties for administration of the product (tonicity). These compounds include proteins, polyhydric alcohols, amino acids, carbohydrates, bulking agents, inorganic salts, and nonionic surfactants. In addition, these excipients may be required for stable lyophilized cake formation. There are special requirements for lyophilized products, such as the control of moisture levels, that generally are defined in the individual USP monograph and that may be important to product stability. Significantly, the assessment of protein stability usually requires the use of multiple analytical methods, each of which may be used to assess a specific mode of protein degradation. The use of accelerated stability studies to predict the shelf life of protein formulations is often complicated by the effects of temperature on protein conformation, resulting in non-Arrhenius behavior. Thus, reliance on real-time, recommended storage condition stability studies is often required for establishing the expiration dating of biotechnology derived products.

Most therapeutic proteins cannot be terminally sterilized and must be manufactured by aseptic processing. The presence of process-related contaminants in a product or device is chiefly a safety issue. The sources of contaminants are primarily the cell substrate (DNA, host cell proteins, and other cellular constituents, viruses), the media (proteins, sera, and additives) and the purification process (process-related chemicals and product-related impurities).

Because of stability considerations, most therapeutic proteins are either refrigerated or lyophilized. Low temperatures and low moisture content are also deterrents to microbiological proliferation. For the validation of aseptic processing of the nonpreserved single dose biopharmaceutical (that is aseptically filled) stored at room temperature as a solution, the limitations of 0.1% media fill contamination rate should be recognized.

Media fill data and validation of the aseptic manufacturing process should be well documented. Some therapeutic proteins may not be very stable and may require gentle mixing and processing. Whereas double filtrations are relatively common for aseptically filled parenterals, single filtration at low pressures is usually performed for therapeutic proteins. It is for this reason that manufacturing directions must be specific, with maximum filtration pressures given.

The environment and accessibility for the batching of the nonsterile therapeutic proteins should be controlled. Because many of these products lack preservatives, inherent bacteriostatic, or fungistatic activity, bioburden before sterilization should be low and this bioburden should be determined prior to sterilization of these bulk solutions and before filling. Obviously, the batching or compounding of these bulk solutions should be controlled in order to prevent any potential increase in microbiological levels that may occur up to the time that the bulk solutions are filtered (sterilized). One concern with any microbiological level is the possible increase in endotoxins that may develop. Good practice for the compounding of these products would also include batching in a controlled environment and in sealed tanks, particularly if the solution is to be stored prior to sterilization. Good practice would also include limitations on the length of manufacturing time between formulation and sterilization.

In-process testing is an essential part of quality control and ensures that the actual, real-time performance of an operation is acceptable. Examples of in-process controls are: stream parameters, chromatography profiles, protein species and protein concentrations, bioactivity, bioburden, and endotoxin levels. This set of in-process controls and the selection of acceptance criteria require coordination with the results from the validation program.

The filling of therapeutic proteins into ampoules or vials presents many of the same problems as with the processing of conventional products. In established companies these issues are addressed using adequate documentation; however, for the new therapeutic proteins facility, attempting to develop and prove clinical effectiveness and safety along with validation of sterile operations, equipment and systems, can be a lengthy process, particularly if requirements are not clearly understood.

The batch size, at least when initially produced, likely will be small. Because of the small batch size, filling lines may not be as automated as for other products typically filled in larger quantities. Thus, there is more involvement of people filling these products, particularly at some of the smaller, newer companies. This can bring quality inconsistencies. Problems during filling include inadequate attire; deficient environmental monitoring programs; hand-stoppering of vials, particularly those that are to be lyophilized; and failure to validate some of the basic sterilization processes. Because of the active involvement of people in filling and aseptic manipulations, the number of individuals involved in these operations should be minimized, and an environmental program should include an evaluation of microbiological samples taken from people working in aseptic processing areas.

Another concern about product stability is the use of inert gas to displace oxygen during both the processing and filling of the solution. As with other products that may be sensitive to oxidation, limits for dissolved oxygen levels for the solution should be established. Likewise, validation of the filling operation should include parameters such as line speed and location of filling syringes with respect to closure to ensure minimal exposure to air (oxygen) for oxygen-sensitive products.

In the absence of inert gas displacement, the manufacturer should be able to demonstrate that the product is not affected by oxygen.

Typically, vials to be lyophilized are partially stoppered by machine. Where an operator places the stopper manually, serious problems can arise. Another major concern with the filling operation of a lyophilized product is assurance of fill volumes. Obviously, a low fill would represent a subpotency in the vial. Unlike a powder or liquid fill, a low fill would not be readily apparent after lyophilization, particularly for a product where the active ingredient may be only a milligram. Because of the clinical significance, subpotency in a vial potentially can be a very serious situation, clinically.

LABORATORY TESTING

The following tests may be applicable to component, in process, bulk, or final product testing. The tests that are needed will depend on the process and the intended use of the product.

- Quality
  - Color/Appearance/Clarity
  - Particulate Analysis
  - pH Determination
  - Moisture Content
  - Host Cell DNA
- Identity: A single test for identity may not be sufficient. Confirmation is needed that the methods employed have been validated. A comparison of the product to the reference preparation in a suitable bioassay will provide additional evidence relating to the identity and potency of the product.
  - Peptide Mapping (reduced/nonreduced)
  - Gel Electrophoresis
  - SDS PAGE
  - Isoelectric Focusing (IEF)
  - Immunoelectrophoresis
  - 2-Dimensional Electrophoresis
  - Capillary Electrophoresis
  - HPLC (Chromographic Retention)
  - Immunoassay
  - ELISA
  - Western Blot
  - Radioimmunoassay
  - Amino Acid Analysis
  - Amino Acid Sequencing
  - Mass Spectroscopy
  - Molecular Weight (SDS PAGE)
  - Carbohydrate Composition Analysis (glycosylation)
- Protein Concentration/Content
  - Tests that may be encountered:
  - Protein Quantitations
  - Lowry
  - Biuret Method
  - UV Spectrophotometry
  - HPLC
  - Amino Acid Analysis
  - Partial Sequence Analysis

- Purity: "Purity" means relative freedom from extraneous matter in the finished product, whether or not harmful to the recipient or deleterious to the product. Purity includes, but is not limited to, relative freedom from residual moisture or other volatile substances and pyrogenic substances. Protein impurities are the most common contaminants. These may arise from the fermentation process, media, or the host organism. Endogenous retroviruses may be present in hybridomas used for monoclonal antibody production. Specific testing for these constituents is imperative in *in vivo* products. Removal of extraneous antigenic proteins is essential to ensure the safety and the effectiveness of the product.
  - Tests for Protein Impurities:
    - Electrophoresis
      - SDS PAGE
      - IEF
    - Dimensional Electrophoresis
    - Peptide Mapping
    - Multiantigen ELISA
    - HPLC Size Exclusion HPLC Reverse Phase HPLC
  - Tests for Nonprotein Impurities:
    - Endotoxin Testing
    - USP Rabbit Pyrogen Test
    - Limulus Amebocyte Lysate (LAL) E
    - Endogenous Pyrogen Assay
- Pyrogen Contamination. Pyrogenicity testing should be conducted by injection of rabbits with the final product or by the limulus amebocyte lysate (LAL) assay. The same criteria used for acceptance of the natural product should be used for the biotech product. The presence of endotoxins in some *in vitro* diagnostic products may interfere with the performance of the device. Also, it is essential that *in vivo* products be tested for pyrogens. Certain biological pharmaceuticals are pyrogenic in humans despite having passed the LAL test and the rabbit pyrogen test. This phenomenon may be due to materials that appear to be pyrogenic only in humans. To attempt to predict whether human subjects will experience a pyrogenic response, an endogenous pyrogen assay is used. Human blood mononuclear cells are cultured *in vitro* with the final product, and the cell culture fluid is injected into rabbits. A fever in the rabbits indicates the product contains a substance that may be pyrogenic in humans.
  - USP Rabbit Pyrogen Test
  - Limulus Amebocyte Lysate (LAL)
  - Assay Endogenous Pyrogen Assay
- Viral Contamination: Tests for viral contamination should be appropriate to the cell substrate and culture conditions employed. Absence of detectable adventitious viruses contaminating the final product should be demonstrated.
  - Cytopathic effect in several cell types
  - Hemabsorption Embryonated Egg Testing
  - Polymerase Chain Reaction (PCR)
  - Viral Antigen and Antibody Immunoassay
  - Mouse Antibody Production (MAP)
- Nucleic Acid Contamination: Concern about nucleic acid impurities arises from the possibility of cellular transformation events in a recipient. Removal of nucleic acid at each step in the purification process may be demonstrated in pilot experiments by examining the extent of elimination of added host cell DNA. Such an analysis would provide the theoretical extent of the removal of nucleic acid during purification. Direct analyses of nucleic acid in several production lots of the final product should be per-

formed by hybridization analysis of immobilized contaminating nucleic acid utilizing appropriate probes, such as nick-translated host cell and vector DNA. Theoretical concerns regarding transforming DNA derived from the cell substrate will be minimized by the general reduction of contaminating nucleic acid.
- DNA Hybridization (Dot Blot)
- Polymerase Chain Reaction (PCR)
- Protein Contamination
  - SDS PAGE
  - PLC
  - IEF
- Foreign Protein Contamination
  - Immunoassays
  - Radioimmunoassays
  - ELISA
  - Western Blot
  - SDS Page
  - 2-Dimensional Electrophoresis
- Microbial Contamination. Appropriate tests should be conducted for microbial contamination that demonstrate the absence of detectable bacteria (aerobes and anaerobes), fungi, yeast, and mycoplasma, when applicable.
  - USP Sterility Test
  - Heterotrophic Plate Count and Total Yeasts and Molds
  - Total Plate Count
  - Mycoplasma Test
  - LAL/Pyrogen
- Chemical Contaminants. Other sources of contamination must be considered (e.g., allergens, petroleum oils, residual solvents, cleaning materials, column leachable materials, etc.).
- Potency (Activity). "Potency" is interpreted to mean the specific ability or capacity of the product, as indicated by appropriate laboratory tests or by adequately controlled clinical data obtained through the administration of the product in the manner intended, to produce a given result. Tests for potency should consist of either *in vitro* or *in vivo* tests, or both, which have been specifically designed for each product so as to indicate its potency. A reference preparation for biological activity should be established and used to determine the bioactivity of the final product. Where applicable, in-house biological potency standards should be cross-referenced against international (World Health Organization [WHO], National Institute of Biological Standards and Control [NIBSC]) or national (National Institutes of Health [NIH], National Cancer Institute [NCI], Food and Drug Administration [FDA]) reference standard preparations, or USP standards. Validated method of potency determination include:
  - Whole Animal Bioassays
  - Cell Culture Bioassays
  - Biochemical/Biophysical Assays
  - Receptor Based Immunoassays
  - Potency Limits
    - Identification of agents that may adversely affect potency
    - Evaluation of functional activity and antigen/antibody specificity
    - Various immunodiffusion methods (single/double)
    - Immunoblotting/radio- or enzyme-linked immunoassays
    - HPLC-validated to correlate certain peaks to biological activity
- Stability: "Stability" is the capacity of a product to remain within specifications established to ensure its identity, strength, quality, purity, safety, and effectiveness as a function

of time. Studies to support the proposed dating period should be performed on the final product. Real-time stability data would be essential to support the proposed dating period. Testing might include stability of potency, pH, clarity, color, particulates, physiochemical stability, moisture, and preservatives. Accelerated stability testing data may be used as supportive data. Accelerated testing or stress tests are studies designed to increase the ratio of chemical or physical degradation of a substance or product by using exaggerated storage conditions. The purpose is to determine kinetic parameters to predict the tentative expiration dating period. Stress testing of the product is frequently used to identify potential problems that may be encountered during storage and transportation and to provide an estimate of the expiration dating period. This should include a study of the effects of temperature fluctuations as appropriate for shipping and storage conditions. These tests should establish a valid dating period under realistic field conditions with the containers and closures intended for the marketed product. Some relatively fragile biotechnically derived proteins may require gentle mixing and processing and only a single filtration at low pressure. The manufacturing directions must be specific with maximum filtration pressures given in order to maintain stability in the final product. Products containing preservatives to control microbial contamination should have the preservative content monitored. This can be accomplished by performing microbial challenge tests (i.e., USP Antimicrobial Preservative Effectiveness Test) or by performing chemical assays for the preservative. Areas that should be addressed are:

- Effective monitoring of the stability test environment (i.e., light, temperature, humidity, residual moisture);
- Container/closure system used for bulk storage (i.e., extractables, chemical modification of protein, change in stopper formulations that may change extractable profile);
- Identify materials that would cause product instability and test for presence of aggregation, denaturation, fragmentation, deamination, photolysis, and oxidation.
- Tests to determine aggregates or degradation products.
  - SDS PAGE
  - IEF
  - HPLC
  - Ion Exchange Chromatography
  - Gel Filtration
  - Peptide Mapping
  - Spectrophotometric Methods
  - Potency Assays
  - Performance Testing
  - 2-Dimensional Electrophoresis
- Batch-to-Batch Consistency: The basic criterion for determining that a manufacturer is producing a standardized and reliable product is the demonstration of lot-to-lot consistency with respect to certain predetermined release specifications.
  - Uniformity: identity, purity, functional activity.
  - Stability: acceptable performance during shelf life, precision, sensitivity, specificity. Like other small molecules, protein drugs are subject to demonstration of stability (providing a predetermined minimum potency) to the time of use and in addition, a safety profile since the degradation products of protein drugs can be immunogenic, compared to small molecules where the concern is mainly creation of toxic molecules. The stability studies for therapeutic proteins are conducted at three levels: preformulation, formulation development, and formal GMP studies. The preformulation studies determine basic stability properties of bulk protein or peptide and the accelerated studies at this stage are primarily intended to establish stability indicating assays and other analytic methods. The formulation development studies are intended for the

candidate formulation and encompass large studies that evaluate the effects of excipients, container/closure systems and where lyophilized, a study of myriad factors that can alter the characteristics of products. The data generated in the formulation development studies are used to select final formulation and to design the studies that follow: formal GMP studies. The formal stability studies are used to support clinical use, IND and then all the way through a Biological License Application (submitted to CDER; effective June 2003, therapeutic proteins are now handled by CDER). When preparing supplies for clinical use, it is important to know that there is no need to demonstrate shelf life for the commercial dosage form and only stability demonstration is required during the testing phase, such as 6 months; many manufacturers use frozen product to assure adequate stability; this may create a logistics problem of ensuring that the clinical sites can store the produce frozen. Obviously, products that may be adversely affected by freezing will not be subject to this method of reducing the clinical startup time. Also, at this stage of initial clinical testing under an IND, the test methods need not be fully validated or have demonstrated robustness; as long as reproducibility and repeatability is demonstrated, this should be acceptable to the FDA. The formal GMP studies monitor commercial lots and clear ICH guidelines are available to follow the protocols of these studies. (See ICH Stability Guidelines for Biologics, *Federal Register* 61, no. 133 (July 10, 1996): 36466–36469.)

LABORATORY CONTROLS

A quality control program for the drug substance and drug product must be defined and acceptance criteria set for each analysis. The setting of acceptance criteria is an ongoing activity throughout development (and scale up) as more and more data become available. A batch is released provided all analytical results are within the specified ranges. A high acceptance rate should be expected if the process is robust and in compliance, implying that both the regulatory authorities and the manufacturer often share identical views. The process designer is advised to carefully consider the above-mentioned issues when designing the purification process (the design in principle). Much of the design can be carried out before entering the laboratory due to the restrictions governing biopharmaceutical processing. The predesign phase is called process modeling, thus preceding the experimental design phase for optimization and testing, which takes place in the laboratory.

In general, quality control systems for biotechnology derived products are very similar to those quality control systems routinely employed for traditional pharmaceutical products in such areas as raw material testing and release, manufacturing and process control documentation, and aseptic processing. Biotechnology derived products for quality control systems incorporate some of the same philosophies applied to the analysis of low molecular weight pharmaceutical products. These include the use of chemical reference standards and validated methods to evaluate a broad spectrum of known or potential product impurities and potential breakdown products. The quality control systems for biotechnology derived products are generally analogous to those established for traditional biologicals with respect to determining product sterility, product safety in experimental animals, and product potency. The fundamental difference between quality control systems for biotechnology derived products and traditional pharmaceuticals is in the types of methods that are used to determine product identity, consistency, purity, and impurity profiling. Furthermore, in biotechnology quality control, it is frequently necessary to use a combination of final product and in-process testing and process validation to ensure the removal of undesired real or potential impurities to the levels suggested by regulatory agencies. Biotechnology derived products generally require a detailed characterization of the production organism (cell), a complete assessment of the means of cell growth/propagation, and explicit analysis of the final product recovery process.

The complexity of the quality control systems for biotechnology derived products is related to both the size and structural characteristics of the product and manufacturing process. In general, the quality control systems required for products produced in prokaryotic cells are less complex than the systems required for products produced in eukaryotic cells. The quality control systems for prokaryotic production organisms usually entail documentation of the origin of the producer strain and encompass traditional testing for adventitious organisms, karyology, phenotyping, and antibiotic resistance. In addition, newer techniques such as DNA restriction mapping, DNA sequence analysis, and routine monitoring that may include measurement of messenger RNA (mRNA) or plasmid DNA levels may be useful. The quality control of the master cell bank and working cell bank for eukaryotic production organisms generally include testing for adventitious organisms, karyology, identity, and stability monitoring. All eukaryotic cell lines (except yeast) are generally tested for the presence of retroviruses, retroviral activity markers, and tumorigenicity, although many of these tests may be of limited value.

The laboratory controls are similar to what is expected in normal cGMP/GLP compliance for all pharmaceutical products with special consideration given to unique materials and their handling:

- Training: Laboratory personnel should be adequately trained for the jobs they are performing.
- Equipment Maintenance/Calibration/Monitoring: Documentation and scheduling for maintenance, calibration, and monitoring of laboratory equipment involved in the measurement, testing, and storage of raw materials, product, samples, and reference reagents.
- Validation: All laboratory methods should be validated with the equipment and reagents specified in the test methods. Changes in vendor or specifications of major equipment/reagents would require revalidation. Raw data should support validation parameters in submitted applications.
- Standard/Reference Material: Reference standards should be well characterized and documented, properly stored, secured, and utilized during testing.
- Storage of Labile Components: Laboratory cultures and reagents, such as enzymes, antibodies, test reagents, etc., may degrade if not held under proper storage conditions.
- Laboratory SOPs: Procedures should be written, applicable, and followed. Quality control samples should be properly segregated and stored.

DOCUMENTATION

The development program comprises a variety of activities such as project planning, cell banking, process development, development of analytical procedures, scale up, manufacture, stability studies, preparation of reference materials, and quality assurance. The work will ultimately lead to a process for the manufacture and control of the licensed product. In order to obtain a license, extensive documentation must be provided (new drug application, biological license application). However, much of the work carried out during development and scale up is not included in the said applications, and it is up to the project owner to provide the development documentation upon inspection from regulatory authorities. The statement "if it is not documented, it has not been carried out" should be taken seriously.

A major part of the documentation required can be planned (e.g., cell banking reports, unit operation descriptions, development report, analytical method descriptions, batch records). Other reports (e.g., summary reports) are written along with the experimental work. Although such reports are not providing a description of the final work, they are very useful for informing coming users about the rationale for decision-making. It is therefore recommended to include summary reports in the tech transfer package.

The drug development program produces hundreds or even thousands of documents written by different people from different departments and often from different companies. Any of these documents may be needed at a later stage and it is necessary to set up an efficient documentation system to ensure document tracking. An important part of the tracking procedure is to ensure efficient authentication of the document comprising information of author, date, version, company, facility, etc.

TECHNICAL PACKAGE

The documents listed above serve as the basis for the technological transfer between laboratory scale, pilot scale up, and non-GMP manufacture and cGMP manufacture.

- According to the Common Technical Document, ICH (www.nihs.go.jp/dig/ich/m4index-e.html), information about the nomenclature and the chemical/physical properties of the target protein should be given.
- The rationale and strategy for the process design should be documented.
- The process development work should be documented in laboratory notebooks, summary reports, unit operation descriptions, a development report, and a process protocol. Batch records should be included for test batches used for process evaluation in small scale.
- It is common practice to include a list of raw materials together with raw material information and qualification documentation.
- The manufacturer must ensure the quality and safety of the drug substance by a series of test procedures with established acceptance criteria to which the drug substance must conform. An important part of the total control strategy is to provide analytical batch data and compare these with the specified acceptance criteria. A complete set of acceptance criteria cannot be disclosed a priori as some acceptance criteria are established and justified during development and production of preclinical and clinical test batches. Acceptance criteria are linked to the total analytical program established as part of the quality control and drug substance characterization program. As more and more data are collected during development and early phase pilot production, the acceptance criteria may be adjusted or changed, thus making it difficult to establish defined batch release procedures in the development phase.
- Updated unit operation documents, raw material lists, and process protocols should be included together with scale-up summary reports and batch records.
- Data collected during development, scale up, and manufacture comprise a valuable repository of information, which can be used for trouble-shooting, comparability, and equivalence studies. Control should be exerted on all levels and should constitute an integrated part of the total quality assurance. Each analytical method used in development and for in-process control, drug substance, and drug product release should be described in an individual report including relevant analytical data. The report will gradually develop into a validation document for the method of choice.
- Short- and long-term stability studies for intermediary compounds, drug substance, and drug product should be documented.
- Reference materials and standards are usually extensively characterized. The process, protocol, analytical methods used and the analytical data must be provided in an accompanying report.

OUTSOURCING IN BIOTECH MANUFACTURING

One of the major bottlenecks in the rapidly growing biotech industry is manufacture of drug products for clinical trials. Demands for safety, robustness, and compliance make it necessary to produce clinical material in highly specialized cGMP facilities making biopharmaceutical drug development and cGMP manufacture a complex multitask operation for experts only. With the steadily increasing number of biotech companies entering this area and the huge costs involved in building cGMP facilities, outsourcing of development activities and manufacture to highly specialized contract research and manufacturing organizations has become common practice. However, one thing that cannot be outsourced is the responsibility for the product, and biotech companies are strongly advised to keep in control by proper management throughout the program. In deciding the nature and extent of outsourcing that can be practiced, several questions must be answered:

- Which contract manufacturer should the biotech company partner with?
- Which research organizations should the biotech company partner with?
- How does the biotech company negotiate the contracts?
- What are the liability issues?
- What does it cost?
- What is the timeline?

ISSUES TO DISCUSS

Area	Items to Discuss
Management	Project plan
	Batch plans
	Budgets
	Work sheets
	Communication
	Gantt chart
Cell work	Cell line optimization
	Establish master cell bank
	Master cell bank sterility
	Master cell bank characterization
	Master cell bank storage and stability
	Establish working cell bank
	Working cell bank sterility
	Working cell bank characterization
	Working cell bank storage and stability
Upstream development	Media, conditions, holding times, etc.
	Process scale
	Critical parameters and interactions
	Production of three consecutive batches in small-scale meeting specifications
Process development	Provide process rationale and strategy
	Process scale
	Process design aiming for cGMP production
	Production of three (consecutive) batches in small-scale meeting specifications
	Critical parameters and interactions
	Protein stability during processing
Non-cGMP production of drug substance from preclinical tests	Amount of drug substance to be produced
	Batch size
	Time schedule
Formulation development	Drug product development

Area	Items to Discuss
Reference material	Amount of reference standard to be produced
	Conditions for storage
In-process control	Protein concentration assays
	1D-SDS PAGE
	High performance IEC
	High performance RPC
	Size exclusion chromatography
	Specific biological activity
Quality control	Protein concentration assays
	1D-SDS PAGE
	High performance IEC
	High performance RPC
	Size exclusion chromatography
	Endotoxins
	Host cell proteins
	DNA
	Bioburden
	Viruses
	Leachables
	Contaminants
	Carbohydrate pattern
	Specific biological activity
	Specific immunological activity
	Toxicity
	Appearance
Drug substance characterization	The following analyses should be discussed:
	Mass spectrometry
	Amino acid sequencing
	Amino acid analysis
	Peptide map
	2D-electrophoresis
	UV-scanning
	IR-spectroscopy
	Optical rotation
	Fluorescence
	Circular dichroism
	NMR
	Diffraction pattern
	FTIR
	Carbohydrate structure
Drug substance stability studies	3, 6, 12, and 24 months' stability study including: HP-IEC, HP-RPC, SEC, biological activity
Drug product stability studies	3, 6, 12, and 24 months' stability study including: HP-IEC, HP-RPC, SEC, biological activity
cGMP production of drug product: Phase I and II	Specifications
	Amount of drug product to be produced
	Batch release procedures
	List of raw materials

Area	Items to Discuss
cGMP production of drug product: Phase I and II (Continued)	Fill and pack
	Documentation
	Data collection and storage
Documentation	Laboratory notebook system
	Cell work reports
	Fermentation reports
	Downstream processing: Strategy and rationale report
	Summary reports
	Unit operation reports
	Analytical reports, QC
	Drug substance characterization reports
	Report on the reference materials
	Development report
	Batch records
	Manufacturing protocols
	List of raw materials
	Change control and deviation reports
	Facility documentation
	Equipment documentation
	Utility documentation
Technology transfer	Discovery to development
	Development to pilot production
	Tech transfer packages
	Tech transfer plan

The level of outsourcing depends to a great deal on the in-house preparedness and can take place at any of the following steps of process of manufacturing:

Molecular Biology (Gene Construct) Fermentation Development (Upstream) Purification (Downstream) Protein Characterization and Analysis Preclinical Testing Regulatory Filing Clinical Supplies (cGMP) Full Scale Manufacturing.

Given below is a list of contract manufacturers for different types of manufacturing of biotech products. The roster of these companies is expanding rapidly and the clients are advised to make a thorough search at the time they are ready to consider these companies for new entries or for any obsolete entries below. Several important sources of information are available including http://www.bioprocessintl.com/ and http://www.bio.org. However, one of the best sources to seek advice on the selection of CMOs and CSOs is the vendors that supply products for the manufacturing of biotechnology products. As suppliers, they often are in a better position to advise you. Here is a list of suppliers that can readily assist.

Company	Website
Ajinomoto	http://www.ajiaminoscience.com/
Amersham Bioscience	http://www.amersham.com
AmProtein & Partners	http://www.rproteinbank.com/
AppliSens	http://www.applisens.com
AppTec	http://www.apptec-usa.com/
ARC Biologics	http://www.biologics.arc.ab.ca/

Company	Website
Asahi Kasei	http://www.planovafilters.com/
BD Biopharm and Industry	http://www.bd.com/industrial
BIA Separations	http://www.biaseparations.com/
BioReliance	http://www.bioreliance.com
Broadley James	http://www.broadleyjames.com/
Cambrex Biopharmaceutical Services	http://www.cambrex.com/
Cardinal Health	http://www.cardinal.com/
Clonex Development Inc.	http://www.clonexdevelopment.com/
Decco Process Solutions	http://www.decco.com/
Diosynth	http://www.diosynthbiotechnology.com/
DSM Pharmaceuticals	http://www.dsmpharmaceuticals.com/
Eden Biodesign	http://www.edenbiodesign.com/
Ertel Alsop	http://www.ertelalsop.com/
Formatech	http://www.fomatech.com
Growcells	http://www.growcells.com
Henogen	http://www.henogen.com
Irvine Scientific	http://www.irvinesci.com
JRH Biosciences	http://www.jrhbio.com
KBI BioPharma	http://www.kbibiopharma.com/
LaureatePharma	http://www.laureatepharma.com/
Millipore	http://www.millipore.com
New Brunswick Scientific	http://www.nbsc.com
NovAseptic	http://www.novaseptic.se
Pall Life Sciences	http://www.pall.com
Pharmenta	http://www.pharmenta.com
ProMetic Biosciences	http://www.prometic.com
Sartorius	http://www.sartorium.com
Serologicals Corporation	http://www.serologicals.com
Sigma-Aldrich	http://www.sigma-aldrich.com
Society of Bioprocessing Professionals	http://www.bioprocessingprofessionals.org/
SPI	http://www.spi.pt/biogmp
Stem Cell Technologies	http://www.stemcell.com/
Swagelok	http://www.swagelok.com
Wave Biotech	http://www.wavebiotech.com

CONTRACT MANUFACTURING ORGANIZATIONS (CMOs)

MICROBIAL CMOs

Company	Website
Abbott	www.abbottcontractmfg.com
Accentus plc	www.accentus.co.uk
Alpha Bioverfahrens Technology	www.alphabvt.com
Asahi Glass company Ltd	www.agc.co.jp/aspex

Company	Website
Avecia	www.avecia.com/biotech
Biochemie GmbH	www.biochemie.com
BioReliance Corporation	www.bioreliance.com
Bio-Technical Resources	www.biotechresources.com
Biotechnology Research Institute/NRC	www.bri.nrc.ca
Biovitrum AB	www.biovitrum.com
Boehringer Ingelheim Austria	www.boehringer-ingelheim.com
Cambrex Bio Science Inc.	www.bscp.com
CAMR (the Centre for Applied Microbiology and Research)	www.camr.org.uk
Cangene Corp	www.cangene.com
Chiron Corporation	www.chiron.com
CMC Biopharmaceuticals A/S	www.cmcbio.com
Cobra Therapeutics Ltd.	www.cobratherapeutics.com
Cobra BioManufacturing	www.cobrabiomanufacturing.com
Diosynth BV	www.diosynth.com
Dow Biopharmaceutical Manufacturing Services	www.dowbcms.com
DSM Biologics	www.dsmbiologics.com
Eurogentec	www.eurogentec.com
Excell Biotech Ltd	www.excellbiotech.com
Formatech Inc.	www.formatech.com
GDS Technology Inc	www.gdstech.com
Icos	www.icosbiologics.com
Indiana Protein Technologies Inc.	www.indianaprotein.com
Intelligene Expressions Inc	www.intelligene.com
IPT (Integrated Protein Technologies) – Monsanto	www.monsanto.com
Lonza Biotec	www.lonzabiotec.com
Marathon Biopharmaceuticals (Cambrex company)	www.marathonbio.com
Pierre Fabre	www.cipf.com
Polymun Scientific Immunbiologische Forschung GmbH	www.polymun.com
Progen Industries Ltd	www.progen.com.au
Qiagen GmbH	www.qiagen.com
Rentschler Biotechnologie GmbH	www.rentschler.de
Rockland Immunochemicals	www.rockland-inc.com
Synco Biopartners	www.synco-biopartners.com
University of Alabama at Birmingham: Fermentation Facility	www.main.uab.edu/show.asp?durki=15811

INSECT CELL CMOS

Company	Website
Accentus plc (formerly AEA)	www.accentus.co.uk
Biotechnology Research Institute/NRC	www.bri.nrc.ca

Company	Website
Biovest International (formerly Cellex Biosciences & Unisyn)	www.biovest.com
Cambrex Bio Science Inc (formerly Bio Science Contract Production Corp)	www.bscp.com
CAMR (the Centre for Applied Microbiology and Research)	www.camr.org.uk
Charles River Laboratories (formerly Primedica)	www.criver.com
	www.primedica.com
Cobra Therapeutics Ltd.	www.cobratherapeutics.com
Cobra BioManufacturing	www.cobrabiomanufacturing.com
Eurogentec	www.eurogentec.com
Excell Biotech Ltd	www.excellbiotech.com
Intelligene Expressions Inc	www.intelligene.com
Progen Industries Ltd	www.progen.com.au

Mammalian CMOs

Company	Website
Abbott	www.abbottcontractmfg.com
Accentus plc	www.accentus.co.uk
Alpha Bioverfahrens Technology	www.alphabvt.com
Bayer Biotechnology	www.pharma-und-chemiepark.de/de/ang_biotech.htm
BioInvent Production AB	www.bioinvent.com
Biotechnology Research Institute/NRC	www.bri.nrc.ca
Biovest International	www.biovest.com
Biovitrum AB	www.biovitrum.com
Boehringer Ingelheim Pharma	www.boehringer-ingelheim.com
Cambrex Bio Science Inc	www.bscp.com
Cangene Corp	www.cangene.com
Charles River Laboratories	www.criver.com
	www.primedica.com
CMC Biopharmaceuticals A/S	www.cmcbiotech.com
Cobra Therapeutics Ltd	www.cobratherapeutics.com
Cobra BioManufacturing	www.cobrabiomanufacturing.com
Cymbus Biotechnology Ltd	www.chemicon.com
Diosynth BV	www.diosynth.com
Dow Biopharmaceutical Manufacturing Services	www.dowbcms.com
Dragon	www.dragonbiotech.com
DSM Biologics	www.dsmbiologics.com
Eurogentec	www.eurogentec.com
Evans Vaccines	www.evansvaccines.com
Excell Biotech Ltd	www.excellbiotech.com
Formatech Inc	www.formatech.com

Company	Website
4C Biotech	www.4c.be
GBF	www.gbf.de
GlaxoSmithKline	www.gsk.com
Goodwin Technology Inc	www.goodwinbio.com
Icos	www.icosbiologics.com/icosbiologics/
Indiana Protein Technologies Inc	www.inprotein.com
Intelligene Expressions Inc	www.intelligene.com
Lonza Biologics Inc	www.lonzabiologics.com
Maine Biotechnology Services Inc	www.mainebiotechnology.com
Marathon Biopharmaceuticals (Cambrex Company)	www.marathonbio.com
Microbix Biosystems, Inc.	www.microbix.com
Orpegen Pharma GmbH	www.orpegen.com
Polymun Scientific	www.polymun.com
Progen Industries Ltd	www.progen.com.au
Rentschler Biotechnologie	www.rentschler.de
Rockland Immunochemicals	www.rockland-inc.com
Sigma-Aldrich Fine Chemicals	www.sigmaaldrich.com
Sorebio	SOREBIO, 1, rue Jacques Monod, Site Montesquieu, Bordeaux Technopolis, 33650 Martillac, FRANCE
Strategic Biosolutions	www.strategicbiosolutions.com
TSD Bioservices Inc	www.taconic.com

TRANSGENIC ANIMAL CMOS

Company	Website
Charles River Laboratories	www.criver.com
Eurogentec	www.eurogentec.com
Genzyme Transgenics Corp	www.genzyme.com
PPL Therapeutics Inc	www.ppl-therapeutics.com

TRANSGENIC PLANT CMOS

Company	Website
Accentus plc	www.accentus.co.uk
Biotechnology Research Institute/NRC	www.bri.nrc.ca
Charles River Laboratories	www.criver.com
Croptech Corporation	www.croptech.com
Dow Biopharmaceutical Contract Manufacturing Services	www.dowbcms.com
Eurogentec	www.eurogentec.com
Intelligene Expressions Inc	www.intelligene.com
Monsanto Protein Technologies	www.mpt.monsanto.com
	www.monsanto.com

Contract Service Organizations (CSOs)

These companies provide services for fill and pack, quality control, formulation, preclinical and clinical trials.

Name	Website
Advion Biosciences	www.advion.com
Alphalyze	www.alphalyse.com
Althea Technologies	www.altheatech.com
Analytical Biochemical Laboratory	www.abl.nl
App Tec Laboratory Service	www.apptecls.com
Associates of Cape Cod	www.acciusa.com
Biopharm	www.biopharm.de
BioReliance	www.bioreliance.com
Cato Research	www.cato.com
CCS Associates	www.ccsainc.com
Charles River Laboratories	www.criver.com
Cirion Biopharma Research	www.cirion.ca
Cobra	www.cobrabio.com
Covance	www.covance.com
Covidence	www.covidence.de
Ecron	www.ecron.com
Endpoint Research	www.endpoint.ca
ERA Consulting	www.eraconsulting.com
Eurogentec	www.eurogentec.com
Exodon Neuroscience Research	www.exodon.com
Harrison Clinical Research	www.harrisoncinical.com
Huntingdon Lifesciences	www.huntingdon.com
ICON Clinical Research	www.iconus.com
IMRO Tramarko International	www.imrotramarko.com
Insmed	www.insmed.com
Inveresk Research International	www.inveresk.com
Kendle International	www.kendle.com
KGK Synergize	www.kgksynergize.com
Kiecana Clinical Research	www.kiecana.com
Microbix Biosystems Inc	www.microbix.com
M-Scan	www.m-scan.com
MDS Pharma	www.mdsps.com
Medeval	www.medeval.com
Medibridge	www.medibridge.fr
Microsafe	www.microsafe.nl
NewLab BioQuality AG	www.newlab.de
OctoPlus	www.octoplus.com
Pharma BioResearch International	www.pbr.nl
Pharmatek Laboratories	www.pharmatek.com
Phylonix	www.phylonix.com

Name	Website
PPD	www.ppdi.com
Research Dynamics Consulting Group	www.resdyncg.com
Ricerca	www.ricerca.com
Scantox	www.scantox.com
Synco Biopartners	www.synco-biopartners.com

OTHER USEFUL LINKS

Name	Website
Bioinformatics	http://www.biolynx.de Links to numerous search engines and a thorough dictionary of biotechnology companies.
Biotechnology Industry	http://www.bio.com Lists biotechnology company profiles with major emphasis on biopharmaceutical companies. http://www.bio.org The homepage for the biotechnology industry organization. Many useful links.
Consultants	http://www.biologicsconsulting.com The Biologics Consulting Group, LLC, provides regulatory affairs and product development advice to manufacturers of biological drugs products. http://www.pharmsci.com: Pharmaceutical Scientist, Inc provides global consulting in biotechnology manufacturing; includes licensing of technology, turnkey setup and regulatory approvals.
Dictionaries	http://www.bumc.bu.edu/www/busm/pharmacology/programmed/glossaryFrame.html Glossary of terms and symbols used in pharmacology. http://www.biotechterms.org http://biotechterms.org/sourcebook/ Glossary of biotech terms.
Literature	http://www.ncbi.nlm.nih.gov/entrez/query.fcgi The Medline/Pubmed literature server. http://www.biosis.org Biosis, database host for biology literature. http://www.embase.com Biomedical and pharmacological information. http://www.dialog.com The Dialog/Datastar server. http://www.fiz-karlsruhe.de STN service center Europe http://www.loc.gov The Library of Congress literature server. http://www.plos.org Public Library of Service. Papers are freely available. PLOS is the publisher of *Plos Biology*, an open-access online, referred journal. http://wwwdoaj.org Directory of open access journals.

Name	Website
Patents	http://www.european-patent-office.org The European Patent Office homepage. http://www.uspto.gov The U.S. Patent and Trademark Office homepage. http://www.wipo.int The World Intellectual Property Organization homepage. http://www.derwent.com The Derwent patent server. http://www.micropatent.com Patent and trademark information. http://ep.espacenet.com Europe's network of patent databases.
Protein Databases	http://www.ebi.ac.uk Databases at the European Bioinformatics Institute for protein searches. http://expasy.hcuge.ch/ Homepage of the ExPASy server. Links to protein databases and software tools. http://www.rcsb.org/pdb Protein Data Bank: The single worldwide repository for the processing and distribution of 3-D biological macromolecular structure data. http://www.ncbi.nlm.nih.gov/Structure/lexington/lexington.cgi?cmd=rps Finds domain architectures. CDART is a way to visualize a protein and its relatives, which takes an accession number or sequence in FASTA format as a query. National Center for Biotechnology information-NCBI. http://www.ncbi.nlm.nih.gov/entrez/batchentrez.cgi?db=Protein Downloads protein sequence data. National Center for Biotechnology information-NCBI. http://www.ncbi.nlm.nih.gov/entrez/query.fcgi?db=Structure The Molecular Modelling Database (MMDB) contains 3-D macromolecular structures, including proteins and polynucleotides. MMDB contains over 10,000 structures and is linked to the rest of the NCBI databases, including sequences, bibliographic citations, taxonomic classifications, and sequence and structure neighbors. National Center for Biotechnology information-NCBI.
Regulatory	http://www.fda.gov Food and Drug Administration, USA. The website for U.S. food and drug regulatory agency. http://www.fda.gov/cber/ctd/ctd.htm The CTD implementation action plan at CBER. http://www.fda.gov/cder/m2/ectd.htm U.S. FDA's draft guidance for CTD electronic submissions. http://www.fda.gov/cber/guidelines.htm Guidance documents on CBER's site. http://www.access.gpo.gov/nara The U.S. Federal Register.

Name	Website
Regulatory (Continued)	http://www.emea.eu.int/
	EMEA, European Union. The website for the central European regulatory agency.
	http://www.nihs.go.jp
	Ministry of Health, Labor and Welfare, Japan. The website for the Japanese regulatory agency.
	http://www.ich.org/ich1.html
	International Conference for Harmonisation (ICH) of the technical requirements for international registration of pharmaceuticals for human use. This organization brings together regulatory authorities and industry experts from Europe, Japan, and the United States to discuss scientific and technical aspects of product registration.
	http://www.ich.org/ich5q.html#Stability
	The ICH guide to quality documents Q1-Q7.
	http://www.pharmweb.net
	PharmWeb is an online community of pharmaceutical and health care-related professionals.
	http://www.ich.org/ich5q.html
	ICH guidelines step 4. An overview with links to Q1-7 guideline documents.
	http://www.ich.org/ichctd.html
	The common technical document section of the ICH website.
	http://dg3.eudra.org/F2/eudralex/vol-2/B/ctdmay02.pdf
	The EU CTD page.
	http://www.accessdata.fda.gov/scripts/cdrh/cfdocs/cfcfr/cfrsearch.cfm
	Search, read, or download any part of the CFR Title 21
	http://pharmacos.eudra.org/F2/eudralex/vol-4/home.htm
	The European Union's Volume 4 GMP guidelines — including annex 13 (revised July 2003).
	http://www.fda.gov/cder/guidance/pv.htm
	The FDA's *Guideline on General Principles of Process Validation* (May 1987).
	http://www.fda.gov/cber/gdlns/pilot.txt
	CBER's *Guidance on the use of Pilot Manufacturing Facilities for the Development and Manufacture of Biological Products* (June 1995).
Scientific Information	http://www.biopharm-mag.com
	Information database from the BioPharm magazine.
	http://www.pharmaportal.com
	Information database from the Advanstar Pharmaceutical Group.
	http://www.biovista.com
	Information database from Biovista.
	http://www.biotech-info.net
	Ag Biotech InfoNet.
	http://www.ncbi.nlm.nih.gov
	National Center for Biotechnology Information.
	http://www.usinfo.state.gov/topical/global/biotech
	An information resource on biotechnology.

Name	Website
Scientific Information (Continued)	http://www.scirus.com/about/ Scirus is the most comprehensive science-specific search engine available on the Internet. Driven by the latest search engine technology, it enables scientists, students, and anyone searching for scientific information to chart and pinpoint data, locate university sites and find reports and articles quickly and easily. It was launched by Elsevier Science, the leading international publisher of scientific information. http://www.cato.com/biotech This directory contains over 2000 links to companies, research institutes, universities, sources of information, and other directories specific to biotechnology, pharmaceutical development, and related fields. It places emphasis on product development and the delivery of products and services.
Transgenic Animals	http://www.lists.ic.ac.uk:80/hypermail/transgenic-list/ Transgenic discussion page from Imperial College, London. http://www.mad-cow.org Useful information and the history of mad cow disease.

4 Genetically Modified Cells

INTRODUCTION

The choice of cell line and the species from where it is derived are the most important strategic decisions in the bioprocess development program. Despite significant developments over the past three decades, the primary choices remain use of bacteria (*E. coli, Bacillus subtilis, Lactococcus lactis*), yeast (*Saccharomyces cerevisiae, Pichia pastoris*), and mammalian cells (Chinese hamster ovary, baby hamster kidney). The baculovirus expression system in insect cells (sf9) is used (e.g., to express beta-glucosidases) but remains to be fully exploited; transgenic animal products are still not approved for human use, though one application for an antibody derived from goat's milk is pending approval.

A master cell bank (MCB) is a homogeneous pool of the production cell line dispensed in multiple containers, by which each aliquot is representative for each other vial, stored under defined conditions (liquid nitrogen). A tested and released MCB provides material for the working cell bank (WCB) using one or more tubes from MCB. The MCB and WCB may differ from each other in certain respects (e.g., culture components and culture conditions), but generally there is no need to extensively characterize WCB unless records indicate wide variability between MCB and WCB. The methods used to characterize cell banks are derived from the WHO requirements for the use of *in vitro* substrates for the production of biologicals (Requirements for biological substances, *Dev. Biol. Stand.* 93, no. 50 [1998]: 141–171; and the ICH guidelines Q5A, B and D [Tables 1 and 2]).

The cell line usually takes a long time to produce the desired products, and strict regulatory demands to cell line history, safety, genetic stability, expression levels, cell densities, and viability must be met in order to ensure its acceptance by the regulatory authorities. Cell line optimization and safety demonstration require additional time. In practice, serially subcultivated cells (the working cell bank) are used as a starting source for each production batch. The WCB derives from the MCB, which is made first, usually from an initial clone or from a preliminary cell bank derived from an initial clone. The MCB and WCB may differ from each other in certain respects (e.g., culture components and culture conditions). The MCB and WCB are also tested differently. The safety issues include testing for adventitious agents, which may be present in the donor cells, serum used to propagate cells, and other culture media components. Especially mammalian cells are prone to contamination because of their complexity and the duration of culture. Mammalian cells may have latent or persistent virus infection or endogenous retrovirus. Alternatively, the virus is introduced into the cells by derivation of cell lines from infected animals, use of virus to establish the cell line, or use of contaminated reagents such as serum. The genetic stability of the cells must be ensured during fermentation, and it must be shown that no mutations or loss of recombinant DNA is taking place during the cell culture period. In the early development phase, the characteristic of expressed proteins is not well understood; other factors like protein stability, batch-to-batch variations, cell mutation rates, fermentation process variables, and process economy are also uncertain. The factors, however, that can be considered at this early stage include intellectual property issues, genetic stability, productivity, quality, impurities, yield, host-cell toxicity, etc.

TABLE 4.1
Test Methods for Microbial Cell Banks (Bacteria and Yeast)

Test	Comments
Auxotrophic markers	Conformation of key markers (yeast).
Characterization	Characterization of insert by Southern Blot and eventually DNA sequence of the integrated expression cassette.
Identity	Phenotyping or genotyping may be used to confirm species and strain. Growth on selective media is considered adequate to confirm host cell identity for most microbial cells. For *E. coli* phage typing should be considered as a supplementary test.
Purity	Freedom from adventitious microbial agents and adventitious cellular contaminants must be assessed (bacteria, bacteriophages, fungi). Visual examination of the characteristics of the isolated colonies using different media is suggested.
Resistance to antibiotics	When antibiotic selection markers have been used.
Stability	It must be demonstrated that the cell line produces the desired product in a consistent quality and quantity. Studies shall be performed to determine whether manipulation of the cell line changes it characteristics significantly.

CELL LINE CHARACTERIZATION

The cell line history includes information about the source and identity of cell line, the nucleotide sequence that code for the target protein, the method used to prepare DNA for genetic engineering, a detailed component map, all inserts and deletions, integration sites, complete sequence of the expression vector used, vector transfer methods, and criteria for selection of cell clones. The cultivation history of the cells should be documented together with information on the culture medium and possible exposure to infectious agents during handling.

- For microbes the species, strain, known genotype and phenotype characteristics, organism, pathogenicity, toxin production, and other biohazard information should be provided.
- For animal cell lines donor characteristics such as tissue or organ of origin, geographic origin, age, sex, species, strains, breeding conditions, and general physiological condition of the original donor should be described.

The International Conference on Harmonisation (ICH) guideline describes characterization of cells used in recombinant DNA work (www.emea.eu.int/pdfs/human/ich/029495en.pdfA). Cell bank characterization is an important step toward obtaining a uniform final product with lot-to-lot consistency and freedom from adventitious agents (Table 4.1 and Table 4.2). Testing to qualify the MCB is performed once and can be done on an aliquot of the banked material or on cell cultures derived from the cell bank. Specifications for qualification of the MCB should be established. It is important to document the MCB history, methods, and reagents used to produce the bank and storage conditions. All the raw materials required for production of the banks, namely, media, sera, trypsin, and the like, must also be tested for adventitious agents.

Testing to qualify the MCB includes: (1) testing to demonstrate freedom from adventitious agents and endogenous viruses and (2) identity testing. The testing for adventitious agents may include tests for nonhost microbes, mycoplasma, bacteriophage, and viruses. Freedom from adventitious viruses should be demonstrated using both *in vitro* and *in vivo* virus tests and appropriate species-specific tests such as the mouse antibody production (MAP) test. Identity testing of the cell bank should establish the properties of the cells and the stability of these properties during manufacture. Cell banks should be characterized with respect to cellular isoenzyme expression and cellular phenotype and genotype, which could include expression of a gene insert or presence of

TABLE 4.2
Test Methods for Insect and Metazoan Cells

Test	Comments
Identity	Phenotyping or genotyping may be used. In most cases isoenzyme analysis is sufficient to confirm the species of origin. Other technologies include banding cytogenetics and use of species-specific anti-sera. An alternative strategy is to demonstrate the presence of unique markers.
Purity	Freedom from adventitious microbial agents and adventitious cellular contaminants must be assessed. Test for the presence of bacteria, fungi, and mycoplasma should be performed. Freedom of contaminating cell lines of the same or different species must be demonstrated.
Purity, viral agents using cell cultures	Mono-layer cultures of the following cell types: • Cultures of the same species an tissue type as the cell line • Cultures of a human diploid cell line • Cultures of another cell line from a different species The polymerase chain reaction (PCR) technology is receiving increasing attention from regulatory authorities especially after new validated quantitative tests have emerged.
Purity, viral agents using animals and eggs	Test for pathogen viruses not able to grow in cell cultures in both animals and eggs (e.g., suckling mice, adult mice, guinea pigs, fertilized eggs). The cell banks are suitable for production if none of the animals or eggs show evidence of presence of any viral agent (European Pharmacopoeia V.2.2.12).
Purity, test for retroviruses, endogenous viruses or viral nucleic acid	Test shall include infective assays, transmission electron microscopy (TEM), and reverse transcriptase (Rtase) of cells cultured up to or beyond *in vitro* cell age. Induction studies have not been found to be useful.
Purity test for selected viruses	Murine cell lines shall be tested species-specific using mouse, rat, and hamster antibody production (MAP, RAP, HAP) tests. *In vivo* testing for lymphocytic choriomeningitis virus is required. PCR techniques may be used as well. Human cell lines shall be screened for human viral pathogens (Epstein-Barr virus, cytomegalovirus, human retroviruses, hepatitis B/C viruses with appropriate *in vitro* techniques.
Stability	It must be demonstrated that the cell line produces the desired product in a consistent quality and quantity. Studies shall be performed to determine whether manipulation of the cell line changes it characteristics significantly.
Serum	Freedom from cultivable bacteria, fungi, mycoplasma, and infectious viruses must be demonstrated. Human serum should not be used and use of bovine serum shall meet specified requirements for biological substances.
Trypsin	Trypsin shall be tested and found free of cultivable bacteria, fungi, mycoplasma, and infectious viruses, especially bovine or porcine parvoviruses, as appropriate.
Viruses	Contaminating viruses are of major concern. Viruses can be introduced into the cell bank by several routes such as derivation of cell lines from infected animals, use of viruses to establish the cell line, use of contaminated reagents (e.g., animal serum), and contaminants during handling of cells. Although continuous cell lines are extensively characterized, viral contaminants will not be cytolytic. However, chronic or latent viruses may be present. Examples of viruses harbored in cell substrates are retroviruses (oncogenic), hantaviruses (CHO cells), hepatitis viruses (human cells), human papilloma virus (human cells), and cytomegalovirus (human cells). Additionally, cell line establishment or cell transformation is achieved using Epstein-Barr or Sendai viruses.

a gene-transfer vector. Suitable techniques, including restriction endonuclease mapping or nucleic acid sequencing, should be used to analyze the cell bank for vector copy number and the physical state of the vector (vector integrity and integration). The cell bank should also be characterized for the quality and quantity of the gene product produced.

Characterization of the WCB is generally less extensive, requiring the following:

- testing for freedom from adventitious agents that may have been introduced from the culture medium,
- testing for RCV, if relevant,
- routine identity tests to check for cell line cross-contamination, and
- demonstration that aliquots can consistently be used for final product production.

CELL LINE SELECTION

Of the currently approved products, the largest numbers of these products are expressed in three hosts: *Escherichia coli*, followed by Chinese hamster ovary cells and *Saccharomyces cerevisiae*. (Table 4.3). There are clear advantages and disadvantages of each of the host system described above. These are summarized in Table 4.4.

Despite the listed disadvantages, the ease of use of *E. coli* and their generally high expression yields for most proteins often have resulted in the continued preferential use of these bacteria, where feasible, with continuous improvements in the bacterial systems to obviate the described disadvantages. The use of yeast strains such as *Saccharomyces cerevisiae* for production has been extensively explored. The production of proteins in yeast offers many theoretical advantages over *E. coli* while raising certain new concerns. Like *E. coli*, yeast can maintain stable plasmids extrachromosomally; however, unlike *E. coli*, yeast possesses the ability to produce glycoproteins.

The development of eukaryotic cell culture for the production of vaccines has long been established in the pharmaceutical industry, and an extensive database has been developed to ensure the suitability of such protein products in humans. The extension of this technology to rDNA products was primarily a response to the limitations in the use of *E. coli*. Particularly with respect to large proteins or glycoproteins, eukaryotic cell expression is an attractive alternative to a bacterial system because eukaryotic cells can secrete proteins that are properly folded and identical in primary, secondary, and tertiary structure to the natural human protein. Concerns about the economics of this production system originally hindered its development. Recent advances, however, in improved expression levels, in large-scale cell culture using Chinese hamster ovary (CHO) cells,

TABLE 4.3
Most Popular Hosts for Approved Drugs Produced by Recombinant Technique in U.S.

Host	Number of Approved Products
Escherichia coli	37
Chinese hamster ovary cell	29
Saccharomyces cerevisiae	11
Baby hamster kidney cells	2
Other mammalian	2
Mouse C 127	2
African monkey kidney cells (COS-1)	1
Lymphocyte activated	1
Mouse myeloma	1
Myeloma NSO	1
Prostate epithelium cell	1

Note: May include repetitive entry for a molecule in case of multiple approvals.

TABLE 4.4
Comparison of Host Systems Advantages and Disadvantages

Host	Advantages	Disadvantages
Bacteria, e.g., *Escherichia coli*	Many reference and experience available, wide choice of cloning vectors, gene expression easily controlled; easy to grow with high yields, product forming up to 50% of total cell protein, can be designed for secretion into growth media allowing for the removal of unwanted N-terminal methionine groups.	No posttranslational modification, biological activity, and immunogenicity may differ from natural proteins; high endotoxin content in Gram negative. The expressed protein product may cause cellular toxicity; inclusion bodies difficult to process.
Bacteria, e.g., *Staphylococcus aureus*	Secretes fusion proteins into the growth media.	Does not express as high levels as *E. coli*; pathogenic.
Mammalian cells, e.g., Chinese hamster ovary cells	Same biologic activity as native proteins, mammalian expression vectors available, can be grown in large-scale cultures.	Cells can be difficult and expensive to grow, cells grow slowly; manipulated cells can be genetically unstable; low productivity as compared to microorganisms.
Yeasts, e.g., *Sacchromyces cervisiae*	Lack detectable endotoxin, generally regarded as safe (GRAS), fermentation relatively inexpensive, facilitates glycosylation and formation of disulfide bonds, only 0.5% native proteins are secreted so isolation of secreted product is simplified, well established large-scale production and downstream processing.	Gene expression less easily controlled; glycosylation not identical to mammalian systems.
Cultured insect cells (Baculovirus vector)	Facilitates glycosylation and formation of disulfide bonds, safe since few anthropods are adequate host for baculovirus; baculovirus vector received FDA approval for a clinical trial, virus stops host protein amplification, high level of expression of product.	Lack of information on glycosylation mechanism, product not always fully functional; few differences in functional and antigenic properties between product and native protein.
Fungi, e.g., *Aspergillis* sp.	Well-established system for fermentation of filamentous fungi; growth inexpensive.	High level of expression not yet achieved; genetics not always characterized.
Fungi, e.g., *A. niger* sp.	This is also generally regarded as safe (GRAS), can secrete large quantities of product into growth media, source of many industrial enzymes.	No cloning vectors available.
Transgenic plants		Low transformation efficiency, long generation time; often commercially not viable.

and in the formulation of more highly defined growth media have combined to dramatically improve the economic feasibility of eukaryotic cell substrates. The number of cell passages required for cloning, selection, amplification, and cell banking prior to production generally necessitates the use of immortal cell lines because nonimmortalized strains (i.e., diploid cultures) cannot be propagated long enough to provide an economically useful time in the production stage. Initial questions regarding the safety of such immortal cell lines were based on concerns over potential oncogenes and potential viral and retroviral contamination. These concerns have been minimized by the exhaustive analysis and characterization of master cell banks for adventitious (accidentally intro-duced) agents, by effective process validation studies, and by the safety data gathered to date for products produced by this method. The resultant thoroughly characterized master cell bank is used for full-scale production. Other eukaryotic cell lines, such as those derived from insect cells, may be useful in achieving many of the conformational and posttranslational advantages that have been described for mammalian cell culture.

A large number of cell lines of animal origin are currently in use. Examples of attachment cell lines include:

- **MRC-5:** Human lung fibroblasts,
- **HELA:** Human cervix epithelial cells,
- **VERO**: African green monkey kidney epithelial cells,
- **NIH 3T3:** Mouse embryo fibroblasts,
- **L929:** Mouse connective tissue fibroblasts,
- **CHO:** Chinese hamster ovary fibroblasts,
- **BHK-21**: Syrian hamster kidney fibroblasts,
- **HEK 293:** Human kidney epithelial cells,
- **HEPG2:** Human liver epithelial cells,
- **BAE-1**: Bovine aorta endothelial cells.

The suspension animal cell lines are mainly composed of:

- **NS0:** Mouse myeloma lymphoblastoid-like cells,
- **U937:** Human hystiocytic lymphoma lymphoblastoid cells,
- **Namalwa:** Human lymphoma lymphoblastoid cells,
- **HL60:** Human leukemia, lymphoblastoid-like cells,
- **WEHI 231:** Mouse B-cell lymphoma lymphoblastoid cells,
- **YAC 1:** Mouse lymphoma lymphoblastoid cells,
- **U 266B1:** Human myeloma, lymphoblastoid cells,
- **SH-SY5Y:** Human neuroblastoma neuroblasts.

Animal cell culture development is faster than transgenics production, and it has a solid regulatory track record. It takes about 1 month (for insect cell processes) to 5 months (for mam-malian cells) to go from genetic engineering to a production culture. Compare this with 6 months to a year for transgenic plants (from inserted genes to harvestable plants) and 1 to 3 years for transgenic animals (from gene to milk-producing mammals, although developing egg-laying hens is faster).

Animal cells by their nature are more fragile, do not have the strong cell wall of microbes, and are much larger than microbes, and as a result, they disrupt too easily, if for example, subjected to the conditions of fermenters, the newer "airlift" designs incorporate forced air and liquid flow designs that replace impellers with pumps for more gentle treatment of animal cells in culture. The complex metabolism of animal cells requires a complex mixture of nutrients. As a result, fetal bovine serum (FBS) obtained as a by-product of the dairy and beef industries has been a common additive to cell culture media. However, recent concerns about transmissible spongiform enceph-alopathies (TSE) and blood-borne pathogens have led to the development of many serum-free, animal-product–free, and even protein-free media formulations. Recombinant insulin, transferrin, bovine serum albumin (usually made by bacterial fermentation), and also human serum albumin made by yeast fermentation take the place of serum in many modern cell culture processes.

Animal cells are also sensitive to culture conditions, often overreacting to small changes in temperature or pH. Animal cells propagate more slowly than microbes do, doubling their numbers during the log phase in 15 to 48 hours They require less oxygen, which is a good thing because getting air to them can be difficult. Stirring the liquid medium by traditional impellers can break up the fragile cells. Even the impellers with rounded blades (based on the three-bladed type used to propel motorboats) designed to produce lower shear forces may be too dangerous. Bioreactors for animal cell culture use forced-air sparging or other means to introduce air into the mixture. Some animal cell lines will proliferate in suspension culture, floating about in their liquid medium. Others require a solid substrate: stuck on the insides of roller bottles, within gas-permeable polymer tubes in "hollow-fiber" bioreactors, or attached to plastic microcarrier beads or flat disks. Anchorage-dependent cells historically exhibited higher protein expression levels, but now optimized cell lines (such as NSO, CHO, HeLa, and HEK-293) are used in suspension culture. Generally, the primary cell lines are attachment dependent and the development scientists are divided on whether it will be possible to create high-yielding suspension cell lines in the future. Other techniques such as hybridomas are immortalized by fusion with myeloma tumor cells to secrete MAbs. With availability of established cell lines such as from American Type Culture Collection (ATCC), cryopreservation allows companies to "bank" cells rather than running all cell lines in constant culture.

Many mammalian cell lines undergo apoptotic death in the bioreactor environment. The high susceptibility to apoptosis partially explains many of the technical problems associated with large-scale animal cell culture. Factors such as nutrient and oxygen deprivation, virus-based protein expression systems, and cytostatic agents have been identified as potent inducers of apoptosis in industrial cultivation. They limit culture duration and productivity. Suppressing apoptosis under such conditions leads to highly robust cell lines with improved production characteristics.

Insect cell culture offers the advantages of cost and ease of culturing over mammalian cells. The expression levels of heterologous proteins achieved using this system are generally variable and fall within the range of 1 to 600 mg/L culture medium. Some collagens have been produced in insect cells at 10 to 40 mg/L. One problem with insect cells is that they tend not to secrete recombinant proteins, maintaining them instead in the intracellular cytoplasm. This is a side effect of the transfection method, and it can complicate downstream processing. Baculovirus (which is not infectious to humans) expression vectors are widely used for expressing heterologous proteins in cultured insect cells. Recent advances include production of multisubunit protein complexes, coexpression of protein-modifying enzymes to improve heterologous protein production, and additional applications of baculovirus display technology. The application of modified baculovirus vectors for gene expression in mammalian cells continues to expand. Kemp Biotechnologies Inc. (www.kempbiotech.com) is working on several insect cell projects. Insect cell lines (with the baculovirus expression vector system [BEVS]), to date, have not produced any approved therapeutics. A number of products are available in advanced clinical trails: Dendreon Corp., Seattle, WA, has a prostate cancer vaccine in Phase III; GSK (London) is developing a human papilloma virus vaccine; Protein Sciences Corporation is working on a flu vaccine (Phase III) and has scaled up their process to 600 L and is looking at a variety of other vaccines. The U.S. Department of Agriculture has developed an immortal insect cell line from *Spodoptera* sp.

CELL LINE CONSTRUCTION

The human body cellular functions are governed by a large number of proteins produced endogenously. Given below is a broad listing of these proteins:

- Chaperones: Proteins involved in protein folding.
- Conjugated proteins: Covalently bonded to prosthetic groups such as glycoprotein and metalloprotein.
- Cytokines: Regulate immunity, inflammation, apoptosis, and hematopoiesis.
  - Interleukins are the cytokines that act specifically as mediators between leukocytes. Table 4.5 shows the major source and effects of various types of interleukins.

TABLE 4.5
Types of Interleukins

	Major Source	Major Effects
IL-1	Macrophages	Stimulation of T cells and antigen-presenting cells B-cell growth and antibody production Promotes hematopoiesis (blood cell formation)
IL-2	Activated T cells	Proliferation of activated T cells
IL-3	T lymphocytes	Growth of blood cell precursors
IL-4	T cells and mast cells	B-cell proliferation IgE production
IL-5	T cells and mast cells	Eosinophil growth
IL-6	Activated T cells	Synergistic effects with IL-1 or TNF
IL-7	Thymus and bone marrow stromal cells	Development of T cell and B cell precursors
IL-8	Macrophages	Chemoattracts neutrophils
IL-9	Activated T cells	Promotes growth of T cells and mast cells
IL-10	Activated T cells, B cells, and monocytes	Inhibits inflammatory and immune responses
IL-11	Stromal cells	Synergistic effects on hematopoiesis
IL-12	Macrophages, B cells	Promotes T_H1 cells while suppressing T_H2 functions
IL-13	T_H2 cells	Similar to IL-4 effects
IL-15	Epithelial cells and monocytes	Similar to IL-2 effects
IL-16	CD8 T cells	Chemoattracts CD4 T cells
IL-17	Activated memory T cells	Promotes T cell proliferation
IL-18	Macrophages	Induces IFN production

- Interferons are the cytokines that can "interfere" with viral growth. They also have the ability to inhibit proliferation and modulate immune responses. Four types of interferons have been identified: IFN-α, IFN-β, IFN-ω, and IFN-γ. The first three are Type I IFNs, which have relatively high antiviral potency. IFN-g is the Type II IFN, also called immune IFN. Type I IFNs are produced by macrophages, neutrophils, and other somatic cells in response to infection by viruses or bacteria.
- Tumor necrosis factors (TNF): Tumor necrosis factors are the cytokines produced mainly by macrophages and T lymphocytes that help regulate the immune response and hematopoiesis (blood cell formation). There are two types of TNF:
  - TNFα: also called cachectin, produced by macrophages.
  - TNFβ: also called lymphotoxin, produced by activated CD4+ T cells.
- Chemokines are the cytokines that may activate or chemoattract leukocytes. Each chemokine contains 65 ~ 120 amino acids, with molecular weight of 8 ~ 10 kD. Their receptors belong to G-protein-coupled receptors. Since the entry of HIV into host cells requires chemokine receptors, their antagonists are being developed to treat AIDS.
- Hormones: Examples: insulin, growth hormone, and prolactin.
- Prions: Toxic proteins that enter brain cells and there convert the normal cell protein PrPC to the prion form of the protein, called PrPSC. When normal cell proteins transform into prions, amino acids that are folded tightly into alpha helical structures relax into looser beta sheets. More and more PrPC molecules transform into PrPSC molecules, until eventually prions completely clog the infected brain cells. Mad Cow Disease is purportedly caused by prions.
- Structural proteins: collagen, myosin.
- Transcription factors regulate gene transcription.
- Ubiquitin: The marker for protein degradation. If a protein binds to ubiquitin, it will be degraded by proteasome.

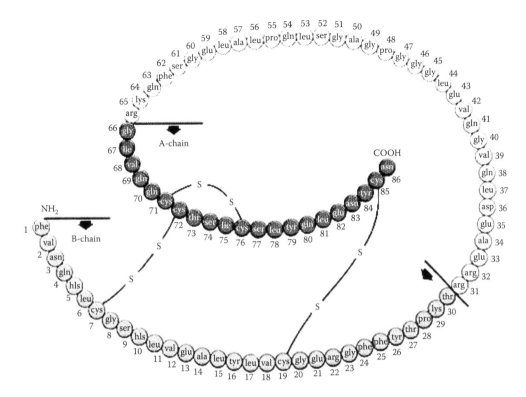

FIGURE 4.1 Amino acid sequence of proinsulin; chains A and B are separated from the third chain to activate insulin.

Several proteins listed above have direct therapeutic application wherein a break in the chain of endogenous production of these proteins produces a disease state. Most relevant proteins include cytokines and hormones. Figure 4.1 shows the structure of the most widely expressed therapeutic protein, human insulin.

On a commercial scale, these therapeutic proteins are manufactured using recombinant DNA (rDNA) techniques. A number of different genetic strategies are available for the design of processes for production of recombinant proteins mostly developed during the past couple of decades. The focus of microbiological processing is to manufacture industrially and pharmaceutically significant substances using organisms that either do not initially have genetically coded information concerning the desired product included in their DNA or (in the case of mammalian cells in culture) do not ordinarily express a chromosomal gene at appreciable levels. To do so, a gene that specifies the structure of a desired polypeptide product is either isolated from a "donor" organism or chemically synthesized and then stably introduced into another organism, which is preferably a self-replicating unicellular organism such as bacteria, yeast, or mammalian cells in culture. Once this is done, the existing machinery for gene expression in the "transformed" or "transfected" microbial host cells operates to construct the desired product, using the exogenous DNA as a template for transcription of mRNA, which is then translated into a continuous sequence of amino acid residues.

The production apparatus to manufacture therapeutic proteins consists of genetically modified cells (GMCs), which include bacteria, yeast, animal-derived cells, etc. The construction of GMCs is a complex process that follows the pathway shown in Figure 4.2.

Whereas the literature is rich in the microbiological techniques and relevant technology used to manufacture recombinant products, the most pertinent information for manufacturers of these drugs can be found in the patents that describe these proprietary methods. This includes the

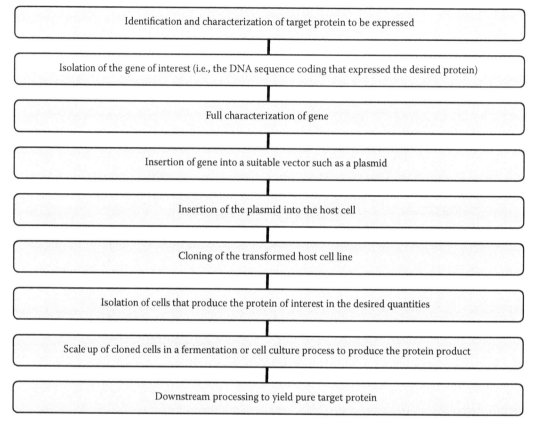

FIGURE 4.2 Process flow of GMC construction.

methodologies for the isolation, synthesis, purification, and amplification of genetic materials for use in the transformation of selected host organisms, which are amply described in various patent instruments. For example, the U.S. Pat. No. 4,237,224 to Cohen et al., describes the transformation of unicellular host organisms with "hybrid" viral or circular plasmid DNA, which includes selected exogenous DNA sequences. The procedures of the Cohen patent first involve manufacture of a transformation vector by enzymatically cleaving viral circular plasmid DNA to form linear DNA strands. Selected foreign ("exogenous" or "heterologous") DNA strands, usually including sequences coding for a desired product, are prepared in linear form through use of similar enzymes. The linear viral or plasmid DNA is incubated with the foreign DNA in the presence of ligating enzymes capable of effecting a restoration process, and "hybrid" vectors are formed, which include the selected exogenous DNA segment "spliced" into the viral or circular DNA plasmid. Transformation of compatible unicellular host organisms with the hybrid vector results in the formation of multiple copies of the exogenous DNA in the host cell population. In some instances, the desired result is simply the amplification of the foreign DNA and the "product" harvested is DNA.

DESIGNING GMCs

GENE CONSTRUCT

The design of a GMC begins with a clear understanding of the genetic material found in the cells. The genetic materials comprise those chemical substances that program and guide the manufacture of natural constituents of cells (and viruses) and direct the normal biological responses of these cells. The elements of genetic material include a long chain polymeric substance known as deox-

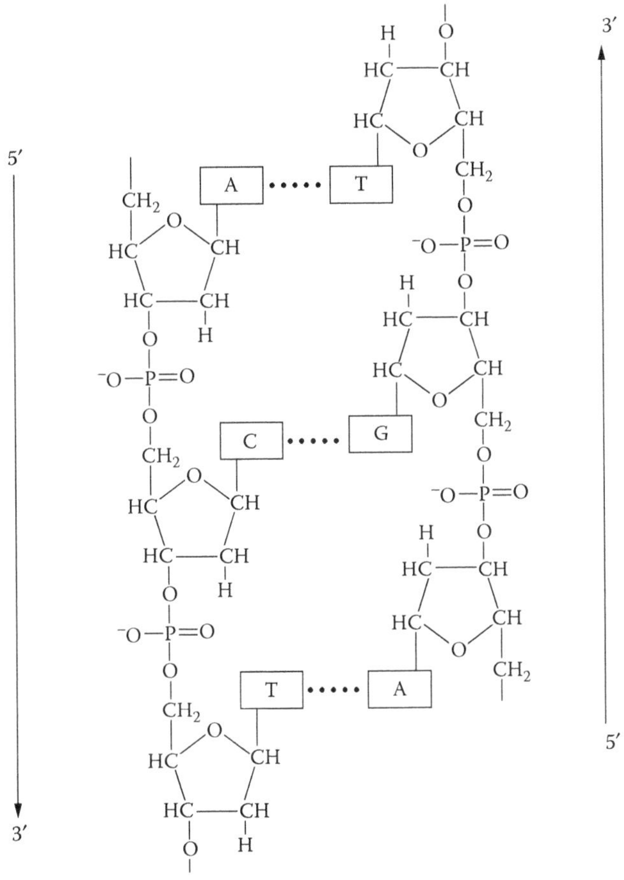

FIGURE 4.3 The two strands of DNA held by hydrogen bonds.

yribonucleic acid (DNA), the genetic material of all living cells and viruses (except for certain viruses that are programmed by ribonucleic acids [RNA] and are thus called RNA viruses). The repeating units in DNA polymers are four different nucleotides, each of which consists of either a purine (adenine or guanine) or a pyrimidine (thymine or cytosine) bound to a deoxyribose sugar to which a phosphate group is attached. Attachment of nucleotides in linear polymeric form is by means of fusion of the 5′ phosphate of one nucleotide to the 3′ hydroxyl group of another. Functional DNA occurs in the form of stable double strands made up of single strands of nucleotides (known as deoxyoligonucleotides) attached to each other by hydrogen bonding between purine and pyrimidine bases [i.e., "complementary" associations existing either between adenine (A) and thymine (T) or guanine (G) and cytosine (C)]. By convention, nucleotides are referred to by the names of their constituent purine or pyrimidine bases, and the complementary associations of nucleotides in double stranded DNA (i.e., A-T and G-C) are referred to as "base pairs." Figure 4.3 shows a drawing of DNA's two strands.

Ribonucleic acid is a polynucleotide comprising adenine, guanine, cytosine, and uracil (U), rather than thymine, bound to ribose and a phosphate group. The programming function of DNA is served through a process wherein specific DNA nucleotide sequences (genes) are "transcribed" into relatively transient messenger RNA (mRNA) polymers. The mRNA, in turn, serves as a template for the formation of structural, regulatory, and catalytic proteins from amino acids. This mRNA "translation" process involves the operations of small RNA strands (tRNA) that transport and align individual amino acids along the mRNA strand to allow for formation of polypeptides in proper amino acid sequences The mRNA "message" derived from DNA provides the basis for

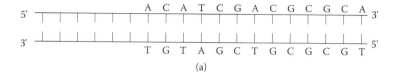

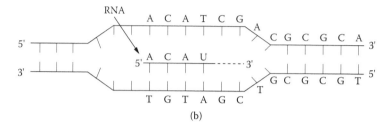

FIGURE 4.4 DNA transcription process. (a) DNA before transcription. (b) During transcription, the DNA unwinds so that one of its strands can be used as a template to synthesize a complementary RNA.

the tRNA supply and orientation of any given one of the 20 amino acids for polypeptide "expression" is in the form of triplet "codons" (sequential groupings of three nucleotide bases). The formation of a protein is the ultimate form of "expression" of the programmed genetic message provided by the nucleotide sequence of a gene. Figure 4.4 shows a typical transcription process.

There are other sequences of importance that control the process of transcription and these include:

- "Promoter" DNA sequences usually "precede" a gene in a DNA polymer and provide a site for initiation of the transcription into mRNA.
- "Regulator" DNA sequences, also usually "upstream" of (i.e., preceding) a gene in a given DNA polymer, bind proteins that determine the frequency (or rate) of transcriptional initiation. Collectively referred to as "promoter/regulator" or "control" DNA sequence, these sequences, which precede a selected gene (or series of genes) in a functional DNA polymer, cooperate to determine whether the transcription (and eventual expression) of a gene will occur.
- "Terminator" DNA sequences follow a gene in a DNA polymer and provide a signal for termination of the transcription into mRNA.

The development of specific DNA sequences for splicing into DNA vectors is accomplished by a variety of techniques, depending to a great deal on the degree of "foreignness" of the "donor" to the projected host and the size of the polypeptide to be expressed in the host. In general terms, three methods are used:

- the "isolation" of double-stranded DNA sequence from the genomic DNA of the donor;
- the chemical manufacture of a DNA sequence providing a code for a polypeptide of interest; and
- the *in vitro* synthesis of a double-stranded DNA sequence by enzymatic "reverse transcription" of mRNA isolated from donor cells. The last-mentioned methods, which involve formation of a DNA "complement" of mRNA, are generally referred to as "cDNA" methods.

Manufacture of DNA sequences is frequently the method of choice when the entire sequence of amino acid residues of the desired polypeptide product is known. Developments in the methods include:

- providing for the presence of alternate codons commonly found in genes, which are highly expressed in the host organism selected for expression (e.g., providing yeast or *E. coli* "preference" codons);
- avoiding the presence of untranslated "intron" sequences (commonly present in mammalian genomic DNA sequences and mRNA transcripts thereof), which are not readily processed by prokaryotic host cells;
- avoiding expression of undesired "leader" polypeptide sequences commonly coded for by genomic DNA and cDNA sequences but frequently not readily cleaved from the polypeptide of interest by bacterial or yeast host cells;
- providing for ready insertion of the DNA in convenient expression vectors in association with desired promoter/regulator and terminator sequences; and providing for ready construction of genes coding for polypeptide fragments and analogs of the desired polypeptides.

When the entire sequence of amino acid residues of the desired polypeptide is not known, direct manufacture of DNA sequences is not possible and isolation of DNA sequences coding for the polypeptide by a cDNA method becomes the method of choice despite its many drawbacks. Among the standard procedures for isolating cDNA sequences of interest is the preparation of plasmid-borne cDNA "libraries" derived from reverse transcription of mRNA abundant in donor cells selected as responsible for high-level expression of genes (e.g., libraries of cDNA derived from pituitary cells that express relatively large quantities of growth hormone products).

Where substantial portions of the polypeptide's amino acid sequence are known and labeled, single-stranded DNA probe sequences duplicating a sequence putatively present in the "target" cDNA may be employed in DNA/DNA hybridization procedures carried out on cloned copies of the cDNA that have been denatured to single stranded form. (See, for example U.S. Patents 4,394,443 and 4,358,535.)

Among the more significant recent advances in hybridization procedures for the screening of recombinant clones is the use of labeled mixed synthetic oligonucleotide probes, each of which is potentially the complete complement of a specific DNA sequence in the hybridization sample including a heterogeneous mixture of single stranded DNAs or RNAs. These procedures are useful in the detection of cDNA clones derived from sources that provide extremely low amounts of mRNA sequences for the polypeptide of interest. Use of stringent hybridization conditions directed toward avoidance of nonspecific binding can allow, e.g., for the autoradiographic visualization of a specific cDNA clone upon the event of hybridization of the target DNA to that single probe within the mixture, which is its complete complement.

The use of genomic DNA isolates is the least common of the three above-noted methods for developing specific DNA sequences for use in recombinant procedures. This is especially true in the area of recombinant procedures directed to securing microbial expression of mammalian polypeptides and is due, principally, to the complexity of mammalian genomic DNA. Thus, although reliable procedures exist for developing phage-borne libraries of genomic DNA of human and other mammalian species origins relating to procedures for generating a human genomic library, commonly referred to as the "Maniatis Library," there have been relatively few successful attempts at hybridization procedures in isolating genomic DNA in the absence of extensive foreknowledge of amino acid or DNA sequences.

VECTOR

The key element in rDNA technology is the recombinant plasmid, which contains the gene that codes for the protein of interest, as described above. Plasmids are simple and small circular extrachromosomal segments of bacterial DNA that are isolated from a bacterium and are self-replicating. The basic technology involves the specific enzymatic cleavage of a plasmid using endonucleases followed by the insertion of a new piece of DNA that contains the gene of interest. The resultant recombinant plasmid is considered the key raw material of rDNA technology. The recombinant plasmid is introduced into the host organism through a process called transformation, where it passes on its new genetic information and results in the production of the protein product.

The vector (plasmid) generally contains a selectable marker that can be used to identify cells that contain this gene. This is in addition to the gene coding for the protein of interest and the regulatory nucleotide sequences necessary for plasmid replication and mRNA transcription (the first step in protein synthesis). Selection of the desired cells is simplified because only properly transformed cells containing the selectable marker gene will survive under the growth conditions used to identify and propagate the transformed cells. Typically, the bacterial and eukaryotic select-able markers may include both antibiotic resistance and genes that complement an auxotrophic host mutation. There are numerous examples of both types of markers in each system.

Significant differences exist in the rDNA production process between prokaryotic and eukary-otic cells. In general, bacterial cells express greater concentrations of protein product and require relatively simple media components. However, prokaryotic cells do not perform many important posttranslational modifications such as glycosylation and, historically, it was not possible to express large proteins in E. coli. These limitations necessitate the use of eukaryotic cells in many cases. The production differences between eukaryotic and prokaryotic host cells have significant impacts that reflect in the requirements for process validation, purification, and analytical methodology.

In order to clone the gene of interest all engineered vectors have a selection of unique restriction sites downstream of a transcription promoter sequence. The host governs the choice of vector family. Once the host has been selected, many different vectors are available for consideration, from simple expression vectors to those that secrete fusion proteins. However, as for the selection of a suitable host system, the final choice of vector should take into consideration the specific requirements of the application and the behavior of the target protein. One key factor that has led to the increased use of fusion protein vectors is that amplification of a fusion protein containing a tag of known size and biological function can greatly simplify subsequent isolation, purification, and detection. In some cases the protein yield can also be increased. Maintenance and cloning protocols are highly specific for each vector and the instructions provided by the supplier should be followed carefully. This topic is further elaborated elsewhere in the book.

The most commonly used vectors include:

- p*Trc* 99 An *E. coli* vector for expression of proteins encoded by inserts lacking a start codon, inducible by IPTG;
- pKK223-3 For overexpression of proteins under the control of the strong *tac* promoter in *E. coli*;
- pSVK 3 For *in vivo* expression in mammalian cell lines;
- PSVL SV40 For high-level transient expression in mammalian cells;
- pMSG For inducible expression in mammalian cells.

The ATCC (http://www.atcc.org/Products/vectors.cfm) provides a large number of vectors (American Type Culture Collection (ATCC), P.O. Box 1549, Manassas, VA 20108). ATCC is also an official depository for the U.S. Patent and Trademark Office; GMCs subject to U.S. patents are deposited here. Figure 4.5 shows a typical scheme how plasmids are made and Figure 4.6 shows a plasmid for *E. coli*.

Host Systems

Several expression host systems are available including bacteria, yeast, plants, filamentous fungi, and insect or mammalian cells grown in culture and transgenic animals. The rDNA products are presently produced in prokaryotic (bacteria) or eukaryotic systems (e.g., yeast, mammalian cell

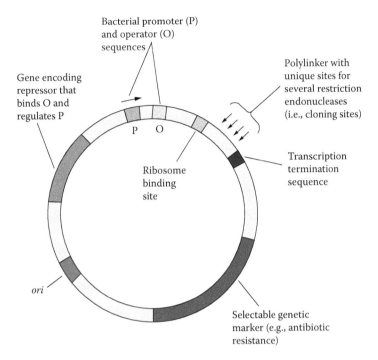

FIGURE 4.5 A typical plasmid design.

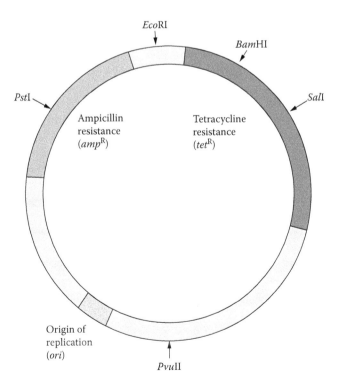

FIGURE 4.6 pBR322 plasmid for use in *E. coli*.

culture). The choice of the production organism is generally a direct function of the molecular complexity of the protein that is to be produced as well as the economics and efficiency of the fermentation or cell culture process. The earliest biotechnology derived products were produced in *E. coli* based on the high degree of understanding of its molecular biology. Within the past few years, however, the use of large-scale eukaryotic cell culture has become relatively commonplace. The choice of host system depends on many factors, such as the size, structure and stability of the product, and the requirements for posttranslational modifications for biological activity, the necessary production yields, acceptable cost, and the quality specifications of the final product also have to be considered. The choice of host generally depends on many factors:

- Properties and the final use of the expressed protein. If the protein consists of multiple subunits or requires substantial posttranslational modifications, the preferred host usually is of higher eukaryotic origin e.g., Chinese hamster ovary cells.
- Regulatory considerations in reducing the immunogenic potential and endotoxin loading. These considerations make yeast the most ideal host.
- Cost considerations dictate that large amounts of proteins (e.g., required in the case of insulin even though it requires multiple subunits) be expressed in bacteria such as *E. coli*, which has been successfully used for production of several relatively complex proteins. The final yield is critical and as a result continuous efforts are made to modify bacterial strains such as deletion of protease genes or engineered for overexpression of rare-codon tRNAs, foldases, or chaperones. Gene-multimerization strategies can be beneficial in improving production yields. In the 1980s, yields approaching 100 mg/L were considered remarkable; now companies like MedImmune® produce 200 to 700 mg/L of an immunoglobulin-M MAb using hybridomas cultured in a hollow-fiber bioreactor. The highest reported CHO cell yields of heterologous proteins 20 years ago were 5 to 50 mg/L, 50 to 500 mg/L 10 years ago, and now we are approaching almost 5 g/L in special circumstances; apparently, we are able to reach a 10-fold increase every 10 years. The question of a workable yield should be considered in light of the regulatory impact of using a new and novel system. For biogeneric drug manufacturers this is an important consideration as they are likely to emulate the approved process, a process that may have been approved decades ago.
- Suitability of extraction of intracellular accumulation of protein versus secretion into periplasm or cell culture medium is important. However, genetic-design approaches are frequently applied to influence the targeting of the gene product. The recent developments in the use of Gram-negative bacteria that secrete the product in the periplasm is of significance. Genetic design are also altered to facilitate the recovery of recombinant proteins by using gene fusion techniques that simplify the recovery process in such a way that it might be possible to integrate several unit operations, increasing the overall efficiency in the downstream purification process. In this realm, affinity fusions are commonly used, as are modified pI or hydrophobic chromatography. A general drawback with fusion strategies is that the fusion partner often has to be removed to release a native gene product. Futuristic techniques like the introduction of combinatorial protein engineering to generate tailor-made product-specific affinity ligands allow highly specific recovery of a recombinant protein that can be expressed in its native form, and this novel type of protein ligand (e.g., the protein A-based affibodies) can be sanitized using common industrial cleaning-in-place (CIP) procedures.

EXPRESSION SYSTEM IN *E. COLI*

In any new development of a host system, *E. coli* remains the primary choice to begin with and alternate systems are tried only if this one fails and the product is biologically inactive after

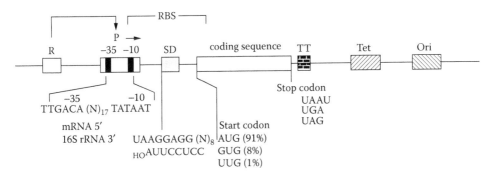

FIGURE 4.7 Sequence elements (not to scale) of a prokaryotic expression vector. (After S. Makrides, "Strategies for achieving high level expression of genes in *E. coli*," *Microbiol. Rev.*, 60, no. 3 (1996): 512–538.)

production due to lack of essential posttranslational modifications, incorrect folding, or when the recovery of the native protein is too low. Successful production of a recombinant protein in *E. coli* involves:

- transcriptional and translational efficiency,
- stability of the expression vector and of the transcribed mRNA,
- localization,
- proteolytic stability,
- folding of the gene product,
- cell growth.

An *E. coli* expression vector (as shown in Figure 4.7) should contain:

- the gene of interest,
- an origin of replication,
- a gene that confers antibiotic resistance (or an alternative selectable marker),
- a promoter, and
- a transcription terminator.

The hybrid *tac* promoter (P) consists of the 35 and 10 sequences, which are separated by a 17-base spacer. In Figure 4.7, the arrow indicates the direction of transcription. The RBS consists of the SD sequence followed by an AT-rich translational spacer that has an optimal length of approximately 8 bases. The SD sequence interacts with the 3 end of the 16S rRNA during translational initiation, as shown. The three start codons are shown, along with the frequency of their usage in *E. coli*. Among the three stop codons, UAA followed by U is the most efficient translational termination sequence in *E. coli*. The repressor is encoded by a regulatory gene (R), which may be present on the vector itself or may be integrated in the host chromosome, and it modulates the activity of the promoter. The transcription terminator (TT) serves to stabilize the mRNA and the vector, as explained in the text. In addition, an antibiotic resistance gene, e.g., for tetracycline, facilitates phenotypic selection of the vector, and the origin of replication (Ori) determines the vector copy number.

CONFIGURATION OF EFFICIENT EXPRESSION VECTORS

The essential architecture of an *E. coli* expression vector is shown in Figure 4.7. The promoter is positioned approximately 10 to 100 bp upstream of the ribosome binding site (RBS) and is under the control of a regulatory gene, which may be present on the vector itself or integrated in the host chromosome. Promoters of *E. coli* consist of a hexanucleotide sequence located approximately 35 bp upstream of the transcription initiation base (35 region) separated by a short spacer from another hexanucleotide sequence (10 region). There are many promoters available for gene expression in *E. coli*, including those derived from Gram-positive bacteria and bacteriophages. A useful promoter exhibits several desirable features: it is strong, it has a low basal expression level (i.e., it is tightly regulated), it is easily transferable to other *E. coli* strains to facilitate testing of a large number of strains for protein yields, and its induction is simple and cost-effective.

Downstream of the promoter is the RBS, which spans a region of approximately 54 nucleotides bound by positions 35 and 19 to 22 of the mRNA coding sequence. The Shine-Dalgarno (SD) site interacts with the 3 end of 16S rRNA during translation initiation. The distance between the SD site and the start codon ranges from 5 to 13 bases (93), and the sequence of this region should eliminate the potential of secondary-structure formation in the mRNA transcript, which can reduce the efficiency of translation initiation. Both 5 and 3 regions of the RBS exhibit a bias toward high adenine content.

The transcription terminator is located downstream of the coding sequence and serves both as a signal to terminate transcription and as a protective element composed of stem-loop structures, protecting the mRNA from exonucleolytic degradation and extending the mRNA half-life.

In addition to the above elements that have a direct impact on the efficiency of gene expression, vectors contain a gene that confers antibiotic resistance on the host to aid in plasmid selection and propagation. Ampicillin is commonly used for this purpose; however, for the production of human therapeutic proteins, other antibiotic resistance markers are preferable to avoid the potential of human allergic reactions. Finally, the copy number of plasmids is determined by the origin of replication. In specific cases, the use of runaway replicons results in massive amplification of plasmid copy number concomitant with higher yields of plasmid-encoded protein. In other cases, however, there appeared to be no advantage in using higher-copy-number plasmids over pBR322-based vectors. Furthermore, increasing the copy number of the plasmid decreases the production of trypsin in *E. coli* and the presence of strong promoters on high-copy-number plasmids severely impaired cell viability.

The origin of replication determines the vector copy number, which could typically be in the range of 25 to 50 copies/cell if the expression vector is derived from the low-copy-number plasmid pBR322, or between 150 and 200 copies/cell if derived from the high-copy-number plasmid pUC. The copy number influences the plasmid stability, i.e., the maintenance of the plasmid within the cells during cell division. A positive effect of a high copy number is the greater stability of the plasmid when the random partitioning occurs at cell division. On the other hand, a high number of plasmids generally decreases the growth rate, thus possibly allowing for cells with few plasmids to dominate the culture, they being the faster growing. Generally there appears to be no significant advantage of using higher-copy-number plasmids over pBR322-based vectors in terms of production yields.

The gene coding for antibiotic resistance is necessary both for identifying transformants and to ensure antibiotic selective pressure, that is, only cells that harbor an expression vector will divide, thus preventing plasmid loss. Genes conferring ampicillin, tetracycline, or kanamycin resistance are commonly used in expression vectors. Ampicillin resistance is mostly used only on a laboratory scale because the lactamase, which confers the resistance, degrades ampicillin and thus the selective pressure is lost after a few generations of cell growth. Furthermore, ampicillin has been thought to be potentially allergenic and is therefore usually not the antibiotic of choice in the production of biotherapeutics intended for human use. Another approach in preventing plasmid loss is to use a mutated *E. coli* strain deficient in a gene encoding an essential protein and include that crucial gene in the plasmid instead.

A number of strong promoters are available for high-level expression in *E. coli*. An important criterion of a promoter is its ability to be efficiently down-regulated under noninduced conditions, i.e., tightly regulated. An early overproduction of the heterologous protein, due to a nonsilent promoter, might impair cell growth. It is therefore desirable to be able to repress the promoter during a cell growth phase to achieve high cell densities, after which the high-rate protein production would be initiated by induction of the promoter. Another important characteristic of a promoter is that it should be simple and inexpensive to induce. For laboratory-scale production, the isopropyl β-D-thiogalactopyranoside (IPTG)-inducible promoters, which are regulated by the product of the *lac*I gene, the lac repressor, are widely used. They include the lac promoter, the lac–trp hybrid promoter tac, and the trc promoter. A disadvantage with these promoters is that they are not completely down-regulated under noninduced conditions, and thus are not suitable if the target-gene product is toxic to the cell. The pET vector has a T7 promoter, which is transcribed only by T7 RNA polymerase and must be used in a strain carrying a chromosomal T7 RNA polymerase gene, which is under the control of a lac promoter. The use of IPTG for induction of these promoters might still not be optimal for the large-scale production of human therapeutic proteins because of the cost of IPTG. Lactose has been shown to be an inexpensive, but somewhat weaker, alternative for induction of the lac promoter in some applications. For large-scale cultivations, either the trp promoter or heat-induced promoters are commonly used. The trp promoter is induced by starvation of tryptophan or by the addition of β-indoleacrylic acid. One potential problem with the trp promoter is that it is difficult to completely down-regulate under noninduced conditions, a problem that can be minimized by the addition of fructose to the cultivation medium. Examples of heat-induced promoters are $P_L(\lambda)$, $P_R(\lambda)$, and the thermosensitive lac promoter lac (TS), which was constructed by mutation of the *lac*I gene. One drawback with these promoters is that the thermal induction could also induce the production of heat-shock proteins, including certain proteases that can cause enhanced degradation. Constitutive promoters, such as the Staphylococcus aureus Protein A (SPA) promoter (P_{SPA}), have also been used for recombinant-protein production. Promoters induced by cultivation conditions such as pH, oxygen levels, stationary growth, and osmolarity as well as weak and moderately strong promoters are also available.

A transcription termination downstream of the coding sequence enhances plasmid stability by preventing transcription through the replication region and through other promoters located on the plasmid. In addition, the transcription terminator enhances the stability of the mRNA transcript by a stem-loop formation at the 3′ end. The tandem T1T2 transcription terminator, derived from the rrnB ribosomal RNA operon of *E. coli*, is an efficient and commonly used transcription terminator.

PROTEIN PRODUCTION

Translation is initiated by the binding of the ribosomes at the Shine-Dalgarno (SD) sequences located within the ribosome binding sites (RBS) in the mRNA sequence. Optimal translation initiation is obtained for mRNAs with the Shine-Dalgarno sequence UAAGGAGG. Also the space between the binding site and the initiation codon, ideally 4 to 8 nucleotides in length, is important for efficient translation initiation. Furthermore, the secondary structure around the RBS and in the sequence immediately downstream of the start codon has been described to influence the translational initiation efficiency, and an enrichment of A and T residues in those regions has been shown to improve the efficiency of translation. It has recently been suggested that the codon that follows the AUG initiation triplet (the + 2 codon) is of particular importance for the translation initiation efficiency, and that there is a preference for adenine residues in this codon in highly expressed gene products.

The frequencies with which the different codons appear in genes in *E. coli* are different from those in genes of human origin. The amount of specific tRNAs is also reflected by the frequency of the codon, which means that a tRNA, which recognizes a rarely used codon, is present in low amounts. Therefore, human genes that contain codons, which are rare in *E. coli*, may be inefficiently expressed. This problem can be solved either by exchanging codons in the target gene for codons, which are more frequently used in *E. coli*, or, alternatively, by coproduction of the rare tRNAs. The most abundant codons in *E. coli* have been determined by examination of sets of genes, and lists of codon usage can be found in several publications. The effect on expression levels by

TABLE 4.6
Advantages and Disadvantages of Different Strategies for the Production of Recombinant Proteins in *E. coli*

Production strategy	Advantages	Disadvantages
Secretion/leakage to the extracellular medium	Disulfide formation possible. Extensive proteolysis might be avoided. Possible to obtain authentic N-terminus. Significantly reduced levels of contaminants. No need for cell disruption.	Secretion to the medium usually not possible. Dilution of the product.
Periplasmic production	Disulfide formation possible. Possible to obtain authentic N-terminus. Reduced levels of contaminants.	Secretion to the periplasma not always possible. No large-scale procedure for selective release of periplasmic proteins available. Periplasmic proteases can cause proteolysis.
Intracellular production as inclusion bodies	Inclusion bodies easy to isolate. Protection from proteases. Protein is inactive and cannot harm host. High production yields usually obtained.	Solubilizing and in vitro folding necessary, which usually give lower yields and higher cost. Normally no authentic N-terminus.
Intracellular and soluble production	No need for solubilization and refolding.	High level of intracellular product can be harmful to the cells. Complex purification. Proteolysis might occur. Disulfide formation usually not possible. Normally no authentic N-terminus.

substitution of rare codons with optimal ones has been extensively studied, but general conclusions have been difficult to draw. The preferred stop codon in *E. coli* is UAA while the prolonged UAAU stop codon can be used for more efficient translational termination.

STRATEGIES FOR PRODUCTION

A major consideration when designing a process for production of a recombinant protein in *E. coli* is whether the gene product should be produced intracellularly or if a secretion system could be used. Different genetic design strategies, together with the inherent properties of the target protein, decide which expression route will be the most successful. Upon intracellular expression, the product can either accumulate as a soluble gene product or precipitate in the form of inclusion bodies. If a secretion system is used, and the product is found to be secretable, the gene product will be accumulated in the periplasm or in some cases even be translocated also through the outer membrane to the extracellular culture medium. Every production strategy has its advantages and disadvantages (see Table 4.6).

PRODUCTION BY SECRETION

The periplasm contains only about 100 proteins as compared with about 4000 proteins in the cytoplasm. Thus, considerable purification and concentration effects are achieved by the targeting of the gene product to the periplasm. Additional beneficial effects achieved through the secretion of the gene product include enhanced disulfide-bond formation, possibility to obtain gene products with authentic N-termini, decreased proteolysis and minimization of harmful action of recombinant proteins, which are deleterious to the cell. The specific release of the periplasmic protein content is simple and commonly used at the laboratory scale by different osmotic-shock procedures. However, on an industrial scale, efficient methods for selective release of periplasmic proteins are lacking. Nevertheless, it has been shown that treatment at an elevated temperature after completed cultivation can improve unspecific leakage to the culture medium. It would be even more attractive to obtain translocation of the gene product to the growth medium, since this would lead to a significantly simplified purification scheme for the gene product. Protection against proteolysis might also be achieved using this strategy, because *E. coli* has very low extracellular proteolytic activity under normal conditions.

SECRETION INTO THE CULTURE MEDIUM

There are no efficient pathways available for specific translocation of proteins through the outer membrane of *E. coli*. Instead, the secretion of some recombinant proteins to the periplasm is suggested to cause a destabilization of the outer membrane, which becomes leaky and allows the protein to diffuse into the extracellular medium in a semispecific manner. Examples of proteins that have been efficiently secreted to the culture medium include different heterologous proteins fused to SPA domains to calmodulin and to the OmpA signal sequence. Another strategy is to use leaky *E. coli* mutants that constitutively release periplasmic proteins into the culture medium due to loss of outer-membrane integrity. However, these mutants are fragile and revert readily to the nonleaky phenotype, which makes these strains unsuitable for large-scale protein production. Alternatives to the use of leaky mutants are coexpression of the bacteriocin release protein or of the third topological domain of the transmembrane protein TolA, whereby a leaky phenotype is induced by disrupting the integrity of the outer membrane, causing periplasmic proteins to leak into the growth medium. Supplementation of the growth medium with glycine has also been shown to enhance the release of periplasmic proteins into the cultivation medium.

SECRETION TO THE PERIPLASMIC SPACE

Many recombinant proteins have been successfully secreted to the periplasm by fusion of a signal sequence or a normally secreted protein N-terminally to the target protein. Frequently used signal sequences include those derived from the *E. coli* periplasmic proteins PhoA and MalE, the outer membrane proteins OmpA and LamB, β-lactamase and DsbA. Interestingly, the Gram-positive signal sequence derived from SPA has been shown to efficiently direct recombinant proteins to the periplasm of *E. coli*.

Proteolysis caused by envelope proteases is one of the most severe problems encountered when directing a recombinant protein to the periplasm of *E. coli*. The proteolysis can be minimized by different approaches, for example by using protease-deficient strains or by genetic design of the gene product. Proteases that degrade many heterologous proteins in the periplasm are DegP, Tsp (denoted Prc in some publications), protease III (also named Pi), and OmpT. *E. coli* strains with single, double, and triple mutants of these proteases have been shown to efficiently decrease the degradation of different heterologous proteins secreted to the periplasm. One problem in using hosts deficient in multiple proteases is that viability, and thus growth, is impaired. Growth condition parameters such as temperature, pH, and medium composition also affect the periplasmic proteolysis. Genetic design approaches include *in vitro* mutagenesis in order to specifically eliminate protease cleavage sites in the target protein gene, and different fusion protein strategies to protect the target protein from proteolysis. For example, the two IgG-binding domains ZZ, derived from SPA (Nilsson et al., 1997), and the albumin-binding protein BB from streptococcal protein G, have successfully been used as fusion partners serving this purpose. They have either been fused to the N-terminus, the C-terminus, or to both termini of the target protein. The most pronounced stabilization effect has been obtained using the dual-affinity fusion strategy, which, in addition, allows recovery of the full-length product by two subsequent affinity-purification steps.

The environment in the periplasm is less reducing than that of the cytoplasm and favors the correct folding of recombinant proteins containing disulfide bonds. The periplasmic space also harbors foldases involved in the formation of disulfide bonds and isomerization of the proline imide bonds.

INTRACELLULAR PRODUCTION

An intracellularly produced recombinant protein can be accumulated in a soluble form in the cytoplasm, precipitate, and form inclusion bodies, or, alternatively, be partly in the form of inclusion bodies and partly in soluble form. It is usually impossible to predict whether the gene product will be soluble or if it will precipitate, and empirical investigations are therefore necessary. Among the most important factors influencing the inclusion-body formation are protein expression rate and presence of disulfide bonds, but hydrophobicity and choice of fusion partner have also been shown to have a significant impact.

PRODUCTION OF SOLUBLE GENE PRODUCTS

If the gene product is stable against proteolysis and not harmful to the host cell, it might be desirable to keep the protein soluble in the cytoplasm, thereby avoiding the solubilization and refolding steps that have to be performed if inclusion bodies are formed. There are several different approaches to minimize the formation of inclusion bodies when producing heterologous proteins intracellularly in *E. coli*. Reduction of the rate of protein synthesis, which can be achieved by using a moderately strong or weak promoter, or partial induction of a strong promoter has been found to result in a higher amount of soluble protein. Other means of reducing the protein-synthesis rate is by growing the culture at a lower temperature or adding nonmetabolizable carbon sources at the time of induction. Substitution of amino acid residues, replacement of multiple hydrophobic phenylalanine residues in respiratory-syncytial-virus (RSV) G protein, or replacement of cysteine residues in S1 dihydrofolate reductase has been shown to dramatically improve the solubility. However, this approach is limited to applications where the substitutions do not alter the desired function or activity of the recombinant protein. Fusion of the target protein to a highly soluble fusion partner, thereby increasing the overall solubility of the fusion protein, is a convenient and efficient method to increase the fraction of soluble gene product in the cytoplasm. Proteins used as solubilizing fusion partners include thioredoxin, ubiquitin, NusA the IgG-binding domains ZZ from SPA, the albumin-binding BB from Protein G, the maltose-binding protein, and a mutant form of DsbA. The overexpression of intracellular chaperones has in many studies resulted in an increased accumulation of soluble gene products. However, as for coexpression of foldases, this approach is protein-specific and is not a universal means of preventing inclusion-body formation. Usually the redox potential in the cytoplasm prevents disulfide formation. In order to generate a less reducing environment in the cytoplasm, thereby facilitating disulfide-bond formation, strains deficient in thioredoxin reductase have been used.

For soluble gene products accumulated intracellularly in the *E. coli* cytoplasm, the first step in downstream processing is the release of the recombinant protein. On a laboratory scale the cells are typically lysed by enzymic treatment, chemical treatment, or by mechanical-disruption techniques such as sonication. High-pressure homogenization or bead mills are used in large-scale processing. Such treatment effectively liberates the desired protein, but it also releases the bulk of host-cell proteins and nucleic acids. If the expressed recombinant protein is thermostable, a convenient method to reduce the amounts of the contaminating host-cell proteins is heat-precipitation. An additional advantage with heat precipitation is the thermal deactivation of the *E. coli* cell and of its proteases, reducing the potential risk of degradation of the target protein. It has also been shown that heat-treatment procedures performed on undisrupted cells efficiently can release recombinant proteins accumulated in a soluble form in the cytoplasm, thus combining the product-release step with the benefits of heat precipitation of host-cell proteins.

Such a heat-treatment procedure was recently successfully used in the recovery of an intracellularly accumulated fusion protein, BB-C7, in a production process for human proinsulin C-peptide, where the heat treatment actually functioned as an initial purification step, giving a purity of approximately 70%, as compared with a purity of 10% obtained after conventional cell-disruption procedures.

PRODUCTION AS INCLUSION BODIES

Many heterologous proteins expressed in *E. coli* are prone to precipitate, which in many cases is an advantage. The formation of inclusion bodies normally protects the gene product from host-cell proteases. The product is inactive and cannot harm the host cell, often giving high expression levels. Furthermore, the dense inclusion bodies can be readily recovered by centrifugation, and a relatively high purity and degree of concentration of the gene product are thus normally obtained after solubilization. The main disadvantage with inclusion-body formation is the need for solubilization and refolding steps, necessary for regaining a correct protein structure and activity. These steps can reduce the yield and be costly, especially on a large scale. Different strategies have been utilized to enhance the tendency for the formation of inclusion bodies, for example, increasing the rate of protein synthesis by using strong promoters such as the T7, trp, or tac promoters, fusion of the target protein to certain other proteins, such as TrpLE, and cultivation at elevated temperatures or at a pH other than 7.0.

In vitro refolding inclusion bodies have an increased density and can easily be recovered by centrifugation after the disruption of the cells. The resulting inclusion-body-containing pellet consists mainly of the overexpressed recombinant protein, but contaminants originating from the host cells are also present. To remove these contaminants, the pellet can be washed with low concentration of denaturants or with detergents. After washing, the inclusion bodies are solubilized by using high concentration of denaturants. If the recombinant protein contains cysteine residues, a reducing and chelating agent should also be included in the solubilization buffer.

Renaturation of the solubilized gene product is initiated by the removal of the denaturant and, where appropriate, also the reducing agent, by dialysis or dilution. During the refolding procedure it is important to limit product aggregation. This can be done by performing the refolding at low protein concentration, typically in the range of 10 to 50 mg/L. However, refolding at such low concentrations requires very large volumes, which becomes difficult and expensive when performed in industrial-scale applications. Therefore, other methods to keep the concentration of the unfolded protein low in the refolding buffer have been developed. Stepwise addition of the denatured recombinant protein and different dialysis approaches are examples of such methods. Different strategies have been developed to increase the refolding yield, either by stabilizing the native state, by destabilizing incorrectly folded molecules, or by increasing the solubility of folding intermediates and of the unfolded state. By performing the refolding at nondenaturing concentrations of denaturant, a high refolding yield has been obtained at high protein concentrations. Other low-molecular-mass additives have also successfully been used to enhance the refolding yield of a variety of different recombinant proteins. Molecular chaperones and foldases, monoclonal antibodies, and specific binding proteins have also been shown to increase the yield of correctly folded protein.

If the recombinant protein contains disulfide bonds, the renaturation buffer also has to contain a redox system, which provides the appropriate redox potential and enables formation and reshuffling of disulfides. The most common redox system is that of GSH and GSSG, but other low-molecular-mass thiol-based redox systems have also been utilized. Typically a 1:1 to 5:1 molar ratio of reduced to oxidized thiol is used. For certain proteins, the yield of renaturation is increased if the thiol groups in the denatured protein are first completely oxidized by formation of mixed disulfides with GSH. Disulfide-bond formation is promoted by addition of catalytic amounts of a reducing agent in a following renaturation step. In another method, the thiol groups in the denatured protein are sulfonated by treatment with Na_2SO_3 and a reducing agent. Under renaturating conditions the protein is thereafter refolded in the presence of small amounts of reducing agent.

PURIFICATION OF THE GENE PRODUCT

After a successful production of a recombinant protein, different purification steps will be needed in order to recover a biologically active protein at high purity. The downstream process for the recovery and purification of a gene product depends on the production strategy used, but it consists typically of product release and clarification steps, an initial purification step, and different chromatographic purification steps. During recent years, the major challenge in designing downstream processes has been to simplify and improve the overall efficiency by combination and elimination of unit operations to cut production costs. This has been achieved both by the development of new separation techniques and by genetic design of the produced recombinant protein.

INITIAL RECOVERY METHODS

The aim of an initial recovery step is to rapidly remove or inactivate proteases that can degrade the product, to remove impurities and particles that have a negative effect on subsequent chromatographic purification steps, and to concentrate the sample. An ideal initial recovery step also gives a high degree of purification. Furthermore, it is essential that the equipment used is compatible with robust cleaning and sanitizing methods when considering industrial-scale production.

The expanded bed adsorption (EBA) technology represents an initial recovery step that allows the capture of proteins from particle-containing feedstock without prior removal of the particulates. EBA has shown to be suitable for industrial production scale, and the technology can also withstand harsh cleaning procedures. Precipitation is another simple approach for recovery of a gene product from a cultivation broth or homogenate. Various methods exist by which precipitation can be achieved: addition of salts, organic solvents, or organic polymers, or varying the pH or temperature. These precipitation methods are nonspecific and give a low degree of purification. By using affinity precipitation, increased specificity can be obtained. Different aqueous two-phase extraction systems have been extensively studied as an initial recovery step. An aqueous two-phase extraction system can also be combined with affinity precipitation combining the benefits of both methods.

GENETIC MANIPULATIONS TO IMPROVE YIELD

In recent years, a number of genetic strategies have been designed to improve production yields, to simplify the recovery processes, to facilitate *in vitro* refolding, to provide site-specific cleavage of gene fusion product, and to create tailor-made product-specific affinity ligands.

GENE FUSION

Currently, there are two types of expression vectors in *E. coli* for expressing mammalian genes. One is the nonfusion expression vector (as described above in detail) and the other is the fusion expression vector. The former is easier to use, however, because certain genes are not expressed well or not expressed at all in nonfusion expression vectors. In such cases, the only choice for expressing genes is to use a fusion expression vector. The features of fusion protein amplification that may influence the final choice of vector are listed in Table 4.7.

Several kinds of fusion expression vectors have been constructed, characterized, and commercialized. The fusion partners include glutathione S-transferase (GST), maltose-binding protein, staphylococcal protein A, and thioredoxin. The greatest advantage of fusion expression vectors is that the inserted genes can usually be expressed well. The major shortcoming of current fusion expression vectors is that chemicals, such as IPTG, are expensive and in short supply. The two

TABLE 4.7
Features of Fusion Tags Used in Recombinant Drug Manufacturing

Fusion proteins	Targeting information can be incorporated into a tag, provides a marker for expression, simpler purification using affinity chromatography under denaturing and nondenaturing conditions, easy detection, refolding achievable on a chromatography column ideal for secreted proteins as the product is easily isolated from growth media.	Tag may interfere with protein structure and affect folding and biological activity, cleavage site is not 100% specific if tag needs to be removed.
Nonfusion proteins	No cleavage steps necessary.	Purification and detection not as simple as reducing potential yield, problem with solubility may be difficult to overcome.

TABLE 4.8
Comparison of GST and HIS Tags

GST Tag	$(His)_6$ Tag
Can be used in any expression system	Can be used in any expression system
Purification procedure gives high yields of pure product	Purification procedure gives high yields of pure product
Selection of purification products available for any scale	Selection of purification products available for any scale
pGEX6P PreScission™ protease vectors enable cleavage and purification in a single step	Small tag may not need to be removed, e.g., tag is poorly immunogenic so fusion partner can be used directly as an antigen in antibody production
Site-specific proteases enable cleavage of tag if required	Site-specific proteases enable cleavage of tag if required. N. B. Enterokinase sites that enable tag cleavage without leaving behind extra amino acids are preferable
GST tag easily detected using an enzyme assay or an immunoassay	$(His)_6$ tag easily detected using an immunoassay
Simple purification. Very mild elution conditions minimize risk of damage to functionality and antigenicity of target protein	Simple purification, but elution conditions are not as mild as for GST fusion proteins. Purification can be performed under denaturing conditions if required. N. B. Neutral pH but imidazole may cause precipitation. Desalting to remove imidazole may be necessary
GST tag can help stabilize folding of recombinant proteins	$(His)_6$-dihydrofolate reductase tag stabilizes small peptides during expression
Fusion proteins form dimmers	Small tag is less likely to interfere with structure and function of fusion partner; mass determination by mass spectrometry not always accurate for some $(His)_6$ fusion proteins

most commonly used tags are glutathione S-transferase (GST tag) and 6 × histidine residues $(His)_6$ tag (Table 4.8). As for the selection of host and vectors, the decision to use either a GST or a $(His)_6$ tag must be made according to the needs of the specific application. Table 4.8 shows the key features of these tags that should be considered.

Polyhistidine tags such as $(His)_4$ or $(His)_{10}$ are also used. They may provide useful alternatives to $(His)_6$ if there are specific requirements for purification.

When choosing an affinity-fusion system, it is important to remember that all systems have their own characteristics, and no single system is ideal for all applications. For example, if secretion of the gene product is desired, it is necessary to choose a system with a secretable affinity tag. If

TABLE 4.9
Examples of Fusion Protein Vectors

Vector Family	Tag
PGEX	Glutathione S-transferase
PQE	6 × Histidine
PET	6 × Histidine
pEZZ 18 (noninducible expression)	IgG binding domain of protein A
pRIT2T(expression inducible by temperature change)	IgB binding domain of protein A

the gene product needs to be purified under denatured conditions, a system with a tag that can bind under those conditions must be chosen, e.g., the polyhistidine affinity tag. The polyhistidine tag is suitable for purification of gene products accumulated as inclusion bodies because the fusion protein can be directly applied to an immobilized metal ion affinity-chromatography (IMAC) column after being solubilized with a suitable denaturing agent. An additional advantage with the small poly-histidine affinity tag is that it can easily be genetically fused to a target protein by PCR techniques. It is also important to choose an affinity-fusion system with elution conditions under which the target protein does not get denatured. For large-scale pharmaceutical production, however, affinity fusions have not been as extensively utilized, despite the ability to replace multiple steps with one step. The main reason is most probably that, for most applications, the affinity tag needs to be removed afterward. Furthermore, proteinaceous ligands may leak from the column during elution, making it necessary to remove the ligand from the eluate. If the ligand originates from a mammalian source, there is also risk of viral contamination. Questions concerning the possibility of column sanitation, and column lifetime, capacity, and cost must also be considered. Table 4.9 lists examples of vectors for fusion proteins together with suggested purification products.

CLEAVAGE OF FUSION PROTEINS

It is necessary to remove the affinity tag after the affinity-purification step. There are several methods, based on chemical or enzymic treatment, available for site-specific cleavage of fusion proteins. Advantages with the chemical cleavage methods are that the reagents used are inexpensive and widely available and the reactions are generally easy to scale up. However, the harsh reaction conditions often required can lead to amino-acid-side-chain modifications or denaturation of the target protein. Furthermore, the selectivity is often rather poor, and cleavage can occur on additional sites within the target protein. Therefore, chemical cleavage methods are usually only suitable for release of peptides and smaller proteins. For many applications, enzymic cleavage methods are preferred to chemical ones because of their higher selectivity and because the cleavage often can be performed under physiological conditions. Disadvantages of enzymic cleavage methods are that some enzymes are very expensive, and that not all enzymes are widely available. Furthermore, if the enzyme is of mammalian origin, virus-removal and virus-clearance validations need to be performed if the target protein is to be used as a pharmaceutical. Recombinant proteases, produced in bacteria or yeast, are for that reason preferred.

IMPROVED RECOVERY

Examples of gene fusions that have been used to improve initial recovery steps include fusions of hydrophobic tails to the target proteins to favor the partitioning into the top phase in aqueous two-phase systems and fusions of aspartic acid residues to the protein to enhance polyelectrolyte precipitation efficiency. Increased efficiency in anion-exchange chromatography in the EBA format was achieved by fusion of the target protein to the ZZ domains from Protein A, whereby the pI was lowered. By fusion of a stretch of arginine residues, glutamic acid residues, and phenylalanine residues, the efficiency of ion-exchange chromatography and hydrophobic-interaction chromatography was increased. One example of a tailor-made fusion partner is the engineered basic variant of the Z domain (Z_{basic}), enabling cation-exchange-chromatography separations to be performed at high pH values. Since almost no other host-cell proteins were found to bind under such conditions, very efficient purification could be achieved. Utilizing the features of the charged Z_{basic}, an integrated production strategy for Klenow DNA polymerase was developed. The Klenow DNA polymerase was produced as a Z_{basic}–Klenow fusion protein that could be efficiently recovered by cation-exchange chromatography in the EBA mode. The Z_{basic}–Klenow fusion was subsequently cleaved to release free Klenow polymerase, with the help of a Z_{basic}-tagged viral protease 3C, whereafter fused Klenow could be recovered from the reaction mix by separating Z_{basic}-protease 3C and Z_{basic} fusion partner using cation-exchange chromatography.

FACILITATED *IN VITRO* REFOLDING

Fusions of target proteins to highly soluble fusion tags have been shown to enhance *in vitro* refolding. For example, a high refolding yield at high protein concentration was obtained by fusion of a moderately soluble target protein to ZZ from protein A. By fusion of a target protein to a histidine tag, immobilization of the fusion protein on an IMAC column can be made under denaturing conditions. A subsequent on-column refolding step typically gives a high yield of renatured target protein. In a related example, in which a hexa-arginine polypeptide extension was fused to the target protein, the fusion protein was immobilized on a cation-exchange column and renatured target protein was obtained after on-column refolding.

GENE MULTIMERIZATION

When expressing peptides in *E. coli*, low yields are often obtained. One reason could be the susceptibility of the peptides to proteolysis. A common strategy to improve the stability is to produce the peptide as a fusion. A major disadvantage with this strategy is that the desired product only constitutes a small portion of the fusion protein, often resulting in low yields of the target peptide. One way of increasing the molar ratio, and hence increasing the amount of peptide produced, is to produce a fusion protein with multiple copies of the target peptide. An additional beneficial effect is often obtained by this strategy, since the gene multimerization has also been shown to increase the proteolytic stability of the produced peptides. When the gene multimerization strategy is employed to increase the production yield, subsequent processing of the gene product to obtain the native peptide is needed. By flanking a peptide gene with codons encoding methionine, CNBr cleavage of the fusion protein, containing multiple repeats of the peptide, has successfully been used for obtaining native peptide at high yield. Takasuga and coworkers produced a pentapeptide multimerized to 3, 14, and 28 copies, fused to dihydrofolate reductase and engineered to be separated by trypsin cleavage. A similar strategy was used to produce a peptide hormone of 28 residues. Eight copies of the peptide gene were linked in tandem, separated by codons specifying lysine residues flanking the peptide, and the construct was fused to a gene fragment encoding a portion of β-galactosidase. Endoproteinase Lys-C, an enzyme that specifically cleaves on the C-terminal side of lysine residues, was used instead of trypsin, together with carboxypeptidase B, to release the native peptide. Similarly, a multimerization strategy was used to improve the yields of the 31-amino-acid human proinsulin C-peptide. The C-peptide was expressed intracellularly in *E. coli* as 1, 3, or 7 copies as parts of fusion proteins. Since it was found that the three different fusion proteins were expressed at equal levels, and that they all were efficiently processed by trypsin/carboxypeptidase B treatment to release native C-peptide, the 7-copy construct was used to generate a recombinant production process.

SIMPLIFIED SITE-SPECIFIC REMOVAL OF FUSION PARTNERS

Genetically designed recombinant proteases have been used to simplify the removal of proteases after site-specific cleavage of fusion proteins. By fusing the protease to the same affinity tag as the target protein, an efficient removal of the affinity-tagged protease, the released affinity tag, and the uncleaved fusion protein can be achieved using affinity chromatography. This principle is commercially available, examples being the systems based on His-tagged tobacco-etch-virus protease and human rhinovirus 3C protease fused to a glutathione S-transferase tag (PreScission™ protease). An affinity-tagged protease can, as an alternative to covalent coupling, also be immobilized to an affinity matrix and be utilized for on-column cleavage. On-column cleavage, in which the produced fusion proteins are site-specifically cleaved while still immobilized on the affinity column, has also been described. An affinity-fusion system, consisting of a protein splicing intein domain from S. cerevisiae and a chitin-binding domain, allows simultaneous affinity purification and on-column cleavage. Different immobilizing approaches are especially important for large-scale applications, since they can reduce the protease consumption and help to avoid additional contamination by the added protease.

TAILOR-MADE PRODUCT-SPECIFIC AFFINITY LIGANDS

Powerful *in vitro* selection technologies, such as phage display, have proven efficient for the isolation of novel binding proteins from large collections (libraries) of peptides or proteins constructed, for example, by combinatorial protein engineering. One example of such binding proteins is the so-called affibodies selected from libraries constructed by random mutagenesis of the Z domain derived from SPA. The Z domain, used as scaffolding during library constructions, is proteolytically stable, highly soluble, small (6 kDa), and has a compact and robust structure devoid of intramolecular disulfide bridges, making it an ideal domain for ligand development. Using phage-display technology, affibody ligands to a wide range of targets have been successfully selected. Recently, such affibody ligands showed selective binding in authentic affinity-chromatographic applications involving the purification of target proteins from E. coli total cell lysates. Such tailor-made product-specific affinity ligands have also been generated and used for highly efficient recovery of recombinant human Factor VIII produced in Chinese-hamster ovary (CHO) cells and a recombinant vaccine candidate, derived from the RSV G protein, produced in baby hamster kidney (BHK) cells.

The obvious advantage of using a ligand selected to bind to the target protein instead of fusing the target protein to an affinity tag is that no cleavage step to obtain the native protein is needed. The disadvantage is that a new high-affinity ligand must be selected and produced for every new recombinant protein needed to be purified. It is nevertheless likely that this strategy will be attractive in recombinant bioprocesses, since highly selective affinity matrices can be created that potentially could discriminate between different folding forms of the target protein and could thus replace several other chromatographic steps in the recovery process. Interestingly, no loss of column capacity or selectivity for the target protein was obtained even after repeated cycles of low pH elution and column sanitation protocols, including 0.5 M NaOH. This might suggest that affinity chromatography using protein ligands could also become increasingly used in industrial-scale recombinant-proteins recovery processes in the future.

MOLECULAR CHAPERONES

It is now well established that the efficient posttranslational folding of proteins, the assembly of polypeptides into oligomeric structures, and the localization of proteins are mediated by specialized proteins termed *molecular chaperones*. The demonstration that efficient production and assembly of prokaryotic ribulose bisphosphate carboxylase in E. coli require both GroES and GroEL proteins led to an increasing interest in the use of molecular chaperones for high-level gene expression in

E. coli. In addition to their utility in purification and detection, specific fusion peptides may confer advantages to the target protein during expression, such as increased solubility, protection from proteolysis, improved folding, increased yield, and secretion. The engineering of specific protease sites in many fusion proteins facilitates the cleavage and removal of the fusion partner(s).

Normally, protein folding proceeds toward a thermodynamically stable end product. Proteins that are drastically destabilized will probably fold incorrectly, even in the presence of chaperones. Thus, the truncation of polypeptides, the production of single domains from multisubunit protein complexes, the lack of formation of disulfide bonds that ordinarily contribute to protein structure, or the absence of posttranslational modifications such as glycosylation may make it impossible to attain thermodynamic stability. Moreover, it is now clear that different types of chaperones normally act in concert. Therefore, the overproduction of a single chaperone may be ineffective. For example, the overproduction of DnaK alone resulted in plasmid instability, which was alleviated by the coproduction of DnaJ. Similarly, the coexpression of three chaperone genes in *E. coli* increased the solubility of several kinases. In some cases, it may be necessary to coexpress chaperones cloned from the same source as the target protein. Still another variable to consider is growth temperature. For example, GroES-GroEL coexpression increased the production of β-galactosidase at 30°C but not 37°C or 42C, whereas DnaK and DnaJ were effective at all temperatures tested. Finally, the overexpression of chaperones can lead to phenotypic changes, such as cell lamentation, that can be detrimental to cell viability and protein production.

CODON USAGE

Genes in both prokaryotes and eukaryotes show a nonrandom usage of synonymous codons. The systematic analysis of codon usage patterns in *E. coli* led to the following observations:

- There is a bias for one or two codons for almost all degenerate codon families.
- Certain codons are most frequently used by all different genes irrespective of the abundance of the protein; for example, CCG is the preferred triplet encoding proline.
- Highly expressed genes exhibit a greater degree of codon bias than do poorly expressed ones.
- The frequency of use of synonymous codons usually reflects the abundance of their cognate tRNAs. These observations imply that heterologous genes enriched with codons that are rarely used by *E. coli* may not be expressed efficiently in *E. coli*.
- The minor arginine tRNA is a limiting factor in the bacterial expression of several mammalian genes, because the codons AGA and AGG are infrequently used in *E. coli*. The coexpression of the *argU* (*dnaY*) gene that codes for tRNA results in high-level production of the target protein. The production of β-galactosidase decreases when AGG codons are inserted before the 10th codon from the initiation codon of the *lacZ* gene. To date, however, it has not been possible to formulate general and unambiguous "rules" to predict whether the content of low-usage codons in a specific gene might adversely affect the efficiency of its expression in *E. coli*. Nevertheless, from a practical point of view, it is clear that the codon context of specific genes can have adverse effects on both the quantity and quality of protein levels. Usually, this problem can be rectified by the alteration of the codons in question, or by the coexpression of the cognate tRNA genes.

5 Upstream Processing

INTRODUCTION

The manufacturing of recombinant DNA products is divided into two distinct steps:

- Upstream processing consists of: a pure *culture* of the chosen organism, in sufficient quantity and in the correct physiological state; *sterilized*, properly formulated media, a seed bioreactor to develop inoculum to initiate the process in the main bioreactor; the production scale bioreactor.
- Downstream processing consists of: equipment for drawing the culture medium in steady state, cell separation, collection of cell free supernatant, product purification, and effluent treatment.

The upstream processing comprises production of target protein in a growth media in one of several forms: secretion to media, inclusion bodies in bacteria, etc. Growing cells in supporting media under optimal conditions results in a wide range of products and process and requires control of precise conditions to provide a commercially feasible yield of the target protein. The fermentation process (or bioprocess) is also used to generate biomass, various amino acids and vitamins, alcohol, or to modify compounds in addition to producing recombinant products, the focus of this book. Microorganisms (prokaryotic) and eukaryotic cell cultures are grown in volumes ranging from a few hundred milliliters to several thousand liters using a variety of cell growth methods and bioreactor designs. The large range of bioreactor sizes is needed because the recombinant protein quantities needed can vary widely, from hundreds of kilograms for albumin, hemoglobin, and insulin to perhaps a few grams for drugs like erythropoietins, interleukins, etc. As a result, it is unlikely that the initial biogeneric therapeutic proteins will be of large volume type, due mainly to the high initial investment required.

BIOREACTORS

A bioreactor is used to grow biological cells and organisms; historically, the word fermenter was used when microorganisms were grown and bioreactor when cells other than microorganisms were grown; however, these terms are now frequently used interchangeably, with preference for bioreactor in the recombinant production industry. A large variety of bioreactors are available such as shake flasks, roller bottles, spinner flasks, flexible cell culture flasks, wave bags, stirred tanks, and airlift reactors to support suspension, microcarrier, and cell encapsulation cultures. Many of these systems work at laboratory scale, yet a large array of them are used in the manufacturing operations if the required growth conditions are not reproduced in larger, more efficient reactors. For biogeneric product manufacturer, another considerations must be made — replicating the system of production used by the innovator and as approved by the regulatory authorities. At times, the biogeneric manufacturer may have to opt for a less efficient system merely to keep from introducing additional variable factors, like using a cube system for cells that require stationary media vis-à-vis the use of roller bottles. The extent to which the biogeneric manufacturer will be able to modify the production technique will depend on the nature of validation required by the FDA in its comparability protocol guidelines for generic manufacturing; these guidelines are not yet released but are likely to be in the coming months. The manufacturer may decide to forgo the original method of production used and instead opt for a more efficient and innovative system to obtain better yields, even though this may require a larger investment upfront.

A newer addition is a simple system with up to 500 L culture with the advantage of using disposable materials. The technology is based on disposable plastic containers with ports to provide media and utility and monitoring probes; the bag rests on a plate that flips back and forth to create a wave motion inside. The wave bioreactor is not free of shear forces and cell damage has been observed, though improvements in the system are appearing rapidly and it is likely that this may turn out to be the premier system for mammalian cells where contamination can be a problem, e.g., using the same suite for multiple products.

The stirred tanks consist of stainless steel containers with rotating impellers of various configurations and devices that maintain constant agitation and control gas transfer, temperature, pH, and fluid level. Most stirred tanks use some form of sintered material or perforated tubing in order to sparge air or specific gas mixtures into the cell suspension. Figure 5.1 shows a typical (and perhaps one of the most popular) bioreactor.

Airlift bioreactors have no moving parts or mechanical seals and offers low hydrodynamic shear forces with a low power input per unit volume (10 to 15 W/m^3). This kind of bioreactor offers gentle gas circulation and good oxygen transfer. However, as the volume of the reactor increases, mixing becomes a limiting factor for the productivity (i.e., the amount of product formed per unit volume per unit time). Table 5.1 summarizes the advantages and disadvantages of the various types of culture processes used.

BATCH CULTURE

A batch culture is a closed system with a fixed culture volume in which the cells grow until maximum cell density, depending on medium nutrients, product toxicity, waste product toxicity, and other essential factors, is reached. When a particular organism is introduced into a selected growth medium, the growth of the inoculum does not occur immediately, but takes a pause, the period of adaptation, called the lag phase. Following the lag phase, the rate of growth of the organism steadily increases, for a certain period, the period of logarithmic or exponential phase. After a certain time, based on a variety of nutritional and cell characteristics, the rate of growth slows down, due to the continuously falling concentrations of nutrients or a continuously increasing (accumulating) concentration of toxic substances. This is called the deceleration phase. After the deceleration phase, growth ceases and the culture enters a stationary phase or a steady state. The biomass (or total quantity of cell mass) remains constant, except when certain accumulated chemicals in the culture begin to lyse the cells (chemolysis). Unless other microorganisms contaminate the culture, the chemical constitution remains unchanged. Mutation of the organism in the culture can also be a source of contamination, called internal contamination. If the desired product is produced in the log phase, it can be prolonged by manipulating the growth conditions but only for a very limited time, and if the desired amount is not produced that quickly, it will be reasonable to choose another culture method. At the onset of the stationary phase, the culture is disbanded for the recovery of its biomass (cells, organism) or the compounds (expressed proteins) that accumulated in the medium. This system of manufacturing is called batch processing or batch culture. A significant advantage of batch processing is the optimum levels of product recovery, control of growth conditions, and better regulatory compliance. The disadvantages are the wastage of unutilized nutrients, high labor costs, and the time lost in batch preparation. Batch cultivation, however, remains the simplest way to produce a recombinant protein. In batch cultivation, all the nutrients required for cell growth are supplied from the start, and the growth is initially unrestricted. However, the unrestricted growth commonly leads to unfavorable changes in the growth medium, such as oxygen limitation and pH changes. Also, certain metabolic pathways in the cell will be saturated,

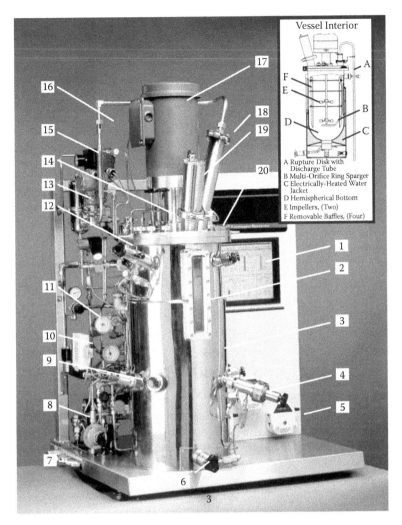

FIGURE 5.1 A typical stirred tank bioreactor: BioFlo 4500® Sterilizable-In-Place Fermentor and Bioreactor (20 and 30 L). (Courtesy of New Brunswick Scientific Company, Edison, New Jersey 08818-4005; http://www.nbsc.com). Key to the labels. 1: Controller with touch-screen interface; 2. Viewing window; 3. Sterilizer-In-Place system; 4. Resterilizable sample valve; 5. Peristaltic pump; 6. Resterilizable harvest/drain valve; 7. Services, water, air, clean and house steam, water return and drain; 8. Steam taps; 9. Ports to allow addition of RTD, pH, DO, and other sensors; 10. Thermal mass flow controller; 11. Open frame piping to facilitate access for cleaning maintenance and servicing; 11. Resterilizable inoculation/addition valves; 13. Filters; 14. Rupture disk to prevent over pressurization; 15. Automatic back pressure regulator. 16. Exhaust line with heat exchanger and view glass; 17. Motor; 18. Exhaust condenser; 19. Combination light and fill port; 20. Headplate ports for sampling, insertion of sensors and other devices.

which potentially leads to the accumulation of inhibitory by-products in the medium. Therefore, only moderate cell densities and production levels can normally be obtained with batch cultivations. To obtain high cell density and high protein production levels, fed-batch cultivation in a bioreactor is commonly used. Acetate is produced when the culture is growing in the presence of excess glucose or under oxygen-limiting conditions. A high concentration of acetate reduces the growth rate, maximum obtainable cell density, and the level of production of the recombinant protein. It is therefore important to maintain the acetate concentration below the inhibitory level. This can be achieved by controlling cultivation in several ways: the growth rate could be controlled by limiting nutrients, such as sources of carbon or nitrogen, by using glycerol or fructose instead of glucose

TABLE 5.1
Comparative Advantages and Disadvantages of Various Culture Systems

Culture	Advantages	Disadvantages
Batch	Well-tested technology, less contamination risk, less expensive.	Limited cell density, downtime between batches, nonhomogeneous product, and variable quality between batches.
Fed batch	High cell densities, longer culture periods using low to medium viscosity.	Nonhomogeneous product due to changing medium, large reactor size required, more susceptible to contamination, difficult to control, needs sophisticated monitoring systems.
Perfusion	Long production phase, short down time, reduced cleaning and sterilization, waste removal, continuous expression, dilution of toxic medium, smaller reactor vessel.	Susceptible to contamination due to frequent handling, difficult to control, requires sophisticated monitoring, nutrient gradients.

as the carbon/energy source, by addition of glycine and methionine or by lowering the cultivation temperature, or by metabolic engineering. Other problems concerning growth to high cell densities are oxygen limitation, reduced mixing efficiency, heat generation, and high partial pressure of carbon dioxide.

CONTINUOUS CULTURE

In continuous processing the growth is limited by the availability of one or two components of the medium. As the initial quantity of a critical component is exhausted, growth ceases, and a steady state is reached; growth is renewed by the addition of the limiting component. A certain amount of the whole culture medium can also be added periodically, after the steady state sets in. These additions increase the volume of the medium in the fermentation vessel, which is arranged so that the excess volume drains off as an overflow, which is collected and used for recovery of products. At each step of addition of the medium, the medium dilutes in the concentration of the biomass and the products. New growth, stimulated by the added medium, increases the biomass and the products, until another steady state sets in; and another aliquot of medium reverses the process. It is called continuous culture or processing since the growth of the organism is controlled by the availability of growth-limiting chemical component of the medium; this system is called a chemostat. The rate at which aliquots are added or the dilution rate determines the growth rate.

Commercial adaptation of continuous processing is confined to biomass production and to a limited extent to the production of potable and industrial alcohol. The production of growth-associated products like ethanol is more efficient in continuous processing, particularly for industrial use.

FED-BATCH CULTURE

In the fed-batch medium, a fresh aliquot of the medium is continuously or periodically added, without the removal of the culture fluid. The bioreactor is designed to accommodate the increasing volumes. The system is always at a quasi-steady state. Fed-batch processing requires a greater degree of process and product control. A low but constantly replenished medium has the advantages of maintaining conditions in the culture within the aeration capacity of the bioreactor, removing the repressive effects of medium components such as rapidly used carbon and nitrogen sources and phosphate, avoiding the toxic effects of a medium component, and providing limiting levels of a required nutrient for an auxotrophic strain. Classically, the fed-batch culture is used in the production of baker's yeast, where biomass is the desired product. Diluting the culture with a batch of fresh medium prevents the production of ethanol, which affects the yield; in the production of yeast, the traces of ethanol were detected in the exhaust gas and the processing steps are adjusted accordingly. Another classic fed-batch process product is penicillin, a secondary metabolite. Penicillin processing has two stages: an initial growth phase followed by the production phase called the iodophase. The culture is maintained at low levels of biomass, and phenyl acetic acid, the precursor of penicillin, is fed into the fermenter continuously, but at a low rate, as the precursor is toxic to the organism at higher concentrations.

In fed-batch cultivation, the carbon/energy source is added in proportion to the consumption rate. Thereby overflow metabolism and the accumulation of inhibitory by-products are minimized. Moreover, the growth rate can be balanced to achieve a maximal production level. The bioreactor should preferentially be equipped to maintain an optimal oxygen concentration, pH, and temperature. Defined media are generally used in fed-batch cultivation. Since the concentrations of the nutrients are known and can be controlled during the cultivation, the cultivation is also more reproducible compared with the use of a complex growth medium. However, the addition of complex media, such as yeast extract, is sometimes necessary to obtain a high level of the desired recombinant protein.

In fed-batch process, neither cells nor medium is leaving the bioreactor, which keeps the sugar levels low for a long time. It is possible to switch from one substrate to another, thus rendering the use of inducible promoters. The process is usually performed at low growth rates while adjusting the feed rate, whose upper limit is dictated by the oxygen transfer limit and cooling strategies available. The feed rate can be subjected to direct feedback control using substrate concentration and indirect feedback control parameters, including cell concentration, culture fluorescence, carbon dioxide evolution rate, pDO and pH-stat; constant, exponential, or increasing rate feeding is fixed and not subject to any feedback control as it is determined in the scale-up stage.

A variation of the classical fed-batch process is the semi-fed-batch process, where nutrients are added in dry form without changing the culture volume. In contrast to the batch mode, the operation of large-scale bioreactors in the fed-batch mode is subject to much variability. The substrate gradients formed may result in overflow metabolism locally in the bioreactor. The resulting product might be inhomogeneous as the cells produce variants of the target protein during different life cycle phases. Product stability might also be challenged by the presence of proteolytic enzymes, as the product cannot be removed from the reactor before the end of production.

A mathematical model of a fed-batch reactor can be derived from a material balance across the reactor. Despite the apparent similarity between the fed-batch reactor model and the continuous culture model, they are very different. The chemostat equation for biomass accumulation is composed of a growth and a removal component:

$$dX/dt = \mu X \text{ (Biomass Growth)} - DX \text{ (Biomass Removal)}$$

The fed-batch equation is composed of a growth and a dilution component (F/V):

$$dD/dt = \mu X \text{ (Growth)} - FX/V \text{ (Dilution)}$$

The fed-batch reactor model contains an additional equation:

$$dV/dt = F$$

The concept of steady state cannot be as easily applied to a fed-batch reactor. The equations must therefore be solved numerically.

PERFUSION CULTURE

In perfusion batch cultivation, a fresh medium is added to the bioreactor and an equivalent amount is removed, with or without cells. A controlled perfusion bioreactor offers tight control of the growth conditions and cells can be kept in their productive phase for several months, if required.

A significant risk in this process is contamination, as the bioreactor is frequently handled in addition to accumulation of nonproducing variants that can affect productivity. The advantages including short harvesting volumes, use of smaller bioreactor vessels, and reduced initial capital costs despite lower yields obtained. Since the cells are maintained in a steady state, the resulting product is often more homogeneous. The isolation of product can be controlled as the harvest can be selected from the steady state production phase of the cell culture, resulting in a more homogeneous product. The higher quality of product obtained from the steady state culture in a perfusion system makes downstream processing more efficient; there is also an option for batch processing of multiple harvests to reduce costs. These differences are often considered in making a choice for the perfusion system when considering the large media volume used in perfusion culture systems.

Suspension Culture

A large variety of cells require adhesion to stationary surface to express proteins, e.g., Chinese hamster ovary (CHO) cells in the production of erythropoietin. Classically, roller bottles are used to immobilize these cells whereby they secrete the protein into the medium, which is frequently harvested. These cells can also be immobilized onto the surface of microcarriers or to macroporous particles, giving two advantages: easier control and high cell densities e.g., upward of 10^8 cells/mL. Microcarrier technology is used both in the batch and perfusion modes. See below for details on the use of microcarrier technology. Several bioreactor systems are based on immobilized cell technology (hollow fiber, ceramic matrix, packed bed, and fluidized bed reactors). Since suspension culture technology is relatively new and the products approved by the FDA decades ago did not have the option of adopting them, many approved processes still rely on validated methods like the use of a roller bottle. There are newer issues with suspension cultures such as cell aggregation and lack of system homogeneity when using hollow fiber systems. These remain to be resolved.

The absence of adventitious organisms in cell cultures is critical. In addition to demonstrating that bacteria, yeast, and molds are not present in cell cultures, the manufacturer must provide evidence for each culture that mycoplasmas and adventitious viruses are not present. It is important to recognize that certain hybridomas used for monoclonal antibody production may contain endogenous retroviruses. However, it must be demonstrated that any viruses present in the culture are removed from the final product. This requires the development of suitable analytical techniques to ensure the absence of contamination by mycoplasmas or human and animal adventitious viruses.

The degree and type of glycosylation may be important in the design of cell culture conditions for the production of glycosylated proteins. The degree of glycosylation present may affect the half-life of the product *in vivo* as well as its potency and antigenicity. Although the glycosylation status of a cell culture product is difficult to determine, it can be verified to be consistent if the culture conditions are highly reproducible.

Cell culture conditions are dependent upon the host system. Before performing large-scale purification, it is important to check protein amplification in a small pilot experiment to establish optimum conditions for expression. The expression is monitored during the growth and induction phases by retaining small samples at key steps in all procedures for analysis of the purification method. The yield of fusion proteins is highly variable and is affected by the nature of the fusion protein, the host cell, and the culture conditions.

MICROCARRIER SUPPORT

Microcarrier culture is a technique that makes possible the high yield culture of anchorage dependent cells. By using macroporous microcarriers it is possible to immobilize semiadherent and suspension cell lines, even in protein-free media. Growing cells on microcarriers can dramatically improve yield, reduce serum and media costs, decrease the risks of contamination, and reduce the number of handling steps. The microcarrier surface supplies focal adhesion sites that support cellular traction, formation of the cytoskeleton, and orientation of organelles. Cells modify and lay down their own extracellular matrix on the microcarrier surface. Cells that form tight junctions can create a uniform cellular sheet around a microporous microcarrier and generate a specific microenvironment inside the carrier. Cells in such sheets are polarized with typical apical and basolateral sides. Microporous carriers allow cell-to-cell communication of low to medium molecular weight media components through the microcarrier. The volumetric cell densities in microcarriers allow use of serum or protein-free media, simplifying downstream processing. There is an additional protection of cells from the shear force stress due to aeration by sparging, spin filters, and impellers. The use of microcarriers allows inoculation and growth of one type of cells inside and another type where necessary, such as in creating "artificial organs." Compared to spin filters, immobilization of cells allows running perfusion cultures, which allows use of serum-free media and switch from growth to production media; high density caused a faster rate of exchange of nutrients, minimizing retention times of secreted products and speeding harvesting of product at lower temperature — this can significantly improve product degradation profile and build up of toxic substances from the cells.

Amersham was the first to produce these microporous microcarriers and it offers several kinds such as Cytodex for use in animal cells; it is a transparent, hydrophilic, and hydrated cross-linked dextran for use in stirred cultures. Cytodex 1 is formed by cross-linking dextran matrix with positively charged diethyl aminoethyl (DEAE) groups, making it more suitable for established cell lines for production from cultures of primary and normal diploid cells. Cytodex 3 is formed by coupling a thin layer of denatured pig skin collagen type 1 to the cross-linked dextran matrix; this is more suitable for difficult to cultivate cells with an epithelial-type morphology. The collagen surface is susceptible to digestion by a variety of proteolytic enzymes, which provide the opportunity to harvest cells from the microcarriers while maintaining maximum cell viability and membrane integrity.

Cytopore (http://www.amersham.com) is a transparent, hydrophilic, and hydrated microporous cross-linked cellulose microcarrier with positively charged N,N-ethyl-aminoethyl groups; it is more rigid than Cytodex. Cytopores can also be used to immobilize insect cells, yeast, and bacteria besides the CHO cells. Cytopore 1 is designed for use in suspension culture systems for growth of recombinant CHO cells with charge capacity of 1.00 meq/g; Cytopore 2 is optimized for anchorage-dependent cells where the optima charge density required is about 1.8 meq/g.

Cytoline has a range of weighted macroporous carriers for use in stirred tank, packed bed, and fluidized bed cultures; it is nontransparent and composed of medical quality polyethylene, which is weighted by silica. Cytoline offers increased protection from shear forces, improves nutrition, and aeration while reducing the need to use serum. Cytoline 1 is optimized for use in fluidized bed cultures of CHO cells; its high sedimentation rate (120 to 220 cm/min) enables a high recirculation rate to allow a better supply of oxygen. Cytoline 2 has a lower sedimentation rate (25 to 75 cm/min) microcarrier for use in stirred cultures, but mainly for the culture of hybridomas and other stress sensitive cells, in fluidized beds. Cytopilot Mini offered by Amersham is a laboratory-scale fluidized bed reactor designed specifically to exploit the potential of Cytoline.

Other suppliers of microporous microcarrier include Cultispher by Percell Biolytica AB (http://www.percell.se/) and Hillex microcarriers by SoloHill (http://www.solohill.com/hillex.html).

Generally, microcarrier cultures can be contained in virtually any type of culture vessel. However, best results are obtained with equipment that gives even suspension of the microcarriers with gentle stirring. The most suitable vessels for general purpose microcarrier culture are those with efficient gassing and mixing systems that do not generate high shear forces and provide a homogeneous culture environment. For really high cell densities a perfusion culture system is needed. However, when selecting a vessel for a perfusion culture some design criteria need consideration. The stirrer should never come in contact with the inside surface of the vessel during culture because it may damage the microcarriers. Similarly, spinner vessels with a bearing immersed in the culture medium are not suitable because the microcarriers can circulate through the bearing and get crushed. Alternatives to fermenters for perfusion culture exist for laboratory, pilot, and production scale applications. Note: *Glass culture vessels should be siliconized before use.*

The exact culture procedure depends on the type of cell and on the culture vessel. Macroporous microcarrier cultures normally contain 1 to 2 g Cytopore l, and are usually inoculated with about 2 $\times$ 10^6 cells/mL. Perfused cultures may contain much higher microcarrier concentrations. In such instances the inoculum should be increased proportionally. Successful microcarrier culture depends on the state of the inoculum and correct operation during the initial stages. Conditions vary with cell type and the culture conditions. Anchorage-dependent cells cannot survive unattached in suspension for very long. The easy access to the interior of the carriers facilitates initiation of the culture at full culture volume and enables continuous stirring at 30 rpm, from commencement of the culture.

For a stationary culture, cover the bottom of a bacteriological petri dish with microcarriers. The suggested starting concentration of microcarriers for a 60 mm–diameter petri dish is approximately 2 mg/mL (about 0.1 cc/mL). For stirred cultures, the optimum concentration varies from cell to cell. The concentration for CHO cells is approximately 1 to 2 mg/mL. However, this very much depends on the feeding strategy for the culture. The high cell density experienced with macroporous carriers means that the culture rapidly consumes any available metabolites. A steady state should be maintained; toxic metabolites should not be allowed to accumulate and pH values should be maintained at the set level. Rapid changes in pH cause cell peeling and a reduction in the final cell yield. CO_2 should also be kept at the desired level. Cell growth can be monitored by glucose consumption and lactate buildup, CO_2 consumption, and cell counting.

ROLLER BOTTLE CULTURE SYSTEM

The roller bottle culture system is the most commonly used method for initial scale up of attached cells, also known as anchorage dependent cell lines. Roller bottles are cylindrical vessels that revolve slowly (between 5 and 60 rph), which bathes the cells that are attached to the inner surface with medium. Roller bottles are available typically with surface areas of 1050cm². The size of some of the roller bottles presents problems since they are difficult to handle in the confined space of a microbiological safety cabinet. Recently roller bottles with expanded inner surfaces have become available, which has made handling large surface area bottles more manageable, but repeated manipulations and subculture with roller bottles should be avoided if possible. A further problem with roller bottles is with the attachment of cells, since some cells lines do not attach evenly. This is a particular problem with epithelial cells. This may be partially overcome by optimizing the speed of rotation, generally by decreasing the speed, during the period of attachment for cells with low attachment efficiency.

SPINNER FLASK CULTURE

The spinner flask culture is the method of choice for suspension lines including hybridomas and attached lines that have been adapted to growth in suspension, e.g., HeLa S3. Spinner flasks are either plastic or glass bottles with a central magnetic stirrer shaft and side arms for the addition and removal of cells and medium and gassing with CO_2 enriched air. Inoculated spinner flasks are placed on a stirrer and incubated under the culture conditions appropriate for the cell line. Cultures should be stirred at 100 to 250 rpm. Spinner flask systems designed to handle culture volumes of 1 to 12 L are available from Techne (http://www.techne.com), Sigma (http://www.sigmaaldrich.com), and Bellco (http://www.bellcoglass.com/).

OTHER SCALE-UP OPTIONS

The next stage of scale up for both suspension and attached cell lines is the bioreactor that is used for large culture volumes (in the range 100 to 10,000 L). For suspension cell lines the cells are kept in suspension by either a propeller in the base of the chamber vessel or by air bubbling through the culture vessel. However, both of these methods of agitation give rise to mechanical stresses. A further problem with suspension lines is that the density obtained is relatively low; in the order of 2×10^6 cells/mL.

For attached cell lines the cell densities obtained are increased by the addition of microcarrier beads. These small beads are 30 to 100 μm in diameter and can be made of dextran, cellulose, gelatin, glass, or silica, and they increase the surface area available for cell attachment considerably. The range of microcarriers available means that it is possible to grow most cell types in this system.

A recent advance has been the development of porous microcarriers, which has increased the surface area available for cell attachment by a further 10- to 100-fold. The surface area on 2 g of beads is equivalent to 15 small roller bottles.

A newly introduced Roller-Cell® system utilizes a rotary system of multiple bottles attached to a central collection duct, avoiding labor costs associated with periodic harvesting of media. It can be used for a simple culture protocol with a "cell harvest" or multiharvest system (i.e., $10 \times$ refeed/harvest). A comparison of the time taken to process the equivalent of 200 standard bottles manually, with a robotic automated system, and the RollerCell 40™ shows that for simple harvesting the total man-hours are 15.5 in regular roller bottles, 5.7 hours in robotic systems, and only 1.5 hours in RollerCell™ system. In multiple harvest system, if the manual hours are 37 in regular roller bottle system and 33.3 in robotic systems, it takes only 6.3 hours. The RollerCell™ system (http://www.synthecon.com/Cellon/rc2.shtml) is certainly worth considering when scaling up production of suspension cell culture systems.

WAVE BIOREACTOR

The newer wave bioreactor system with a completely disposable bioreactor has many advantages including no cleaning, cross-contamination, or validation issues. Cells stay in contact with a disposable sterile biocompatible plastic, which conforms to USP Class VI and ISO 10993. Bioreactors, including all fittings and filters, are delivered sterile and ready for use. These are ideal for cGMP applications and no biosafety cabinet is required in their use. These can be use in an incubator or on the bench with an integral heater and optional CO_2/air mixing unit. For suspension, microcarrier, or perfusion culture, spinners, roller bottles, and similar systems are not scalable due to inherently limited mass transfer surface area. The Wave Bioreactor® has no such limit and operation up to 580 L has been demonstrated, with cell densities over 6×10^7 cells/mL. Studies have shown excellent validation for CHO cells from 1 to 500 L capacity wave bioreactors (see Figure 5.2) (http://www.wavebiotech.com).

The biogeneric recombinant protein manufacturers are advised to consider this system as their choice system to avoid many cGMP issues that are inevitable in any bioprocess scaling. The Wave Bioreactor system is an excellent option for suspension clones or attachment-dependent lines using microcarriers. It is not usually a good option for attachment-dependent cell lines that have hitherto been grown on rigid surfaces in roller bottles (e.g., currently available erythropoietin cell line). The surface of the bag is usually not designed for attachment. The Waver Bioreactor provides still too much disturbance during periodic harvesting, which can cause a high degree of stress on the cells and probably cause them to slough off the surface and clump rather than maintain the confluent monolayer. Given below are some of the present applications of Wave Bioreactors:

- Monoclonal Antibodies: The Wave Bioreactor has been used extensively for monoclonal antibody production. Culture can be started at low volume and then fresh media is added whenever the cell count is sufficiently high. This enables inoculum scale up without transfers. In batches ranging from 100ml to 580 liters have been run with cell densities over 6×10^6 cells/mL, the productivity was comparable to stirred tank bioreactors. Dissolved oxygen concentrations were not limiting and remained above 50% saturation.

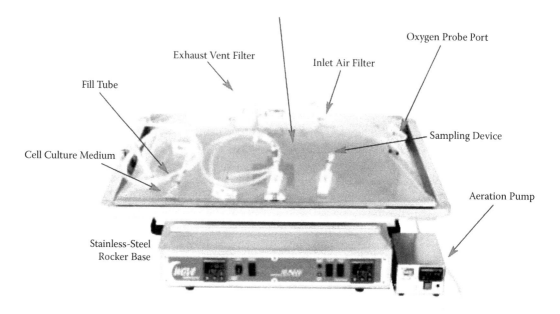

FIGURE 5.2 Essential features of Wave Bioreactor® System 500/1000. (Courtesy Wave Biotech LLC Bridgewater, New Jersey; http:/www.wavebiotech.com.)

- Insect Cells/Baculovirus: The high oxygen supply capability of the Wave Bioreactor makes it ideal for insect cell culture. Ten L batch volumes are routine with cell densities over 9×10^6 cells/mL. Baculovirus yields are higher than with conventional bioreactors. The Wave Bioreactor system is extremely easy to operate and inoculum scale up and infection can be made inside the bioreactor, reducing the need for transfers.
- Anchorage Dependent Cells: Agitation in the Wave Bioreactor is powerful enough to mix and aerate the culture, yet it is gentle enough to cultivate anchorage-dependent cells on various microcarriers. Some reports indicate displacement and rupture of cells not specifically designed for the purpose.
- Perfusion Culture: Unique internal perfusion filter equipped Cellbags make perfusion culture easy. Bioreactors can be operated for weeks, and cell densities up to 6×10^7 cells/mL have been reported. Applications include high-density culture and patient-specific cell therapy. Wave Bioreactors are in use in GMP applications, producing inoculum for large conventional bioreactors and also for clinical and commercial production of human therapeutics. Reduced cleaning and validation requirements make this an ideal system for GMP applications.
- Other Uses: The Wave Bioreactor has many other uses, for example, keeping in-process inoculum pools agitated and aerated prior to use; bead-to-bead transfer; thawing, and media mixing. Custom Cellbags can be provided for special applications.

CELL CUBE TECHNOLOGY

The CellCube® System offered by Corning (http://www.corning.com/lifesciences/news_center/press_releases/electronic_e-cube.asp) provides a fast, simple, and compact method for the mass culture of attachment dependent cells. Disposable CellCube modules have a polystyrene tissue culture–treated growth surface for cell attachment where the production can range from module with 8500 cmΣ cell growth surface to one with 340,000 cmΣ using the same control package. The system continually perfuses the cells with fresh media for increased cell productivity. The CellCube

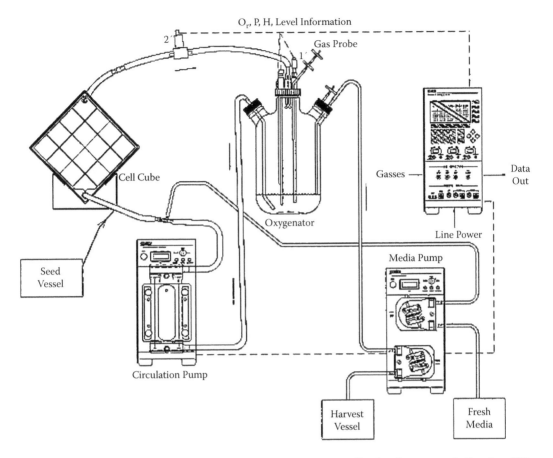

FIGURE 5.3 Layout of the CellCube® Culture System. (Courtesy Corning Incorporated, Corning, NY; http://www.corning.com.)

System is comprised of four pieces of capital equipment — the system controller, oxygenator, circulation pump, and media pump. The cell cubes consist of a series of parallel rigid plates designed for attached monolayers. One set of the plates has the equivalent area to 200 roller bottles. The media is contained in a large reservoir, which could be replaced on a daily basis (Figure 5.3).

ROTARY CULTURE SYSTEM

A newer entry to culture systems is the Rotary Cell Culture System™ (e.g., Synthecon's RCCS™; http://www.synthecon.com), which is different from all other cell culture systems. The cylindrical culture vessel is filled with culture fluid and the cells or tissue particles are added. All air bubbles are removed from the culture vessel. The vessel is attached to the rotator base and rotated about the horizontal axis. Cells establish a fluid orbit within the culture medium in the horizontally rotating cylindrical vessel. They do not collide with the walls or any other parts of the vessel and often appear as if embedded in gelatin. As cells grow in size the rotation speed is adjusted to compensate for the increased settling rates of the larger particles. The tissue particles do move enough within the fluid culture medium to exchange nutrients, wastes, and dissolved gases and make contact with other tissue particles. The cells or tissue particles often join to form larger tissue particles that continue the differentiation process.

Oxygen supply and carbon dioxide removal is achieved through a gas permeable silicone rubber membrane, which acts very much as lung membranes. Since the Rotary Cell Culture System has no impellers, airlifts, bubbles, or agitators, tissue damage from impact and turbulence is significantly decreased as compared to conventional bioreactors. Shear stress and damage is so low that it is essentially insignificant. Under these conditions, cells communicate and synthesize tissue as they would in the body rather than concentrate their energy on repair.

Unlike cell and tissue cultures grown in two-dimensional flat plate systems, cells grown in the Rotary Cell Culture System are functionally similar to tissues in the human body. You will be able to grow three-dimensional tissues *in vitro* that mimic the structure and function of the same tissue *in vivo*.

MEDIA

The integral component of upstream processing is the medium used; its selection depends on the type of bioreactor used and type of culture system adopted. Whereas a large volume of data are available in the scientific literature on the selection of media, the best advise is available from the patent applications that described the original product as well as the information available from the media suppliers. Several environmental and regulatory considerations have changed the selection of media, and the manufacturers are strongly advised to develop a good working relationship with media suppliers, who are more than cooperative in offering advice and frequently offer to run test batches to optimize the selection process. The search for media should begin with the following companies:

www.bd.com
www.cambrex.com
www.specialtymedia.com
www.hynetics.com
www.invitrogen.com
www.jrhbio.com
www.irvinesci.com
www.cellgro.com
www.pharma-ingredients.questint.com
www.serologicals.com
www.sial.com

The composition of the cell growth medium is very important as it significantly affects both the cells and the protein expression. For example, the translation of different mRNAs is differentially affected by temperature as well as changes in the culture medium. Nutrient composition and fermentation variables such as temperature, pH, and other parameters can affect proteolytic activity, secretion, and production levels. Specific manipulations of the culture medium have been shown to enhance protein release into the medium. Thus, supplementation of the growth medium with glycine enhances the release of periplasmic proteins into the medium without causing significant cell lysis. Similarly, growth of cells under osmotic stress in the presence of sorbitol and glycyl betaine causes more than a 400-fold increase in the production of soluble, active protein.

SCALING AND PRODUCTION COSTS

The upstream process is linked to downstream process and the selection of each step in the two phases is determined based on cost optimization considerations, even though the expertise required in each of these steps is highly specialized. The downstream processing adds 80 to 90% of the total cost of production; compare this with the cost of recovery in other biological fermentation productions: 5% for whole-cell yeast biomass, 10 to 50% for bulk chemicals, 10% for extracellular enzymes, 20 to 50% for antibiotics. The high cost of recombinant DNA (rDNA) products arises from the low yields in aqueous fermentation broths and high purification regulatory requirements. As a result, it is not unusual to find market price for rDNA products in the range of $100,000 plus, while the biomass and chemicals can be bought for pennies per kg.

Cost reduction in the manufacturing of recombinant products is an integrated approach wherein the upstream and downstream processing are developed to minimize waste and use of raw materials, capital, and energy. The large-scale process development for the upstream process takes into consideration several key factors, such as:

- Organism selection, with regard to substrate versatility, by-product formation characteristics, robustness of the organism, e.g., to process upsets, viability with regard to cell recycling, physiological characteristics (maximum growth rate, aeration requirements, etc.), and genetic accessibility.
- Metabolic and cellular engineering to improve existing properties of the organism, to introduce novel functions, for example, by simplifying product recovery, expanding substrate and product ranges, and enabling fermentation to occur under nonstandard conditions.

Fermentation process development should achieve culture and media optimization (from complex to defined minimal media), optimization of cultivation parameters that take into account product recovery and purification (minimize by-product formation, minimize chemical inputs, and develop high-cell-density cultivation), and incorporation of cell retention/recycling. Several specific steps can be taken to minimize cost:

- Simplification of broth to remove whatever is nonessential, albeit at reduced efficiency, is a good general rule; inevitably, any added component burdens the downstream processing.
- Select an alternate product form that is easier to separate in downstream processing. Reusing broth components, e.g., recycling cells, although a technical challenge, holds promise for improving fermentation efficiency. The CHO cells show declining yield over a 7-day period; however, adding fresh cells to already present cells may present a cost-reducing possibility. This cannot be done for processes where the drug is contained as an inclusion body. Another strategy is reusing some or all of the broth after product separation. Often, optimum product synthesis and biomass growth take place when medium nutrients are present in excess. However, this results in nutrients being left over at the end of fermentation.
- Removing the product during fermentation improves the yield as the possible inhibitory effects of the product on production are reduced. Using continuous extraction, a side-stream, can be routed out of the unit and the extracted broth returned to conserve broth as well. Further, two-phase fermentations have been developed to extract the product from a biomass-containing aqueous phase into an organic phase, which can then be removed on-line.
- Reducing the water content, which is typically as high as 90%, reduces downstream processing cost as well as the cost of purified water. This is accomplished by increasing the biomass concentration (i.e., high-cell-density [HCD] fermentation), engineering the organism to tolerate higher product concentrations, and removing inhibitory elements from the fermentation media composition.
- Use of microcarriers in bioreactors for cells that requires stationary surface is an excellent approach to improve overall yield.
- Introduction of downstream unit operations within a fermentation process reduces cost substantially, e.g., extractive fermentation, electrodialysis, and in-line membrane separation technologies.

PROBLEM RESOLUTION IN EXPRESSION

A large expense should be budgeted for problem resolution during scale up of upstream processes. The inherent nature of cells, how they interact with media, the role of contamination, etc. make it almost impossible to predict the fate of any scale-up batch. It is this knowledge and experience that the innovator companies purportedly adduce as the reason why a biological product cannot be produced as a generic equivalent. It is therefore imperative that the scale up should be fully validated. Table 5.2 lists some of the noted problems that may arise in the expression of fusion proteins and their solutions.

Table 5.2
Problems and Solutions in the Expression of Fusion Proteins

Problem	Solution
Too high a level of expression	Add 2% glucose to the growth medium. This will decrease the basal expression level associated with the upstream *lac* promoter but will not affect basal level expression from the *tac* promoter. The presence of glucose should not significantly affect overall expression following induction with IPTG. Basal level expression (i.e., expression in the absence of an inducer, such as IPTG), present with most inducible promoters, can affect the outcome of cloning experiments for toxic inserts; it can select against inserts cloned in the proper orientation. Basal level expression can be minimized by catabolite repression (e.g., growth in the presence of glucose). The *tac* promoter is not subject to catabolite repression. However, with the pGEX vector system there is a *lac* promoter located upstream between the 3′-end of the *lac*Iq gene and the *tac* promoter. This *lac* promoter may contribute to the basal level of expression of inserts cloned into the pGEX multiple cloning site, and it is subject to catabolite repression.
No protein detected in bacterial sonicate	Check DNA sequences. It is essential that protein-coding DNA sequences are cloned in the proper translation frame in the vectors. Cloning junctions should be sequenced to verify that inserts are in-frame.
	Optimize culture conditions to improve yield. Investigate the effect of cell strain, medium composition, incubation temperature, and induction conditions. Exact conditions will vary for each fusion protein expressed.
	Analyze a small aliquot of an overnight culture by SDS-PAGE. Generally, a highly expressed protein will be visible by Coomassie™ blue staining when 5 to 10 μL of an induced culture whose A600 is ~1.0 loaded on the gel. Nontransformed host *E. coli* cells and cells transformed with the parental vector should be run in parallel as negative and positive controls, respectively. The presence of the fusion protein in this total cell preparation and its absence from a clarified sonicate may indicate the presence of inclusion bodies.
	Check for expression by immunoblotting. Some fusion proteins may be masked on an SDS-polyacrylamide gel by a bacterial protein of approximately the same molecular weight. Immunoblotting can be used to identify fusion proteins in these cases. Run an SDS-polyacrylamide gel of induced cells and transfer the proteins to a nitrocellulose or PVDF membrane (such as Hybond™-C or Hybond-P). Detect fusion protein using anti-GST or anti-His antibody.
Most of fusion protein is in the postsonicate pellet	Check cell disruption procedure. Cell disruption is seen by partial clearing of the suspension or by microscopic examination. Addition of lysozyme (0.1 volume of a 10 mg/mL lysozyme solution in 25 mM Tris-HCl, pH 8.0) prior to sonication may improve results. Avoid frothing as this may denature the fusion protein.
	Reduce sonication since over-sonication can lead to copurification of host proteins with the fusion protein.
	Fusion protein may be produced as insoluble inclusion bodies. Try altering the growth conditions to slow the rate of translation, as suggested below. It may be necessary to combine these approaches. Exact conditions must be determined empirically for each fusion protein.

Continued.

Table 5.2 (Continued)
Problems and Solutions in the Expression of Fusion Proteins

Problem	Solution
Most of fusion protein is in the postsonicate pellet	Lower the growth temperature (within the range of +20 to +30°C) to improve solubility.
	Decrease IPTG concentration to < 0.1 mM to alter induction level.
	Alter time of induction.
	Induce for a shorter period of time.
	Induce at a higher cell density for a short period of time.
	Increase aeration. High oxygen transport can help prevent the formation of inclusion bodies. It may be necessary to combine the above approaches. Exact conditions must be determined empirically for each fusion protein.
	Alter extraction conditions to improve solubilization of inclusion bodies.

6 Manufacturing Systems

INTRODUCTION

Over the past quarter century, manufacturing systems have been developed around the various cells — bacterial, yeast, animal, and insect — and whole animals. A system comprises the target cell, the host, and the means to isolate or create gene sequence, a means to insert the sequence in the host, and elaborate methods to remove and purify the target protein. Whereas a large number of canned commercial systems are available, making the entire process relatively straightforward, there remains a need to custom design a system.

BACTERIAL EXPRESSION SYSTEMS

The typical protein to be expressed in Gram-negative bacteria comprises 100 to 300 amino acids, has no posttranslational modifications, and possesses a restricted number of cysteine residues to make *in vitro* refolding possible. Whereas in this chapter, the discussion on bacteria pertains mainly to Gram-negative bacteria, a discussion of how the Gram-positive bacteria are viewed with great interest should be made. The problems of methionine blocking the N-terminus and the intracellular formation of inclusion bodies that add host cell impurities in the use of Gram-negative bacteria can be resolved by using Gram-positive bacteria such as *Bacillus subtilis* and *Lactococcus lactis*. Also, the presence of endotoxin is of little concern in Gram-positive bacteria. On the negative side, while using *Bacillus,* endogenous proteolytic degradation can be significant, a drawback not found in *Lactococcus.* The extra-cellular expression of the folded target protein in the use of Gram-positive bacteria additionally eliminates significant problems in the use of *E. coli* expression system: the requirements of *in vitro* folding and performing cleavage of the N-terminal tag. This results in simpler process design comprised of harvest, capture, intermediate purification, polishing, concentration, and finishing, as described below for Gram-negative bacteria. The rest of the chapter refers to the expression system comprising Gram-negative bacteria, particularly *E. coli*.

Although bacteria cannot be used to express some large, complex proteins (with eukaryotic posttranslational modifications including glycosylation, acetylation, and amidation), other proteins such as interferons, interleukins, colony stimulating factors, growth hormones, growth factors, and human serum albumin have been successfully produced. Marketed products produced include human growth hormone, human insulin, α, β, and γ-interferon, and interleukin 2. This chapter deals with the upstream and downstream processing for the manufacturing of therapeutic proteins using bacteria, particularly the Gram-negative bacteria such as *E. coli*. This system is most popular because of its low fermentation cost and high expression yields. The most common form of bacterial expression is cytoplasmatic or intracellular expression, where inclusion bodies contain the target protein, which is in an inactive form and thus harmful to bacteria; the yield is generally high and the system requires simpler plasmid construct. The disadvantages include the need for *in vitro* folding, expression of Met-protein, and complex purification steps. The cell disruption to recover inclusion bodies releases a large volume of host cell proteins, nucleic acids, and proteolytic enzymes that can damage target protein. Measures to reduce this proteolysis include use of thioredoxin deficient strains, processing at low temperatures, and coexpression of chaperones, coexpression of PDI, and fusion partners; unfortunately, none of the methods have been developed far enough to be useful in commercial processing operations. Cytosolic expression in *E. coli* also produces methionine blocking of the N-terminus, requiring a specific enzymatic cleavage step to produce the native molecule. To eliminate expression of Met-protein, N-terminally extended protein constructs are expressed followed by an enzymatic cleavage step in which the extension is cleaved with an endo-peptidase or removed step by step with and exo-peptidase. Typical extensions are fusion proteins, histidine tags, or, if proline is the second amino acid in the protein, a few amino acids. These disadvantages, particularly the inability of Gram-negative organisms to express folded proteins to the periplasm or to the medium, have resulted in attempts to use other forms of expression, namely, periplasmic and secretion. Attention has been focused on Gram-positive bacteria, e.g., *Bacillus* species, which naturally secretes large amounts of protein to the medium, but where endogenous proteolytic degradation is of general concern. *Lactococcus*, traditionally used in the dairy industry, has no detectable extra-cellular proteases or toxins and also offers direct expression to the medium. The periplasmic expression has the advantage of producing native protein with correct N-terminal structure, requiring simpler purification and less extensive incidence of proteolysis. The disadvantages include inefficient translocation through the inner membrane and the fact that inclusion bodies may still form. The extracellular secretion system would be idea for it results in least extensive proteolysis, provides for simpler purification, and corrects N-terminus situation; however, there is little secretion that results in very low yields; one exception being the expression of β-glucanase.

GENETICALLY MODIFIED BACTERIA

The genetically modified bacteria are prepared by introducing a recombinant gene into the bacteria on a plasmid, modified to optimize heterologous protein expression comprising complete genetic elements to enhance transcription and translation and to stabilize mRNA. A plasmid is a double strand circular DNA, small (2 to 25 Kbp, some bigger), bacterial artificial chromosome that has the characteristics of autonomous replication. Plasmid vectors are very useful as a quick way to introduce genes to the cell and are much more easy to manipulate than the chromosome. Components of a gene include promoter, operator, RBS, CDS, and start and stop codon. All vectors comprise an origin of replication (Ori) that determines the vector copy number. The stability of the expression cassette has a high impact on productivity. Loss of the cassette during the course of the fermentation (the cell tends to minimize the stress by getting rid of the plasmid) results in formation of nonproductive, plasmid free cells, which usually outgrow plasmid carrying cells in fermentation unless selective pressure can be effectively employed. Plasmid stability is increased by using vectors that confer an antibiotic resistance (e.g., ampicillin) to the host or complement some auxotrophic feature of the host strain. If periplasmic or extracellular expression is desired, the vector must also include a signal sequence for the transport of the protein.

Great advances have been made in the availability of commercial systems that help resolve some of the problem related to expressed protein harming the host, formation of inclusion bodies, target proteins appearing translationally, and complex purification procedures. The popular commercial systems provide supporting materials and reagents in kit to cone, express, and purify recombinant proteins with a fair amount of ease. These support systems are broadly classified as promoters; stabilizing and optimizing elements; ribosome binding sites; and transcriptional and translational termination sequences.

PROMOTERS

Promoters are DNA sequences to which the endogenous bacterial RNA polymerase will bind to initiate transcription. The promoter has an important function in that it determines the polarity of the transcript by specifying which strand will be transcribed. More important, how tightly regulated a promoter/operator is will greatly affect the ability to express proteins. Most bacterial promoters used in expression vectors consist of two elements located (−35) and (−10) from the actual transcriptional start. These elements comprise the consensus sequences that are bound by a specific transcription factor and the RNA polymerase. One of the most commonly encountered promoters is the trc promoter.

DNA sequences that act in conjunction with promoters and bind repressor molecules regulate the induction of transcription. One of the most commonly used in *E. coli* is the lacO/lacIq repressor system. In this system, transcription is virtually shut off until the promoter is derepressed by the addition of IPTG. At this point, the promoter is freed (i.e., the repressor no longer physically blocks transcription) and transcription is turned on. Inducible elements provide the ability to keep expression of the target gene off, should it produce a product that might be toxic to the host strain. There are a number of different methods of regulation that are available in commercial expression systems. Although most are capable of inducing tremendous levels of expression, even slightly leaky expression during culture expansion can limit final product yield.

TERMINATORS

In prokaryotic systems, antitermination elements are incorporated into vectors to stabilize the RNA polymerase on the DNA template. These elements help ensure optimal transcript elongation during message synthesis. Transcription terminators are used to signal the active RNA polymerase to release the DNA template and halt transcription of the newly transcribed RNA. These terminators are ordinarily positioned downstream of the multicloning site and act to prevent pausing, prevent premature termination, and limit read-through of transcription, which adversely affects plasmid replication. Use of transcription terminators such as rrnB T1 and T2 from *E. coli* 5S rRNA are especially important for use with strong promoters.

RIBOSOME BINDING SITES

Ribosome binding sites (RBS) are small, open reading frames upstream of the coding sequence of interest engineered to encourage ribosomes to bind and translate the sequence of interest. An RBS (Shine-Dalgarno sequence) is required just upstream of the translational start to provide the context for efficient translation initiation. RBS sequences are engineered into vectors to enhance and stabilize ribosome binding. Often RBS elements may be "borrowed" from different sources or are the native RBS for the fusion species. Frequently used RBS elements are obtained from either the *lacZ* gene or the gene 10 of the bacteriophage T7.

Several commercial systems are now available with more appearing on the scene regularly; what used to be a great deal of science and art has been practically reduced to a kit approach with remarkable consistency and proven results. Given below are some of these systems; the Novogen pET system remains one of the best systems that we have used.

Arabinose-Regulated Promoter (Invitrogen pBAD Vector)

This system generates very low levels of uninduced expression through glucose-catabolite-dependent repression. The pBAD promoter is induced by arabinose. Adding arabinose into the medium in increasing concentrations induces transcription in a dose-dependent manner.

T7 Expression Systems (Novagen, Promega, Stratagene)

The pET-based vectors utilize the T7 RNA polymerase-based expression vector of Moffat and Studier (*J. Mol. Biol.* 189 [1986]: 113–130) to achieve very high levels of protein expression. The power of the pET system is that the T7 RNA polymerase is specific for its own promoter, which is found only on the expression plasmid. During growth and culture expansion, the T7 promoter is under tight control of the lacIq gene, repressing any expression that might adversely affect bacterial growth. When induced with IPTG, rather than directly inducing the T7 promoter 5′ to the target gene, a T7 RNA polymerase is expressed in host *E. coli*, allowing transcription from the T7 promoter. Transcription and translation can be accomplished in only a few hours, with the expressed protein often comprising the most abundant cellular component. It is important to know that some of these commercial systems are sold under intellectual property rights that may require royalty agreements. For example, the Invitrogen's pET system is licensed from Brookhaven Institute that has no fee when used for development in the laboratory, $5000 if used to test products in humans, and a royalty of 1% if the product derived from using the T7 pET system results in a commercial product used in humans in U.S. The licensing agreement is signed directly with Brookhaven and requires the manufacturer to carry liability insurance.

Trc/Tac Promoter Systems (Clontech, Invitrogen, Kodak, Life Technologies, MBI Fermentas, New England BioLabs, Amersham, Biotech, Promega)

Trc promoters are IPTG-inducible hybrid promoters. The Trc promoter is a trp/lac fusion, where the (−35) position is derived from trp and the (−10) position is obtained from lacUV5 promoter elements. Although extremely strong, some low-level expression of the recombinant protein may occur during growth.

P$_L$ Promoters (Invitrogen pLEX, and pTrxFus Vectors)

P$_L$-based systems place the protein of interest under the tight transcriptional control of the Lambda cI repressor protein. The repressor protein must be engineered into the *E. coli* host or be incorporated into the vector itself. The repressor protein is placed under the control of an inducible promoter. Expression of the cI repressor binds to the operator of the P$_L$ promoter to prevent transcription of the recombinant gene. Induction occurs with the addition of tryptophan, which prevents expression of the repressor, allowing transcription for the P$_L$ promoter.

Phage T5 Promoter (Qiagen)

The phage T5 promoter provides a strong recognition site for *E. coli* RNA polymerase and can direct the expression of targets to levels up to 50% of total cellular protein. The promoter is regulated by two lactose operator elements.

tetA Promoter (Biometra pASK75 Vector)

The tetA promoter is induced by the addition of anhydrotetracycline in concentrations that are not antibiotically effective. This promoter is not regulated by any endogenous cellular mechanisms and therefore is not influenced by catabolic repression.

FUSION PROTEINS AND TAGS

One-step purification of the recombinant protein by high-affinity binding can be accomplished in some situations using vectors engineered with DNA sequences encoding a specific peptide fused to the expressed protein. One of the most popular systems is the 6xHis system in which six histidine residues enable the tagged-recombinant protein to be purified by a nickel-chelating resin. Often, an endopeptidase recognition sequence is also engineered between the affinity tag and the protein of interest to allow subsequent removal of the leader sequence, peptide-tag, or fusion sequences by enzymatic digestion.

　　Tags serve several functions, providing purification and stabilization of the expressed protein; fusion may act as a tag with the generation of antibodies.

Calmodulin-Binding Peptide (CBP) Tag (Stratagene pCAL Vectors)

pCAL Expression Vectors contain a sequence encoding a CBP. The CBP tag allows the hybrid recombinant protein to bind to a calmodulin resin in the presence of low concentrations of calcium. Elution is accomplished in the presence of 2 mM EGTA and neutral pH. The conditions are milder than in other tag systems. The cyclase associated protein (CAP) tag is one of the smaller tags, encoding a 4kDa tag. Smaller tags have potentially less impact on the protein of interest than larger tags.

Glutathione S-Transferase (GST) Tag (Amersham pGEX Vectors)

Vectors containing the GST fusion tag allow encoded proteins to be efficiently purified from bacterial lysates, utilizing an affinity matrix containing glutathione. Elution of the purified protein is accomplished under mild, nondenaturing conditions. The GST fusion adds a 26kDa tag to the recombinant protein, which can be removed when an endopeptidase cleavage site sequence is incorporated between the tag and the protein.

6xHIS Tag (Invitrogen, Kodak, Life Technologies, New England BioLab, Pierce, Amersham [GE], Promega, Qiagen, Novagen)

6xHis-tagging vectors fuse a six histidine-peptide to the recombinant protein. This small addition rarely affects protein structure to a significant degree and therefore usually does not require removal following purification of the protein. The 6-His residues impart a remarkable affinity for matrices containing nickel. The fact that binding can occur under native as well as under denaturing conditions distinguishes this affinity purification method from the others. Recombinant proteins, frequently encountered in inclusion bodies in bacterial expression systems, can be solubilized under denaturing conditions using urea or guanidine hydrochloride. The solubilized 6xHis-tagged proteins can then be purified by binding to nickel ions on the matrix. The strong affinity of the 6xHis tag tolerates denaturing conditions that facilitate the removal of nonspecific contaminants often associated with recombinant proteins expressed in bacteria. Elution is accomplished under mild conditions by either reducing the pH or adding imidazole as a competitor. With great advances taking place in the field of commercial kits and systems, the reader is referred to market leaders to obtain information on a system suitable for their use.

Dihydrofolate Reductase (QIAGEN)

Short peptide sequences from the murine DHFR are fused to target proteins to increase stability of the target protein, as well as enhance its antigenicity.

Thioredoxin Fusion Sequences (Invitrogen, pTrxFUS and pThioHis Vectors, Novagen pET-32 Vectors)

Designed to maximize the accumulation of fusion proteins in the soluble fraction, a number of additional advantages are imparted when recombinant proteins are fused with sequences encoding thioredoxin. Fusion with thioredoxin helps overcome insolubility encountered with some bacterial systems. Additionally, in *E. coli*, thioredoxin accumulates in adhesion zones, which can be selectively released by rapid osmotic shock. The temperature stability of thioredoxin also allows temperatures as high as 80°C to be tolerated during purification. These features can be exploited to simplify purification of expressed fusion proteins. Finally, thioredoxin possesses a unique active dithiol, which directs high-affinity binding to phenylarsine oxide, allowing rapid purification of expressed proteins.

Protein A (Amersham pEZZ 18 and pRIT2T)

The ability of Protein A to bind to IgG immunoglobulins continues to be a workhorse in biotechnology. pEZZ 18 contains two synthetic "Z" domains of the "B" IgG binding domains of Protein A and pRIT2T contains the natural IgG binding domains of Protein A. Fusion proteins are easily purified using IgG Sepharose resins. The two Z domains add a 14kDa peptide to the recombinant protein.

Biotinylation (Promega PinPoint™ Vector)

Biotinylation-based epitopes encode peptide sequences that become biotinylated *in vivo* during expression. Relying on the strong affinity of streptavidin for biotin, the biotinylated peptide acts as a purification tag for the fusion protein. Promega provides a unique monomeric avidin that allows elution of the fused proteins under mild nondenaturing conditions (5mM biotin), not possible with native avidin.

Cellulose Binding Domain (CBD) (Novagen, pET CBD Vectors)

CBDs allow for the purification of expressed proteins with cellulose or chitin matrices. These materials are generally very low cost and quite stable and may be found in a variety of forms including beads, powders, fibers, membranes, filters, and sheets. Additionally, the CBD fusion often increases thermostability of the recombinant protein, which may be useful in purification strategies or in simply increasing the stability of expressed proteins.

Maltose Binding Protein (MBP) (New England BioLabs, pMAL Vectors)

The malE gene encodes the MBP, which has the capability to bind tightly to amylose. The MBP is separated from the desired expressed sequence by a polylinker encoding 10 asparagine residues. The linker is designed to ensure that the MBP can adequately bind amylose, which is immobilized on resin. In addition to aiding in expression and purification, the MBP fusion partner also helps keep proteins soluble and provides a choice of folding pathways.

S-Peptide Tag (Novagen, selected pET Vectors)

The 15 amino acid peptide (S-Tag) encoded by these vectors is a small, hydrophilic tag that has a strong affinity (Kd = 109M) for a 104 amino acid protein (S-protein) derived from pancreatic ribonuclease A. When associated, the S-protein:S-peptide complex possesses ribonuclease activity (ribonuclease S). This strong association and activity have been exploited to measure S-Tag fusion protein (ribonuclease assay, which can detect as little as 5 fmol target) and can be used with reagents and resins for detection and purification purposes. For example, the S-Protein itself can be directly conjugated to alkaline phosphatase or horseradish peroxidase and used as a probe to detect S-Tag fusion protein by Western blot.

Strep-tag (Biometra pASK75 Vector)

A C-terminal fusion tag, the Strep-tag encodes a 10 amino acid sequence and binds streptavidin. Affinity of the tag for streptavidin allows purification of recombinant proteins under mild conditions. Along with affinity-purification applications, the strep-tag can be utilized to directly detect recombinant proteins by Western blot or ELISA assays using streptavidin-enzyme (alkaline phosphatase) conjugates.

Intein Mediated Purification with Affinity Chitin-Binding Tag (New England BioLabs, pCYB Vectors/IMPACT System)

This chimeric system produces a C-terminally tagged protein in which a small 5kDa chitin-binding domain (CBD) from Bacillus circulans is physically separated from the target protein by the protein splicing element derived from the Saccharomyces cerevisiae VMA gene 1. The splicing element, or Intein, has been modified such that it undergoes a self-cleavage reaction at its N-terminus at low temperatures in the presence of thiols. The fusion protein is purified by passing extracts through a chitin column; the purified protein is then induced to undergo the Intein-mediated self-cleavage on the column by overnight incubation at 4°C in the presence of DTT or b-mercaptoethanol. The target protein without additional residues is released, while the chitin-binding fusion domain remains adhered to the resin.

Immunoreactive Epitopes (Invitrogen, Novagen, Kodak)

Although many vectors utilize fusion or epitope tags for multifunctional purposes, some vectors encode fragments that are essentially immunoreactive epitopes. Immunoreactive tags provide a rapid means of detecting tag-hybrid proteins with high specificity and affinity without needing to generate specific antisera to each protein of interest. The monoclonal anti-myc antibody detects recombinant proteins containing the myc epitope (GluGlnLysLeuIleSerGluGluAspLeuAsn). An alternative is the 11 amino acid epitope tag (GlnProGluLeuAlaProGluAspProGluAsp) derived from herpes simplex (HSV) glycoprotein D, which can be recognized by an anti-HSV monoclonal antibody.

Kinase Sequences for *in vitro* Labeling (Stratagene, Amersham)

To enable rapid *in vitro* labeling of proteins with 32P, some vectors incorporate the recognition sequence for the catalytic subunit of cAMP-dependent protein kinase as a fusion epitope. The site encoding the sequence (ArgArgAlaSerVal) is usually located between a primary fusion sequence and the sequence for the gene of interest. Expressed proteins can be directly labeled using protein kinase and (gamma 32P)-ATP (W. G. Kelin et al., *Cell*, 70 [1992]: 351).

Protein A Signal Sequence (Amersham pEZZ18)

The Protein A signal sequence of this vector results in the secretion of the expressed protein into the aqueous culture.

ompT and ompA Leader Signal Peptides (Biometra, New England BioLabs, Kodak)

The ompT and ompA leader sequence directs secretion of proteins into the periplasmic space. This periplasmic localization can simplify recovery of expressed proteins since osmotic shock treatments can enrich for proteins localized within the periplasm.

malE Signal Sequence (New England BioLabs pMAL-p2)

The normal malE signal sequence contains residues that direct the expressed fusion protein through the cytoplasmic membrane to the periplasm. This provides an alternate folding pathway that particularly helps in the formation of disulfide bonds.

T7 gene 10 Leader Peptide (Novagen, Stratagene, Promega, Invitrogen)

An 11 amino acid leader peptide (MetAlaSerMetThrGlyGlyGlnGlnMetGly) derived from the T7 major capsid protein (gene 10) is incorporated into vectors to provide an ATG source for fused proteins. This leader peptide is often used in T7 expression systems. Antibodies generated against this epitope can be used to detect the production of expressed protein in Western or immunoprecipitation assays.

FUSION AND TAGGED PROTEIN CLEAVAGE SYSTEMS

Whereas the use of tagged or fusion proteins allows for rapid quantitation and purification of recombinant proteins, this requires an addition to the vector-derived epitope to provide a cleavage system. Although some epitopes such as the 6xHis tag are small and may be inconsequential, others are significantly larger and may affect the downstream use of the recombinant protein. By incorporating site-specific protease cleavage sites between the epitope/fusion and the target protein, these sequences can be removed. One complication arises when the recombinant protein has proteolytic cleavage site within its own sequence, making it difficult for the protease to recognize its intended target site. Using a protease to mediate cleavage eventually requires that the protease itself be removed following the reaction in order to obtain a truly purified recombinant protein. To address this issue, some manufacturers have incorporated novel methods of releasing the target protein from the fusion product while simultaneously including a strategy of immobilizing the protease on a resin through use of an engineered tag on a recombinant endopeptidase. The PreScission Protease from Amersham is a genetically engineered fusion protein consisting of the 3C protease of the human rhinovirus type 14 and glutathione S-transferase. This protease can be used either following purification of the recombinant protein, or while the target protein is bound to glutathione sepharose. Since the protease itself contains a GST tag, it remains bound to the sepharose matrix, allowing rapid purification of the target away from the protease. New England BioLabs has recently introduced a vector that relies on Intein-mediated self-cleavage rather than proteolytic cleavage of the fusion. The Intein sequence mediates self-cleavage between the tag-epitope and the target sequence and liberates the target protein from the fusion species without the introduction of additional proteins. The affinity tag can remain immobilized, and purification of the target is relatively easy.

Some commonly encountered protease/cleavage sites are:

Thrombin (KeyValProArg/GlySer)
Factor Xa Protease (IleGluGlyArg)
Enterokinase (AspAspAspAspLys)
rTEV (GluAsnLeuTyrPheGln/Gly): a recombinant endopeptidase from the tobacco etch
    virus
Intein-mediated self-cleavage (New England BioLabs)
3C human rhino virus Protease (Amersham Biotech) (LeuGluValLeuPhe Gln/GlyPro)

Polylinkers or MCSs are synthetic DNA sequences encoding a series of restriction endonuclease recognition sites that are engineered for convenient cloning of DNA into a vector at a specific position. MCS sites can range in size from two restriction sites and up. To accommodate reading frame differences with translational start sequences, many vectors are offered in an "A, B, C" format, meaning there is a single base shift between each vector, allowing easy cloning into each of the three reading frames. Additionally, some vectors are provided where the MCSs are in opposite orientations. For sequences where the amino terminus has not been precisely defined, Kodak has developed a FLAG-Shift vector. These vectors contain a "shift" sequence that allows expression of an open reading frame without regard to the reading frame in which it was originally cloned. This shift is facilitated by ribosomal slippage caused by a run of A/Ts.

LIC vectors (ligation-independent cloning, Novagen, Stratagene) allow directional cloning of PCR products without restriction digestion or ligation reactions of the amplified products. LIC vectors rely on sequence complementarity between the primer used for amplification and the ends of the vector. These overhangs, following treatment with T4 polymerase, allow specific and efficient annealing and subsequent transformation directly into bacteria. Primers for the overhang can also be engineered to accomplish additional tasks. Novagen, for example, uses primers that encode the recognition site for Enterokinase. All vectors must contain a DNA sequence that directs binding of DNA polymerase and associated factors in order to maintain copies of the vector. Most vectors utilize elements from pBR322. Many vectors also provide an M13 origin of DNA replication (f1) allowing the production of single-stranded DNA for sequencing and mutagenesis.

SELECTION PRESSURE

All vectors contain sequences that provide a means to select only those cells containing a vector. As a selection pressure an antibiotic is usually added to the medium. The following markers function by either conveying drug resistance on the host or enabling the host to compensate for the absence of an essential component in the media (auxotrophic markers):

- Ampicillin: interferes with a terminal reaction in bacterial cell wall synthesis. The resistance gene (bla) encoding beta-lactamase cleaves the beta-lactam ring of ampicillin. Ampicillin is rapidly degraded by the extracellular enzyme β-lactamase secreted by the plasmid-carrying cells. This can be a major problem decreasing yields significantly due to the outgrowth of plasmid carrying cells by noncarrying ones. This problem has been addressed adding ampicillin during the fermentation or using carbenicillin, which is more stable but expensive.
- Tetracycline: prevents bacterial protein synthesis by binding to the 30S ribosomal subunit. The resistance gene (tet) specifies a protein that modifies the bacterial membrane and prevents transport of the antibiotic into the cell.
- Kanamycin: binds to the 70S ribosomes and causes misreading of messenger RNA. The resistant gene (Km) modifies the antibiotic and prevents interaction with the ribosome.

With the ever-increasing rate of discovering new genes comes the equal challenge of understanding how the products of these genes are used and regulated, when they appear, and how they interact within cells. Although much attention has been given to high-throughput PCR and sequencing, numerous advancements have been made in lower profile areas such as developing tools to rapidly express and purify proteins.

PROCESS OPTIMIZATION

Commercial success of a bacterial cell production system depends on a large number of factors, from the cell density to type of media to the conditions of process; optimization remains trial and error based, though some basic principles help us avoid obvious pitfalls.

CELL DENSITY AND VIABILITY

As most proteins are intracellular accumulated in *E. coli*, productivity is proportional to the final cell density and the specific productivity, i.e., the amount of product formed per unit cell mass per unit time. High cell densities require sufficient oxygen supply to avoid formation of acetate, lactate, or pyruvate when *E. coli* is grown under anaerobic or oxygen-limiting conditions (mixed acid fermentation). A further complication of *E. coli* growth on glucose under aerobic conditions is incomplete glucose oxidation, resulting in accumulation of acetate, sometimes referred to as the bacterial "Crab-tree" effect; therefore, excess glucose in the medium should be avoided.

Proteolysis is often a major problem especially when the microorganism is stressed, where a high proteolytic protein turnover can be expected. Variations between shake flasks and large-scale bioreactors have been observed, challenging the scale up and limiting the value of down-scale studies.

Higher cell densities are also obtained when using *E. coli* by separating growth and production phases, taking advantage of regulated promoters to achieve high cell densities in the first phase (promoter off) and high rate of target protein expression in the second phase (promoter on). Inducers such as 3,β-indolacrylic acid (IAA), isopropyl-β-D-thiogalactoside (IPTG), and lactose are used to turn the promoter on (trp and lac promoters respectively).

High cell density growth is inevitably faced with problems of oxygen supply, formation of toxic products, high carbon dioxide, and heat generation; one way to resolve this would be to switch to modes other than batch mode since merely increasing the concentration of nutrients is not advised. For example, the maximum concentration of glucose in media should not exceed 50 g/L; ammonia by 3 g/L, Iron(II) by 1.15 g/L; magnesium by 8.7 g/L; manganese by 68 mg/L; phosphate by 10 g/L; zinc by 0.038 g/L; molybdenum by 0.8 g/L; boron by 44 mg/L; and cobalt by 0.5 mg/L. Even in fed-batch mode and in some situations of perfusion mode the longevity of continuous culturing causes accumulation of nonproducing variants of the microbial cells, resulting in decreasing productivity.

Cell density is calculated from OD_{470} on the basis of a calibration curve or by laser turbidimetry and expressed as unit g/L. The viscosity of culture broth increases sharply when the cell concentration exceeds 200 g/L, which is regarded as the maximum attainable cell density of *E. coli*. The cell dry weight is calculated from OD_{470} or OD_{500} on the basis of a calibration curve or by centrifugation and weight of the pellet. Viable cells can be identified by spread out of the cell suspension on nutrient agar plates with or without kanamycin or like selection markers. Cell lysis can be measured from the DNA content in the supernatant following centrifugation. Plasmid instability influences the productivity. Instability may result from defective partitioning during cell division (loss) or undesired modifications (insertion, deletion, rearrangement of DNA). Most plasmids of industrial interest are lost at frequencies of 10^{-2} to 10^{-5} per cell generation. The plasmid free cells will have a higher specific growth rate and they will, over time, reach a higher concentration. Plasmid instability is influenced by plasmid construction, plasmid copy number, cultivation conditions, and the bioreactor configuration. The stability can be estimated by replica plating to ampicillin, kanamycin, or like selection marker agar plates. The method sensitivity is 1% of the number of plasmid molecules per genome in a single cell. The plasmid copy number (PCN) is a criterion for the strength of the expression system on the DNA level. The production of target protein depends on the PCN. The PCN is calculated from measurement of the total DNA content and the plasmid DNA content of the biomass by quantitative DNA assays (e.g., agarose slab gel electrophoresis, capillary electrophoresis) after cell disintegration.

MEDIA

The common media include:

- Complex systems containing chemically undefined nutrients such as yeast extract, peptone, tryptone, and casamino acids; it typically comprises tryptone, yeast extract, mineral salts (e.g., sodium choride, potassium hydrogen phosphate, magnesium sulfate), glucose, and an antibiotic (e.g., kanamycin, ampicillin, chloramphenicol).
- Defined media comprising solely defined nutrients; it typically comprises mineral salts including ammonium sulfate, trace elements, foam controlling agents, glucose, and eventually additional components such as thiamine and ampicillin.
- Semicomplex media, which is a combination of the above two types.

CONTROL PARAMETERS

The in-process control parameters have well-defined lower and upper parameter limits and measurement of a variety of output parameters (responses):

- pH is typically set at 6.9; repeated sterilization of probe may delay response time.
- Dissolved oxygen must exceed 20%; because of low solubility in media (approximately 7.6 mg/L), the oxygen transfer rate is a limiting factor when scaling up bacterial cultures. The dissolved oxygen is measured by a polarographic oxygen electrode 32.
- Temperature lowering to 26 to 30°C reduces nutrient uptake and growth rate as well as inclusion bodies, but also reduces toxic by-product formation. Heat generation during culture in large-scale fermenters requires cooling.
- Agitation rate is adjusted to keep dissolved oxygen above critical value; generally, 300 to 1000 rpm are maintained.
- Aeration rate of 1vvm at 30 to 70 kPa proves optimal.
- Ammonia feed is maintained to keep ammonium concentrations below 170 mM; Ammonia is determined by Kjeldahl analysis.
- Glucose feed is adjusted not to exceed optimal glucose levels using feedback mechanisms. The levels of glucose are measured by HPLC, RI, or commercial kits.
- Acetate forms in complex and defined media when the specific growth rate exceeds 0.2 and 0.35 h^{-1}, respectively; pCO_2 > 0.3 atm decreases growth rate and stimulates acetate formation, which is reduced by using glycerol as a carbon source instead of glucose and by using the exponential feeding method. A concentration of less than 20 mM of acetate maintains an exponential growth. Acetate concentration is monitored by gas chromatography or with an acetate kit.
- Foam level should be minimized by adding antifoam agents.
- By-products are routinely monitored; ethanol detected by gas chromatography (flame ionization detector) or ethanol sensor; propionate and lactate detected by gas chromatography (flame ionization detector); amino acids detected by HPLC and the product by specific assay (see BP, EP, or USP for assay methods).

DOWNSTREAM PROCESSING

The downstream process comprises harvest, capture, *in vitro* refolding, intermediary purification, enzymatic cleavage, and polishing after the step of generating starting material from fermentation and extraction. The most commonly used techniques in downstream processing include chromatography, filtration, microfiltration, ultrafiltration, active filtration, centrifugation, precipitation, and crystallization. The downstream process is designed for effective and efficient removal of cell debris, host cell proteins, nucleic acids, and endotoxins that arise from the disruption of the cells. It is also important to remove the closely related target protein derivates such as cleaved forms, deamidated forms, oxidized forms, and scrambled forms as much as possible. As a result of these considerations, a minimum of three different chromatographic steps is generally required. In most instances, the last step would be size exclusion chromatography (and thus four steps). Virus removal is required (in instances where animal-derived raw materials are used), this would add an additional step to the total processing scheme.

The biogeneric manufacturing client should make a thorough search of the intellectual property infringement in using any technique since a large number of patents often protect the innovator's molecules. (See Chapter 12 on Intellectual Property Issues.)

HARVEST

The harvesting step generally uses techniques like centrifugation, filtration, microfiltration, or ultrafiltration. The purpose of the harvest step is to isolate the inclusion bodies from cell culture impurities such as cell debris and to condition the sample for the following chromatographic capture step. Generally, centrifugation separates the cells from media; the cells are washed and their disruption is a mechanical (e.g., french press), chemical (e.g., urea and cysteine), or enzymatic nature (e.g., lysozyme) process to release host cell proteins (and therefore also proteolytic enzymes) to the medium. If the cells are exposed directly to the extraction buffer, cell debris is removed by centrifugation. It is recommended to use urea (7 to 8 M) as the denaturing agent and cysteine (50 to 100 mM, of nonanimal origin) as the reducing agent. Note that urea solution must be free of cyanate to prevent carbamylation of primary amino-groups (for further information see the car-bamylation document). EDTA is often added to the extraction buffer in 1 to 2 mM concentrations in order to inhibit metalloproteases. The typical result of the harvest and extraction procedure is a viscous sample at 4°C with high levels of target protein, host cell proteins, DNA, and endotoxins in a 7 to 8 M urea, 50 to 100 mM cysteine, 1 to 2 mM EDTA buffer at pH 7.5 to 9.0. The use of expanded bed adsorption technique recovers proteins directly from preparations of broken cells, saving one or several centrifugation or filtration steps. Since, during cell lysis and extraction, the recombinant product is exposed to a variety of proteolytic enzymes, enzyme inhibitors should not be used at this stage. The enzymatic activity can be reduced by using protease negative mutant hosts, low temperatures, and fast procedures. Inevitably, the presence of denaturing agents leads to the formation of minor amounts of cleaved products, such as split and truncated forms.

CAPTURE

The capture step follows the harvesting and generally uses chromatographic techniques like AC, IEC, IMAC; expanded bed, or packed bed. The purpose of the capture step is to remove cell culture and process-related impurities and to prepare for *in vitro* folding. The nature of the capture step depends on the protein construct expressed. For example, histidine tags are exceptional, binding to metal chelating matrices under denaturing conditions. Affinity chromatography can be used for fusion proteins if *in vitro* refolding has been carried out prior to the capture step. For nontagged proteins with short N-terminal extensions, ion exchange chromatography can be used under dena-turing conditions provided urea is used as the denaturant. The particle size of media should be in the range of 100 to 300 nm. It may be an advantage to use expanded bed technology. The typical result of the capture procedure is a purified sample comprising the target protein (1 to 5 mg/mL) and low to medium levels of impurities in 7 to 8 M urea, 50 to 100 mM cysteine, 1 to 2 mM EDTA buffer at pH 7.5 to 9.0.

IN VITRO REFOLDING

As mentioned above, inclusion bodies do not produce target protein in its natural form, requiring refolding that is often chaotrope mediated, cosolvent assisted, requires dilution, desalting, use of hollow fiber, SEC, or immobilized protein. In some instances, prior to refolding of the proteins, some purification can be made by means of dilution, size exclusion chromatography, dialysis, or immobilization techniques prior to adding refolding buffer. The purpose of the *in vitro* folding step is to bring the denatured target protein into its native biological active form. From a regulatory point, it is important to keep this procedure as a separate unit operation, as random *in vitro* refolding is very difficult to control and impossible to document. Note that whereas the inclusion bodies from different subbatches can be pooled, the refolding step requires use of single container and uniform conditions. The *in vitro* refolding comprises transfer from the initial denaturation buffer (e.g., in 7 to 8 M urea, 50 to 100 mM cysteine, 1 to 2 mM EDTA buffer at pH 7.5 to 9.0) by means of dilution, desalting, dialysis, size exclusion chromatography, or immobilization technologies to the renaturation buffer (e.g., 1 to 5 mM cysteine, 1 to 2 mM EDTA, cosolvent, buffer pH 7 to 9.5), which is also the composition of the sample for intermediary purification. The sample should be

directly taken to intermediate purification column avoiding excessive handling to prevent aggregation of the newly folded target protein.

The refolding is always carried out at low protein concentration (0.1 to 0.5 mg/mL) to prevent
protein aggregation; as a result, the volume of buffer used at this stage is large. Additionally this
may require use of cosolvents added to the folding buffer, typically salts, sugars, detergents,
sulfobetaines, or short chain alcohols. The most difficult refolding, formation of disulfide bonds
between cysteine residues, is managed by adjusting the redox potential, pH, temperature, conductivity, and protein concentration. Whereas refolding is often spontaneous when the environment is
more oxidizing, a validated system is needed to reduce the loss of proteins at this stage. It is not
uncommon to lose 50% of protein at this stage, and, therefore, to make a commercial yield possible,
this step must be most carefully monitored.

ENZYMATIC CLEAVAGE

The purpose of the cleavage procedure is to remove the N-terminal extension. The enzyme used
to remove the tag must be of nonanimal origin. The enzyme may be immobilized in order to reduce
its amount in the final product. If immobilized folding is being used, the cleavage enzyme may be
added after refolding, thus combining the two operations. A specific immobilized refolding method
using the FXa cleavage site has been described and used in small scale. The folded protein is eluted
from the column by means of FXa, leaving the tag immobilized to the column. The composition
of the sample for polishing depends on the cleavage procedure used. Typical tags are fusion proteins
or repeated histidine sequences. If the second amino acid (N-terminally) is proline, this amino acid
will act as a stop codon for specific di-amino acid exo-peptidases and the tag can be removed
without the enzymatic cleavage site insert. There are several types of cleavage sites, for example,
where there is an enzymatic cleavage site insert between a fusion protein or tag and the mature
protein and thus the cleavage is performed with an endopeptidase, such as Factor Xa (FXa), which
recognizes the sequence -Ile-Glu-Gly-Arg-, resulting in a correct N-terminal sequence of the mature
protein as FXa cleaves after the arginine residue. More than 10 eukaryotic proteins have been
expressed by this method. Another construct type makes use of the exopeptidase, dipeptidyl amino
peptidase I (DPPI), which cleaves every second peptide bond from the N-terminal end of the
molecule except for the amino acid residues Glu or Pro, which act as terminators for proteolytic
degradation. The Glu stop terminator is used in constructs where the second amino acid residue is
not proline. The N-terminal extension, be it a fusion protein, a His-tag, or a few selected amino
acids, must be removed using specific bioprocess grade enzymes of recombinant origin. Well-
characterized bioprocess enzymes for this purpose are rare (an exception is DPPI), limiting the
number of protein constructs to be used in biopharmaceutical processes.

INTERMEDIARY PURIFICATION

The intermediary purification step utilizes techniques like IEC, IMAC, HAC, HIC, or packed bed
to remove cell culture and process-derived impurities and to prepare the sample for polishing.
Anion exchange, cation exchange, or hydroxyapatite chromatography will apply for the purification
step following *in vitro* folding. Chromatography based on hydrophobic interaction should be
avoided, as the renatured protein tends to aggregate during such procedures. The particle size of
media should be in the range of 50 to 120 nm. An important part of the process design is to ensure
a smooth transfer between unit operations, making use of the ability of ion exchangers to bind
proteins at low salt concentrations and hydrophobic interaction media to bind proteins at high salt
concentrations. However, in certain cases buffer exchange or sample concentration is required. It
is recommended to use chromatographic desalting as the buffer exchange principle (no shear forces)
and ultrafiltration (or precipitation) for sample concentration. Note that variations in the composition

of eluted samples (e.g., protein concentration, conductivity, pH) may influence the proceeding sample application and thus interfere with process robustness.

POLISHING

Polishing typically uses techniques like RPC, IEC, or packed bed. This is the most refined step in purification to remove host cell and process and product-related impurities. Powerful chromatographic methods (high performance HP-RPC or HP-IEC) should be used to separate the protein from its derivatives (enzymatic cleaved forms, des-amido forms, oxidized forms, scrambled forms, etc.). To obtain optimal resolution, the particle size of the media should be in the range of 15 to 60 nm.

CONCENTRATION

In most instances, the eluant from the polishing step would provide the final product in a concentrated form. However, in some instances reduction of volume may be required. This can be accomplished by ultrafiltration. See comments under intermediate purification relating to buffer exchange.

FINISHING

This is generally the final step using SEC, desalting, or packed bed. SEC (packed bed) removes di- and polymer forms, small molecules (e.g., endotoxins, cosolvents, leachables), and prepares the drug substance for formulation into drug product. Whereas the host cell proteins are removed all along, DNA is removed by means of anion exchange or hydroxyapatite chromatography (DNA binds strongly to both types), and endotoxins are removed by binding to anion exchange matrices, polymyxin, Sepharose, or histamine-Sepharose; additionally, endotoxins are removed by ultrafiltration, gel filtration, or phase separation with the detergent Triton X114, the final step of finishing ensures that the drug substance is ready to be used in the drug product formulation.

MAMMALIAN CELLS MANUFACTURING SYSTEMS

The main disadvantage in the *de novo* synthesis of recombinant eukaryotic proteins in a prokaryotic system is the improper protein folding and assembly and the lack of posttranslational modification, principally glycosylation and phosphorylation. This leads to utilization of eukaryotic cells, wherein viruses are used as vectors. Eukaryotic expression systems fall into four distinct classes based upon host type: yeast, *Drosophila*, insect (nondrosophila), and mammalian. This chapter highlights the use of mammalian eukaryotic cells; for other types see other chapters.

GENETICALLY MODIFIED CELL LINES

Mammalian cell culture systems offer the distinct advantages of extracellular expression in native form including complex posttranslational modified proteins; the expression vectors are commercially available with large-scale production batches (2 to 5000 L), and the track record for FDA and other regulatory body approvals has been very good. On the negative side, mammalian cells take longer (4 to 6 months) to develop from introduction of gene to protein production; they grow slowly with density not exceeding 100 million cells/mL, and the culture media used is expensive, provides low yields (generally less than 100 mg/L; recently, systems have begun to yield gram quantities per liter), and may contain bovine products, allergens, and low yields; the ICH requirements for characterization are elaborate and extensive as there is a possibility of carrying virus contamination; the process is subject to shear stress and thus difficult to use as suspension culture or even in Wave bioreactors; cell lines are also sensitive to osmolarity changes; and finally there are safety issues in the management of cell lines.

The most popular cell lines used include Chinese hamster ovary (CHO), human cervix (HeLa), African green monkey kidney (COS), baby hamster kidney (BHK) cells, and hybridomas. Well-characterized cell lines can be obtained from the American Type Culture Collection (ATCC) and the European Collection of Cell Cultures (ECACC). These continuous cell lines have the potential of an infinite life span and can usually be cultivated as perfusion cultures. A cell bank system, comprising the master cell bank and the working cell bank, provides the means for production of well-characterized and standardized cells.

The establishment of cell banks for newly developed cell lines is critical to the successful development of many biological products. The cell bank system ensures that the cell line is preserved, its integrity is maintained, and a sufficient supply is readily available. A well-characterized cell bank is the consistent source of production cells throughout the life of the product. Worldwide regulatory authorities require screening cell cultures for the presence of contaminating agents by testing for adventitious viral or microbial agents using both *in vivo* and *in vitro* methodologies. The cGMP compliant preparation of MCBs and MWCBs is performed in a class 100 environment with in-phase testing for mycoplasma and sterility. Cell banks are stored in validated and continuously monitored liquid nitrogen dewars. Given below are suggestions for testing MCBs and end of production cells:

- Microbial Contamination: Sterility (USP 24): Determines the presence of aerobic and anaerobic bacteria and fungi, mycoplasma (1993 PTC CBER/FDA)
- Cell Line Authenticity: Karyology and Isoenzyme analysis determines the species of origin of the cell line
- Transmission Electron Microscopy (TEM): Determines cellular morphology, presence of microbial contaminants, enumeration of retroviral, and retrovirus-like particles
- Endogenous Retroviruses: Reverse transcriptase assays and retroviral infectivity assays detect the presence of retroviruses
- *In vitro* and *in vivo* Adventitious Virus Testing
- Mouse, Rat, and Hamster Antibody Production Assays (MAP, RAP, & HAP): Detects species-specific viruses in rodent cell lines.
- Bovine and Porcine Virus Assays (9 CFR).
- Human Viruses HIV-I and -II, HTLV-I and -II, HAV, HBV, HCV, CMV, EBV, HSV-2, HHV-6, AAV-2, and B-19.
- Primate Viruses SIV, STLV, Foamy Agent, and SMRV.

The following tests are required for the working cell banks:

- Microbial Contamination: Sterility (USP 24) determines the presence of aerobic and anaerobic bacteria and fungi, mycoplasma (1993 PTC CBER/FDA).
- *In vitro* Adventitious Virus Testing.

Eukaryotic expression vectors are of two basic types: virion or virion-plasmid hybrids. Virion-type vectors are most commonly used for the delivery of foreign genes, or a replacement for a defective host gene, into mammalian cell hosts. The virion-plasmid hybrid vectors are used to facilitate the overexpression of protein in native form. Additionally, the availability of authentic pure protein has hastened the development of structure-dependent epitope-specific antibodies to native proteins, the crystallization, and subsequent X-ray/NMR analysis of proteins in their native, correctly folded, posttranslationally modified state, the characterization of gene products for genes whose phenotype may or may not be known, and the isolation of proteins whose native form is in such low abundance that they are very difficult to purify from the original natural organism or tissue. The main features of eukaryotic expression vectors include various sequence elements that explicitly define the level of expression, the transcriptional start and stop points, postprocessing (transcript splicing, poly-adenylation, etc.) transport, selectable markers, and in some cases a peptide tag to facilitate isolation and purification of the gene product. The earliest expression vector, pSV2, is a composite of sequence elements from the papova virus, Simian Virus 40, and the prokaryotic cloning vector, pBR322. SV40 sequence provided transcriptional enhancers, promoter (early region), splicing signal (small t-antigen gene), and the polyadenylation signal element, and pBR322 provided the origin of replication (ori) element. The presence of a selectable marker, pBR322 AmpR gene, completes this model's eukaryotic expression vector. Practically all modern eukaryotic expression vectors possess one or more of these elements. Other viruses used include cytomegalovirus (CMV), Murine sarcoma virus (MSV), Rous sarcoma virus (RSV), Mouse mammary tumor virus (MMTV), and Semliki Forest Virus (SFV).

Generally, recombinant proteins are expressed in a constitutive manner in most eukaryotic expression systems and frequently with inducible promoters such as heat shock protein, metallothionein, and human and mouse growth hormone, MMTV-LTR, and inducible enhancer elements ecdysone, muristerone A, and tetracycline/doxycycline.

Two principal strategies have been employed to increase cell productivity: gene regulation and gene amplification. Gene regulation aims to increase the number of times a single gene is transcribed and then translated into product. Gene amplification aims to increase the number of genes that are available for transcription to produce the product (e.g., use of BPV virus, use of DNA amplifying drugs such as methotrexate).

Commercial systems that incorporate the entire gene sequence to support the expression of desired proteins are available from Clontech, Invitrogen, Novagen, Life Technologies, Promega, Pharmacia Biotech (GE), Strategene, Quantum Biotech, and many more. Selectable markers generally are either recessive or dominant; the recessive markers are usually genes that encode products that are not produced in the host cells (cells that lack the "marker" product or function). Marker genes for thymidine kinase (TK), dihydrofolate reductase (DHFR), adenine phosphoribosyl transferase (APRT), and hypoxanthine-guanine phosphoribosyl transferase (HGPRT) are in this category. Dominant markers include genes that encode products that confer resistance to growth-suppressing compounds (antibiotics, drugs) or permit growth of the host cells in metabolically restrictive environments. Commonly used markers within this category include a mutant DHFR gene that confers resistance to methotrexate; the gpt gene for xanthine-guanine phosphoribosyl transferase, which permits host cell growth in mycophenolic acid/xanthine containing media; and the neo gene for aminoglycoside 3'-phosphotransferase, which can confer resistance to G418, gentamycin, kanamycin, and neomycin. Practically all eukaryotic expression vectors used today possess at least one marker from either or both of these categories, although dominant markers are the most common.

Host-range specificity for virion vectors is determined primarily by the presence of recognizable host cell surface receptors, whereas for virion-plasmid hybrid vectors, the determinant is the degree to which the host's cellular machinery recognizes the transcriptional control signals of the hybrid vector. Transcriptional enhancers appear to be the primary determinants of cell-type specificity.

After the target gene has been engineered into the appropriate cloning vector, the vector will need to be introduced into the host cell. Given the infectious nature of the viruses from which most eukaryotic expression vectors are derived, it would seem that the introduction of the vector into the host would be rather straightforward. Unfortunately, this process can be complicated.

The introduction of the vector into mammalian cells can be effected by microinjection, electroporation, and calcium phosphate-, DEAE-dextran-, polybrene-, DMSO-, or cationic lipid-mediated transfection. Although the method of choice usually depends on the cell type and cloning application, cationic lipids or liposome-mediated transfection protocols generally yield the highest and most consistent transfection efficiencies in mammalian cell systems. Thus, many corporate suppliers of expression systems recommend a lipid-based transfection protocol, with many providing proprietary liposome reagents (for example, Clonetech's Clonfectin Transfection Reagent, Novogen's GeneJuice, Invitrogen's PerFect Transfection Kit, Promega's Transfection and Tfx-50 reagents, or Life Technologies Lipofectin Reagent).

TABLE 6.1
Principles of Techniques Used to Remove Various Adventitious Agents

Principle	Endotoxins	Nucleic Acids	Viruses	Note
Anion exchange	++	+++	+++	Strongly basic IgGs and IgMs form stable complexes with DNA, especially at low conductivity reducing clearance.
Cation exchange	+	+++	++	Nucleic acids do not bind to cation exchangers.
HIC	+	+++	++	Nucleic acids do not bind to HIC media. Antibody-nucleic acid complexes are dissociated at high salt concentrations. Endotoxins may form micelles or higher secondary structures in aqueous solutions, especially at high salt concentrations and thus get excluded from the matrix.
Hydroxyapatite	+	+	+	Nucleic acid clearance is variable in phosphate gradients.
IMAC	++	++	+++	Assuming similar purification properties as for Protein A.
Protein A	++	++	+++	Complexes between monoclonal antibodies and nucleic acids are dissociated at high salt concentrations tolerated in the Protein A application.
Size exclusion	+	+	+	Nucleic acids form complexes with monoclonal antibodies at low conductivity resulting in a reduced clearance factor. The endotoxin clearance factor is less for IgM.

MONOCLONAL ANTIBODIES PRODUCTION

Monoclonal antibodies are expressed in mammalian cells and also in mouse ascites. This section refers to special considerations involved in the production of monoclonal antibodies using mammalian cells. The typical expression level of the target protein is from 50 to 1000 mg/L. The protein purification strategy takes into consideration the poor stability at pH below 4.5 and irreversible structural changes that may result in loss of immunoactivity. This consideration is different from the manufacturing of other classes of therapeutic proteins where the goal is to keep the protein as nonimmunogenic as possible through structural modifications. IgM tends to precipitate at low conductivity where the protein is in its pentameric form. Generally, IgMs are less stable than IgGs. Most IgGs are stable and soluble at medium to high pH and low conductivity, a condition often used in application samples for chromatographic procedures. However, some mAbs (up to 20% of IgMs) are cryoglobulins with reduced solubility below 37°C. MAbs being highly basic, form stable ionic complexes with polyvalent anions (phosphate, citrate, sulfate, borate). The complexes easily aggregate. MAbs also form complexes with nucleic acids; the reaction can be reversed in presence of 0.3 to 1.0M NaCl. MAbs strongly bind to divalent metal ions; the result in the net charge of the molecule leads to destabilization. Table 6.1 lists the principles used to remove adventitious agents in the manufacturing of human monoclonal antibodies. Many of these principles apply to removal of adventitious agents in general as well.

UPSTREAM PROCESS OPTIMIZATION

Commercial-scale manufacturing is carried out in closed reactors with no or limited supply of medium (batch or rarely fed-batch mode) or in bioreactors allowing media throughput with cell retention (perfusion systems). Immobilized cells can be utilized in both modes resulting in cell densities from 10^6 cells/mL (suspension cultures) to 10^8 cells/mL (immobilized cells). The productivity of batch cultures is often relatively high (up to 2 g/L for antibodies), but product stability, toxicity, and bioreactor volume reduction make perfusion bioreactors fairly competitive. The total process yield following downstream processing may be better using the perfusion mode (less purification problems due to higher quality of the starting material), despite the slightly lower productivity.

There are two types of media used, one as a growth media to support multiplication of cells and production media to maintain cells in the most productive phase. The culture media used for establishing master cell banks still uses serum; but the fact that MCB is extensively characterized, the use of serum is justified. However, the rest of the media used should be free of adventitious agents (e.g., viruses, prions), which restricts use of fetal calf serum, peptones of animal origin, and porcine trypsin. Several commercial suppliers distribute these types of media and the claims made regarding their suitability should be evaluated vis-à-vis the process requirements. The serum-free media consist of salts, vitamins, amino acids, and carbohydrates supplemented with specific growth and attachment factors such as insulin, IGF-1, transferrin, epidermal growth factor, somatostatin, fibronectin, and collagen. In addition, cells often need steroid-type hormones such as dexamethasone, testosterone, progesterone, and hydrocortisone and lipid-based factors including phospholipids, cholesterol, and sphingomyelin. Protein additives (e.g., albumin, transferrin, growth factors, peptones) are often of recombinant or plant origin. Albumin, which is the most important protein of all animal sera, is included in many serum-free media. It exhibits a number of functions (transport, detoxification, buffering, mechanical protection against shear forces). However, the growth stimulatory effect seems to be associated with a factor not present in the recombinant form, indicating that recombinant albumin can only partially replace the natural source. Transferrin, which transports Fe-ions to the cells, is used in almost any serum-free medium or is replaced with iron complexes (e.g., ferri-sulfate, iminodiacetic acid complexes, ferri-sulfate-glycine-glycine-complexes, ferri-citrate, ferri-tropolone, phosphate compounds). Peptones are often produced from Soya by enzymatic degradation. Typical concentrations of additives are 5 mg/L of insulin, 5 to 35 mg/L of transferring, 20 µM of ethanolamine, and 5 µg of selenium. Sometimes sodium carboxymethyl cellulose (0.1%) is added to prevent mechanical damage to cells. Pluronic F68 (0.1%) is used to reduce foaming and to protect cells from bubble shear forces in sparged cultures.

Cell detachment has been achieved by the use of trypsin or trypsin/EDTA derived from porcine or bovine pancreas. Serum-free media are devoid of the antitrypsin activity of serum, and trypsin has been sought to replace dispase I/II, papain, or pronase or by use of thermo-responsive polymer surfaces.

N-linked glycosylation is a posttranslational modification commonly performed on proteins by eukaryotic cells and it can significantly alter the efficacy of a human therapeutic protein. The use of mammalian cells, such as Chinese hamster ovary (CHO) cells, for the commercial production of recombinant human proteins, is often attributed to their ability to impart desired glycosylation features on proteins. An essential step in N-linked glycosylation is the transfer of oligosaccharide from a lipid in the endoplasmic reticulum membrane to an asparagine residue within a specific amino acid consensus sequence on a nascent polypeptide. In cultured cells, this reaction does not occur at every identical potential glycosylation site on different molecules of the same protein. The resulting variation in the extent of glycosylation for a given protein is known as site occupancy heterogeneity. Although current regulatory practice permits product heterogeneity, demonstration of specific and reproducible glycosylation is required. Hence, heterogeneity in protein glycosylation presents special challenges to the development and production of a candidate therapeutic with consistent properties. In view of the inevitable occurrence and significance of glycosylation heterogeneity in protein therapeutics derived from mammalian cells, much research has been directed toward understanding factors that influence glycosylation heterogeneity during a bioprocess. When using CHO cells, there occurs a gradual decline in glycosylation site occupancy over the course of batch and fed-batch cultures of recombinant CHO cells: the proportion of fully glycosylated molecule can decrease by 9 to 25% during the exponential growth phase. This deterioration in glycosylation does not arise from extracellular degradation of product, nor could it be overcome by supplementation of the cultures with extra nutrients, such as nucleotide sugars, glucose, and glutamine. Certain lipid supplements can minimize the glycosylation changes; since lipid-linked oligosaccharides (LLOs) are the oligosaccharide donors in N-linked glycosylation, their availability may be a key regulatory mechanism for controlling the extent of protein glycosylation. Inadequate formation or excessive degradation of LLOs can result in LLO shortages and consequently limit cellular glycosylation capacity. Under subsaturating LLO levels, a gradual decrease in the intracellular pool of LLOs would lead to a corresponding decrease in protein glycosylation. The CHO cells glycosylate their proteins to a gradually increasing extent as culture progresses, until the onset of massive cell death (15 to 25%). The glycosylation site occupancy of different proteins may undergo distinct changes over the length of culture even though the net glycosylation efficiency in CHO cells improves with cultivation time. The glycosylation pattern of each individual glycoprotein product needs to be tracked over the course of the culture because different proteins may exhibit different glycosylation variations with time, even when the same culture method is used.

Process parameters of importance in optimizing mammalian cell yields include:

- pH, which is optimal at 6.8 to 7.2; lower pH inhibits growth; since CO_2 is generated, control of pH throughout fermentation may be needed due to formation of lactic acid. pH must be controlled to compensate lactic acid formation by adjusting supply of CO_2. The problems associated with deterioration of pH measuring devices as described in bacterial cell culture applies here as well.
- Redox potential optimal value is +75 mV, which equals a pO_2 of 8 to 10%, which is approximately 50% of air saturation. The redox potential depends on the concentration of reducing and oxidizing agents, the temperature, and the pH of the solution. The redox potential falls under logarithmic growth and is at its lowest 24 h before the onset of stationary phase.
- Dissolved oxygen should be in the range 0.06 to 0.3 μmol oxygen/106 cells/h. As oxygen solubility in aqueous solutions is very low (7.6 μg/mL) the oxygen transfer rate (OTR) is a main limiting factor when scaling up cell cultures.
- The optimal temperature range is from 33 to 38°C. The relative low level of metabolic activity makes it easier to control temperature in animal cell bioreactors.
- Osmolality in culture medium used with lepidopteran cell lines is 345 to 380 mOsm/kg.
- Agitation rate ranging from 50 to 200 rpm are common but need optimization depending on the size of equipment.
- Ammonia production rate (mmol/106 cells/h) is an indicator of metabolic rate and should be continuously measured and kept under control. The specific ammonia production rate (mmol/10^6 cells/h) is an indicator of metabolic rate. Analysis of ammonia can be performed using a BioProfile 100 analyzer or similar instrument. Ammonia may also be determined using an enzyme based assay kit.
- Glucose levels should be analyzed to monitor glucose utilization (mmol/106 cells/h) as an indicator of metabolic rate.
- Glutamine, an essential amino acid for cell growth, should not be used as an energy source. The metabolic product, ammonia, which is toxic to the cells, should be controlled. The glutamine concentration should be kept in the range of 2 to 8 mM.
- Lactate is formed by conversion of glucose — a balance between glycolysis and oxidation of glucose is maintained.
- pCO_2 is used to adjust the CO_2 flow to regulate the pH of the cell culture, and the flow is maintained only as long as the pH is above the set point. In late stage cultures the CO_2 to HCO_3 buffer system is no longer sufficient to maintain pH and sodium hydrogen carbonate or NaOH is used instead.
- Foam level is controlled by addition of antifoam agents.

Growth rates are measured in terms of cell density (using a hematocytometer); cell viability is tested using trypan blue, erythrosine staining, or electronic counting (e.g., Coulter counter) and specific production rates are monitored using a cell-hour approach, which expresses the relationship between protein productivity and cell population dynamics. LDH activity reflects the extent of cell lyses, since LDH is not secreted by mammalian cells. The concentration of the reduced form of nicotinamide adenine dinucleotide or its phosphorylated form correlates with cell mass during the lag phase and exponential growth phase and provides information of the physiological state of the culture. The reduced form fluoresce at 460 nm when irradiated with light at 340 nm, while the oxidized form does not fluoresce. Various amino acids can be analyzed by HP-RPC after derivatization with o-phthaldehyde, 3-mercaptopropionic acid, and 9-fluorenylmethylchloroformate using a fluorescence detector. Glutamine can be analyzed using a BioProfile 100 analyzer or similar instrument.

Adventitious agents are tested at the end of the cell culture in the unprocessed bulk and where multiple harvest pools are prepared at different times, the culture is tested at the time of the collection of each pool. The test program should include tests for bacteria, fungi, mycoplasma, and viruses. Tests for adventitious viruses in continuous cell line cultures used for expression of recombinant proteins should include inoculation onto mono-layer cultures of the same species and tissue type as that used for production of human diploid cell line, or another cell line from a different species. If appropriate, a PCR test or another suitable method may be used. When cells are readily accessible (e.g., hollow fiber), the unprocessed bulk would constitute harvest from the fermenter.

DOWNSTREAM PROCESS OPTIMIZATION

Since the target protein is typically expressed directly to the medium, the typical procedures of harvest, capture, intermediary purification, and polishing are used, in addition to viral clearance steps where required (when used, it is advisable to clear virus as early as possible despite the difficulties in handling early samples of media due to their viscosity etc.). Since mammalian cell lines are subject to shear, milder bioreactor conditions are used; roller bottles are still widely used despite the high cost; similarly the downstream processes chosen should be of such nature as to maintain the structural integrity of protein. For example, the use of chromatographic desalting as the buffer exchange principle (no shear forces) and ultrafiltration (or precipitation) for sample concentration are recommended. The process design should ensure a smooth transfer between unit operations, making use of the ability of ion exchangers to bind proteins at low salt concentrations and hydrophobic interaction media to bind proteins at high salt concentrations fully coordinated.

Harvest

Harvesting conditions the sample for the capture step. Cells and cell debris are typically removed by means of centrifugation, microfiltration, or expanded bed technology. The expanded bed technology may prove impractical due to cell aggregation. Several new membrane technologies obviate the problems of cell aggregation and improve the efficiency of tangential flow filtration. Mammalian cell cultures are sometimes carried out as continuous cultures running over several weeks (typically from 4 to 8 weeks). The harvest is collected into subbatches at regular intervals and sometimes even processed further before pooling. It should be emphasized that each subbatch must undergo testing before being added to the pool of batches in order to demonstrate process control.

Capture

Capture removes cell culture and process-derived impurities and prepares the sample for intermediary purification. Both packed bed and expanded bed technology are used. The typical chromatographic capture procedure used is ion exchange chromatography, although affinity or hydrophobic interaction chromatography work for some proteins. Presence of antifoam agents in the harvest may eliminate use of HIC due to their relative high hydrophobicity. The particle size of chromatographic media is ideally in the range of 100 to 300 nm.

Several purification principles are suited for capture purification of IgG. Protein A affinity chromatography has been used in a number of cases, but the less common Protein G or IMAC technology should offer advantages such as many monoclonal antibodies bind strongly to metal affinity matrices. Note that monoclonal antibodies bind to nucleic acids and divalent metal ions. Protein A binds to all subclasses of human IgG (except for IgG class 3) in the Fc region at neutral to alkaline pH with low to high conductivity. Generally, only slight adjustment of the culture medium is needed for application and binding, although high ionic strength increases the binding capacity of the column. The binding is unaffected by the nature and variations of the glycosylation pattern. The mAb is eluted by decreasing pH, but the instability at low pH must seriously be taken into consideration. Addition of cosolvents, such as 30 to 60% ethylene glycol or 1 to 2 M urea to the buffer, is sometimes used to elute the protein at a higher pH. Further, a stabilizing effect is obtained if the mAb is eluted into a neutral pH buffer. If fetal calf serum has been added to the culture medium, bovine IgG may amount to up to 50% of the IgG eluted. Several IgMs bind to Protein A, but elution often requires lower pH than 4.5, which seriously challenges the protein stability. Leakage of the Protein A ligand is a serious drawback and specific analytical assays must be introduced to prove efficient removal. IMAC is a very attractive capture purification principle for IgGs, which binds to metal chelating columns at neutral to alkaline pH (buffers containing chelating agents, free ammonium ions, free amino acids, amines, or aminated zwitterion should not be used). The binding is relatively independent of salt concentration and the presence of nonionic detergents and urea in low concentrations. The cell culture medium can therefore be applied to the column with little or no conditioning. Elution is performed by decreasing pH in the range of 8 to 4, mainly reflecting titration of histidyl residues or with chelating agents such as EDTA displacing the metal from the column. Leakage of Ni^{++} or similar metal ions must be expected, and thus further purification is needed in subsequent steps. Although IMAC can be used virtually anywhere in the downstream process with only minor adjustment of the application sample, the capture features dominate because there is little or no adjustment of the large volume of cell culture application sample required, the majority of contaminants pass through the column at loading conditions, and metal ions can be removed in later steps. IMAC binds IgG from more species and subclasses than do Protein A and it operates under far milder conditions. It is less expensive and does not leach cytotoxic biological material into the product. IMAC will selectively recover intact IgG from supernatants in which the light chain is in surplus. It should be emphasized that the expanded bed technology offers the advantages of very gentle isolation of the expressed mAb, saving at least one centrifugation or filtration step.

Virus Inactivation

Inactivation is typically (but not necessarily) performed after the capture step, where the sample volume has been severely reduced. The virus inactivation program should be linked to the infectious viruses used for transfection of the cells.

Intermediary Purification

This step removes cell culture and process-derived impurities and prepares the sample for polishing. The intermediary purification step offers a wide range of chromatographic principles (IMAC, HIC, IEC, HAC). The particle size of chromatographic media should be in the range of 50 to 120 nm. Both cation and anion exchange chromatography (IEC) are suited purification principles for all mAbs, although the former is restricted in that very few mAbs are soluble at low pH and low conductivity. Binding conditions and choice of ion exchange depend on the pI of the antibody and thus some IgG class 3 mAb may be too basic to support high binding capacities on anion exchangers. Hydrophobic interaction chromatography (HIC) is applicable to all mAbs. Application in highly concentrated salt solutions and elution in low conductivity buffers may result in precipitation of the antibody, and care should therefore be taken to investigate the stability of the mAb under these conditions. Mixed mode ion exchangers, such as hydroxyapatite, are suited to the purification principle, also for IgM. However, chelating agents cannot be tolerated in the application buffer and the matrix does not withstand acidic pH buffers.

VIRUS FILTRATION

The techniques used for virus filtration include pH modification, addition of detergents, and use of microwave heating. Membrane filtration can contribute to the overall virus reduction in a reliable and controlled manner without damaging the target protein. In many cases large viruses could be removed to the detection limit of the assay used. Small viruses (e.g., parvoviruses) may require filtration through special membranes that have limited protein transmission. cGMP facilities are typically divided into an area where viruses are expected to be present (harvest and capture) and nonvirus areas potentially free of viruses. An early virus filtration step is recommended if the viscosity and particulates levels would allow an effective process (Table 6.1).

POLISHING

Polishing removes host cells and process and product-related impurities. Powerful chromatographic methods (HP-IEC) should be used to separate the protein from its derivatives (enzymatic cleaved forms, des-amido forms, oxidized forms, scrambled forms, etc.). The polishing step makes use of the most highly developed purification methods to obtain optimal resolution. The particle size of chromatographic media should be in the range of 15 to 60 nm.

FINISHING

Finishing removes di- and polymer forms and small molecules (e.g., endotoxins, cosolvents, leachables) and allows for easy reformulation of the drug substance. Techniques used include SEC, desalting, and packed bed. The high molecular weight of IgM at 900 KDa makes SEC a powerful purification tool for IgM antibodies

YEAST CELL EXPRESSION SYSTEM

The use of nonmammalian hosts has a distinct generic advantage that these hosts are generally regarded as safe since they are not pathogenic to humans. Yeasts are particularly attractive as they can be rapidly grown on minimal (inexpensive) media. Recombinants can be easily selected by complementation, using any of a number of selectable (complementation) markers. Expressed proteins can be specifically engineered for cytoplasmic localization or for extracellular export. And finally, yeasts are exceedingly well suited for large-scale fermentation to produce large quantities of heterologous protein. Classical studies in yeast genetics have generated a wide array of potential cloning vectors and, in the process, defined which plasmid and host genomic sequences are important in expression technology.

    In summary, the yeast culture system has many significant advantages such as it is easy and cheap to grow in large scale, it has a good regulatory track record, the genetics of yeast is well understood, it allows some posttranslational modifications, there is a short doubling time, high cell densities and yield are achievable, there is no endotoxin release from host cell organism, extra-cellular expression to low viscosity medium is possible, there is only minor secretion of host cell proteins, no specialized bioreactor is required, and it is safer than working with mammalian tissue or cell lines.

The disadvantages of yeast system include problems with correct glycosylation, overglycosylation can ruin protein bioactivity, glycosylation is not identical to mammalian glycosylation, extensive proteolysis of target protein, nonnative proteins are not always correctly folded, fewer cloning vectors are available, gene expression is less easy to control, and *S Saccharomyces cerevisiae* is unable to excise introns in gene transcripts of higher eukaryotes.

The use of yeast expression systems involves an entirely different set of techniques and principles than those used for other eukaryotic or prokaryotic systems. Commonly used yeast hosts are *S. cerevisiae*, *Schizosaccharomyces pombe*, *Pichia pastoris*, *Hansela polymorpha*, *Kluyveromyces lactis*, and *Yarrowia lipolytica*. Newer research tools like lithium acetate and electroporation-mediated transformation of intact yeast cells and the creation of 2μ yeast episomal plasmids have helped yeast rise to the most favorite list of expression systems.

Wild-type yeasts are prototrophic, that is, they are nutritionally self-sufficient, capable of growing on minimal media. Classical genetic studies have created auxotrophic strains — those that require specific nutritional supplements to grow in minimal media. The nutritional requirements of the auxotrophic strains are the basis for selection of successfully transformed strains. By including a gene in the plasmid expression cassette that complements one or more defective genes in the host auxotroph, one can easily select recombinants on minimal media. Hence, strains requiring leucine will grow on minimal media if they harbor a plasmid expressing the LEU2 gene. The most commonly used selectable markers found in yeast are for leucine, uracil, histidine, and tryptophan deficiencies.

Although the number and variety of *S. cerevisiae* and *S. pombe* strains possessing nutrition selectable markers make these yeasts attractive hosts, their limitations include hyperglycosylation; weak, poorly regulated promoters; and biomass fermentation. Many of these and other problems are circumvented using *P. pastoris. K. lactis,* and *Y. lipolytica* that have been extensively utilized in the industrial-scale production of metabolites and native proteins (for example, β-galactosidase). Vector-host genetic incompatibilities and a relatively undefined biology have limited their use as heterologous expression hosts.

The methylotrophic yeast, *H. polymorpha*, and to a greater extent *P. pastoris* — unique in that they will grow using methanol as the sole carbon source — are becoming a favorite expression host alternative for many researchers. *P. pastoris* has produced some of the highest heterologous protein yields to date (12 g/L fermentation culture), 10- to 100-fold higher than in *S. cerevisiae*. In *P. pastoris*, growth in methanol is mediated by alcohol oxidase, an enzyme whose de novo synthesis is tightly regulated by the alcohol oxidase promoter. The enzyme has a very low specific activity. To compensate for this, it is overproduced, accounting for more than 30% of the total soluble protein in methanol-induced cells. Thus, by engineering a heterologous protein gene downstream of the genomic AOX1 promoter, one can induce its overproduction. This is the basis for the *P. pastoris* expression system. *H. polymorpha* produces the methanol oxidase (MOX) protein under control of the MOX1 promoter. A complete *P. pastoris* expression system is available from Invitrogen.

Most yeast vectors for protein expression contain one or more of these basic elements: the *S. cerevisiae* 2μ plasmid origin of replication, a ColE1 element, a antibiotic resistance "marker" gene (to aid development and screening of plasmid constructs in *E. coli*, a heterologous (constitutive or inducible) promoter, a termination signal, signal sequence (encoding secretion leader peptides), and occasionally fusion protein genes (to facilitate purification).

Constitutive gene expression by the yeast plasmid cassette is commonly mediated (in *S. cerevisiae* and *S. pombe*) by the promoters for genes to the glycolytic enzymes: glyceraldehyde-3-phosphate dehydrogenase (TDH3), triose phosphate isomerase (TPI1), or phosphoglycerate isomerase (PGK1). Protein expression can also be regulated (induced) using the alcohol dehydrogenase isozyme II (ADH2) gene promoter (glucose-repressed), glucocorticoid responsive elements (GREs, induced with deoxycorticosterone), GAL1 and GAL10 promoters (to control galactose utilization pathway enzymes, which are glucose-repressed and galactose-induced), the metallothionein promoter from the CUP1 gene (induced by copper sulfate), and the PHO5 promoter (induced by phosphate limitation). Most native yeast gene termination signals, when included in the plasmid expression cassette, will provide proper termination of RNA transcripts. The most commonly used are terminator signals for the MF-alpha-1, TPI1, CYC1, and PGK1 genes.

Complete packaged system for quickly developing yeast expression systems are available from Clontech, Invitrogen or Stratagene, and others. For example, Invitrogen sells an expression vector for *S. cerevisiae* and a complete system for *P. pastoris* expression cloning. The Easy Select Pichia Expression Kit includes vectors (pPICZ series), *P. pastoris* strains, reagents for transformation, sequencing primers, media, and a comprehensive manual. Researchers can clone their protein gene into any reading frame contained in each of three different vectors, select recombinants by Zeocin resistance, induce protein expression with methanol (sole carbon source), and identify expression using antibody to a C-terminal c-myc peptide tag. These vectors also harbor an *S. cerevisiae* alpha-factor secretion gene and polyHIS-encoding element, thus expressed protein is easily recovered from culture extract supernatant and purified using metal-chelate chromatography (for example, ProBond resin packaged in Invitrogen's Xpress Purification System).

The yeast species *S. cerevisiae* and *P. pastoris* are the most widely used species for therapeutic protein manufacturing as they offer high efficiency, lower cost, and large yields (10G+/L). The development time from introduced gene to protein is about 14 days (in comparison *E. coli* is 5 days and mammalian cells from 4 to 5 months). In contrast to *E. coli*, yeast can express correctly folded proteins directly to the medium, which greatly facilitates purification (low level of host cell proteins, nonviscous solution, low DNA level). The rigid cell wall renders the use of all sorts of bioreactors possible regardless of stirring and shaking mechanisms. Yeast cell cultures have been widely used for the production of biopharmaceuticals such as insulin, streptokinase, hirudin, interferons, tissue necrosis factor, tissue plasminogen activator, hepatitis B vaccine, and epidermal growth factor.

Large-scale operations are associated with a number of restrictions related to host strain physiology and fermentation technology. Many promoter systems that work well in small scale cannot be implemented in production processes demanding a substantial number of generations. Use of low-expression cassettes reduces the loss of plasmid to some extent, but a profound effect on productivity may be observed due to lack of stability. Expression systems characterized by a high specific rate of product formation at low specific growth rates are highly favorable for large-scale operations. Oxygen demand and temperature control are key factors in controlling yeast fermentations, which are mainly carried out as fed-batch cultivations. Proteolysis of the target protein can be a major problem.

CELL SUBSTRATES

S. CEREVISIAE

The baker's yeast *S. cerevisiae* is the most extensively studied yeast strain. Its genetics are well known and it has obtained a generally regarded as safe (GRAS) status. Protease deficient strains such as BT150, deficient in proteases A and B, carboxypeptidase Y, and carboxypeptidase S, are available. *S. cerevisiae* exhibit alcoholic fermentation under aerobic conditions, unless the sugar supply rate is low. This response occurs at glucose concentrations of 0.15 g/L, hence, the demand for low sugar supply rate (which is growth limiting). To prevent this, the use of nonrepressing substrates, such as raffinose or continuous culture, are employed. It is common practice to measure the ethanol concentration or the respiratory quotient (RQ). An indirect feedback control of RQ data has been applied to ensure effective production (RQ < 1.3), but it must be kept in mind that the low growth rate may affect target protein expression.

A commonly employed strategy when expressing recombinant proteins in yeast is to put the gene of interest under the control of an inducible promoter. The use of inducible promoters (e.g., GAL1 induced by galactose) provides for the separation of growth and recombinant protein production. There is no strong inducible promoter available in *S. cerevisiae*, and the expression of recombinant protein will only amount to about 1 to 5% of total cellular protein, as compared to 35% in *P. pastoris*. An example is the expression of recombinant Hirudin, a thrombin inhibitor and therapeutic for cardiovascular diseases. If separation of growth and production is not desired (e.g., if protein expression is growth associated) the use of a constitutive promoter such as PHO5 can be employed.

The stability of the expression cassette has a high impact on productivity. Loss of the cassette during the course of the fermentation results in formation of nonproductive, plasmid free cells, which usually outgrow plasmid-carrying cells in fermentation unless selective pressure can be effectively employed. More than 30 generations are required from stock culture to the final stage, and if the expression cassette is lost during the process, this will result in loss of productivity.

To target the recombinant protein for secretion a signal sequence is needed. This can be derived directly from the protein of interest if it is recognized and correctly processed in yeast. If not, the signal sequence of the *S. cerevisiae*-mating pre-pro leader sequence or invertase may be used. This signal directs the recombinant protein to the endoplasmatic reticulum for further processing and secretion.

Although *S. cerevisiae* has been fermented in several different ways, the fermentation protocol of *P. pastoris* cultures is, broadly speaking, nearly always the same — generating biomass by growing on excess glycerol then inducing protein production with methanol. It is a three-stage combination of batch and fed-batch modes. The first stage is a 24-hour glycerol batch usually conducted with 4% v/v glycerol. The end of this stage is indicated by a sharp rise in dissolved oxygen (DO) after which a glycerol fed-batch phase is started, typically with a 50% v/v glycerol solution at a feed rate of 15 ml/L. This phase de-represses the AOX1 promoter and must last for at least one hour. Examples of glycerol fed-batch stages lasting all the way up to 32 h have been employed. The third stage, a methanol fed-batch, is initiated either with a 100% methanol feed when the last batch of glycerol is exhausted or by slowly adapting the cells to growing on methanol typically on 5% v/v methanol while still feeding glycerol. This induction phase triggers the production of heterologous protein and usually lasts about 80 to 90 h. Tight control of the methanol concentration is obtained by regularly performing "spike tests" to make sure the methanol is present at limiting amounts. The rapid proliferation of *P. pastoris* cells set high demands to oxygen supply and cooling.

The nutritional needs of yeast are simple and depend on the yeast species, strain, and growth conditions. The main culture media components are: a carbon source (which also functions as the energy source), salts, trace elements, nitrogen, and growth factors.

For *S. cerevisiae* fermentations, glucose is often chosen as the carbon source because of its inexpensiveness and relative high solubility, whereas for *Pichia pastoris* fermentations glycerol and methanol are used. The growth factor requirements vary in a case-to-case manner. *S. cerevisiae* has in some cases a requirement for inositol, pantothenate, pyridoxine, thiamine, nicotinic acid, and biotin, whereas *P. pastoris* has been reported to require biotin.

P. PASTORIS

P. pastoris is a methylotrophic yeast, which means that it can grow on methanol as the only carbon source. The knowledge of this yeast's genetics stems from the extensive research on the production of single-cell protein (SCP). It is characterized as glucose insensitive yeast. *P. pastoris* has a high oxygen demand, and the fermentation of this yeast generates considerable amounts of heat. It has the advantage of a very strong inducible promoter, the AOX1 promoter. The AOX1 gene encodes one of two alcohol oxidases expressed in the presence of methanol. When growing on glucose, transcription from the AOX1 promoter is completely repressed even in the presence of methanol. Growth on glycerol allows for induction with methanol, but the total effect of glycerol is not completely understood. It has become evident that glycerol, even at low levels, also inhibits expression from the AOX1 promoter, though not as pronounced as glucose. The availability of the strong AOX1 has provided for protein expression levels as high as 22 g/L for intracellular expressed proteins and 11 g/L for secreted ones. In contrast to *S. cerevisiae* this species exhibits a relatively short glycosylation chain length, and the major problem is enzymic deglycosylation and varying glycosylation patterns.

CELL CULTURES

Yeast can grow both anaerobically and aerobically. In anaerobic growth, most of the carbon substrate is metabolized into inorganic substances, like ethanol and carbon dioxide, making this growth less desirable for protein production. The preferred large-scale aerobic fermentation yields more biomass. However, the presence of high levels of readily metabolically available sugars (e.g., glucose) represses aerobic respiration (the Crab-tree effect) in certain yeast species (e.g., *S. cerevisiae*) and it can be difficult in practice to completely suppress the anaerobic growth. The use of a nonrepressing substrates (e.g., raffinose) or continuous culture is often employed to overcome this problem.

Basically the fermentation of yeast can be divided into two modes: batch systems with its different variants, and continuous systems. The classical batch systems offer minor risks, relative inexpensiveness, and well-tested procedures. The Crab-tree effect of *S. cerevisiae* and other limiting factors of batch fermentations have led to the development of fed-batch systems, and this is now the most commonly employed fermentation strategy. Continuous modes offer the possibility of prolonged fermentation, high productivity, and greater flexibility than do batch modes. However, the higher risk of contamination and greater expense make it less amenable. When choosing fermentation mode, the volumetric productivity, final product concentration, stability, and reproducibility must be considered in a case-to-case manner.

BATCH CULTURE

The batch culture is a closed system with a definite amount of nutrients and one single harvest. The cells follow classic kinetics with a log phase of rapid proliferation where some products are produced and a stationary phase where the amount of cells does not change and where other products are produced. If the desired product is produced in the log phase, it can be prolonged by manipulating the growth conditions but only for a very limited time. If the desired amount is not produced that quickly, it will be reasonable to choose another culture method. When fermenting *S. cerevisiae,* the cells will start by producing ethanol due to the Crab-tree effect and will not enter the log phase of aerobic respiration until the sugar level is low enough. The osmotic sensitivity of yeast cells puts another constraint on the initial sugar concentration. In addition to these disadvantages, batch culture does not allow for control of the growth rate and the culture becomes rapidly limited by oxygen. Altogether these factors restrict the duration of batch fermentations. Higher yield of biomass can be achieved in batch fermentations by keeping the sugar level low, using a glucose insensitive yeast like *Candida*, or replacing glucose with a nonrepressive substrate such as acetate, galactose, or glycerol.

FED-BATCH CULTURE

Another solution to the problems with the Crab-tree effect and osmotic sensitivity is to conduct the fermentation in a fed-batch mode. Medium is added in fixed volumes throughout the process, thus increasing the volume of the cell culture with time. Neither cells nor medium are leaving the bioreactor. In this way the sugar levels can be kept low for a long time and it is possible to switch from one substrate to another, thus rendering the use of inducible promoters possible. The process is usually performed at low growth rates with the key control parameter being the feed rate whose upper limit is dictated by the oxygen transfer limit and cooling strategies available. The feed rate is often subjected to feedback control strategies, using, for example, measurement of the RQ, biomass production, or heat generation. In *S. cerevisiae* this feedback includes on-line analysis of glucose and ethanol, whereas *P. pastoris* fermentations often are controlled by either direct on-line measurement of methanol but more frequently by "spike tests." The "spike tests" confirm that the compound in question (e.g., methanol, glycerol, glucose) is the rate-limiting factor. Variants of the classical fed-batch strategy, such as semi-fed-batch where nutrients and vitamins are added in dry form but do not change the culture volume, have also been employed with success.

PERFUSION CULTURE

An alternative approach to batch cultivation is to continuously add fresh medium to the bioreactor and to remove equivalent amounts of medium with cells. Continuous cultures are performed at low dilution rates usually up to 0.3 h^{-1}. It has been reported that higher dilution rates cause washout even though successful fermentation has been performed with dilution rates up to 0.6 h^{-1} after a time of adaptation. Low dilution rates usually promote a high yield of biomass and a RQ of about 1. In *S. cerevisiae* fermentations, high dilution rates promote a switch to anaerobic fermentation because of too much accessible sugar. Continuous cultures are conducted in chemostats having all the sophisticated monitoring and control apparatus necessary to maintain a successful continuous culture. In the chemostat, the cell density will not be as high as in batch fermenters, resulting in a lower productivity, but the long-term continuous expression of product will in many cases be advantageous to the batch mode. In contrast to batch cultures, a steady state is reached, where the cell density, the substrate concentration, and the product concentration are constant. The disadvantages of continuous cultures are high risk of contamination with faster growing organisms and demand for very complex and expensive apparatus. The longevity of continuous culturing can cause accumulation of nonproducing variants of the yeast cells, resulting in decreasing productivity.

CELL IMMOBILIZATION STRATEGIES

It has been shown that immobilizing cells increases the achievable cell density and plasmid stability, enabling longer cultivation time and higher productivity. The reason for this is not yet clear. Conventional immobilizing methods such as chemical cross-linking or entrapment of cells in a gel matrix can alter cell physiology, increase contamination risks, and decrease efficiency, reasons why these methods have not become very widespread. However, it has been reported that immobilization of *S. cerevisiae* strain XV2181 cells in a fibrous bed bioreactor promoted a stable long-term production of GM-CSF with a relatively high volumetric productivity (0.98 mg/L h) performed for 4 weeks without any contamination or cell physiology alteration. The specific protein production and total product yield was, however, much lower than the control batch fermentation with cells in suspension.

MEDIA

Media can be divided into two categories — complex and defined. The complex media are rich broths comprising yeast extract or yeast nitrogen base along with the carbon source and can be supplemented with biotin and peptone. They can be buffered with potassium phosphate. Typical concentrations are 1% yeast extract, 2% peptone, and 0.00004% biotin, and the carbon source can be 2% glucose, 1% glycerol, or 0.5% methanol. The defined media comprise salts, trace elements, and optionally amino acids. Often the trace elements are added after sterilization along with the carbon substrate and the required vitamins. Commonly used additives are casein hydrolysates, which can prevent proteolytic degradation of the final product by inhibiting extracellular proteases, and antifoam agents.

IN-PROCESS CONTROL

In-process control is becoming an increasingly important part of the safety measurements taken in biopharmaceutical development and manufacture. The control program comprises strict parameter control using defined lower and upper parameter limits and measurement of a variety of output parameters (responses). Critical parameters and interactions should be identified from the data collected. The aim is to ensure a robust and reproducible process. Table 6.2 lists a number of important parameters and responses related to bacterial cell cultures. The responses monitored during yeast culture are listed in Table 6.3.

The regulatory issues relating to yeast systems are relatively simpler. The risk related directly to the cells fall into three categories:

- viruses and other transmissible agents,
- cellular DNA, and
- host cell proteins (e.g., growth factors).

The potential introduction of adventitious agents such as fungi, bacteria, viruses, and prions in cell culture media is of major concern and has led the biotech community to constantly search for safe media and raw materials. Thus, raw materials possessing high contamination risk (e.g., hydrolysates and peptones produced from animals or by means of animal derived enzymes) should be avoided. Use of antibiotics is discouraged. Yeast is generally regarded as a safe expression system (GRAS status). Its use is not associated with release of endotoxins and adventitious agents such as viruses or prions, which are not present. The major concern is presence of DNA and host cell proteins in the final product.

DOWNSTREAM PROCESSING

In contrast to the bacterial expression systems, yeast does express proteins with the correct N-terminal amino acid residue. Consequently, use of tagged proteins is rarely observed with this expression system. The protein is normally expressed to the medium in its native form, although disulfide rearrangement or reduction may appear due to the low redox potential of the fermentation broth. Proteins are often expressed in yields ranging from 50 to 300 mg/L. Besides being regarded as generally safe to use, the yeast expression system does not raise any concerns related to endotoxin release from cell walls and possible virus infections. The cell wall is rigid and separation of cells from the medium is relatively easy using centrifugation or expanded bed technology.

The purification techniques generally used are similar to those used for bacterial expression systems, except there are no refolding and cleavage steps involved. There are no specific purification methods for removal of host cell proteins, but use of three to four different chromatographic methods during downstream processing will, in most cases, result in an acceptable level. Unintended glycosylation products may be coexpressed with the target protein (e.g., mono- and di-glycosylated forms). They can be difficult to separate from the target molecule even during polishing. Table 6.4 lists the major steps in the downstream processing of yeast-derived proteins.

INSECT CELLS SYSTEMS

The nonmammalian hosts like insect cells have several advantages:

- The protein is secreted to the medium in its native form.
- Expresses posttranslational modified proteins including glycosylation, phosphorylation, palmitoylation, myristoylation, and glycosyl-phosphatidylinositol anchors.

TABLE 6.2
Important Parameters to Control when Using Yeast Culture Systems

Parameter	Comments
Aeration rate	The aeration rate is commonly set to a fixed value or to increase as the biomass increases. Typical values are 1 to 2 vvm (liter oxygen per liter of culture per minute).
Agitation rate	The stirrer speed is either fixed on a value known to be sufficient to keep the dissolved oxygen (DO) above the critical 20% (common values are 500 to 600 rpm) or established empirically in response to the DO9.
Dissolved oxygen	The dissolved oxygen must exceed 20% and is most commonly set to 30%. Since oxygen solubility in aqueous solution is very low (7.6 µg/mL) the oxygen transfer rate (OTR) is a main limiting factor when scaling up yeast cultures. The oxygen level can be controlled via the aeration rate, vessel top pressure, and agitation rate. The DO is a valuable tool for analyzing the actual culture composition via the "spike test." The "spike test" confirms that the compound in question (e.g., methanol, glycerol, glucose) is the rate-limiting factor. The feeding of the said compound is stopped and the DO is measured. If the response time is long (1 to 2 min) or the rise in DO is small (~10%), the fermentation is not limited by the compound. A typical rate limited culture will have spike times of 15 to 30 sec.
Foam level	The foam level is controlled by addition of antifoam agents.
Glucose and glycerol feed	These carbon substrates can be determined on-line with a near infrared analyzer or off-line with HPLC. Glucose is often determined off-line using an enzymatic analytical kit. Spike tests are used to see if these substrates are present at limiting amounts.
Methanol and ethanol	Since high levels (2 to 3%) of methanol are toxic to the cells, it is important to keep strict control with the concentration in the cell culture and adjust the feed rate often. Traditionally, the culture is kept methanol limited by performing spike tests regularly. Since a limiting concentration of methanol may not be optimal, it can be advantageous to perform on-line control with an alcohol sensor in the exhaust gas or a near infrared analyzer. Alternatively the alcohol content can be analyzed off-line with gas chromatography. It has been reported that a methanol concentration of 1% is optimal for *P. pastoris* fermentations. The same analytical methods apply to ethanol measurement in *S. cerevisiae* fermentations.
pCO_2	It is not certain, that pCO_2 have any effect on yeast cultures, but a negative effect on cell growth has been observed at pressures above 350 mbar1. pCO_2 is used to calculate the respiration quotient (RQ), an important parameter, as described below.
pH	Yeast grow well at pH 5 to 6, although it has been reported that lowering pH to 4 has no effect on the growth of *S. cerevisiae*. A pH decrease to 3 has been employed to reduce the action of proteases. pH 4 has been reported to increase plasmid stability, and thereby protein production, and has been employed to lower the risk of bacterial contamination. The metabolism of actively growing yeast will result in a decrease in pH; this is opposed by the automatic addition of ammonia hydroxide, which can also be a nitrogen source. pH is measured with permanently sealed gel-filled glass combination electrodes or with pressurized electrodes. They are standardized against commercially available standard solutions. Repeated sterilization over a prolonged period of time depletes the outer gel layer of the glass membrane, increasing the response time. Pilot-scale and larger vessels are sterilized with steam *in situ*. NaOH or HCl is often used to adjust pH. Care should be taken to avoid locally high pH during addition. It is recommended to use less concentrated NaOH solutions (0.1 M).
RQ	The RQ is defined as the ratio of CO_2 production to oxygen consumption. It is a valuable guide to the metabolic state of the yeast cell culture. Aerobic growth yields RQ values above one, whereas values below one indicate a switch to anaerobic fermentation with the concomitant decrease in biomass. For *S. cerevisiae* BT150 a RQ of 1 is optimal for biomass production. The optimal value for protein production must be determined from case to case.
Temperature	The optimal temperature is 30°C. Temperature is sometimes shifted to 28°C or lower to prevent overheating. Respiration generates heat and especially *P. pastoris* fermentations, demanding high amounts of oxygen, generate substantial heat.

TABLE 6.3
Important Responses or Outcome when Using Yeast Culture Systems

Response	Comments
Amino acids	Detected by HPLC.
Ammonia	Can be determined by Kjeldahl analysis.
Biomass and cell density	The biomass states the amount of wet cell weight (WCW) that can be converted to the dry cell weight (DCW). DCW can be measured gravimetrically. DCW has a linear relationship with the absorbance at a given wavelength (A_{590} to A_{660}) over a certain range, a relationship that must be established case by case, since it varies with the size and shape of the cells. For a typical diploid strain $A_{660} = 2 = 10^7$ cells and for a typical haploid strain $A_{660} = 2 = 2 \times 10^7$ cells. The linear range is often very short (usually within 0,1-0,3 absorbance units at 660 nm). The actual cell number can be calculated electronically (Coulter counter) or visually by coupling a hemocytometer to a light microscope. The normal convention with budding yeast cells is to consider a daughter cell only an individual cell when completely separated from the mother cell. A brief sonication of the cells before counting will separate cells that have completed cytokinesis. Cell aggregations should not be a frequently encountered problem since the yeast strains used in the industry usually aggregate only when contaminated with bacteria or fungi. In addition, indirect methods measuring the metabolic activities such as glucose or oxygen consumption, RQ, and increase in product formation can be applied.
Cell viability	A vide variety of marker genes is currently available. Use of marker genes that encode resistance against antibiotics is generally not recommended.
Methanol and ethanol	Since high levels (2 to 3%) of methanol are toxic to the cells, it is important to keep strict control with the concentration in the cell culture and adjust the feed rate often. Traditionally the culture is kept methanol limited by performing spike tests regularly. Since a limiting concentration of methanol may not be optimal, it can be advantageous to perform on-line control with an alcohol sensor in the exhaust gas or a near infrared analyzer. Alternatively the alcohol content can be analyzed off-line with gas chromatography. It has been reported, that a methanol concentration of 1% is optimal for *P. pastoris* fermentations. The same analytical methods apply to ethanol measurement in *S. cerevisiae* fermentations.
Product	Specific assay.

- Expression vectors are commercially available.
- The system is suited for expression of cell toxic products since the cells can be grown in a healthy state before infection
- The baculovirus vectors are harmless to humans.
- Safer to handle.
- Provide high yields (1 to 600 mg/L).
- Easy to develop (taking about a month to prepare and purify a recombinant virus, compared to more than 6 months for mammalian cells).
- Less expensive to operate.

The main drawbacks include:

- Minimal regulatory track record; FDA is yet to approve the first product.
- Semiexpensive culture media.
- Cell line stability.
- Cells are killed during infection releasing intracellular proteins (*Lepidopteran* species).
- Inactivation of the secretory pathway results in low expression yields due to aeration requirements not met.
- Presence of immunogenic host cell proteins due to release of proteolytic enzymes upon cell disruption.

TABLE 6.4
Unit Operations in Manufacturing Recombinant Drugs Using Yeast-Derived Systems

Harvest (centrifugation, filtration, microfiltration, ultrafiltration)	The purpose of the harvest step is to condition the sample for the capture step. Cells and cell debris are typically removed by means of centrifugation or expanded bed technology. The latter may in some cases prove difficult to operate due to cell aggregation. Several new membrane technologies have been developed to improve the efficiency of tangential flow filtration. The redox potential of the solution may be close to reducing conditions (< 100 mV) resulting in cleavage of the disulfide bonds. This parameter should therefore be closely monitored during operation.
Capture (AC, IEC, IMAC; expanded bed, packed bed)	The purpose of the capture step is to remove cell culture and process derived impurities and to prepare the sample for intermediary purification. Both packed bed and expanded bed technology will apply. The typical chromatographic capture procedure is ion exchange chromatography, although affinity or hydrophobic interaction chromatography may apply for some proteins. Presence of antifoam agents in the harvest may eliminate use of HIC due to their relative high hydrophobicity. The particle size of chromatographic media should be in the range of 100 to 300 nm. The sample composition depends on the chromatographic principle used.
Intermediary purification (IEC, IMAC, HAC, HIC; packed bed)	The purpose of the intermediary purification step is to remove cell culture and process derived impurities and to prepare the sample for polishing. The intermediary purification step offers a wide range of chromatographic principles (IMAC, HIC, IEC, HAC). The choice of media does not only include the protein purification ability, but also the ability to "receive" pooled fraction from the capture step and to "deliver" a suitable application sample to the polishing step. The particle size of chromatographic media should be in the range of 50 to 120 nm. The nature of the sample for polishing depends on the chromatographic principle used.
Polishing (RPC, IEC, HIC; packed bed)	The purpose of the polishing step is to remove host cell and process and product-related impurities. Powerful chromatographic methods (high performance HP-RPC or HP-IEC) should be used to separate the protein from its derivatives (enzymatic cleaved forms, desamido forms, oxidized forms, scrambled forms, etc.). The polishing part of the process makes use of the most highly developed purification methods to obtain optimal resolution. Minor amounts of glycosylated products may be present from the fermentation broth and specific care should be taken to remove these products during polishing. The particle size of chromatographic media should be in the range of 15 to 60 nm.
Concentration (ultrafiltration)	This step may be required to concentrate the output to meet the product formulation requirements.
Finish (SEC, desalting; packed bed)	The purpose of the SEC step is remove di- and polymer forms, small molecules (e.g., endotoxins, cosolvents, leachables) and to allow for easy reformulation of the drug substance.

- Inability to produce eukaryotic glycoproteins with complex N-linked glycans.
- Inability to properly process proteins that are initially synthesized as larger inactive precursor proteins (e.g., peptide hormones, neuropeptides, growth factors, matrix metalloproteases).
- Risk of infection with mammalian viruses.
- Sensitive to shear forces.
- Difficulties in scale up.

The classical strategy for production of proteins in insect cells involves the distinct stages of growing insect cells (*Lepidopteran* species) to midexponential growth phase, infecting the cells with the vector, *Autographa californica* nuclear polyhedrosis virus (AcNPV) or *Bombyx mori* nuclear polyhedrosis virus (BmNPV), containing the gene cloning for the target protein, and finally harvest and purification of the expressed protein. The reason for using the AcNPV infection step is the ability of baculovirus to replicate in established insect cell lines, where the polyhedrin gene is replaced with a gene of choice (under the control of the strong polyhedrin promoter). The result is high-level expression of the gene insert and the accumulation of the target protein. In contrast to other microbial or mammalian cell expression systems, the host cells are killed during each infection cycle.

Eukaryotic expression systems employing insect cell hosts are based upon one of two vector types: plasmid or plasmid-virion hybrids. Although the latter is most commonly used, plasmid-based systems offer methodological advantages. The typical insect host is the common fruit fly, *Drosophila melanogaster*. Other insect hosts include mosquito (*Aedes albopictus*), fall army worm (*Spodoptera frugiperda*), cabbage looper (*Trichoplusia ni*), salt marsh caterpillar (*Estigmene acrea*), and silkworm (*Bombyx mori*). In most all cases, heterologous protein overexpression occurs in suspension cell cultures. The exception, and one of the advantages of plasmid-virion systems, is that the recombinant virus may also be injected into larval host hemocel or literally fed to the mature host. Three basic options are available for protein expression in insect cells: vectors that enable high-level transient expression; vectors that enable continuous expression from stably trans-fected cells; and the lytic baculovirus system.

TRANSIENT EXPRESSION SYSTEMS

Transient expression is the most rapid method requiring simple transfection of insect cell expression vectors containing appropriate promoters (e.g., ie1 and gp64 promoters) in the absence of selection. Expression when optimized peaks between 24 and 48 hours after transfection. Novogen's Insect-Direct® System (http://www.novogen.com) is a complete system based on several vectors featuring an enhanced ie1 promoter. The plasmid-based vector systems provide a mechanism for both transient and long-term expression of recombinant protein. This expression system is exemplified by the Drosophila Expression System (DES) available from Invitrogen. The transfection of competent *D. melanogaster* cells with engineered plasmid will mediate the transient (2 to 7 days) expression of heterologous protein.

CONTINUOUS EXPRESSION SYSTEMS

Continuous expression using stably transfected insect cells lines is useful for the study of glyco-proteins, secreted proteins, and membrane proteins such as receptors. An alternative to the discontinuous insect cell system (cells are killed by the baculovirus infection; see below) is continuous culture of permanently transfected cells. Cell cultures of the fruit fly, *Drosophila melanogaster* grown to cell densities of 5.7×10^7 cells/mL in a low-cost media makes this system a promising candidate for future recombinant protein expression.

The gene of interest is cloned into a vector that utilizes a promoter recognized by the insect cell transcription machinery (e.g., baculovirus ie1 or gp64 promoters). The majority of resistant cells will express the target protein at various intervals. Such cell lines maintain stable expression for many passages (more than 50), enabling long-term culture for the accumulation and study of expressed protein. Establishing transformed cells that will express protein for longer time periods requires that the host cells be cotransfected with a "selection" vector, which results in the stable integration of the expression cassette into the host genome. This system offers two advantages over plasmid-virion systems: methodological simplicity, saving the researcher time, effort, and materials; and a choice of expression regimes, constitutive or inducible. Constitutive expression is mediated using the Ac5 Drosophila promoter, whereas a metallothionein promoter guides copper-inducible expression. The DES vectors are designed with multiple cloning sites for insertion of the heterol-ogous protein gene in any of three reading frames. A choice of vectors also provides for the expression of a variety of C-terminal fusion tags: V5 epitope for identification of expressed protein with V5 epitope antibody, polyhistidine peptide for simplified purification with metal chelate affinity resin, and the BiP secretion leader peptide. The DES system also includes media for maintenance of the host cell line and expression of protein, as well as reagents to facilitate transfection. The commonly used stable cell lines include: *Aedes aegypti*, *Aedes albopictus*, and *Anopheles gambia*; in addition, the following lines can be stable cell lines or used with baculovirus system (see below): *Drosophila melanogaster* (Schneider S2 and S3), *Spodoptera frugiperda* (Sf9), *Spodoptera frugiperda* (Sf21), *Trichoplusia ni* (High Five), *Trichoplusia ni* (BTI-TN-5B1-4).

BACULOVIRUS EXPRESSION SYSTEMS

The baculovirus expression cassette contains all the genetic information needed for propagation of progeny virus, so no helper virus is needed in the transfection process. The biology of the virus provides a simple means, using plaque morphology to identify transformed host cells. The virus does not appear to be transmissible to vertebrate species; therefore, this virus-based system is safe for human handlers. Since with many virus vectors, heterologous protein genes are under the control of the late-stage baculovirus p10 and polyhedrin promoters, recombinant protein is, in most cases, the sole product produced. Hence, cells harboring the baculovirus expression cassette integrated in their genomes can produce relatively high amounts of heterologous protein. Most of this protein is easily extracted from the cytoplasm (no inclusion bodies characteristic of prokaryotic systems) or harvested from extracellular culture filtrate (when the expression cassette includes a secretory leader fusion peptide engineered to the recombinant protein). However, the cell machinery may be starting to shut down late in infection, which can impact, in particular, proteins requiring processing. Hence, some companies have introduced viral vectors with hybrid early/late promoters that permit the still functioning cell to process glycosylated or secreted proteins. The commonly used cell lines are: *Drosophila melanogaster* (Schneider S2 and S3), *Spodoptera frugiperda* (Sf9), *Spodoptera frugiperda* (Sf21), *Trichoplusia ni* (High Five), and *Trichoplusia ni* (BTI-TN-5B1-4; HighFive™).

Baculovirus expression system provides one of the highest levels of target protein expression using baculovirus expression vector system such as BacVector offered by Novogen. In this system, insect cells are infected with a recombinant baculovirus bearing the gene of interest. The infected cells undergo a burst of protein expression, after which the cells die and may lyse. High-level expression is obtained by the very late baculovirus promoters (e.g., polh and p10 promoters), which are only active during the final stages of the infection cycle. Expression at earlier times can be advantageous to allow more complete protein modification such as glycoprotein processing and is obtained by using alternative baculovirus promoters, e.g., ie1 and gp84 promoters. The process of creating and expressing heterologous protein with the plasmid-virion system is rather straight-forward, in theory, but does require a bit of technical finesse and close attention to detail. The process begins with the engineering of the heterologous protein gene into a "transfer plasmid." This plasmid contains all the elements for autonomous replication in *E. coli*, a bacterial selection marker (usually an ampicillin resistance gene), and elements of the baculovirus genome. The heterologous protein gene is inserted in a specific orientation and location into the plasmid so it is flanked by elements of the baculovirus genome. Successfully engineered plasmids are then cotransfected with viral expression vector (essentially wild-type baculovirus DNA with p10 or polyhedrin genes removed) into permissive host cells. Cell-mediated double recombination between viral sequences flanking the heterologous protein gene and the corresponding sequences of the viral expression vector results in the incorporation of the heterologous protein gene into the viral genome. Hence, recombinant progeny viruses will produce heterologous protein late in their life cycle. Novagen's pIE vectors are based on the baculovirus immediate early promoter ie1. These plasmids can be used with G418 selection to generate stable cell lines from Sf0 or Sf21 cell lines. Other suppliers of vectors and complete baculovirus systems are Clontech, Invitrogen, Life Technologies, Novagen, Pharmingen, Quantum Biotechnologies, and Stratagene. (Check out the vendors offering as these are upgraded frequently.)

The baculovirus system has several drawbacks:

- The cyclic killing and lysis of the host cell releases intracellular proteins to the medium, adversely affecting the purification of the target protein.
- The production can only be achieved in batches or at best, semicontinuously.
- The expression yield is often much lower than expected due to inactivation of the secretory pathway during the late phase of infection.
- Inactivation of secretory path affects posttranslational events such as glycosylation (the sugar chain will end in a mannose and not contain galactose or terminal sialic acid) rendering the expressed protein unsuitable for *in vivo* applications.
- Baculovirus infected cells do not efficiently excise introns from expressed genomic DNA, thus limiting foreign protein expression from cDNAs. Recent developments to obviate these disadvantages novel expression vectors have been used to transform *Lepidopteran* insect cells into high-level expression systems using both the Bm5 and the HighFive™ transfected cell lines to achieve high yield and complex glycosylation under the control of the enhanced actin promoter system; a yield of 27 mg/L has been possible using this system for GM-CSF in suspension cultures. Though currently not significant, insect cell technology is likely to produce many dramatic advances in the near future.

PROCESS OPTIMIZATION

Large-scale insect cell cultures are processed in a batch or fed-batch suspension culture grown in a serum-free medium to a cell density of $1–3 \times 10^6$ cells/mL before the viral infection is conducted at early or middle exponential phase. Late exponential phase infection can be done if cells are resuspended in fresh medium leading since production is limited either by depletion of nutrients or by accumulation of toxic compounds. Give below are some of the highlights of the optimization process for insect cells:

- Suspension cultures are the preferred choice for large scale insect cell processes although in some cases relative higher yields have been reported in static cultures. Growing the culture to higher cell densities in spinner flasks ($2–3 \times 10^6$ cells/mL in uninfected cells) often results in decreased target protein expression due to an unusually high oxygen demand; as a result, culture volumes above 500 mL requires additional oxygen sparging that can damage the shear-sensitive insect cells. As a result, airlift fermenters are recommended that provide good agitation at low shear. Polymers (e.g., 0.1% w/v Pluronic polyol F-68) are added to reduce foam formation and thus provide protection of the cells. Typical doubling times are 20 to 40 h.
- If the fed-batch mode is used, addition of nutrients such as yeastolate ultrafiltrate, lipids, amino acids, vitamins, trace elements, and glucose is done under controlled conditions. The recombinant baculovirus is generated by homologous recombination to stock solution of a titer of 1×10^7 to 1×10^8 pfu/mL, which is used to infect the insect cells around day 40 to 47. Protein expression usually takes place shortly after infection. The product yield decreases sharply when cultures are infected later than an optimal time of infection (TOI), which is in the early- or mid-exponential phase of a culture.
- Replacement of growth media prior to infection and feeding with glucose, glutamine, and yeastolate in later stages of the infection improves yield.
- Addition of human nerve growth factor also improves yield if the cells are grown in the fed-batch mode feeding with a mixture of glutamine, yeastolate, and lipids.
- When using the efficient medium like YPR for *sf*9 and HighFive™ cells, ensure that all components, oxygen, glucose, and glutamine, of feeding are available in ample supply during protein synthesis and also viral replication stages.
- Microemulsions are often used to introduce lipids to the culture to avoid presence of insoluble lipid droplets in the culture medium.

- Where serum-free media cannot be used, ensure that it is free of TSE; serum-free media may contain discrete proteins or bulk protein fractions but not of animal origin; also there should be no components of unknown origin.
- pH range of 6.0 to 6.4 is optimal for most *Lepidopteran* cell lines.
- Dissolved oxygen (DO) corresponding to 10 to 50% of air saturation is needed in large-scale bioreactors. Supply of pure oxygen may be needed for high-density cell cultures. A standard oxygen probe (e.g., Ingold) is used for oxygen measurements.
- Temperature range is from 25 to 30°C for optimal operations; lower temperatures (20°C) are useful for keeping the cells as a slower growing stock.
- Osmolality is optimally maintained at 345 to 380 mOsm/kg for culture medium used with lepidopteran cell lines.
- Agitation rates are determined empirically; range of 50 to 200 rpm are most common.
- Ammonia production rate (mmol/10^6 cells/h) is an indicator of metabolic rate.
- Glucose utilization (mmol/10^6 cells/h) is an indicator of metabolic rate.
- pCO_2 is monitored through pH changes; the CO_2 flow is used to regulate the pH of the cell culture, and the flow is maintained only as long as the pH is above the set point. In late stage cultures the CO_2–HCO_3 buffer system is no longer sufficient to maintain pH and sodium hydrogen carbonate or NaOH is used instead.
- Lactate dehydrogenase activity reflects the extent of cell lysis, since LDH is not secreted by insect cells.
- Multiplicity of infections (MOI) has a limited effect on the maximum achievable yield, it is generally in the interval between 0.1 and 1.0 pfu/cell for most efficient operation; lower MOI are used for fed-batch production.
- TOI is typically initiated at cell densities of 1–3 × 10^6 cells/mL.
- Adventitious agent contamination is best detected at the end of the cell culture in the unprocessed bulk (if multiple harvest pools are prepared at different times, the culture should be tested at the time of the collection of each pool). The test program should include tests for bacteria, fungi, mycoplasma, and viruses.

DOWNSTREAM PROCESSING

The use of the standard baculovirus system requires cyclic killing and lysis of the host cell that releases intracellular proteins to the medium and complicates the purification of the target protein; as a result, alternate systems like transfection with appropriate plasmids are often preferred. The typical expression level of the target protein is from 50 to 500 mg/L and tags are not necessary. Insect cells are sensitive to shear forces, a factor that is not relevant when using baculovirus systems. Since there is a release of proteolytic enzymes, harvesting and capturing should be done under conditions where the enzymatic activity is decreased (low temperature and fast procedures) without using any enzyme inhibitors. The standard procedures of harvesting, capturing, intermediate purification, and polishing apply to insect cells as well as they to other systems described above and additionally a step of virus decontamination is introduced. It is recommended to use this virus inactivation step early in the purification process despite the difficulties in the filtration in the early stages of processing.

HARVEST

Most insect cell cultures are run as batch or fed-batch cultures; hollow fiber modules prove useful.

CAPTURE

The typical chromatographic capture procedure is ion exchange chromatography, although affinity or hydrophobic interaction chromatography may apply for some proteins. Presence of antifoam agents in the harvest may eliminate use of HIC due to their relative high hydrophobicity. The particle size of chromatographic media should be in the range of 100 to 300 nm.

Virus Inactivation

Since pathogenic or infectious viruses are not used to transform, it is difficult to define a suitable inactivation program. Generic inactivation methods (e.g., microwave) may be considered, but it may be enough to highlight inactivation measures taken as part of the downstream process (e.g., low pH, presence of cosolvents).

Intermediary Purification

The intermediary purification step offers a wide range of chromatographic principles (IMAC, HIC, IEC, HAC).

Virus Filtration

Small viruses (e.g., parvoviruses) may require filtration through special membranes that have limited protein transmission. Harvest and capture are the areas where viruses can be expected; use early viral filtration where possible, taking into account viscosity and particulate load.

Polishing

Chromatographic methods (high performance HP-RPC or HP-IEC) are used to separate the protein from its derivatives (enzymatic cleaved forms, des-amido forms, oxidized forms, scrambled forms, etc.).

Finishing

SEC removes di- and polymer forms, small molecules (e.g., endotoxins, cosolvents, leachables). DNA is removed by means of anion exchange or hydroxyapatite chromatography (DNA binds strongly to both types).

TRANSGENIC ANIMAL SYSTEMS

A transgenic animal is one that carries a foreign gene that has been deliberately inserted into its genome. The foreign gene is constructed using recombinant DNA (rDNA) methodology. In addition to a structural gene, the DNA usually includes other sequences to enable it to be incorporated into the DNA of the host and to be expressed correctly by the cells of the host. Transgenic sheep and goats have been produced that express foreign proteins in their milk. Transgenic chickens are now able to synthesize human proteins in the white of the eggs. These animals should eventually prove to be valuable sources of proteins for human therapy. In July 2000, researchers from the team that produced Dolly reported success in producing transgenic lambs in which the transgene had been inserted at a specific site in the genome and functioned well. Transgenic mice have provided the tools for exploring many biological questions.

Until recently, the transgenes introduced into sheep were inserted randomly in the genome and often worked poorly. However, in July 2000, success at inserting a transgene into a specific gene locus was reported. The gene was the human gene for alpha 1-antitrypsin, and two of the animals expressed large quantities of the human protein in their milk. The method used to create transgenic sheep is as follows. Sheep fibroblasts (connective tissue cells) growing in tissue culture are treated with a vector that contained the segments of DNA: 2 regions homologous to the sheep *COL1A1* gene. This gene encodes Type 1 collagen. This locus is chosen because fibroblasts secrete large amounts of collagen and thus one would expect the gene to be easily accessible in the chromatin. Also inserted is a neomycin-resistance gene to aid in isolating those cells that successfully incorporate the vector and the human gene encoding alpha1-antitrypsin. The vector further contains promoter sites from beta lactoglobulin gene to promote hormone-driven gene expression milk-producing cells and also binding sites for ribosomes for efficient translation of the mRNAs. Successfully transformed cells are then fused with enucleated sheep eggs and implanted in the uterus of a ewe (female sheep). The offspring secrete milk containing large amounts of alpha1-antitrypsin (650 μg/mL; 50 times higher than previous results using random insertion of the transgene). This project has now been abandoned because of its high cost despite remarkable success.

Chickens grow faster than sheep and large numbers can be grown in close quarters. Also chickens synthesize several grams of protein in the whites of their eggs. Two methods have succeeded in producing chickens carrying and expressing foreign genes: infecting embryos with a viral vector carrying the human gene for a therapeutic protein, and the promoter sequences that will respond to the signals for making proteins such as lysozyme in egg white. This is followed by transforming rooster sperm with a human gene and the appropriate promoters and checking for any transgenic offspring. Initial results from both methods indicate that it may be possible for chickens to produce as much as 0.1 g of human protein in each egg that they lay, and these proteins are likely to have correct sugars to glycosylate proteins, something not possible when using *E. coli*.

Transgenic pigs have also been produced by fertilizing normal eggs with sperm cells that have incorporated foreign DNA. This procedure, called sperm-mediated gene transfer (SMGT), may someday be able to produce transgenic pigs that can serve as a source of transplant organs for humans. Progress is being made on several fronts to introduce new traits into plants using recombinant DNA. The genetic manipulation of plants has been going on since the dawn of agriculture, but until recently this has required the slow and tedious process of cross-breeding varieties. Genetic engineering promises to speed the process and broaden the scope of what can be done. There are several methods for introducing genes into plants, including infecting plant cells with plasmids as vectors carrying the desired gene and shooting microscopic pellets containing the gene directly into the cell. In contrast to animals, there is no real distinction between somatic cells and germline cells. Somatic tissues of plants, e.g., root cells grown in culture, can be transformed in the laboratory with the desired gene and grown into mature plants with flowers. Therapeutic protein genes can be inserted into plants and expressed by them with glycosylation, reducing dangers inherent in tissue culture techniques and offer simple purification potential. Corn is the most popular plant for these purposes, but tobacco, tomatoes, potatoes, and rice are also being used. Some of the proteins that being produced by transgenic crop plants are: human growth hormone with the gene inserted into the chloroplast DNA of tobacco plants; humanized antibodies against such infectious agents as HIV, respiratory syncytial virus (RSV), sperm (a possible contraceptive), and herpes simplex virus (HSV), the cause of "cold sores"; protein antigens to be used in vaccines and other useful proteins like lysozymes and trypsin.

Transgenic animals are one of the most promising recombinant protein expression systems, making it possible to produce plasma proteins, human antibodies, and other proteins not easily derived from other sources; however, the development process is long as it takes 18 to 33 months from introduction of gene to production at usable levels. The FDA is about to approve its first transgenic product, a human antibiotic expressed in milk.

The target protein is usually expressed in the mammary gland, often at high protein concentrations (50 mg/mL), resulting in a yearly production of 10 to 100 kg per animal (cows). The animal husbandry and milking procedures are known technologies upgraded to good agricultural practices (GAP). The whey fraction can be processed by known chromatographic procedures, resulting in high-quality pathogen-free drug substance bulk materials — a prerequisite for preclinical and clinical trials. For large-scale production (> 100 kg/yr), the costs of raw products are approximately 10 times lower for transgenic animals compared to mammalian cell cultures, mainly because of reduction in capital investment.

Examples of major products undergoing clinical trials are Alpha-1 antitrypsin (Cystic fibrosis), Alpha-glucosidase (Pompe's disease), and Antithrombin III (Coronary artery bypass grafting).

The considerations in the use of transgenic animals are different from those of cell culture techniques:

- Need to redefine the master/working cell bank concept.
- Consider the variation of milk composition with lactation period.
- Control of sick animals and use of medications.
- Presence of pathogenic agents in the expressed proteins.
- Virus inactivation and documented clearance is required. There is a link between bovine spongiform encephalopathy (BSE) and Creutzfeldt-Jakob disease (CJD). Both types of CJD and other forms of transmissible spongiform encephalopathy (TSE) are probably caused by aberrant protein agents, named prions.
- Prions are notoriously difficult to inactivate without denaturing the protein product, but specific filters are entering the market. Prions have not been found in milk from bovine spongiform encephalopathy (BSE) infected cows, and use of good breeding practice and pathogen free purification facilities should reduce the risk of infections to a minimum.
- Strategic methodologies such as milking pigs and rabbits can be very arduous besides other problems of herd control.
- Coexpression of the animal protein in milk, often possessing close physical and chemical properties with the target protein (bovine serum albumin has for example 76% homology with serum albumin); process design should include powerful purification procedures for removal of the coexpressed protein.
- Regulatory controls are poorly defined.
- High bioburden (levels up to 10,000 cfu/mL are common) can affect stability; raw milk cannot be stored for more than 12 h, and some expressed proteins may not tolerate pasteurization; freezing and low temperature storage is therefore required.

DOWNSTREAM PROCESSING

Assuming the starting material is raw milk, it is normally converted to skim milk by centrifugation using techniques common in the dairy industry. After removal of casein the capture, intermediary purification, and polishing concept can be applied using the same purification principles as for cell culture harvests. Special attention should be paid to proteases and to separation of the target protein from its animal counterpart coexpressed in milk.

HARVEST

Here harvesting consists of removing fat micelles and casein; centrifugation, filtration, microfiltration, and possibly use of expanded bed. Variation in the starting material composition is associated with the lactation cycle, presence of subclinical infections, etc., requiring testing after each milking to establish conditions of separation of therapeutic proteins. The most dominant proteins present in cow or sheep milk is α- and β-lactoglobulin, immunoglobulin, and serum albumin, but a number of plasma proteins may also be found. Skimming removes 95 to 98% of lipid, still enough fat to affect the useful life of chromatographic capture column and to block filters used.

CAPTURE

Capture removes cell culture and process derived impurities to prepare the sample for intermediary purification. The shear bulk of casein (40 g/l) can be removed by precipitation at pH 4.5 or by adding precipitating agents such as polyethylene glycol. Use of low pH should be avoided as many proteins lose their biological activity, such as glycoproteins that can lose sialic acid residues. The casein micelles are solubilized by chelation of the calcium with EDTA or citrate prior to chromatography. Ceramic and organic membranes are used to remove casein micelles by micro- or ultrafiltration. Finally, clarification of skim milk using EDTA followed by addition calcium phosphate-based particles has been used to reform casein micelles away from the target protein. Many proteins such as Protein C bind to the casein micelles, and if the micelles are not dissolved, the Protein C can be lost. The process is suitable for expanded bed or big bead technology in the capture step assuming that the protein does not bind to casein micelles. In a simple two-step procedure (decreaming and capture), the protein solution is made ready for virus inactivation and purification. The typical chromatographic capture procedure is ion exchange chromatography, although affinity or hydrophobic interaction chromatography may apply for some proteins. The particle size of chromatographic media should be in the range of 100 to 300 nm.

VIRUS INACTIVATION

Inactivation is typically (but not necessarily) performed after the capture step, where the sample volume has been severely reduced. Details provided for virus inactivation in other chapters on cell cultures apply here as well.

INTERMEDIARY PURIFICATION

Intermediary purification removes cell culture and process-derived impurities to prepare the sample for polishing. The intermediary purification step offers a wide range of chromatographic principles (IMAC, HIC, IEC, HAC).

VIRUS FILTRATION

Membrane filtration can contribute to the overall virus reduction in a reliable and controlled manner without damaging the target protein.

POLISHING

Polishing removes host cells and process and product-related impurities. Powerful chromatographic methods (HP-IEC) are used to separate the protein from its derivatives (enzymatic cleaved forms, des-amido forms, oxidized forms, scrambled forms, etc.). Reversed phase chromatography is probably not an option taking the type of molecules expressed in transgenic animals into consideration (monoclonal antibodies, complex proteins). The particle size of chromatographic media should be in the range of 15 to 60 nm.

FINISHING

The use of SEC removes di- and polymer forms, small molecules (e.g., endotoxins, cosolvents, leachables). The coexpressed animal target protein must be efficiently removed.

7 Downstream Processing

INTRODUCTION

Whereas upstream process generates the crude protein depending on the genetically modified cell, the downstream processing defines the final product.

Downstream processing schemes comprise several distinct unit operations and stages (Figure 7.1), each serving a specific function; primarily this consists of capture, intermediate purification, and polishing or final purification. Highest efficiency and cost reduction are achieved when the number of steps is reduced to minimum, without appreciably affecting the final yield and certainly not the fitness of the product. The methods used in downstream processing are crucial to the safety of the product and as a result the processing area is required to be of a higher air quality standard than the upstream area (10,000 vs. 100,000). For recombinant proteins intended for use as human drugs, the purity must often exceed 99%, and some impurities, such as endotoxins and DNA, are limited to an upper level in the range of parts per million. Chromatographic methods available provide adequate purification and the purity levels required and are easily scalable. The most frequently used chromatographic methods are ion-exchange chromatography, size-exclusion chromatography, hydrophobic-interaction chromatography, reversed-phase chromatography, and affinity chromatography.

A careful selection of the processes in any downstream processing begins with an understanding of the characteristics of the protein in question, its stability profile, and the factors that may alter its structure. The most important criteria in the design of downstream process are the physical and chemical properties of the protein manufactured (Table 7.1).

Capture

Capture includes a number of different unit operations such as cell harvesting, product release, feedstock clarification, concentration, and initial purification. Expanded bed adsorption technology is specifically designed to address the problems related to the beginning of the downstream sequence and may serve as the ultimate capture step since it combines clarification, concentration, and initial purification into one single operation. Details of expanded bed operations are provided later in the chapter.

The overall purpose of the capture stage is to rapidly isolate the target molecule from critical contaminants such as proteases, glycosidases, remove particulate matter, concentrate, and transfer to an environment that conserves the potency or the product. At this stage, high throughput (i.e., capacity and speed) and short process times are very important. Processing time is critical because the fermentation broths and crude cell homogenates contain proteases and glycosidases that reduce product recovery and produce degradation products that may be difficult to remove later. Adsorption of the target molecule on a solid adsorbent as done in expanded bed systems, and adsorption chromatography decreases the likelihood of interaction between degradative enzymes and susceptible intramolecular bonds in the target molecule. The first step is a capturing step, where the product binds to the adsorbent while the impurities do not. The product is often eluted with a step gradient, giving a high concentration of the product but a moderate degree of purification. The main requirements of this first step are high capacity, high degree of product recovery, and high

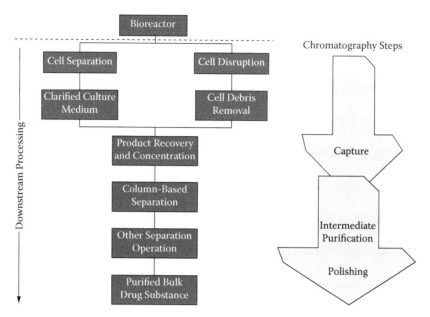

FIGURE 7.1 Stages in downstream processing.

chemical and physical stability. Ion-exchange chromatography, and to some extent hydrophobic-interaction chromatography, are frequently used as the first chromatographic step.

Intermediate Purification

After the capturing step, the bulk of impurities, such as host-cell proteins, nucleic acids, and endotoxins, are typically removed with high-resolution techniques such as hydrophobic-interaction chromatography, ion-exchange chromatography, reversed-phase chromatography, or affinity chromatography. Lower flow rates, gradient elution, and matrices with particles of smaller size are used for enhanced resolution. After these steps, the product purity is typically at a level of 99%.

Polishing

The last step is a polishing step to remove any aggregates, degradation products, or target protein molecules that may have been modified during the purification procedure. It also serves to condition the purified product for its use or storage. Commonly used techniques for the final step are size-exclusion chromatography and reversed-phase chromatography.

System Suitability

The purification schemes should enable the eluted sample from one step or stage to be applied directly to the next step, avoiding buffer changes and concentration steps. It is also important to keep the number of steps as low as possible, since the total recovery decreases rapidly with the increasing number of steps. A convenient way to reduce the number of steps in the purification scheme without reducing the purity is to include a step with high selectivity, such as affinity chromatography, at each stage. Finally, the sanitization and cleanability of equipment is important. Cleaning chromatography columns is particularly challenging because of the inability to achieve the recommended linear velocities necessary to efficiently clean bioprocess equipment. Consequently, the mechanical design of the column plays a large role in its cleanability. The column's internal flow geometries and seal configurations must prevent dead flow areas that allow liquid to remain static during normal operation. All areas of the column must be swept with sufficient and

TABLE 7.1
Protein Properties and Choice of Downstream Processing Systems

Property	Affects
Charge	Choice of purification methods, precipitation, crystallization, and chromatography.
Cofactors	Choice to add cofactors to stabilize proteins.
Cosolvents	Choice of cosolvents depends on function of pH, ionic strength, temperature, and redox potential on stability and solubility.
Detergent requirement	Choice and concentration of detergents depends on hydrophobicity of proteins during separation and purification.
Disulfide bonds	Control of redox potential; a shift of one pH unit results in a 60 mV change in redox potential (toward the reducing side when pH is raised); use of reducing agents such as dithiothreitol or cysteine to reduce the cystin residues to cysteine conversion.
Free cysteines	Control of reducing agents and condition (mM amounts of reducing agents are added to the buffer to prevent air oxidation) to maintain free cysteine residues.
Hydrophobicity	Use of detergents to the buffers to prevent aggregation and binding to surfaces. Hydrophobic proteins are sticky and tend to bind to surfaces and to other proteins and hydrophobic cosolvents (detergents); choice of reverse phase chromatography depends on hydrophobicity.
Ionic strength	The solubility of the protein depends on the ionic strength of the solution.
Isoelectric point	pH adjustment to prevent unintended precipitation, particularly at low ionic concentration, during elution from chromatographic columns.
Metal ion sensitivity	Addition of EDTA to remove divalent metal ions.
Molecular weight	Selection of ultra- and microfiltration membranes and chromatographic columns.
Posttranslational modifications	Choice of methods including translation medium to control glycosylation and phosphorylation as essential properties for regulatory approvals.
Protease sensitivity	Storage of the harvest, or during downstream processing, to prevent protease activity.
Solubility	Conditions that cause unintended precipitation by electrostatic interaction at low ionic strength, especially at pH values close to the isoelectric point (isoelectric precipitation), hydrophobic interactions under conditions of high salt concentration (salting out) in the preparation of feed stock for hydrophobic interaction chromatography. (Precipitation of even small particles blocks filters, columns and valves in preparative loadings to chromatographic columns.)
Stability	Control of pH, conductivity, temperature, redox potential, protein concentration, divalent metal ions, proteolytic enzymes, cofactors and presence of cosolvents to prevent degradation and aggregation. Biologic activity correlates with stability.

consistent velocity to ensure effective cleaning and sanitization. The prospective manufacturer is advised to seek from the manufacturer certification that the column is sanitizable and the regulatory authorities do accept this claim. Examples of sanitizable column include the QuikScale® biochromatography column, which is designed to distribute the solution evenly across the packed media bed to prevent any areas of stagnant liquid. This column can be easily and consistently sanitized and cleaned to FDA guidelines using typical sanitization protocols employing sodium hydroxide. As an example, the BioProcess™ HPLC columns from Amersham comprise a family of stainless steel, high-pressure chromatography columns with a wide range of bed heights and inner diameters and feature dynamic axial compression that uses solvent as the compression medium; these columns are of GMP grade. In addition, dynamic axial piston pressure eliminates the formation of voids or channels in packed beds. Together with a specially designed flow distribution system fitted at both the piston and the bottom of the column, this ensures a uniform distribution of the mobile phase across the whole bed. These columns comply with the technical performance demands placed on equipment operated at pressures up to 100 bar in industrial bioprocessing. In addition, they withstand temperatures up to 50°C, which allows effective cleaning with warm water. Construction is in stainless steel AISI 316 L, and the sanitary design includes Quick connections. Sealing materials are resistant to organic solvents and a leakage detection system is included.

TABLE 7.2
Commonly Used Downstream Buffers and the Conditions of Their Use

Buffer	pKa	dpKa/dT	Comments
Acetic acid	4.76	−0.0002	Supplied as glacial acetic acid (d = 0 1.058 g/ml at 20°C). Acetic acid is corrosive and fumes irritant.
Ammonia	9.25	−31	Volatile. Fumes are harmful. Buffers are often prepared of ammonium hydrogen chloride or bicarbonate.
Boric acid	9.23	−0.008	Often used in combination with Tris and not so often as a stand-alone buffer.
Carbonic acid	6.35	−0.0055	CO_2 exchange with environment. Carbonate buffers are commonly used in cell
	10.33	−0.009	cultures to sustain CO_2 levels. Work above pH 7.5 to avoid release of CO_2.
Citric acid	3.14		Commonly used buffer in the pH range 3 to 7.
	4.76		
	6.39		
Ethanolamine	9.50	−0.029	Smelly harmful liquid. Reacts with many amine modifying agents.
Glycine	2.35	−0.002,	Make sure the amino acid is not of animal origin. It is a zwitterions reactive
	9.78	−0.025	primary amine. Also used as a carbon and nitrogen source in cell cultures.
HEPES	7.66	−0.014	4-(2-hydroxyethyl)piperazine-I-ethanesulphonic acid. Low UV absorbance, commonly used in cell culture media.
Phosphoric acid	2.15	0.0044	Reacts with divalent metal ions. pH changes may occur if freezing samples
	7.20	−0.0028	stored in phosphate buffers.
	12.33		
Tris	8.06	−0.028	Tris(hydroxymethyl)-aminomethane. High temperature sensitivity, reactive primary amine, influences pH measurements, undesirable effects on some biologic systems.

Source: After Beynon RJ, Easterby JS. Properties of common buffers. In *Buffer solutions: The basics.* IRL Press at Oxford University Press, Oxford, 1996: 67–82.

DOWNSTREAM PROCESSING SYSTEMS

The choice of process equipment, chemicals used, columns selected, and the conditions under which processing is made are all critical. This section provides a general discussion of these elements. Details of processing can be found in the discussion of cell-specific processes described elsewhere in the book.

BUFFERS AND SOLVENTS

A large number of buffers and solvents are used in the various unit operations associated with downstream processing. The largest range for buffers should normally is pKa ± 1. The solvents are selected based on their incompatibility with the proteins and the resins used. Table 7.2 lists the most commonly used buffers and Table 7.3 lists the cosolvents, along with the general conditions of their use.

SAMPLE PREPARATION

Each unit operation processes a prepared sample, which is generally a solution of target protein with variable levels of impurities and has specific chemical and physical properties suitable for the processing desired. Conditioning of samples includes such steps as centrifugation, filtration, micro-filtration, ultrafiltration, desalting, and precipitation (Table 7.4).

An optimized sample preparation will include the least number of steps; for samples prepared for initial handling, use of expanded bed technology is advised (described later in the chapter).

TABLE 7.3
Commonly Used Downstream Solvents and the Conditions of Their Use

Cosolvent	Conditions for Use	Comments
Ammonium sulfate	1–3 M	Precipitating and stabilizing agent at concentrations above 0.5 mg/ml and to increase ionic strength in HIC.
Benzonase		Enzyme used to degrade DNA and RNA.
Cysteine	1–100 mM	Reducing agent. Used in low mM concentrations in protein refolding, and in 50–100 mM concentrations in reduction of protein disulfide bonds. Relatively cheap.
Dextran sulfate	10%	Precipitates lipoproteins.
1,4-Dithiothreitol (DTT)	1–100 mM	Reducing agent. Used in low mM concentrations in protein refolding, and in 50–100 mM concentrations in reduction of protein disulfide bonds. Relatively expensive.
Ethylenediaminotetraacetic acid (EDTA)	1–10 mM	Binds strongly to divalent metal ions.
EGTA	1–10 mM	Binds strongly to divalent metal ions.
Dodecyl-β-D-maltoside	0.5–1.0% v/v	Nonionic detergent for membrane protein solubilization. May absorb at 280 nm. Expensive.
Glucose	20–50 mM	Protein stabilizer.
Glycerol	5–50% v/v	Protein stabilizer.
Guanidinium hydrochloride	1–6 M	Protein denaturant used to dissolve inclusion bodies. Expensive.
Mannose	20–50 mM	Protein stabilizer.
NaCl	0.1–1 M	Maintains ionic strength. Corrosive to stainless steel.
Nonidet P40	0.05–2.0%	Nonionic detergent. May absorb at 280 nm. Expensive.
Octyl-β-D-glucoside	0.05–1.5%	Nonionic detergent for membrane protein solubilization. May absorb at 280 nm. Expensive.
Polyethylene glycol	Up to 20% v/v	Precipitating agent with no denaturing effect. Mr usually less than 6000. Complete removal may be difficult; does not affect AC or IEC.
Polyethylene imine	0.1% v/v	Precipitates aggregated nucleoproteins.
1-propanol	0.05–1.0%	Organic modifier.
Protamine sulfate	1%	Precipitates aggregated nucleoproteins.
Sodium dodecyl sulfate (SDS)	0.1–0.5%	Ionic detergent and denaturant. Expensive.
Sucrose	20–50 mM	Protein stabilizer.
Tris	0.01–0.2 M	Maintains pH.
Triton X-100	1–2% v/v	Nonionic denaturing detergent absorbing at 280 nm. Expensive.
Urea	1–8M	Protein denaturant used to dissolve inclusion bodies. Cheap.

Any of these processes can significantly affect sample stability (Table 7.5). Of greater importance is the physical stability of the sample, comprising aggregation and precipitation that change in the secondary and tertiary structures of protein. Ideally, the protein should retain its biologically active form throughout the processing, though it is often not practical. The sample stability is monitored by the biological activity of sample (e.g., IU/mg) throughout the process development stages. A comprehensive stability assurance plan would include testing to study the effects of overnight storage of sample, changes in pH (2 to 10), ionic strength (0.05 to 2.0 M), solvents, temperature (1° to 40°C), and sheer force. A factorial design is most optimal to evaluate these data. The stability of samples is further affected by the presence of cosolvents and other impurities (Table 7.6).

TABLE 7.4
Techniques Used for Sample Conditioning at Different Unit Operation Steps

Technique	Comments
Filtration	To clarify the sample; the sample must pass a 0.45 μm filter before being applied to the column. Filtration should be done just prior to chromatography as its composition may change with time due to precipitation or viscosity changes. These steps must be properly validated.
Ultrafiltration	For buffer exchange or to concentrate the sample. Sheer forces may result in protein destabilization.
Microfiltration	To remove cells or cell debris. Sheer forces may result in protein destabilization.
Centrifugation	To remove cells, cell debris, or particulate matter.
Dilution	To reduce conductivity or viscosity when sample volume is not extremely large.
Removal of divalent metal ions	With EDTA or similar chelating agents.
Desalting	Chromatographic desalting is a very efficient buffer exchange method; used for removal of GuHCl or urea.
Hollow fiber dialysis	For buffer exchange.
Bioprocessing aids	Normally added batch-wise to crude protein solutions in order to remove particulate matter and hydrophobic compounds.
Benzonase	Enzyme used to degrade DNA and RNA.
Precolumn	Safety device to protect the main column.
Cyclodextrins	Bind strongly to detergents; used to remove detergents from protein surfaces.
Precipitation	Separation and concentration step; better to use other newer techniques allowing continuous operations.

TABLE 7.5
Sample Characteristics and Their Effect on Protein Stability

Parameter	Comments
Concentration	Very low protein concentration may limit the equilibrium capacity in adsorption chromatography.
Conductivity	The ionic strength of the solution affects protein solubility and binding to ion exchangers. Precipitation may occur slowly over time, gradually transforming the clear solution to a filter-blocking sample.
Holding times	The sample stability is a function of time. Note that holding times in large-scale operations are much longer than in laboratory scale.
pH	The pH of the solution will affect the solubility of the protein, its ability to bind to ion exchangers, and protein stability. pH will also influence the redox potential of the solution.
Redox potential	The redox potential of the solution influences disulfide bond stability. At reducing conditions, the disulfide bonds will open up, resulting in free cystinyl residues. The redox potential is a function of pH.
Temperature	The temperature influences pH, ionic strength, and the redox potential. The protein stability is a function of temperature. Proteolytic enzymes are less active at low temperatures.
Viscosity	Viscous samples are difficult to filter and apply to chromatographic columns.
Volume	When working with SEC or other isocratic techniques, a large volume will call for a larger column to satisfy throughput.

PROTEIN FOLDING

When using *E. coli*, the protein is retained in the inclusion bodies, as a result of overexpression, which is brought into solution prior to downstream processing; at this stage the protein is likely to have an incorrect disulfide pattern as *E. coli* does not carry out the intracellular folding of the cloned protein. The amino acid cysteine plays a dominant role in protein folding. Under oxidizing conditions, this amino acid will form a disulfide bridge to another cysteine residue, making the

TABLE 7.6
Cosolvents and Impurities that Can Affect Sample Stability during Manufacturing

Cosolvent and Impurities	Comments
Cell debris	Increases column back pressure and blocks of filters.
Nucleic acids	Increase viscosity.
Enzymes	Proteolytic enzymes degrade the target protein.
Divalent metal ions	Bind to proteins and ion exchangers and affect *in vitro* renaturation. EDTA binds strongly to divalent metal ions.
Salts	Increase the conductivity (ionic strength) of the solution, which may produce salting-in and salting-out effects; significantly affects affinity, ion exchange, and hydrophobic interaction chromatography, etc.
Nonionic detergents	Affects affinity, hydrophobic interaction, reversed phase chromatography. Bind strongly to the protein.
Ionic detergents	Affects ion exchange, hydrophobic interaction, reversed phase and affinity chromatography. Bind strongly to the protein.
Zwitterionic detergents	Affects ion exchange, hydrophobic interaction, reversed phase, and affinity chromatography. Bind strongly to the protein.
Organic solvents	May cause precipitation. Affects hydrophobic and reversed phase chromatography. Large volumes require costly explosion proof facilities.
Poly-alcohols	May cause precipitation.
Antifoam agents	Reduces formation of foam. These agents are hydrophobic in nature and bind to hydrophobic matrices.
Carbohydrates	Are present from the fermentation process. Rarely affect the subsequent purification step.
Lipids/lipoproteins	Hydrophobic in nature. May affect all forms of chromatography due to irreversible binding to the matrix.
Colored compounds	Very often bind irreversibly to chromatographic matrices.
Urea	Is present from *E. coli* inclusion body extraction buffers. Does not affect ion exchange chromatography.
GuHCl	Is present from *E. coli* inclusion body extraction buffers. Does affect ion exchange chromatography.

redox potential of the solution an essential (but rarely measured) parameter in protein folding. It is a difficult task to reestablish the secondary and tertiary structures of proteins with disulfide bonds. Carefully designed folding buffers and fine-tuned parameter intervals (protein concentration, pH, conductivity, temperature, and redox potential) are needed to ensure even reasonable yields and to reduce the amount of incorrectly folded (scrambled) forms, which are often very difficult to separate from the native form.

During the renaturation process, proteins tend to aggregate either due to electrostatic or hydrophobic interactions or as a result of intermolecular disulfide formation. As the intramolecular folding reaction is of first order and the intermolecular aggregation reaction is of second order, it is often necessary to carry out the folding at low protein concentrations (0.05 to 0.2 mg/mL), resulting in large tank volumes when folding takes place in an industrial environment. The composition of the buffer used to extract proteins produces first a denaturation (and reducing), and the buffer used to refold the protein (producing oxidation) is different. The final buffer used is of the greatest importance and final yields can often be improved by adding specific cosolvents; if detergent assisted renaturation is used, the detergents are later removed by addition of cyclodextrins. The protein refolding generally takes place at alkaline pH (usually the interval 7.5 to 9.5 is used), as the deprotonated form of cysteine is required.

There are several methods for transfer from the initial denaturing or reducing buffer to the folding or oxidizing buffer. Dialysis in the bag is a common laboratory method, not suited for manufacturing scale production. Use of dilution in large-scale manufacturing requires larger tanks and careful addition of denatured protein to the folding buffer to ensure proper mixing to obtain low protein concentrations uniformly throughout the tank. Dilution folding can also be accomplished using a method of pulse renaturation where aliquots of the denatured protein are added at successive time intervals. Desalting ensures a very efficient transfer to the folding buffer, thus ensuring well-defined folding conditions. If aggregation can be prevented by means of additional cosolvents, the method can be very efficient (moderate protein concentrations). The size exclusion chromatography allows high protein concentrations in the application sample as polymeric protein is removed from the folding zone due to size exclusion. The fast removal of aggregates will decrease the rate of the second-order aggregation reaction. Ultrafiltration is used for buffer exchange by using methods like hollow fiber dialysis, which operates at low protein concentrations; the high capacity of hollow fiber devices makes this technique suited for industrial scale. The application sample is dialyzed against the folding buffer. In the technique of immobilized folding, the protein is immobilized to a chromatographic matrix in the presence of the initial buffer. Freedom for structure formation is facilitated by binding through N-terminal extensions (His-tags or cellulose tags), which are later removed by enzymatic cleavage. Folding is achieved by applying the renaturation buffer to the column. Aggregation is severely reduced and *in situ* purification can be achieved before eluting the protein.

The first buffer system used is for the purpose of denaturing a protein prior to renaturing. Commonly used denaturants are urea, guanidinium chloride, or detergents.

- Urea is cheap, but presence of cyanate contaminant in urea will result in carbamylation of free amino groups. Therefore, cyanate must be removed (using a mixed anion exchange matrix) before use of the urea solution. The temperature of solution is often kept at 4 to 8°C during the operation to prevent formation of cyanate and a concentration of 7 to 8 M urea is recommended.
- Guanidinium chloride is a strong denaturant, but very expensive. A concentration of 4 to 6 M is recommended.
- Most detergents are also very efficient denaturants at 1 to 2% solutions. They may bind strongly to the protein and certain chromatographic techniques cannot be carried out in the presence of detergents.
- EDTA is often added to the buffer (to bind divalent metal ions) in order to prevent oxidative side reactions during folding. A concentration of 1 to 5 mM is recommended.
- Dithiothreitol (DTT) or cysteine is commonly used as the reducing agent. Cysteine is the cheaper of the two and does not smell. A concentration of 50 to 100 mM is recommended.
- A recommended buffer for denaturation includes 7 M urea or 6 M GuHCl or 0.1 to 2.0% detergent, 1 to 5 mM EDTA, 50 to 100 mM reducing agent (dithiothreitol or cysteine), 50 mM buffer in the pH interval 7.5 to 9.5 (Tris or glycine). The buffer should have a pH range 7.5 to 9.5; protein concentration 1 to 50 mg/mL; conductivity 10 to 50 mS/cm; temperature (urea) 4 to 8°C; temperature 4 to 25°C; redox potential −300 to −100 mV.

In the oxidation step or renaturation step, the typical conditions are low protein concentration, alkaline pH, low to medium denaturant concentration, presence of reducing or oxidizing disulfide agent, presence of EDTA, and often a specific cosolvent to facilitate folding. The folding is a slow process and up to 24-h reaction time should be expected for folding of proteins with disulfide bonds. Specific enzymes (protein disulfide isomerase) are rarely used in industrial scale. Refolding strategies depend on whether or not there is a concomitant disulfide bond formation. Where such a bond is formed, the most common methods include air oxidation, the use of mixed disulfides, and the use of low molecular weight thiols. The latter method is well suited for large-scale operations partly because of its simplicity and partly because of the few side reactions observed. The cystinyl amino acid residue will form a disulfide bond with another cystinyl residue at oxidizing conditions (some disulfide bonds form at a redox potential of –50 mV). The reagents used are 2-mercaptoethanol, glutathione, or cysteine, which is added to the reaction mixture. It may be useful to take advantage of the presence of oxygen (approximately 0.4 mM) in normal aqueous buffers and add instead the reduced mercapto reagents. Cysteine is a cheap, nonsmelling, reagent well suited for large-scale operations (make sure the amino acid is of nonanimal origin). It has been common practice to make use of a specified ratio between the reduced and oxidized form of the mercapto reagent. However, in industrial application, it is strongly recommended to adjust the ratio between the reduced and oxidized form by controlling the redox potential of the solution. A typical folding buffer comprises 50 to 100 mM Tris or glycine, 0 to 3 M of denaturant, 1 to 5 mM EDTA, 2 to 5 mM mercapto reagent, a cosolvent. The conditions of reaction should be at pH 9.0 to 9.5, protein concentration of 0.1 to 0.5 mg/mL (G25 or hollow fiber), 3 to 15 mg/mL (GPC), conductivity 10 to 30 mS/cm, temperature 4 to 25°C, and redox potential of –50 to +50 mV. Several cosolvents have been used to facilitate protein folding mainly by suppressing aggregation in the inhibition of intermolecular hydrophobic interactions. These include: acetamide, albumin, L-arginine hydrochloride, Brij 30, 35, and 58, carboxymethylcellulose, cetyltrimethylammonium bromide, CHAPS 3-(3-chloramidopropyl)dimethylammonia-1-propane sulfonate, CHAPSO, CTAB cetyltrimethylammonium bromide, cyclodextrins, cyclohexanol, deoxycholate, dodecyl maltoside, dodecyltrimethyl ammonium bromide, ethanol, ethylurea, formamide, glycerol, n-hexanol, hexadecyldimethylethyl ammonium bromide, hexadecylpyridinium chloride monohydrate, laurylmaltoside, methylformamide, methylurea, myristyltrimethyl ammonium bromide, NP40, n-pentanol, POE(10)L ($CH_3(CH_2)_{11}(OCH_2CH_2)_{10}OH$), potassium sulfate, SB3-14 (N-tetradecyl-N,N-dimethyl-3-ammonio-1-propane sulfonate), SB12, sodium dodecyl sulfate, sodium sulfate, sorbitol, sulfobetaines, tauro cholate, tetradecyl trimethyl ammonium bromide, Tris, Triton X-100, Tween 20, 40, 60, 80, and 81, and ZW3-14 ($CH_3(CH_2)_{13}(N(CH_3)_2CH_2CH_2SO_3)$).

Another cosolvent approach, called the dilution additive strategy, has been to employ small molecules to promote protein folding in which the interaction between the small molecule and the protein is transient. In another cosolvent approach, named artificial chaperone assisted folding, aggregation is prevented by the formation of protein-detergent complexes. In the second step, the detergent is removed with cyclodextrins having a higher binding constant for the detergent than that of the protein. The stripping of the protein facilitates intramolecular folding. The naturally occurring chaperones GroEL and GroES are rarely used in industrial applications. Compounds used for chaperone-assisted refolding include cycloamylose, cyclodextrins, and linear dextrins.

In those instances where folding of proteins does not involve formation of disulfide bonds, an optimization for disulfide formation is omitted. Further, those conditions that promote disulfide formation such as a correct redox potential are important. As most proteins comprise cystinyl residues, it is common practice to add from 1 to 10 mM reduced mercapto reagent to the folding mixture in order to prevent unintended disulfide bond formation.

Table 7.7 and Table 7.8 show the typical initial and final buffer conditions for two proteins, lysozyme and IGF-1.

FILTRATION

Filtration unit process is used for:

- Harvesting, washing, or clarification of cell cultures, lysates, colloidal suspensions; microfiltration of cell cultures (prior to the capture operations) is an alternative to centrifugation or expanded bed technology.
- Removal of aggregates and precipitated proteins.
- Removal of particulate matter.

TABLE 7.7
Example of Buffer Conditions: Lysozyme

Parameter	Initial Conditions	Final Conditions
Protein concentration	50 mg/mL	0.2 mg/mL
Denaturant	6M GuHCl guanidinium hydrochloride	30 mM GuHCl guanidinium hydrochloride
Buffer	0.1 M Tris-sulfate pH 8.5	0.1 M Tris-sulfate pH 8.5
EDTA		2 mM EDTA
Reducing agent	30 mM dithiothreitol	
Oxidizing agent		4 mM GSH glutathione/GSSG oxidized glutathione
Cosolvent		4 mM detergent
Cyclodextrin		16.5 mM methyl-beta-cyclodextrin

Source: After Rozema, D., Gellman, S.H., Artificial chaperone-assisted refolding of denatured-reduced lysozyme: modulation of the competition between renaturation and aggregation. *Biochemistry* 35, no. 49 (1996): 15760–15771.

TABLE 7.8
Example of Buffer Conditions: IGF-1

Parameter	Initial Conditions	Final Conditions
Protein concentration	1.5 mg/ml	
Denaturant	7 M urea	
Buffer	50–100 mM Tris	50 mM Tris
EDTA (ethylenediaminotetraacetic acid)	1–2 mM	2 mM EDTA
Reducing agent	50–100 mM cysteine	
Oxidizing agent		2 mM Cys/Cys-Cys
Cosolvent		25% v/v ethanol

Source: After Obukowicz, M. G., M. A. Turner, E. Y. Wong, and W. C. Tacon. Secretion and export of IGF-1 in Escherichia coli strain JM101. *Mol. Gen. Genet.* 215 (1988): 19–25.

- Prechromatographic clarification to remove colloidal particles (chromatographic columns act as filters; a medium of particle size 50 to 100 μm is equivalent to a 0.45 μm filter); use a prefilter to columns to prolong their life.
- Buffer filtration.
- Sterile filtration and depyrogenation of small molecules.
- Specific virus removal.
- Buffer exchange; diafiltration can be used and tangential flow or hollow fibers are commonly used in parallel with chromatographic desalting procedures; force applied here can affect protein stability.
- Concentration, clarification, and desalting of proteins; ultrafiltration is used for sample concentration (e.g., prior to size exclusion chromatography or precipitation).

Alternatives to filtration unit process are the techniques like expanded bed, precipitation, or desalting. The choice of filtration vis-à-vis other techniques is made by comparing the losses of target protein with the losses incurred in using other methods. The common losses during filtration consist of retention (0.4 to 10%), adsorption (0.02 to 2%), aggregation (0.1 to 20%), and hold-up volumes (0.2 to 10%). The wide range of losses is carefully optimized by choosing membranes with appropriate retention characteristics and adjusting various chemical and physical parameters such as pH and ionic strength. The adsorption depends on the membrane area vis-à-vis the amount of protein present in the sample feed and the volume passed; generally, hydrophilic membranes will exhibit lower protein binding than hydrophobic membranes. Hold-up volumes can be reduced by careful piping design, optimization of membrane area, and flushing the system (and thereby diluting the filtrate or retentate). Aggregation in micro- and ultrafiltration affects protein stability by inducing aggregation.

Filtration is a pressure-driven separation process that uses membranes to separate components in a liquid solution or suspension based on their size and charge differences: prefiltration (5 μm), clarification (1 μm), filtration (0.45 μm), and sterilization (0.22 μm).

In *conventional flow*, the fluid is pushed across the membrane; in *tangential flow* filtration, the fluid is pumped tangentially along the surface of the membrane such as microfiltration and ultrafiltration.

Microfiltration is usually used upstream in the recovery process to separate intact cells or cell debris from the harvest. Membrane pore size cut-off values are typically in the range from 0.05 to 1.0 μm. Ultrafiltration is used to separate protein from buffer components (buffer exchange), sample concentration, or virus filtration. Depending on the protein to be retained, the nominal molecular weight limits are from 1 to 1000 kD or even up to 0.05 μm (virus filtration). In tangential flow filtration, the liquid is divided into two streams, namely permeate and concentrate, the latter is too large to pass. The microfiltration technique is used early in the process to separate cells or cell debris from the harvest in order to clarify the sample before the first chromatographic capture unit operation.

The ultrafiltration technique has traditionally been used to separate solutes that differ by more than 10-fold in size, making it ideal for buffer exchange and protein concentration. The low selectivity offered has mainly been attributed to the wide pore size distributions in commercial membranes, the presence of significant bulk mass transfer limitations, and membrane fouling phenomena. However, by proper selection of solute wall concentrations, in combination with the intrinsic sieving coefficients, the separation characteristics of the system can be altered toward better separation of the protein solute molecules. Ultrafiltration may be used throughout the downstream process with the purpose of buffer exchange or protein concentration. However, the sheer forces applied to the target protein may affect its stability, and tangential flow operations should always be carefully controlled. It is common practice to use ultrafiltration as the final downstream unit operation in order to ensure correct bulk buffer composition, but protein stability may be affected. Alternatively, desalting using size exclusion chromatography should be considered.

The most commonly used types of membranes are:

- Flat membranes in a cartridge where the feed is applied tangential to the membrane. The incoming solution flows in the channels between the elements (filter surfaces) and the permeate filters through the elements. The channels can be open or equipped with a turbulent promoter (net). The concentrate, which is recycled, flows through the cartridge or modular elements. The system is easy to clean.
- Tubular membranes are used with a porous support assembly, which is perforated inside and supports the tube. The input feed flows through the tube, and the permeate flows through the membrane outside the tube. It has a greater surface area than flat plate and high capital costs.
- Spiral membranes are rolled up flat sheets. Alternate layers of membrane, porous support, membrane, and a spacer are wound around a perforated tube. The surface is greater than tubular and flat plate. It may be difficult to clean deposited material on the surface of the spacer.
- Hollow fiber filters are small porous fibers bundled together and sealed in a chamber. The feed is pumped through the fibers and the permeate flows through the tubing in the chamber. Hollow fibers filters have a very large surface area; however, they cannot handle solids in the feed stream.

Filtration Optimization Considerations

The tangential flow filtration is controlled by adjusting the constant cross-flow rate to adjust changes in viscosity of the sample; the pressure drop is maintained when cross-flow rates are adjusted, through the adjustment of retentate pressure and the transmembrane pressure, which is often kept constant. The process conditions that affect these adjustments include:

- Configuration of the membrane is important to obtain correct flux and pressure. The flux depends on the membrane configuration, where the energy input per membrane unit area may vary considerably. Typically filtration is run at flux of 25 to 250 L/m^2 and pressure of 0.2 to 4 bar. The selection of the optimal membrane material/type is not straightforward and depends on fouling, membrane rejection, flux, pressure, time, energy consumption, etc.
- Molecular weight cutoff of the membrane must match the need. A membrane with a higher molecular weight cutoff has a higher permeability and flux. Sometimes, the difference in rejection is not significant and there can be considerable economical advantages in optimizing the cutoff range.
- Intact cells/cell debris are retained on 0.05 to 1μm membrane passing colloidal material, viruses, proteins, and salts.
- Viruses are retained on 100kD to 0.05 μm membrane passing proteins and salts.
- Proteins are retained on 10kD to 300kD or 1kD to 1000kD membrane passing other proteins including small peptides and salts.
- Physicochemical characteristics such as: pH and ionic strength, which affects protein solubility; precipitation of proteins reduces permeability of membrane.
- Temperature increases the diffusivity and decreases the viscosity. The effect is significant resulting in an increased flux. If the temperature is not adjusted, an increase in temperature should be expected as the filtration proceeds due to the energy input. Note that the protein stability might be affected by the temperature change.
- Protein concentration is a limiting factor for flux decreases with increasing protein concentration in the retentate; there is always a maximum concentration to which the feed can be concentrated.
- Diffusivity directly but not linearly determines process flux; higher diffusivity results in a higher flux, because solids are removed from the gel layer at a faster rate.
- Viscosity increased decrease flux.
- Transmembrane pressure increases compress the gel, lowering its permeability. At low protein concentrations, the flux is a function of the transmembrane pressure, while at high protein concentration, the flux becomes less dependent on transmembrane pressure. Membranes with relatively high water fluxes, such as polysulfones, are less pressure dependant than membranes that have low water fluxes (e.g., cellulose based membranes).
- Fouling of membranes results from adsorption of solutes to the membrane surface or polymerization of solutes, which is an irreversible process leading to decreased flux.
- Cross-flow velocity (tangential flow) increases flux at equal transmembrane pressure but it can also affect protein stability.
- Filtrate velocity is normally uncontrolled (the operation depends on cross-flow velocity and transmembrane pressure); transmembrane pressure can be controlled by filtrate velocity.

PRECIPITATION

It is often advantageous to precipitate the protein:

- As an intermediary product for storage
- As final drug substance bulk material.
- For buffer exchange or protein concentration.

The advantages of protein precipitation include mainly the volume reduction, removal of specific impurities, and enhanced stability when using certain cosolvents. The main drawbacks in using this unit process are that the precipitated protein may be difficult to redissolve, disposal of waste may create environmental issues, the high cost (large space, labor intensive, the use of explosion-proof environment when solvents are used, inefficiency at low protein concentration), and decreased protein stability when some solvents are used. A volume reduction remains the primary reason for using precipitation techniques.

Protein precipitation depends on the distribution of hydrophobic and charged patches on the surface and the properties of the surrounding aqueous phase. The most common technique of precipitation is salting out using high concentrations of salts, largely depending on the hydrophobicity of the protein (Table 7.9). The nature of the salt is of importance, and salts, such as ammonium sulfate, which encourage hydration of polar regions and dehydration of the hydrophobic regions without interacting with the protein surface, are favored. The salting-out effect of anions follows the Hofmeister series (phosphate > sulfate > acetate > chloride) and the most effective cations are ammonium > potassium > sodium. The heat of solution and change in solvent viscosity should be taken into account when choosing a precipitating salt, as should the presence of other contaminants in the salts that can also affect protein structure and stability (e.g., heavy metals in ammonium sulfate).

A globular protein will exhibit minimum solubility near its isoelectric point, as an overall charge close to zero minimizes the electrostatic repulsion between the solute molecules. This is called isoelectric precipitation, which is often carried out in the presence of polyalcohols in order to enhance the precipitation yield.

Addition of organic solvents (e.g., acetone, ethanol) to the aqueous phase reduces the water activity and decreases the dielectric constant of the solvent. It has been suggested that the precipitating forces are electrostatic in nature, much in the same way as under isoelectric precipitation,

---

TABLE 7.9
Precipitation Agents Used in Downstream Processing

Precipitating Agent	Typical Conditions for Use	Comments
Acetone	0–80% v/v at 2–8°C	Denatures irreversibly; explosion-proof area (10 L+) required; volume contraction calculations required.
Ammonium sulfate	1–3 M	May damage proteins; solid use produces uncontrolled precipitation locally; use saturated solution only; ideally protein concentration of 1 mg/mL is required to obtain acceptable yields.
Caprylic acid	Sample volume/15 gram	Precipitates bulk of proteins from sera and ascites, leaving IgG in solution.
Dextran sulfate	0–0.5% v/v	Precipitates lipoproteins.
Ethanol	0–60% v/v	Denatures irreversibly; explosion-proof area (10 L+) required; volume contraction calculations required.
Polyethylene glycol (3000–20,000)	0–20 w/v	Rarely denatures; difficult to remove. the residual polymer will rarely interfere with the purification procedures used in industrial downstream processing.
Polyethylene imine	0–0.1% w/v	Precipitates aggregated nucleoproteins.
Polyvinylpyrrolidine	0–3% w/v	Precipitates lipoproteins. Alternative to dextran sulfate.
Protamine sulfate	0–1% w/v	Precipitates aggregated nucleoproteins.

rather than through hydrophobic interaction. Larger proteins tend to precipitate at lower concentrations of organic solvent.

Polyethylene glycol (PEG) of molecular weight 4000 to 20,000 is used to precipitate proteins (in concentrations up to 20% w/v). The mechanism is similar to that of organic solvents and PEG can be regarded as a polymerized organic solvent. It should be noted that PEG is not easy to remove from the protein, although its presence rarely affects chromatographic techniques.

EXPANDED BED ADSORPTION (EBA) SYSTEM

The initial purification of the target molecule in the downstream processing scheme is traditionally treated with adsorption chromatography using a packed bed of adsorbent. However, this requires clarification of the crude feed before application to the chromatography column. The cells or cell debris are removed by centrifugation or microfiltration. Both of these traditional methods of separation have several disadvantages. For example, the efficiency of a centrifugation step depends on particle size, density difference between the particles and the surrounding liquid, and viscosity of the feed-stock. When handling small cells, such as *E. coli*, or cell homogenates, small particle size and high viscosity reduce the feed capacity during centrifugation and sometimes make it difficult to obtain a completely particle-free liquid. To obtain a particle-free solution centrifugation is usually combined with microfiltration. Although microfiltration yields cell-free solutions, the disadvantages of this combination system include:

- Reduction in the flux of liquid per unit membrane area due to fouling of membrane,
- Long process times,
- Use of large units and thus large capital costs,
- Recurrent cost of equipment maintenance,
- Product loss due to degradation.

The EBA technology provides a fluidized adsorption resin; adsorption of the target molecule to an adsorbent in a fluidized bed also eliminates the need for particulate removal by centrifugation or microfiltration. The properties of EBA make it the ultimate capture step for initial recovery of target proteins from crude feed-stock. The process steps of clarification, concentration, and initial purification can be combined into one unit of operation, providing increased process economy due to a decreased number of process steps, increased yield, shorter overall process time, reduced labor cost, and reduced running cost and capital expenditure. Successful processing by EBA has been reported in many commercial processes, e.g., *E. coli* homogenate, lysate, inclusion bodies, and secreted products; yeast cell homogenate and secreted products; whole hybridoma fermentation broth; myeloma cell culture; whole mammalian cell culture broth; milk; animal tissue extracts, etc. The EBA technology has been pioneered by Amersham (GE Healthcare) through their Streamline® product line, which is fully scalable and widely used in the manufacturing of therapeutic proteins.

The adsorbent in the EBA system is expanded and equilibrated by applying an upward liquid flow to the column, hence the title of the technology. A stable fluidized bed is formed when the adsorbent particles are suspended in equilibrium due to the balance between particle sedimentation velocity and upward liquid flow velocity. The column adaptor is positioned in the upper part of the column during this phase. Crude, unclarified feed is applied to the expanded bed with the same upward flow as used during expansion and equilibration. Target proteins are bound to the adsorbent while cell debris, cells, particulates, and contaminants pass through unhindered. Weakly bound material, such as residual cells, cell debris, and other type of particulate material, is washed from the expanded bed using upward liquid flow.

When all weakly retained material has been washed from the bed, the liquid flow is stopped and the adsorbent particles quickly settle in the column. The column adaptor is then lowered to the surface of the sedimented bed. Flow is reversed and the captured proteins are eluted from the

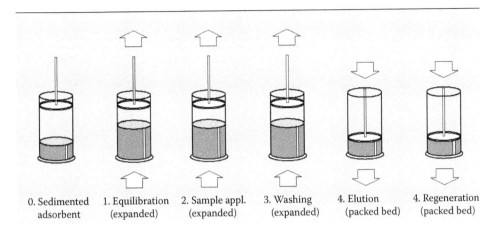

| 0. Sedimented adsorbent | 1. Equilibration (expanded) | 2. Sample appl. (expanded) | 3. Washing (expanded) | 4. Elution (packed bed) | 4. Regeneration (packed bed) |

FIGURE 7.2 Schematic presentation of the steps of expanded bed adsorption.

sedimented bed using suitable buffer conditions. The eluate contains the target protein, which is clarified and partly purified, ready for further purification by packed bed chromatography. After elution, the bed is regenerated by washing it with downward flow in sedimented bed mode using buffers specific for the type of chromatographic principle applied. This regeneration removes the more strongly bound proteins that were not removed during the elution phase (see Figure 7.2).

Finally a cleaning-in-place (CIP) procedure is applied to remove nonspecifically bound, precipitated, or denatured substances from the bed and restore it to its original performance. During this phase, a moderate upward flow is used with the column adaptor positioned at approximately twice the sedimented bed height.

Tailoring the chromatographic characteristics of an adsorbent for use in expanded bed adsorption includes careful control of the sedimentation velocity of the adsorbent beads. The sedimentation velocity is proportional to the density difference between the adsorbent, and the surrounding fluid is multiplied by the square of the adsorbent particle diameter. To achieve the high throughput required in industrial applications of adsorption chromatography, flow velocities must be high throughout the complete purification cycle. Most EBA systems are based on adsorbent agarose, a material proven to work well for industrial scale chromatography. The macroporous structure of the highly cross-linked agarose matrices combines good binding capacities for large molecules, such as proteins, with high chemical and mechanical stability. High mechanical stability is an important property of a matrix to be used in expanded bed mode to reduce the effects of attrition when particles are moving freely in the expanded bed. Agarose is also modified to make it less brittle and to improve performance. The column also has a significant impact on the formation of stable expanded beds. The columns are equipped with a specially designed liquid distribution system to allow the formation of a stable expanded bed.

The need for a specially designed liquid distribution system for expanded beds derives from the low pressure drop over the expanded bed. Usually, the flow through a packed bed generates such a high pressure drop over the bed that it can assist the distributor in producing plug flow through the column. Since the pressure drop over an expanded bed is much smaller, the distributor in an expanded bed column must produce a plug flow itself. Consequently, it is necessary to build an additional pressure drop into the distribution system. Besides generating a pressure drop, the distributor also has to direct the flow in a vertical direction only. Any flow in a radial direction inside the bed will cause turbulence that propagates through the column. Shear stress associated with flow constrictions also requires consideration when designing the liquid distributor. Shear stress should be kept to a minimum to reduce the risk of molecular degradation. Another function of the distribution system is to prevent the adsorbent from leaving the column. This is usually accomplished by a net mounted on that side of the distributor that faces the adsorbent. The net

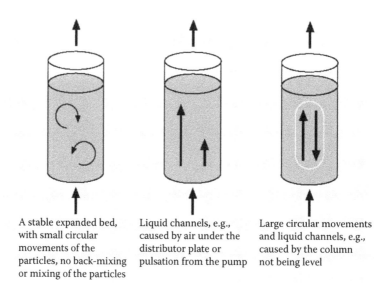

A stable expanded bed, with small circular movements of the particles, no back-mixing or mixing of the particles

Liquid channels, e.g., caused by air under the distributor plate or pulsation from the pump

Large circular movements and liquid channels, e.g., caused by the column not being level

FIGURE 7.3 Visual patterns of movement of adsorbent beads in an expanded bed.

must have a mesh size that allows particulate material to pass through and yet at the same time confine the adsorbent to the column. The distributor must also have a sanitary design, which means that it should be free from stagnant zones where cells/cell debris can accumulate.

Understanding the hydrodynamics of the expanded bed is critical for the performance of an expanded bed adsorption operation. The hydrodynamics of a stable expanded bed, run under well-defined process conditions, are characterized by a high degree of reproducibility, which allows the use of simple and efficient test principles to verify the stability (i.e., functionality) of the expanded bed before the feed is applied to the column. The same type of test principles used to verify functionality of a packed chromatography column is used in expanded bed adsorption. The bed is stable when only small circulatory movements of the adsorbent beads are observed. Other movements may indicate turbulent flow or channeling, which leads to inefficient adsorption. Large circular movements of beads in the upper part of the bed usually indicate that the column is not in a vertical position. Channeling in the lower part of the bed usually indicates air under the distributor plate or a partially clogged distribution system. These visual patterns are illustrated in Figure 7.3.

Besides visual inspection, bed stability is evaluated by the degree of expansion and number of theoretical plates before each run. The degree of expansion is determined from the ratio of expanded bed height to sedimented bed height, H/H0. If the degree of expansion differs from the expected value, it may indicate an unstable bed. Absolute values for the degree of expansion can be compared only if the buffer system (liquid density and viscosity) and temperature are constant between runs. A significant decrease in the degree of expansion may indicate poor stability or channeling due to trapped air under the distributor plate, infection or fouling of the adsorbent, the column not being in a vertical position, or a blocked distributor plate.

The residence time distribution (RTD) test is a tracer stimulus method that can be used to assess the degree of longitudinal axial mixing (dispersion) in the expanded bed by defining the number of theoretical plates. A dilute acetone solution is used as a tracer input into the fluid entering the column. The ultraviolet absorbance of the acetone is measured in the exit stream from the column. The number of theoretical plates is calculated from the mean residence time of the tracer in the column and the variance of the tracer output signal, representing the standard band broadening of a sample zone. The RTD test is a simple but efficient tool for function testing complete systems. If used to test systems before feed application, the risk of wasting valuable feed is reduced considerably. The test should be performed with the buffer and flow rate that are to be used during process operation. Note that when using a small tracer molecule (such as acetone) with a porous adsorbent, the measurement of RTD is a function of tracer permeation in the matrix pores in addition to the actual dispersion in the liquid phase. A plate number of 170 to 200 N/m should be easily reached.

The critical parameters in expanded bed adsorption can be divided into chemical parameters, physical parameters, and the nature of feedstock.

Chemical parameters relate to the selectivity and capacity of the separation process and include pH, ionic strength, types of ions, and buffers used. The influence on separation performance of these parameters is virtually the same in expanded bed adsorption as in traditional packed bed chromatography. For example, high conductivity feed-stock applied directly to an ion exchange adsorbent would reduce capacity, requiring dilution prior to application. If conductivity is minimized at the end of the fermentation step, dilution is unnecessary. This results in less feed volume and shorter feed application time. In an intracellular system, conductivity of feed-stock can be reduced by running the homogenization step in water or a dilute buffer. The pH range defined during method scouting should also be verified in expanded bed mode since reduced pH in some systems may cause aggregation of biomass. This aggregation can block the column distribution system, causing poor flow distribution and an unstable bed.

Physical parameters relate to the hydrodynamics and stability of a homogeneous fluidization in the expanded bed. Some physical parameters are related to the broth composition, e.g., cell density, biomass content, and viscosity. Others are related to operating conditions such as temperature, flow velocity, and bed height. Cell density and biomass content both affect viscosity, which may reduce the maximum operational flow rate by overexpanding the bed. Temperature also affects the viscosity and, hence the operational flow rate in the system. Increased temperature can improve binding kinetics. Optimization experiments are usually carried out at room temperature, but a broth taken directly from the fermentor may have a higher temperature. This difference in temperature must be considered when basing decisions on results from small-scale experiments.

Feedstock characteristics widely determine the application and efficiency of EBA systems (Table 7.10). Secretion systems generate dilute, low viscosity feed-stock that contains rather low amounts of protein and intracellular contaminants, thus providing favorable conditions for downstream processing. Intracellular systems, on the other hand, generate feed-stocks rich in intracellular contaminants and cell wall/cell membrane constituents. Along with the nutrient broth, these contaminants pose a greater challenge during the optimization phase of expanded bed adsorption. Much of the nutrient broth and associated contamination can be removed prior to cell lyses by thorough washing of the cells, but such steps introduce additional costs to the process. The main source of contaminants in feed-stock where the target molecule is located within the host cell is the complex cell membrane that has to be disrupted to release the target molecule. Bacterial and yeast cell walls have a high polysaccharide content that can nucleate into larger structures that foul solid surfaces. Proteins and phospholipids are other integral parts of such cell walls that will be released upon cell disintegration. Bacterial cell walls are particularly rich in phospholipids, lipopolysaccharides, peptidoglycans, lipoproteins, and other types of large molecules that are associated with the outer membrane of a bacterial cell. These contaminants may complicate downstream processing by fouling the chromatographic adsorbent.

Contaminant may also be present as charged particulates that can act as ion exchangers and adsorb proteins, especially basic ones, if the ionic strength of the homogenate is low. This problem is, however, not specifically related to expanded bed adsorption and should be addressed when selecting conditions for cell disruption.

The main concern when processing a feed based on a secretion system would be to maintain intact cells, thereby avoiding the release of cell membrane components and intracellular contaminants such as DNA, lipids, and intracellular proteins that may foul the adsorbent or block the inlet distribution system of the column. Release of intracellular proteases is a further concern since it will have a negative impact on the recovery of biologically active material.

TABLE 7.10

Characteristics of Feed-Stocks According to the Location of the Product in the Recombinant Organism

E. coli	Yeast	Mammalian Cells
Secreted — Dilute, low viscosity feed containing low amounts of protein. Proteases, bacterial cells, and endotoxins are present. Cell lysis often occurs with handling and at low pH. DNA can be released and cause high viscosity.	Secreted — Dilute, low viscosity feed containing low amounts of protein. Proteases and yeast cells are present.	Secreted — Dilute, low viscosity feed containing low amounts of protein. Proteases and mammalian cells are present. Cell lyses often occurs with handling and at low pH. DNA can be released and cause high viscosity. Cell lysis can also release significant amounts of lipids. Agglomeration of cells can occur.
Cytoplasmic — Cell debris, high content of protein. Lipid, DNA and proteases are present. Very thick feedstock that needs dilution. Intact bacterial cells and endotoxins are present.	Cytoplasmic — Cell debris, high content of protein. Lipid, DNA and proteases are present. Very thick feedstock that needs dilution. Intact yeast cells are present.	Cytoplasmic — Unusual location for product accumulation.
Periplasmic — Cell debris, high content of protein. Lipid and proteases are present. Thick feedstock which needs dilution. DNA is present if cytoplasmic membrane is pierced. Intact bacterial cells and endotoxin are present.	Periplasmic — Not applicable to yeast cells.	Periplasmic — Not applicable to mammalian cells.
Inclusion body — Cell debris, high content of protein. Lipid and proteases are present. Very diluted solutions after renaturation. Intact bacterial cells, DNA, and endotoxin are present. Precipitation of misfolded variants occurs in a time-dependent manner.	Inclusion body — Not applicable to yeast cells.	Inclusion body — Not applicable to mammalian cells.

Animal cells lack a cell wall, which makes them more sensitive to shearing forces than microbial cells. The mammalian cell membrane is composed mainly of proteins and lipids. It is particularly rich in lipids, composing a central layer covered by protein layers and a thin mucopolysaccharide layer on the outside surface. Due to the high membrane content of mammalian cells, lysis can complicate the downstream process by causing extensive lipid fouling of the adsorbent. Another consequence of cell lysis is the release of large fragments of nucleic acids, which can cause a significant increase in the viscosity of the feedstock or disturb the flow due to clogging the column inlet distribution system. Nucleic acids may also bind to cells and adsorbent, causing aggregation in the expanded bed. These types of contamination also lead to problems in traditional processing where they cause severe fouling during microfiltration.

Hybridoma cells are generally considered to be particularly sensitive to shear forces resulting from vigorous agitation or sparging. In contrast, CHO cells have relatively high resistance to shear rates and a good tolerance to changes in osmotic pressure.

The use of expanded bed adsorption reduces the amount of cell lysis that occurs, as compared with traditional centrifugation and cross-flow filtration unit operations, since the cells are maintained in a freely flowing, low shear environment during the entire capture step. Nevertheless, it is important to actively prevent cell lysis during processing, for instance by avoiding exposure to osmotic pressure shocks during dilution of the feed-stock and by minimizing the sample application time.

Nonsecreted products sometimes accumulate intracellularly as inclusion bodies, which are precipitated protein aggregates that result from overexpression of heterologous genes. Inclusion bodies are generally insoluble and recovery of the biologically active protein requires denaturation by exposure to high concentration of chaotropic salts such as guanidine hydrochloride or dissociants such as urea. The subsequent renaturation by dilution provides very large feed-stock volumes. Expanded bed adsorption can be advantageous since precipitation of misfolded variants increases with time, which usually causes problems for traditional packed bed chromatography. Even after extensive centrifugation of the feed-stock, precipitation continues and may finally block a packed chromatography bed.

When a nonsecreted product accumulates in the periplasmic compartment, it can be released by disrupting the outer membrane without disturbing the cytoplasmic membrane. Accumulation in the periplasmic space can thus reduce both the total volume of liquid to be processed and the amount of contamination from intracellular components. However, it is usually very difficult to release the product from the periplasmic space without piercing the cytoplasmic membrane and thereby releasing intracellular contaminants such as large fragments of nucleic acids, which may significantly increase the viscosity of the feed-stock.

Method scouting, i.e., defining the most suitable adsorbent and the optimal conditions for binding and elution, is performed at small scale using clarified feed in packed bed mode. Selection of adsorbent is based on the same principles as in packed bed chromatography. The medium showing strongest binding to the target protein while binding as few as possible of the contaminating proteins, i.e., the medium with the highest selectivity or capacity for the protein of interest will be the medium of choice. Regardless of the binding selectivity for the target protein, adsorbents are compatible with any type of feed material. The flow velocity during method scouting should be similar to the flow velocity used during the subsequent experiments in expanded mode. The nominal flow velocity for EBA is 300 cm/h. This may need adjustment during optimization, depending on the properties of the feed-stock.

Elution can be performed step-wise or by applying a gradient. Linear gradients are applied in the initial experiments to reveal the relative binding of the target molecule versus the contaminants. This information can be used to optimize selectivity for the target molecule, i.e., to avoid binding less strongly bound contaminants. It can also be used to define the step-wise elution to be used in the final expanded bed.

When selectivity has been optimized, the maximum dynamic binding capacity is determined by performing breakthrough capacity tests using the previously determined binding conditions. The breakthrough capacity determined at this stage will give a good indication of the breakthrough capacity in the final process in the expanded bed.

The purpose of the method optimization in expanded mode is to examine the effects of the crude feed on the stability of the expanded bed and on the chromatographic performance. If necessary, adjustments are made to achieve stable bed expansion with the highest possible recovery, purity, and throughput.

The principle for scale up is similar to that used in packed bed chromatography. Scale up is performed by increasing the column diameter and maintaining the sedimented bed height, flow velocity, and expanded bed height. This preserves both the hydrodynamic and chromatographic properties of the system.

In any type of adsorption chromatography, the washing stage removes nonbound and weakly bound soluble contaminants from the chromatographic bed. In expanded bed adsorption, washing also removes the remaining particulate material from the bed. Since expanded bed adsorption combines clarification, concentration, and initial purification, the particulate removal efficiency is a critical functional parameter for the optimal utilization of the technique. Washing may also be performed with a buffer containing a viscosity enhancer such as glycerol, which may reduce the number of bed volumes needed to clear the particulates from the bed. A viscous wash solution follows the feed-stock through the bed in a pluglike manner, increasing the efficiency of particulate removal. Even if the clarification efficiency of an expanded bed adsorption step is very high, some interaction between cell/cell debris material and adsorbent beads can be expected, which retain small amounts of cells or cell debris on the adsorbent. Such particulates may be removed from the bed during regeneration, for instance when running a high salt buffer through an ion exchanger, or during cleaning between cycles using a well-defined CIP protocol.

Cells retained on the adsorbent may be subjected to lysis during the washing stage. Such cell lysis can be promoted by reduced ionic strength when wash buffer is introduced into the expanded bed. Nucleic acids released due to cell lysis can cause significant aggregation and clogging owing to the "glueing" effect of nucleic acids forming networks of cells and adsorbent beads. If not corrected during the washing stage, wash volume/time may increase due to channeling in the bed. Other problems may also arise during later phases of the purification cycle, such as high back pressure during elution in packed bed mode and increased particulate content in the final product pool. If such effects are noted during washing, a modified wash procedure containing Benzonase (Merck, Nycomed Pharma A/S) can be applied to degrade and remove nucleic acids from the expanded bed.

Step-wise elution is often preferred to continuous gradients since it allows the target protein to be eluted in a more concentrated form, reduces buffer consumption, and gives shorter cycle times. Being a typical capture step, separation from impurities in expanded bed adsorption is usually achieved by selective binding of the product, which can simply be eluted from the column at high concentration with a single elution step.

The efficiency of the CIP protocol should be verified by running repetitive purification cycles and testing several functional parameters such as degree of expansion, number of theoretical plates in the expanded bed, and breakthrough capacity. If the nature of the coupled ligand allows it, an efficient CIP protocol would be based on 0.5 to 1.0 M NaOH as the main cleaning agent. If the medium to be cleaned is an ion exchange medium, the column should always be washed with a concentrated aqueous solution of a neutral salt, e.g., 1 to 2 M NaCl, before cleaning with NaOH.

Occasionally, the presence of nucleic acids in the feed-stock is the cause of fouling the adsorbent and in such a case, treating the adsorbent with a nuclease (e.g., Benzonase, Merck, Nycomed Pharma A/S) could restore performance. Benzonase can be pumped into the bed and be left standing for some hours before washing it out. Where the delicate nature of the attached ligand prevents the use of harsh chemicals such as NaOH, 6 M guanidine hydrochloride, 6 M urea, and 1 M acetic acid can be used.

VIRUS INACTIVATION AND REMOVAL

Mammalian cell cultures and monoclonal antibodies derived from hybridoma cell cultures pose an essential risk of contamination with retroviral particles or adventitious viruses. Despite the preventive actions (master cell bank characterization, use of raw materials of nonanimal origin, end of production procedures), viral contamination remains a problem for all recombinant products as adventitious viruses can also be introduced during production (e.g., raw materials, cross contamination) with the risk of contaminating the final product. Virus inactivation and virus removal during protein purification are important steps, particularly in insect cells, mammalian cells, or transgenic animals. Whereas it is possible to inactivate the viruses without appreciably affecting the target protein, only prevention and partial inactivation techniques suitable for maintaining the purity of proteins are viable choices. Besides inactivation, chromatographic and filtration procedures are used to clear viruses during downstream processing. The overall level of clearance is the ratio of the viral contamination per unit volume in the pretreatment suspension to the concentration per unit volume in the posttreatment suspension. It is usually expressed in terms of the sum of the logarithm of the clearance found for individual steps possessing a significant reduction factor. Reduction of the virus titer of one $\log_{10}$ or less is considered negligible. Clearance should be demonstrated for viruses (or viruses of the same species) known to be present in the master cell bank (*relevant viruses*), or when a relevant virus is not available a *specific model virus* may be used as a substitute to challenge the samples and calculate clearance ratios. The choice of the viruses selected should be fully justified.

The accepted methods for virus clearance are virus inactivation and virus removal; inactivation is the irreversible loss of any viral infectivity, while virus removal is the physical reduction of viral particles in number achieved by such methods as depth and ultrafiltration and chromatography techniques exploiting electrostatic, hydrophobic, and hydrophilic surface characteristics. Inactivation of virus is achieved by:

- Radiation: γ- and UV-irradiation destroy the virus genome; short wave-length UV-treatment can course the formation of free radicals leading to protein damage. This can be minimized by the use of antioxidants or filters excluding the 185 nm wave length),
- Heat inactivation: Contributes significantly to the inactivation of viruses. The introduction of high temperature short time (HTST) heat treatment offers substantial inactivation of small nonenveloped viruses while fully maintaining the integrity of the protein product. This method features the unique opportunity to spike and recollect a virus sample of a volume as low as 20 to 30 mL into the fluid pathway using a designed sample applicator under operational conditions for the manufacturing process (flow rate 35 to 80 Lh^{-1}, peak temperature 60 to 165°C) at full scale. The complete pathway is disposable, hence offering an extraordinary validation opportunity as well as a multiproduct use and avoiding any potential cross contamination
- pH: acid treatment results in destruction in the nucleocapsid and genome. Acid treatment works well with larger virus particles. Particles < 40 nm may require a combination of pH < 3 and 3 M urea. Acid treatment at pH > 3 does not inactivate nonenveloped viruses. Enveloped viruses are not inactivated in a reliable manner.
- Pressure: High-pressure procedures at near-zero temperatures may be useful in inactivation of viruses.
- Cosolvents: Organic solvents dissolve the virus envelope or disintegrate the nucleocapsid.
- Detergents: Detergents dissolve the virus envelope or disintegrate the nucleocapsid. The method is very efficient for lipid-enveloped viruses, but is ineffective against nonenveloped viruses.
- Denaturation: The method selected for inactivation depends to a great degree on the nature of virus. It results in disintegration of the nucleocapsid. Urea treatment does not inactivate small nonenveloped viruses. Large enveloped viruses are inactivated to some extend. Urea treatment works well with larger virus particles. Particles < 40 nm may require a combination of pH < 3 and 3 M urea. Chaotropic agents dissolve the virus envelope or disintegrate the nucleocapsid.
- Fatty acids: Treatment with caprylate is a useful approach to remove the risk of lipid-enveloped viruses from protein pharmaceuticals.
- β-propiolactone: An effective virucidal agent; 3.5 to 5 log reduction of viral infectivity is observed, but it is toxic and removal must be ensured by analytical testing validation.
- Inactine: The technology is based on disruption of nucleic acid replication while preserving the integrity of lipids and protein.
- Biosurfactants: Surfactin, a cyclic lipopeptide antibiotic with a molecular weight of 1036, possessing antiviral effect (enveloped RNA and DNA viruses) and antimycoplasma properties. The activity decreases with increasing protein concentration and the reagent is not effective in solutions of high protein concentration. The *in vivo* toxicity is low.

- Imines: 0.05% v/v N-acetylethylenimine (AEI) inactivates infectious units of polio-virus and foot-and-mouth disease virus at 4 or 37°C without damaging a variety of proteins tested.
- Quaternary ammonium chloride: 3-(trimethyloxysilyl)-propyldimethyl-octadecylammo-nium chloride (Si-QAC) covalently binds to alginate and removes viruses from protein solutions.

Because of the differences in the nature of viruses and their *in vitro* reactivity, it is difficult to adopt general methods for their clearance, for example, solvent-detergent treatment is highly effective for inactivation of enveloped viruses, but has no or little effect on nonenveloped viruses. Low pH is effective in mammalian cell systems but has little effect on parvoviruses. It is important to include at least one virus inactivation step in the downstream process scheme. The process should be properly validated, keeping in mind that the inactivation is a biphasic process. The sample is ordinarily spiked with virus in small amounts so as not to change the sample characteristics (e.g., buffer composition, protein concentration, conductivity). Parallel control assays should be included to assess loss of infectivity due to dilution, concentration, or storage. Buffers and products should be evaluated independently for toxicity or interference in assays used to determine the virus titer, as these components may adversely affect the indicator cells. Virus escaping a first inactivation step may be more resistant to subsequent steps (e.g., virus aggregates).

Most downstream processes include at least three different chromatographic procedures that also help remove adventitious agents. The virus capsid is a shell consisting of different proteins and the virus particle might behave as any other protein present in the sample to be purified. Also the envelope of enveloped viruses contains a variety of proteins. Given the diversity in the nature of viruses, these methods cannot be relied upon to definitely remove viruses. Generally, anion exchange chromatography at basic pH and low conductivity proves most useful.

Filtration works through two mechanisms — size exclusion and absorptive retention of partic-ulates. Size exclusion, which occurs due to geometric or spatial constraint, provides a predictable method of particle removal, as it is not directly influenced by process and filtration conditions. In contrast, a number of process-dependent factors (e.g., charge, hydrophobicity, pH, ionic strength) influence the absorption of particulates in a much less controlled manner. Size exclusion and adsorptive filtration are not mutually exclusive. Depth-filters with anion exchanging characteristics are very efficient virus removers.

The viruses of interest, such as retroviruses (100 to 140 nm) and small viruses (about 30 nm), can be removed by use of nanofiltration or by ultrafiltration. Nanofilters featuring pore sizes in the range of 20 to 70 nm utilize the classical depth structures, which are typical for commercial microfiltration membranes. Tighter pore sizes results in high back pressure (> 0.3 MPa). Nanofilters are inexpensive in practical use and can be used anywhere in the downstream process as long as the load solution is 0.1 μm prefiltered. A significant feature of nanofilters is the possibility of measuring their integrity. Complete clearance (to the limits of detection) is easily accomplished in the removal of viruses above 35 nm from human globulin by 35 nm nanofiltration.

Ultrafiltration offers the possibility to operate at much smaller pore sizes (> 1kDa cut off) more or less depending on the strokes radius of the protein. A cut off of 200 kDa allows for the passage of IgG-type antibodies (Mw around 150 kDa), resulting in excellent clearance factors for virus particles > 40 nm. Depending on process parameters, even a 100 kDa filter can be used successfully with significant retention of particles <40 nm³.

Membrane filtration is an effective, reliable, and controllable technique to remove viruses. In many cases large viruses could be removed to the detection limit of the assay used. Small viruses (e.g., parvoviruses) may require filtration through special membranes that have limited protein transmission. cGMP facilities are typically divided into an area where viruses are expected to be present (harvest and capture) and nonvirus areas potentially free of viruses. An early virus filtration step is therefore of advantage, but is challenged by the composition (viscosity, particulates) of the sample material in early downstream processing. Virus filtration should also be used whenever cell culture media or buffers are believed to include a virus contamination risk.

PROCESS FLOW

The entire downstream process is presented in a process flow diagram that specifies the details of processes in a logical order, properly sized to meet the requirements of each operation. Table 7.11 is a process flow for the manufacturing of erythropoietin (X stands for a quantity, volume, or size, redacted for proprietary reasons) (Table 7.11; see also Figure 7.4).

Table 7.11
A Typical Process Flow Chart for Erythropoietin

Equipment Used	Process and Material	Process Description
XX L S.S. vessel Sartorius membrane filter 2.0 μm and 0.45 μm	Growing media preparation: Using fetal bovine serum, gentamicin, DMEM, high glucose	Add X L of DMEM, high glucose in XX L vessel. Add X L fetal bovine serum and X g gentamicin, mix until dissolved. QS to XX L with high glucose. Filter the solution and keep at X°C for XX h.
X L sterile S.S. vessel Sartorius membrane filter 2.0 μm and 0.45 μm	Harvesting media preparation: using human insulin gentamicin DMEM, high glucose	Add X L of DMEM, high glucose in XX L sterile vessel. Add XX mg human insulin and X g gentamicin, mix for XX min. QS to XX L with high glucose. Filter the solution and keep at X°C for XX h.
Water bath Centrifuge CO$_2$ Incubator Rolling bottle apparatus	Cell subculture for XX frozen vials of CHO EPO	Thaw the vials at X°C in water bath, wash vials with X% ethanol, transfer the contents of each vial into XX mL centrifuge tube. Wash the cell by centrifugation at XX rpm for X min. with X–Y mL growing media for X times. Disperse the cellular pellets in X mL of growing media in X mL flask and divide the dispersion into X flasks and complete the volume to X mL with growing media. Repeat the above steps for all vials. Incubate all flasks at X°C for X days. Split the contents of each flask into X flasks and complete the volume to XmL with growing media. Incubate all flasks at X°C for X days. Split the contents of each flask into X roller bottles and complete the volume to X mL with growing media.
Centrifuge Sartorius membrane filter 2.0 μm and 0.45 μm	Harvesting for X days	Transfer the contents of each bottle to a centrifuge flask and wash the cell by centrifugation two times with PBS 15–20 mL. Inoculate the cell dispersion of each flask with harvesting medium into roller bottles. Media containing EPO collected every 24 h, filtered through 2.0 μm and 0.45 μm. Collected medium replaced with new medium for X d.
Column XXX	Purification: affinity chromatography	Filtered cellular supernatant rh-EPO is purified through an affinity column. Filtered collected media is loaded in the column equilibrated in PBS.

Continued.

Table 7.11 (Continued)
A Typical Process Flow Chart for Erythropoietin

Equipment Used	Process and Material	Process Description
		The column is then washed with X column volumes with PBS and elute the bounded protein with PBS-1.4M NaCl (X g of NaCl/L of PBS). The sample obtained are stored at –4°C.
		After the EPO elution the column is washed first with X mL of NaOH 0.1 M and later with 2 column volume of PBS-X M NaCl. Finally the column is equilibrated in PBS for the next day.
Column XXX	Desalting	The rh-EPO recovered from previous step is desalted using column.
		The column is equilibrated in X mM Tris-HCl pH X with an increasing flow going from X mL/min to XmL/min with a limit pressure of X MPa. The maximum volume loaded is around X mL.
		The elution of the protein is controlled at X nm and the salts concentration is followed by the conductimeter in line.
		The column is cleaned with X column volumes of X M NaOH and reequilibrated with XmM Tris-HCl pH X for the next day.
Column XXX	Anion exchange	The desalted fraction containing the rh-EPO is purified using XXX.
		The column is equilibrated with X volumes of XmM Tris-HCl pH X and later with X volumes of 50 mM Tris-HCl pH X — XmM NaCl (X% Buffer B, XmM Tris — HCl pH X — NaCl XM).
Column XXX	Desalting	The rh-EPO recovered from previous step is desalted using column XX.
		The column is equilibrated in X mM NaAC pH X at XmL/min. The maximum volume loaded in the column is X mL.
		The solution is monitored at X nm controlling the elution of the protein and of the salt with the conductimeter line. The flow through is collected and the salt is left to complete its elution.
		The column is cleaned with X volumes of XM NaOH and re-equilibrated with X mM NaAC pH 6.0 for the next day.
Column XXX	Cation exchange	The rh-EPO containing fractions eluted from the XX column and desalted is loaded in a XXX column.
		This SP-column retains isoforms of incomplete glycosylation enriching the specific activity and another high molecular weight contaminant products.
		The fraction containing the EPO molecules with high glycosylation elute with the flow through (FT) of the column using X mM NaAC, pH X.
		The column is first equilibrated with 10 volumes of X mM NaAC pH X.
		The fraction containing the rh-EPO is loaded in the column at X mL/min.
		Measure the optical density with a spectrophotometer to determine the quantity of protein present in the sample.
		Measure the volume obtained.
		Filter the flow through in a Millipore Stericup 0.22 μ.
		Store the product obtained at 2–8°C
		The column is then washed with X volumes of X mM NaAC, pH X- X M NaCl and reequilibrated in X mM NaAC, pH X.

Table 7.11 (Continued)
A Typical Process Flow Chart for Erythropoietin

Equipment Used	Process and Material	Process Description
Gel filtration column, Superose	Gel formation	The final polishing of the purified rh-EPO is performed using a gel filtration column. The fraction is loaded at X mL/min. following the spectrum at X nm, collecting the peak containing the purified rh-EPO.
Polyethylene storage container	Final product	Erythropoietin concentrated solution has a concentration of X mg/mL to X mg/mL and potency of not less than 100,000 international units (IU) per milligram of active substance determined.

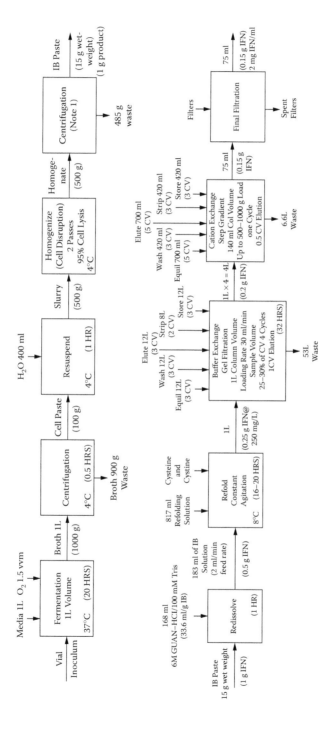

FIGURE 7.4 Block diagram for process flow for interferon.

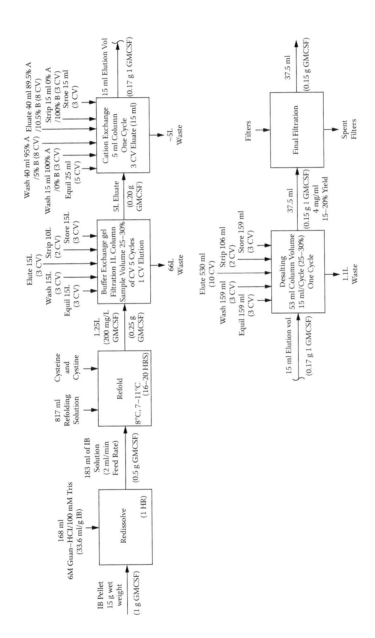

FIGURE 7.4 Continued.

8 Purification Techniques

INTRODUCTION

The downstream purification steps comprise the most important part of the manufacturing of therapeutic proteins. The upstream process accumulates a large number of impurities including viruses, electrolytes, and other uncharged degradation products and structurally related molecules. Cleaning out these unwanted components to a level where it can comply with compendial requirements where available is accomplished in the purification steps. The chromatography techniques used can add contaminants of their own, causing protein degradation or modification of protein structure. Additionally, the yield obtained through the purification process is critical in making the system commercially feasible. Establishing optimal separation on a cost-effective basis requires a good understanding of the physicochemical nature of the target protein, particularly its physical and chemical stability profile. The first part of this chapter deals with the properties of protein that can have a significant effect on its separation potential; this is followed by a description of the most commonly used chromatography techniques.

PROTEIN PROPERTIES

All proteins are made up of amino acids and may contain other molecules as well. Amino acid contain amino group (-NH2), a carboxyl group (-COOH), and an R group with a general formula, R-CH(NH2)-COOH. The R group differs among various amino acids. In a protein, the R group is also called a side chain. There are over 300 naturally occurring amino acids. There are 20 of interest to humans. The type of R attached determines if they would at neutral pH retain a negative charge (acidic, aspartic, and glutamic acid), positive charge (basic, lysine, arginine, and histidine), or are aromatic in nature (tyrosine, tryptophan, and phenylalanine), contain sulfur (cysteine and methionine), are uncharged hydrophilic (serine, threonine, asparagines, and glutamine), are inactive hydrophobic (glycine, alanine, valine, leucine, and isoleucine), or have special structures (proline, where amino acid groups are not directly connected and thus appearing at the end of the peptide chain). These classifications are important in imparting certain properties to proteins, besides the charge, that should be evaluated in the selection of an appropriate separation procedure. For example, interaction between positive and negative R groups may form a salt bridge, which is an important stabilizing force in proteins. The disulfide bond formed between two cysteine residues provides a strong force for stabilizing the globular structure. A unique feature about methionine is that the synthesis of all peptide chains starts from methionine. Hydrophilic groups can form hydrogen bonds. The inactive hydrophobic amino acids are found inside the protein interior and do not form hydrogen bonds and rarely interact.

The amino acids are designated specific symbols to represent them in a complex structure. One of the most significant properties of proteins derives from their hydrophobicity imparted by the component amino acids. Table 8.1 lists the hydrophobicity indices of the 20 amino acids found in proteins. The hydrophobicity index, as given below, tells the relative hydrophobicity among amino acids. A higher value means higher hydrophobicity and it is more likely to be found in the protein interior. Table 8.1 arranges amino acids in the increasing order of hydrophobicity except for praline.

Table 8.1
Structure and Hydrophobicity of Amino Acids

Name	Symbol 3 Lett.	Symbol 1 Lett.	R Group	Hydrophobicity
Aspartate	Asp	D		−3.5
Glutamate	Glu	E		−3.5
Lysine	Lys	K		−3.9
Arginine	Arg	R		−4.5
Histidine	His	H		−3.2
Tyrosine	Tyr	Y		−1.3
Tryptophan	Trp	W		−0.9
Phenylalanine	Phe	F		2.8
Cysteine	Cys	C		2.5

Table 8.1 (Continued)
Structure and Hydrophobicity of Amino Acids

Name	Symbol		R Group	Hydrophobicity
	3 Lett.	1 Lett.		
Methionine	Met	M	$CH_3-S-CH_2-CH_2-\overset{\overset{H}{\mid}}{\underset{\underset{+}{NH_3}}{C}}-COO^-$	1.9
Serine	Ser	S	$HO-CH_2-\overset{\overset{H}{\mid}}{\underset{\underset{+}{NH_3}}{C}}-COO^-$	−0.8
Threonine	Thr	T	$CH_3-\underset{\underset{OH}{\mid}}{CH}-\overset{\overset{H}{\mid}}{\underset{\underset{+}{NH_3}}{C}}-COO^-$	−0.7
Asparagine	Asn	N	$\underset{O}{\overset{NH_2}{\diagdown}}C-CH_2-\overset{\overset{H}{\mid}}{\underset{\underset{+}{NH_3}}{C}}-COO^-$	−3.5
Glutamine	Gln	Q	$\underset{O}{\overset{NH_2}{\diagdown}}C-CH_2-CH_2-\overset{\overset{H}{\mid}}{\underset{\underset{+}{NH_3}}{C}}-COO^-$	−3.5
Glycine	Gly	G	$H-\overset{\overset{H}{\mid}}{\underset{\underset{+}{NH_3}}{C}}-COO^-$	−0.4
Alanine	Ala	A	$CH_3-\overset{\overset{H}{\mid}}{\underset{\underset{+}{NH_3}}{C}}-COO^-$	1.8
Valine	Val	V	$\overset{CH_3}{\underset{CH_3}{\diagup}}CH-\overset{\overset{H}{\mid}}{\underset{\underset{+}{NH_3}}{C}}-COO^-$	4.2
Leucine	Leu	L	$\overset{CH_3}{\underset{CH_3}{\diagup}}CH-CH_2-\overset{\overset{H}{\mid}}{\underset{\underset{+}{NH_3}}{C}}-COO^-$	3.8

Table 8.1 (Continued)
Structure and Hydrophobicity of Amino Acids

Name	Symbol 3 Lett.	Symbol 1 Lett.	R Group	Hydrophobicity
Isoleucine	Ile	I		4.5
Proline	Pro	P		−1.6

For Isoleucine, the R group structure:

$$CH_3-CH_2-\underset{\underset{CH_3}{|}}{CH}- -\underset{\underset{\overset{+}{N}H_3}{|}}{\overset{\overset{H}{|}}{C}}-COO^-$$

For Proline, the R group structure shows a ring with CH_2, CH_3, CH_2 groups connected to $C-COO^-$ and N with H.

AFFINITY CHROMATOGRAPHY

Molecules are separated in affinity chromatography (AC) through structure-specific interactions with ligand. AC is preferably used for capture operations, where high selectivity ensures good separation between the protein and cell culture components and impurities. The advantages of AC include its high specificity and mild elution conditions; the disadvantages include its inability to separate derivatives from target protein, inability to use sodium hydroxide for cleaning, and the overall cost of operation. In the elution stage, the adsorption is carried out using a specific substrate ion in combination with one of the above-mentioned principles. To be effective, the dissociation constant must be in a range of 10^{-5} to 10^{-7} M to allow efficient elution of the protein generally accomplished by changing pH, ionic strength, polarity, or by addition of specific cosolvents. The commonly available affinity interactions used are: antibody-antigen, enzyme-substrate, inhibitor-enzyme, lectin-polysaccharide, hormone-receptor, protein A-IgG, triazine-protein, peptide-protein, metal ion-protein, and glutathione-glutathione-S-transferase. As a result, this chromatographic technique is highly selective but offers poor resolution of related derivative products, making it an ideal unit operation for initial capture of product where the pass through volumes may be very large and where step-elution of target protein is made after washing away impurities.

The advantage of using affinity chromatography in large-scale capture operations has resulted in the availability of several generic options based on ligand screening technology such as the use of:

- Small organic triazine-based ligands, which are identified by screening against the target protein, immobilized to a matrix, and optimized in a column mode.
- Aminimide molecules as molecular recognition agents.
- Fusion protein capture.

Ligands Protein A and Protein G for antibody purification or from the cell culture harvest. Protein A binds effectively to the human IgG subclasses IgG_1, IgG_2, IgG_4, and Protein G binds effectively to the human IgG subclasses IgG_{1-4}. Ligands are chosen to take into account their toxicity and environmental impact, if these are not already in wide use. Commonly used ligands are antibodies, antigens, cofactors, Protein A, metal chelators, miomimetic triazine compounds, and structural peptides. Both expanded bed and packed bed technology are used for capture operations.

The elution techniques used in AC include:

- Isocratic elution (not very practical in large-scale productions).
- Stepwise elution, one of several isocratic elutions to remove bound impurities by passing one or two bed volumes at each step. This process is more robust than gradient operations.
- Gradient elution, where the concentration of the eluting buffer is increased continuously by mixing starting and final buffer so that the percentage of final buffer pumped into the column is gradually increased.
- Gel filtration, which should be evaluated during elution. If used, the nonbinding solutes will be fractioned according to size, as in size exclusion chromatography, and some molecules may be affected (delayed elution) by the pore size of the particles. The sample molecules cannot migrate ahead of the eluting buffer since they encounter conditions that favor their rebinding to the matrix.

The column size is usually not a critical parameter and it is determined by the capacity of the adsorbent. Short bed heights (10 to 30 cm) and wide columns will allow for high throughput of the often large volumes handled during capture. Some of the common media used that comply with cGMP purification qualification include: Blue Sepharose 6 FF, Chelating Sepharose FF, Heparin Sepharose 6 FF, Streamline Heparin, Protein A Sepharose 4 FF, Protein A Sepharose 6 FF, Streamline rProtein A, rProtein A Sepharose FF, rmp Protein A Sepharose FF, MabSelect, Protein G Sepharose 4 FF, Chelating Sepharose FF, and Streamline Chelating, all from Amersham.

The operating conditions are optimized through adjustment of pH where variations affect the affinity between the protein and the ligand due to a change of surface properties of the protein. An increase in pH will mostly result in enhanced binding, and thus the elution is done at lower pH values, though high pH may be necessary in some instances. The ionic strength is adjusted by adding salt (typically 0.15 M) to the buffer to suppress nonspecific electrostatic interactions. This may be unnecessary in situations where the ligand interacts predominantly by electrostatic forces where higher ionic strength (1 to 3 M) is used, such as in the binding to dye resins. When the binding is dominated by hydrophobic interactions, high salt concentrations enhance binding (e.g., binding of IgG to Protein A resins). The binding capacity should not be exceeded to avoid precipitation; for example, the theoretical binding capacity of a protein with M_r 60,000 is approximately 80 mg/mL on a 4% agarose-based affinity matrix. The polarity is important where binding is a result of hydrophobicity and where elution is not easily achieved through changes in pH or ionic strength; this requires reduction of polarity or inclusion of a chaotropic salt, denaturing agent, or detergent in the eluting buffer. Useful detergents are Lubrol, Nonidet P-40, octylglycosides, and Triton X-100 (note that it causes high UV absorption) at concentrations below the critical micelle concentration. Chaotropic salts, such as KSCN and KI (1-3 M), are typical. Polarity reducing agents such as ethylene glycol and dioxan often promote desorption at concentrations of 20 to 40% (v/v) and 10% (v/v), respectively. Denaturants such as GuHCl or urea, used at moderate concentrations, affect the structure of the protein and thereby the ability to bind to the ligand. Other displacers include monomeric (e.g., imidazole) and polymeric displacers (e.g., vinyl imidazole and vinyl caprolactam). The common buffers used in elution in AC on A and G resins depend on the target proteins. For example, for most IgGs, the starting buffer would be sodium phosphate at pH 7, but the elution buffer can be glycine-HCl, ammonium acetate, sodium citrate, or sodium phosphate.

IMMOBILIZED METAL AFFINITY CHROMATOGRAPHY

The immobilized metal affinity chromatography (IMAC) is a special type of affinity chromatography where the target protein is captured based on its affinity to metal ions complexed with a chelating group (e.g., iminodiacetic acid). Since the strength of binding is highly dependent on the protein structure, IMAC provides a high selectivity. To be bound to metal ions, the protein must exhibit certain amino acid residues such as histidine, cysteine, or tryptophan; since histidine-tagged proteins are widely expressed in *E. coli,* the use of IMAC is common. The binding potential remains viable even when proteins are denatured, such as by using 7 to 8 M urea or 6 M GuHCl; ionic adsorption is obviated using high ionic strength buffers. The binding is influenced by pH, where low pH often leads to desorption. Clearance of viruses is performed often in some instances; however, this must be thoroughly validated.

Briefly, the main advantages of IMAC are high selectivity and mild elution conditions, they are effective in the presence of denaturants, detergents, glycol, and ethanol, and binding at high ionic strength is possible. The main disadvantages are that it cannot separate derivatives from the protein of interest, and there is a potential leakage of metal ions. IMAC is preferably used for capture or first intermediary purification operations, where good separation between the protein, cell culture components, and impurities is needed.

IMAC is highly useful for purification of IgGs as they bind to metal chelating columns at neutral to alkaline pH, the binding being relatively independent of salt concentration and the presence of nonionic detergents and urea in low concentrations. As a result, the cell culture medium can be applied to the column with no required conditioning. Elution is performed by decreasing pH in the range of 8 to 4, mainly reflecting titration of histidyl residues or, by using competitive elution with imidazole, providing a more gentle technique in case the target molecule shows limited stability at low pH. Since the leakage of metal ions is inevitable, further purification is needed in subsequent steps.

The capture feature of IMAC is highly desirable because there is little or no adjustment of the large volume of cell culture application sample required, the majority of contaminants pass through the column at loading conditions, and the divalent metal ions can be readily removed in simple additional steps. The elution techniques in the use of IMAC are similar to those described above for affinity chromatography. The same holds true for column dimensions. The most common media used in IMAC are Chelating Sepharose FF and Streamline Chelating from Amersham Biosciences. The most optimal binding conditions are obtained at neutral to slightly alkaline pH, and pH variation is a good tool to discriminate binding to histidyl residues. A decrease in pH will generally lead to desorption of the protein. Most proteins elute between pH 6.0 and 4.2. High concentrations of salt in the buffer do not appreciably affect the adsorption of protein, and as a result it is common to include sodium chloride (0.1 to 1.0 M) in buffers used in IMAC in order to suppress ion exchange effects as well as formation of electrostatic complexes between the contaminants and target protein. Loading considerations are similar to those observed for AC. The choice of metal ion depends on the relative stability of complexes formed with iminodiacetic acid, and for divalent metal ions it is in the following order: $Cu^{2+} > Ni^{2+} > Zn^{2+} > Co^{2+} > Ca^{2+}, Mg^{2+}$. Some proteins bind only to Cu^{2+}; the use of weakly binding Zn^{2+} is often made to enhance selectivity. When using Ni^{2+}, generally for polyhistidine-tagged proteins, the choice must be balanced with the possibility that remnants of nickel may produce allergic reactions. Additives that alter polarity have only a minor effect. And denaturants only slightly affect the performance of IMAC. Most suitable elution solvents are ammonium chloride, glycine, histamine, histidine, Tris, or imidazole, EDTA with affinity for the chelated metal at high ionic strength as they strip the metal ions from the column. A milder elution system comprises solutes such as ammonium chloride and glycine for competitive elution from the column. EDTA is used to recover very tightly bound proteins, but it also strips metal ions. Buffers used in IMAC are phosphate, borate, or acetate for initial screening, as they do not interfere with binding. If the protein:metal affinity is high, a buffer that tends to reduce the binding strength can be used (e.g., Tris-HCl). However, amine-based buffers may affect both metal leakage and binding capacity. The most commonly used starting buffers are Tris-HCl, Tris, sodium borate, sodium acetate, and phosphate, and the common elution buffers are likely to be the starting buffer with histidine, sodium acetate with sodium chloride, phosphate-acetic acid, EDTA, sodium acetate, imidazole, histidine, or phosphate.

ANION EXCHANGE CHROMATOGRAPHY

The most widely used purification technique in the manufacturing of therapeutic proteins is some form of ion exchange chromatography because of their system robustness, excellent scalability, high resolution power, and capacity. They are used widely for capture, intermediary purification, and polishing; high resolution is possible only surpassed by RPC; organic solvents, urea, and detergents do not affect the efficiency; it is highly flexible; and low protein concentration samples can be applied directly without significant loss. The disadvantages of anion exchange chromatography (AEC) include poor binding at medium to high ionic strength, high ionic strength in eluted fractions when salt desorption is used, localized pH extremes during elution that can affect protein stability, uncontrolled pH during elution that may cause precipitation in the column, and some glycoproteins may exhibit a very complex purification pattern.

Although the science behind the binding of protein to charged surfaces is not well understood, the use of protein characteristics like pI, and M_r the charge, the matrix used, and the pH and conductivity of solvent provide good predictability of separation. Anion exchangers are basic ion exchangers containing positive ligands binding negatively charged proteins (or counter ions, anions). They are traditionally divided into two groups: weak or strong anion exchangers based on the pKa of the charged group. The trend is toward the use of the strong anion exchangers (quaternary amines) capable of binding proteins in the pH range 2 to 12 depending on the pI of the protein (a protein of pI 3.1 is expected to bind at pH 4.1, while a protein of pI 6.1 is expected to bind at pH 7.1). A pH change in the interval of 2 to 12 will consequently not affect the net charge of a strong anion exchanger. The corresponding pH interval for a weak anion exchanger is 2 to 9.

Seven out of 20 amino acid residues contain charged groups affecting binding to ion exchangers. The simplest model will assume the protein net charge to be the dominant binding force (the more highly charged a protein is, the more strongly it binds), but local charge distributions on the protein surface should be taken into consideration. It is the chromatographic contact region of the protein surface that determines the chromatographic behavior illustrated in binding of proteins at their pI to ion exchangers. The number of charged sites of the protein interacting with the ion exchanger is called the Z value. An increase in Z indicates increasingly stronger binding. The Z value depends on pH, protein conformation, solvent, amount of protein bound, and ion exchanger properties. There is little relation between the protein net charge and the Z value.

Most proteins have an isoelectric point at pH below 7, expanding the range in which anion exchange chromatography can be used. A rule of thumb is that the protein will bind to the ion exchanger one pH unit from the isoelectric point, which should be the starting point before going into experimental design (a protein with pI of 5.5 is expected to bind at pH 6.5 and over).

As a rule, a negatively charged protein will bind to the anion exchanger, making adsorption strongly pH dependent. At pH values far from the isoelectric point, proteins bind strongly. Near the isoelectric point, weaker binding may be expected, and, at the isoelectric point, local charge distributions may occur even if the net charge is neutral. The pH of the solution is therefore a very essential parameter in ion exchange chromatography, and a decrease in pH may be used to elute the protein.

Negatively charged ions (chloride, acetate, citrate, phosphate) are used as counter ions to replace the protein during elution. The protein competes with those ions for binding to the ion exchanger. To ensure high binding capacity, low buffer concentrations are used during column equilibrium and sample application (0.01 to 0.05 M), which makes it important to use buffers with a pKa close to the pH working range (± 0.5 units) to ensure sufficient buffer capacity. Note that pKa varies with temperature. The effect of ions on chromatographic behavior has been studied extensively, but safety, economy, robustness, and large-scale considerations very often restrict industrial applications to a few well-characterized buffer systems, such as acetate, citrate, phosphate, carbonate, and ammonia. Generally, the steric factors only affect the separation of charged solutes as a result of their influence on the available capacity for each substrate.

There are several different elution techniques utilized. In isocratic elution, which is rarely used, the solvent composition is constant and all components move simultaneously. A stepwise elution is a serial application of several isocratic elutions. At each step, typically one to two bed volumes of eluent are passed through the column. Column wash procedures are often step elutions used to remove bound impurities. Stepwise elution of the target protein is often a good alternate to gradient elution as it provides a more robust system. In gradient elution, the concentration of the eluting buffer is increased continuously by mixing starting and final buffer so that the percentage of final buffer pumped into the column is gradually increased. The elution process depends on the stage at which AEC is applied; in the capture stage, the ionic strength may be too high, requiring an additional ultrafiltration step that will increase process volume; though one can use high-resolution procedures (gradients) at capture, it is recommended to make use of simple elution techniques (on/off) and use the column in a similar way to affinity columns. At the intermediate stage, an ion exchanger may be used where sample conductivity is low (e.g., after a HIC step) to keep sample handling to a minimum. In the polishing stage, the use of such high separation media as the mono-dispersed small particle (15 and 30µ) ion exchangers (e.g., Source30Q) helps separate even closely related compounds (e.g., des-amido and oxidized forms and target protein).

In the capture mode, the column dimensions may be defined to obtain maximum throughput of the broth. If ion exchange is used for intermediary purification or polishing, the bed height is a critical parameter. The normal range is between 10 and 30 cm bed height. Columns used for isocratic elution should have a larger bed height than columns used for gradient elution. Some of the most popular media used include: ANX Sepharose 4 FF, DEAE Sepharose FF, Q Sepharose FF, Q Sepharose Big Beads, Q, Sepharose High Performance, Q Sepharose XL, Source 15Q, Source 30Q, Streamline DEAE, and Streamline Q XL from Amersham Biosciences. Only marginal gains are made from choosing a weak ion exchanger over a strong ion exchanger. The more important considerations include the size of particle; larger proteins require media with large pore sizes and it must be ensured that the protein is not excluded from the inner part of the particle due to a pore size being too small. This will considerably lower the capacity. The pore size of the particles is an important consideration, as size exclusion effects may occur following elution. To protect media, the sample should be filtered with a 0.45 µm filter prior to application, which may result in increased back pressure. Filtration is not necessary if expanded bed technology is used (see elsewhere in the book).

Typically the pH of the application sample should be at least one pH unit above the isoelectric point of the target molecule. A pH farther away from the isoelectric point will increase the net charge of the target molecule, inducing stronger binding but also increased capacity. The choice of optimal pH will always be a balance between binding capacity and selectivity, and this must be defined by experimental work. An increase in pH will result in desorption from the column as pH becomes closer to pI. Electrophoretic titration curves allow optimization of the charge-pH relationship and are particularly useful for predicting suitable conditions for an ion exchange separation.

As a rule, the ionic strength of the sample and the mobile phase should be low to ensure firm binding of the target molecule. Typical buffer concentration should be within 0.01 to 0.05 M (resulting in an ionic strength of around 5 mS/cm) in order to ensure maximum binding capacity. Increasing the ionic strength of the solution will lead to desorption of the protein. It is possible to influence both resolution and the elution pattern by changing the nature of counter ions, as proteins respond differently to the said changes (in a nonpredictable way). Commonly used anions are acetate, citrate, sulfate, and phosphate. Chloride may also be used, but due to its corrosive effect on stainless steel, chlorides are often exchanged with acetate counter ions in large scale. There is also a concern due to the buffering effect of some of the counter ions (e.g., acetate). Polyvalent anions are better displacers (less retention) of small molecules from an anion exchanger than monovalent ions (compared at the same ionic strength). The elution strength of different anions is acetate < formate < chloride < bromide < sulfate < citrate.

The reason temperature is important in ion exchange chromatography is not because of its effect on ion behavior but for the change in pKa brought about by changes in temperature, particularly as samples are subjected to a wide range of transition from cold room to work areas.

Though the capacity of ion exchange matrices is generally high, precipitation can occur inside the column during elution at high local protein concentration.

Polarity of solvents due to the presence of nonionic detergents and organic solvents (such as ethanol or ethylene glycol) does not affect the protein binding significantly; zwitterions, such as betaine and taurine, decrease aggregate formation and strength of binding to the ion exchanger, thus increasing the resolution. PEG, a neutral polymer, increases the interaction with the ion exchanger, resulting in increased resolution.

The chaotropic effects of anions increase in the order sulfate, phosphate, acetate, carbonate, and chloride. Presence of chaotropic salts (e.g., thiocyanate) or denaturing agents (e.g., urea) increases the solubility of the protein; urea does not influence the binding of protein to the ion exchanger.

Examples of common and elution buffers used in AEC include ammonium acetate, sodium phosphate, and Tris (for elution Tris will contain additional sodium chloride). It is important to ensure optimal buffer capacity (pKa ± 1 pH unit) in sufficient concentration (usually in the interval of 25 to 50 mM). The charged form of the buffer species should be of the same sign as the ligand on the adsorbent (e.g., NH_4^+, Htris$^+$) to prevent these ions from becoming part of the ion exchange process and inducing localized pH changes.

CATION EXCHANGE CHROMATOGRAPHY

The advantages and disadvantages of selecting and using cation exchange chromatography (CEC) are similar to those described above for AEC and are not repeated in this section. Cation exchangers are acidic ion exchangers containing negative ligands binding positively charged proteins (or counter ions, cations) that can be weak or strong based on the pKa of the charged group. The stronger cation exchangers, such as sulfopropyl or methyl sulfonate, which can bind proteins in the pH range 4 to 13, depending on the pI of the protein, are more popular. Weak cation exchangers will work to a lower pH of 6. Most proteins have an isoelectric point at a pH below 7, restricting the range in which CEC can be used, for example, a protein with a pI of 5.5 is expected to bind at pH 4.5 and under, which might exclude strong cation exchangers. Positively charged ions (sodium, ammonium, potassium) are used as counter ions to replace the protein during elution. The protein competes with those ions for binding to the ion exchanger. To ensure high binding capacity, low buffer concentrations are used during column equilibrium and sample application (0.01 to 0.05M), which makes it important to use buffers with a pKa close to the pH working range (± 0.5 units) in order to ensure enough buffer capacity.

The media commonly used in CEC include: CM Sepharose FF, SP Sepharose FF, SP Sepharose BigBeads, SP Sepharose XL, SP Sepharose High Performance, Source 15S, Source 30S, Streamline SP, and Streamline SP XL by Amersham.

As a general rule, the ionic strength of the sample and the mobile phase should be low to ensure firm binding of the target molecule. Typical buffer concentration should be within 0.01 to 0.05 M (resulting in an ionic strength of around 5 mS/cm) in order to ensure maximum binding capacity.

Increasing the ionic strength of the solution will lead to desorption of the protein. It is possible to influence both resolution and the elution pattern by changing the nature of counter ions, as proteins behave differently to the said changes (in an unpredictable way). Commonly used anions are acetate, citrate, sulfate, and phosphate. Chloride may also be used, but due to its corrosive effect on stainless steel, chlorides are often exchanged with acetate counter ions in large scale. One should be aware of the buffering effect of some of the counter ions (e.g., acetate). The elution strength of different anions is acetate < formate < chloride < bromide < sulfate < citrate. Examples of common starting and elution buffers are ammonium acetate and water (for starting buffer).

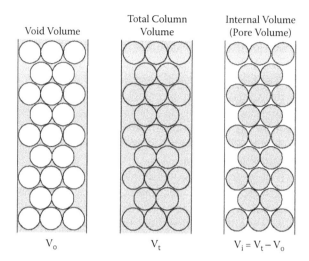

FIGURE 8.1 Description of volume parameters in gel chromatography.

SIZE EXCLUSION CHROMATOGRAPHY

Size exclusion chromatography (SEC) (gel filtration, gel permeation chromatography, molecular sieving chromatography) is a high-resolution separation process used to separate molecules based on the difference in molecular size (e.g., polymeric and dimeric compounds), to desalt, where low molecular compounds are exchanged, for group separations (e.g., removal of low molecular weight impurities), and to facilitate refolding of denatured proteins. The main advantages of SEC are the effective removal of di- and polymers (highly desirable in finishing or polishing operations), its fast method development, that it does not affect protein stability, and that the buffer can be exchanged independent of the chromatographic technique. The disadvantages include its low capacity (the application sample volume should not exceed more than 5% v/v of the column volume; as a result SEC is rarely used in capture and intermediary operations), high cost of columns, long cycle times due to long beds and low flow velocities, and the dilution of sample (or increase in volume).

The solute molecules are separated on the basis of the pore volume of media. Large molecules, which cannot enter the intraparticle volume, are not retained, while small molecules, able to enter the particles and diffuse into a larger volume, are retained. The elution volume of a nonretained solute is equal to the interparticle volume (the void volume, V_0). The ratio between the intraparticle volume (V_i) and V_0 is called the permeability of the chromatographic medium (Figure 8.1).

As the sample moves down the bed of media under elution medium, the small molecules, which diffuse into the bed (including the buffer components of the sample), are delayed compared with the large molecules, which cannot diffuse (or only partly diffuse) into the gel particles. The result is separation according to molecular size (or approximately molecular weight) (Figure 8.2).

The resolution is determined by the size difference between the solutes, the selectivity of the gel, and parameters such as load, flow rate, particle size, and column dimensions. The application sample should be highly concentrated in order to reduce its volume. Ultrafiltration is a commonly used technique to achieve concentrated samples. The capacity can be improved by concentrating the sample prior to application. This may cause an increase in viscosity and may lead to precipitation. The costs included in introducing an extra step should be balanced against the increased capacity.

Gel filtration separates mixtures of biomolecules according to size. Large molecules elute either in the void volume or early in a chromatographic separation. Smaller molecules elute later, depending on their degree of penetration of the pores of the matrix. Gel filtration is a simple and mild technique that complements ion exchange, hydrophobic interaction, and affinity chromatography.

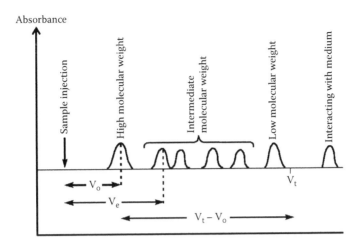

FIGURE 8.2 Isocratic elution in gel filtration.

In process-scale chromatography, gel filtration is principally used for desalting the product, for buffer exchange, for rapid removal of reagents to terminate a reaction, or for specific removal of contaminants with molecular weights above or below that of the desired product. Typically, molecules must differ in size by twofold to yield a good separation, although other adsorptive effects can augment some separations where molecules are similar in size. Gel filtration is useful at the polishing stage, where volumes are much lower than at the capture or intermediate stage, where there is a need to remove dimers or aggregates. Gel filtration separates mixtures of biomolecules according to size. Large molecules elute either in the void volume or early in a chromatographic separation. Smaller molecules elute later, depending on their degree of penetration of the pores of the matrix.

Gel filtration is performed in three principally different modes, depending on the size differences of the solutes to be separated: (1) group separation, (2) fractionation, and (3) determination of molecular mass (distributions) When the size difference is large, i.e., a factor of more than 10, this is referred to as group separation (e.g., desalting, buffer exchange), and when the size difference is small, i.e., a factor of 2 to 5, it is called fractionation. The third mode is analytical gel filtration, e.g., determination of molecular mass distributions, where an array of molecular masses is to be separated. These different modes put different requirements on the equipment and media used and will yield widely different productivity in terms of information or material processed. Amersham provides excellent guidelines on selection of media for gel filtration.

Desalting and buffer exchange of protein samples are two examples of group separation. The large size difference between the protein and the low molecular solute make it possible to select a gel filtration medium that will exclude the protein from the porous network while allowing full permeation of the low molecular weight solute such as when using HiPrep™ 26/10 desalting column. The separation takes place over a volume equal to the pore volume. In desalting the gel filtration, medium is used to selectively exclude the large molecular weight solute, e.g., protein or DNA from entering the porous gel phase. Thus, a rational choice of matrix will allow the protein to be eluted in the void, or interstitial, volume of the column. As a result the protein zone will be diluted to a minimum, as caused by eddy dispersion only (e.g., nonequilibrium effects are eliminated). This also means that the zone broadening, or dilution of the protein zone, is rather insensitive to fluid velocity, and high velocities (e.g., exceeding 500 cm/h) may be employed for fast desalting (since the zone broadening of low molecular weight solutes is also generally small unless extreme velocities are used). Low molecular weight impurities, e.g., salt, will permeate the pore volume and will have a retention volume equal to the total liquid volume of the column (provided the size of the molecule is small as compared to the pore size of the gel filtration medium). If the impurities have an intermediate size they will only permeate part of the pore volume, giving a less favorable situation.

As a result of the mechanism of separation, the characteristics of the gel filtration medium that should be considered in the selection of media include pore size, pore volume, particle size, and matrix rigidity. The pore size is chosen so that the large molecular weight solute is excluded from the gel matrix. However, the pore size must not be too small since the low molecular weight impurities will then not elute at the total volume, limiting the applicable sample volume. The pore volume is a very important characteristic of the gel filtration medium and will directly influence the sample volume that is applicable. Therefore, the matrix volume of a desalting gel filtration medium for preparative use should be kept as low as possible. However, this is contradictory to the demand of high matrix rigidity, which generally is increased with increased matrix volume. A small pore volume may of course be compensated for by using a larger bed volume, but this will be at the expense of lower productivity. The particle size will influence the sample dispersion in the bed. Since the large molecular mass solute will not enter the porous phase, the main cause of zone broadening in gel filtration (i.e., due to nonequilibrium) is not present and only eddy dispersion contributes. This effect may be small compared to dispersion from sample application and column dead volumes (e.g., at inlet and outlet).

The influence of particle size in the range 50 to 300 µm on the bed dispersion is rather small for column lengths above 15 cm. However, for shorter columns bed dispersion reduces the sample volume that can be applicable, especially for media of large particle size. In addition to the effect from the dispersion of the bed, a contribution from column dead volumes may be anticipated, the extent being dependent upon the column design. This will reduce the relative influence of the particle size to some degree. The effect will be largest for small particles since these yield lower dispersion than larger particles. If the sample volume is very small, a column of small size is recommended. If dilution of the sample must be kept to a minimum, a small particle size gel filtration medium should be selected. The particle size has a large influence on the pressure drop over the packed bed. In principle the pressure drop is inversely proportional to the particle size squared. This is because smaller intraparticle channels are formed by smaller particles. The higher liquid velocities in these smaller channels will result in higher friction forces acting on the particles, yielding higher pressure drops but also leading to higher stress, which may result in compaction of the bead. The reduced size of the flow channels with lower particle size will also lead to a higher sensitivity to viscous fingering effects, i.e., the distortion of highly concentrated sample zones due to hydrodynamic instability of the rear part of the zone. A high matrix rigidity will allow high flow rates to be employed for fast desalting, but this may be at the expense of the maximum sample volume that can be applied, and these factors need to be considered simultaneously. If large sample volumes are to be quickly desalted, it may be better to use a larger particle of low matrix volume.

The productivity is expressed as the amount of product purified per unit of time and unit bed volume. The amount of purified product is equal to the concentration times the sample volume times the yield. The yield for desalting (and gel filtration in general) is very high and may be set to 100%. The maximum concentration of proteins that may be applied is restricted by the relative viscosity of the sample compared to eluent and a sample concentration of 50 mg/mL of a protein having a molecular mass of 50,000 seems to be the upper limit in simple aqueous eluents. The productivity decreases with increasing column length. Thus, it is advantageous to use "short and fat" columns as long as the column construction minimizes column dead volumes. In order to utilize the entire pore volume for desalting, it is important that the pore size is not too small since this will lead to low molecular weight impurities being eluted too early. A gel filtration medium of larger pore size, which still excludes the protein of interest, should be used, or the sample volume must be reduced to allow for separation (the sample volume may not exceed the difference in elution volume of the impurity and the void volume).

The mobile phase is selected based on desired outcome. Preparative SEC includes buffer exchange and fractionation. Buffer exchange, or desalting, is the exchange of low molecular components of the sample (typically salt molecules) with another buffering substance. In fractionation, the solute is separated from other solutes according to their molecular size, typically separation of polymers and dimmers from the monomeric target protein.

Commonly used SEC media are Sephadex (based on cross-linked dextran), Superdex (based on highly cross-linked agarose), Superose (based on highly cross-linked agarose), and Sepharose (based on cross-linked agarose) from Amersham. The SEC media are not inert and can induce electrostatic, hydrophobic, hydrogen bonding, and biospecific interactions. The resolution is proportional to the square root of the bed height. The effective column length may be increased by adding columns in series (column stacking). The sample volume is the single parameter having the greatest impact on resolution. The sample volume should not exceed 5% v/v of the column volume. (Even smaller loads are often necessary in order to obtain the desired resolution.) In desalting mode, up to 30% v/v of the total bed volume may be applied without disrupting the separation effect.

The sample concentration is restricted by the protein precipitation and the viscosity of the sample plug compared to that of the mobile phase. The general rule is that the viscosity of the sample should be less than 1.5. This corresponds to a sample concentration of 70 mg/mL of a globular protein such as albumin. At lower temperature the viscosity is increased by a large factor, often doubling the back pressure and slowing the diffusion rate of the solute molecules. The resolution decreases with increasing flow velocity relative to the viscosity of the eluent. Typical flow velocities at large scale are in the range of 30 to 50 cm/h. In desalting mode (e.g., Sephadex G-25), it can be as high as 200 cm/h depending on the bed diameter and height. An increase in bed height increases the resolution. The increase in resolution relates directly to the square root of the increase in bed height. The application sample should be filtered with a 0.45 μm filter prior to application in order to protect the column against particles, aggregates, etc., which may result in increased back pressure.

The common buffers used include ammonium acetate and sodium phosphate (alone or in combination with ammonium sulfate). To avoid precipitation due to change of pH, ionic strength, presence of cosolvent, or changes in temperature, ensure that the application sample complies with the equilibration buffer.

The problems of later or earlier elution are readily solved by adjusting a large number of parameters available. When elution is later than expected, it can be caused by:

- Ionic adsorption due to negatively charged groups on the support (Carboxyl-, Sulfate-) and positively charged groups on sample molecules. It is resolved by including 150mM NaCl (or other salt) in buffer.
- Hydrophobic adsorption. It is resolved by adding 10 to 20% ethanol or other organic solvents to buffer or decrease salt concentration in high ionic strength buffer.
- More compact shape of the sample molecule due to hydrogen bridge bonds. It is resolved by including 8M urea or 6M guanidine hydrochloride in buffer.
- Digestion by proteases. It is resolved by adding protease inhibitors to buffer.

When elution is earlier than desired, its causes and remediation are:

- Ionic aggregates and complexes due to carbohydrate chains (glycoproteins). It is changed by including 150mM NaCl or up to 10% betaine in buffer.
- Complexes associated via SH-groups. It is resolved by adding a reducing agent (e.g., DTT) to buffer.
- Hydrophobic aggregates are removed by adding 10 to 20% ethanol or other organic solvents to buffer.

- Gel filtration of micelles/protein aggregates is resolved by decreasing buffer detergent concentration until below CMC or use a different detergent (stay below its CMC).
- Exclusion of molecules due to ionic repulsion of negatively charged groups on sample and support is resolved by including 150mM NaCl or 0.1% TFA in buffers.

REVERSED PHASE CHROMATOGRAPHY

Reversed phase chromatography (RPC) is one of the most widely used chromatography methods in downstream processing as well as in the analytical testing of therapeutic proteins. Whereas other methods rely on the size of molecule, RPC is governed by the hydrophobic interaction between the solute molecules (in the mobile phase) and the ligand (in the stationary phase). This should not be confused with HIC (hydrophobic interaction chromatography), where the ligands interact individually with the solutes; in RPC, the stationary phase is a continuous hydrophobic phase with the solute molecules partitioning between the mobile phase and the stationary phase. The separation occurs by a reversible dynamic absorption/desorption onto a matrix of hydrophobic ligand, which is chemically attached to a porous, insoluble matrix generally composed of silica or a synthetic organic polymer, such as polystyrene. The unattached silanol groups on silica (when used) interact with the solute molecules (an undesirable situation reduced by blocking the groups with alkyl silane reagents—known as end-capping), which makes the media support an important element. Whereas silica-based matrices are chemically stable at acidic pH, synthetic organic polymers are stable throughout the pH range from 1 to 12. The unattached surface of polymers is also strongly hydrophobic, in contrast to the unattached ends on silica. The selectivity in separation is determined by the type of ligand attached to the medium, such as n-alkyl hydrocarbon or aryl hydrocarbon compounds; if the solute is highly hydrophobic, the ligands must be less hydrophobic (or they will elute). Proteins bind C4 to C8 columns. If impurities present are charged they can bind to the ligand, which can be reduced by a proper selection of the mobile phase.

The mobile phase is generally a mixture of water, organic modifier (e.g., water-ethanol), and a buffering substance to ensure that the solutes are uncharged during separation. The organic modifier is often present in concentrations from 0 to 60% v/v such as 2-propanol, acetonitrile, methanol, and ethanol (listed in decreasing elution strength order). (The use of organic solvents in large-scale operations requires explosion-proof equipment and facilities.) The concentration of modifier is important and often a gradient system is used to improve separation where the initial binding conditions are designed to favor adsorption of the solute from the mobile phase (aqueous solution with little or no organic modifier present). In this case, adsorption is considered the extreme equilibrium state where the distribution of solute molecules is essentially 100% in the stationary phase. This is followed by desorption where the solute is essentially 100% distributed in the mobile phase achieved by decreasing the polarity (increasing the concentration of organic modifier). Several elution techniques are used with RPC: isocratic, stepwise, gradient, affinity elution, gel filtration, etc. Common media include Source 15RPC or Source 30RPC from Amersham.

The primary advantages of RPC are its very high resolution, even with closely related molecules, and its tolerance of high ionic strength solutions; RPC is a perfect polishing technique, but rarely used in intermediary purification and not in the capture mode. Presence of organic solvent in the eluted fractions often makes it necessary to introduce a subsequent buffer exchange step. The disadvantages in using RPC include the mandatory use of organic solvents, which often denature the target or affect their solubility, and that the ligand may also denature the proteins; RPC is also not suitable for proteins with molecular weight above 25 kD.

The common mobile phase solvents include hydrochloric acid, phosphoric acid, trifluoroacetic acid, triethylammonium phosphate, and ammonium acetate. The PRC matrix is stable at wide pH ranges (silica unstable at alkaline pH). At low pH the silanol groups of silica-based matrices will be uncharged reducing binding of ionic impurities. When using low pH, basic proteins show a tail when eluted; this can be obviated by increasing pH. The competition between carboxyl and basic groups is eliminated at low pH, where the carboxyl group ionization and the amino groups are essentially fully protonated. Generally, higher selectivity is seen when running below the pI of the protein (the mechanism is not well explained). In the absence of ions that stabilize secondary and tertiary structures, lowering of pH results in loss of resolution; since ionic strength does not have any significant direct effect, RPC offers great flexibility; however, where ion pairing agents are involved, it results in increased hydrophobicity of the solute molecules and thus its resolution on the columns; examples of ion pairing agents include TFA, PFPA, HFBA, ammonium acetate, phosphoric acid, tetramethylammonium chloride, tetrabutylammonium chloride, and triethylamine. Before any of these agents can be used, their toxicity must be considered. Presence of denaturing agents does not affect the capacity of the column.

Elevated temperatures expedite mass transfer of the solutes, more rapid unfolding/refolding, and interactions with ions and solvents, all improving efficiency of system; however, protein denaturation at high temperatures should be the controlling factor.

Whereas much higher loading can be done compared to ion exchange chromatography, generally more than 30% of maximum capacity would lead to losses in resolution and chemical deterioration as irreversible adsorption, denaturation, or conformational alterations. When the samples are very dilute, losses are minimal.

HYDROXYAPATITE CHROMATOGRAPHY

Hydroxyapatite matrix (poly-calcium phosphate $[Ca_{10}(PO_4)_6(OH)_2]$) is both the support and ligand where positively charged pairs of crystal calcium ions and clusters of six negatively charged oxygen atoms associated with triplets of crystal phosphates bind proteins through nonspecific and by specific complexing of protein carboxyls with calcium loci on the mineral. At low pH (5 or below) or in the presence of chelating agents, the crystal structure and efficiency is lost; however, hydroxyapatite media are resistant to sodium hydroxide, detergents, organic solvents, and denaturing agents. The major advantages in the use of hydroxyapatite chromatography (HAC) are its applicability during capture, its intermediary purification and polishing stages, often offering unique separation of even closely related compounds, and its effectiveness with different buffers and organic solvents, allowing mixed mode purification. HAC is applicable to all antibodies, providing good fractionation regardless of the production medium, species, class, or subclass. The disadvantage relates to stability of matrix at low pH and in the presence of chelating agents; matrix can degrade due to microbial secretion of acidic contaminants (this can be obviated using 50 to 60% methanol, though it represents a hazardous situation). The availability of different size uniform stable particles in the range from 10 to 100 μm is suitable for intermediate purification and polishing operations, as an alternate to IMAC, IEC, HIC, and RPC.

Proteins are eluted either as a result of the nonspecific ion screening of charges or by specific displacement of protein groups from the sites of the column with which they have been complexed. The good results obtained using HAC are surprising in the absence of a solid theory of how it works. It is particularly useful for the purification of medium- to large-size proteins with a well-defined tertiary structure; low molecular weight solutes and denatured proteins show lower affinity to hydroxyapatite. The adsorption depends on pH and ionic strength. The elution behavior is a function of the isoelectric point of the protein; basic proteins elute at moderate concentrations of phosphate, fluoride, chloride, or thiocyanate (0.1-0-3 M), with alternately low concentrations (< 0.003 M) of Ca^{2+} or Mg^{2+}; acidic proteins elute at equally moderate concentrations of phosphate and fluoride but do not elute with Ca^{2+} and usually not with chloride; neutral proteins elute with phosphate, fluoride, and chloride and not with Ca^{2+} or thiocyanate.

The elution techniques used are isocratic, stepwise, gradient, gel filtration, etc. The common media are the Macro-prep ceramic hydroxyapatite I and II from BioRad. Generally, an increase in pH would result in decreased binding capacity at a given ionic strength, and the matrix is unstable below pH 5. In general, low ionic strength favors protein adsorption and moderate to high salt concentrations may be workable depending on protein and salt. However, increasing phosphate concentration (even at low concentration) results in desorption of the protein. All proteins elute at moderate phosphate ion concentrations. Basic proteins elute at less than 3 mM Ca^{++} or Mg^{++} and with moderate Cl^-. Neutral proteins do not elute with Ca^{++} or other divalent metal ions. Acidic proteins do not elute with Ca^{++} or other divalent metal ions and do not usually elute with chloride. Likewise, 0.005 M $MgCl_2$ or 1 M NaCl/KCl is recommended to elute basic proteins, 1.0 M $MgCl_2$ to elute protein with pI between 5.5 and 8.0, and 0.3 M phosphate to elute acidic proteins. The load capacity of HAC is high but there remains a possibility of localized precipitation of target protein at high local concentration. Organic solvents (such as ethanol, ethylene glycol) do not affect the protein binding significantly and are even desired to keep hydrophobic proteins in solution or to keep the protein in its monomeric form. Proteins usually do not bind in the presence of detergents or denaturing agents, such as urea. Because only native proteins bind to hydroxyapatite, binding of weakly interacting basic proteins can be strengthened by inclusion of 1 mM phosphate in the buffer. The common starting buffers are potassium phosphate, sodium phosphate, sodium chloride, and magnesium chloride, and the elution buffers are mainly phosphates.

HYDROPHOBIC INTERACTION CHROMATOGRAPHY

Hydrophobic interaction chromatography (HIC) is based on interaction between hydrophobic patches on the protein surface and hydrophobic ligands of the matrix and is a result of the solvophobic effect, a solute-avoiding solvent. As a result, the high ionic strength of the solvent favors binding or the presence of salts that imparts the solution higher surface tension. (Balance this with the risk of salting out of proteins.) Unlike RPC, where the absorbent was a continuous phase, the ligands interact individually with the solutes in HIC, which is a much stronger chromatographic method with lesser risk of protein denaturation compared to RPC. The factors of importance are the type of ligand and base matrix, the solvent properties, temperature, and the type and concentration of salt. Retention is proportional to the length of the alkyl ligand chain (hydrophobic character); ligands containing from 4 to 10 carbon atoms are suited for most purposes. Aryl ligands, showing both aromatic and hydrophobic interactions, offer a mixed mode. Solvent additives (alcohols, detergents, chaotropic salts) that decrease the surface tension of water weaken the hydrophobic interaction, leading to desorption of the bound protein. Different salts give rise to differences in hydrophobic interaction and combinations of strong ligand-weak salt, medium ligand-medium salt and weak-ligand-strong salt can be used in the unit operation optimization. In summary, the HIC has an advantage of using both high and low salt concentrations and giving high recovery with high binding capacity, and it makes an excellent complementary technique to IEC. The conductivity of fermentation samples is often relatively high (10 to 30 mS/cm), making HIC an excellent capture step for hydrophobic proteins. Additionally, the binding capacity often decreases in the presence of antifoam agents added during fermentation. The disadvantages include protein precipitation at high salt concentrations and the environment risk considerations in large-scale operations (high salt consumption and disposal). (If used in intermediate purification, it is an excellent step following ion exchange chromatography, where high salt concentrations have been used to elute the target protein.). HIC is used in the polishing mode, but the resolution cannot be compared to that of IEC and RPC.

In the capture mode, the column dimensions are generally short (heights from 5 to 20 cm). The common media used are Butyl Sepharose 4 FF, Octyl Sepharose 4 FF, Phenyl Sepharose 6 FF (high sub), Phenyl Sepharose FF (low sub), Phenyl Sepharose High Performance, Source 15ETH, Source 15SO, and Source15PHE from Amersham. Since there is a correlation between increase in pH and weakened hydrophobic interaction, binding capacity must be tested at various pH values. Adsorption of proteins to HIC columns is favored by high salt concentrations (typically from 0.5 to 3 M concentrations are used). The strength of interaction depends on the salt used following the series (Hofmeister) ammonium sulfate > ammonium chloride > sodium sulfate > sodium chloride

> sodium bromide > sodium thiocyanate, with ammonium sulfate as one of the most utilized salts. The concentration of salt needed for protein binding may vary considerably from protein to protein. The HIC medium of choice should bind the protein of interest at relatively low salt concentration (< 1 M). The effect of salts in HIC can be accounted for by reference to the Hofmeister series for the precipitation of proteins or for their positive influence in increasing the molal surface tension of water. Elution is carried out with salt free buffers of low ionic strength. Less hydrophobic matrix is used if nonpolar solvents are needed for elution. Elution is achieved by a linear or stepwise decrease in the concentration of salt in the mobile phase. Temperature significantly affects HIC, a lower temperature reducing interaction. Presence of polarity-decreasing solvents (low levels of alcohols, detergents, ethylene glycol) decreases the binding of the target protein; these can be added after the salt has been removed from the column. Presence of chaotropic ions (e.g., Gu^{2+}, SCN^-) or urea decreases the binding of the target protein with risk for protein denaturation. Charged molecules containing short alkyl or aryl groups can be used as displacers in HIC.

The common starting buffers are potassium phosphate, sodium phosphate with aluminum sulfate, Tris with ammonium sulfate, Tris with EDTA and ammonium sulfate, sodium phosphate with sodium chloride, sodium succinate with ammonium sulfate, glycine, and sodium acetate with ammonium sulfate. The elution buffers include potassium phosphate, sodium phosphate, Tris with EDTA, sodium phosphate with sodium chloride, sodium succinate with ammonium sulfate, glycine, and ethylene glycol.

SCALE UP AND OPTIMIZATION

Scale up requires an in-depth understanding of parameters prior to establishing a scale-up plan. These parameters include: chromatography medium type, sample concentration, protein load/mL gel (adsorption techniques), sample volume/mL gel (gel filtration), linear flow rate, productivity (g/h/l of gel), column bed height, back pressure, buffer type and allowed variations in pH and conductivity, feed-stock and buffer storage stability, acceptable materials in contact with liquid, protein sensitivity to shear forces, recovery based on a well-defined product quality assay, washing procedures, gel life length, buffer consumption, product volumes, number of product fractions to be collected, and monitoring parameters.

There are several approaches to scale up; for example, we can maintain bed height, linear flow rate, gradient volume:media volume, sample concentration and composition, and sample volume:media volume. Another choice will be to increase column diameter, volumetric flow rate, sample volume proportionally, and gradient volume proportionally. In scale up of adsorption techniques the diameter is increased but the bed height is maintained. When using gel filtration we can increase diameter, maintain bed height, and additionally use columns in series. Most parameters that can be changed hover around the column used wherein the wall support and wall effects determine the choice of which parameter to change and which one to keep constant. The wall support affects distribution system, handling/packability, chemical resistance, pressure rating, and hygienic design (referring to cGMP compliance). The wall effects include pressure/flow curves in columns with different diameters; the system considerations include extra column zone spreading, accuracy (flow rate, gradient), chemical resistance, pressure rating, and hygienic design. The nonchromatographic factors that can affect performance upon scale up include changes in sample composition, changes in sample concentration, longer holding times, and buffer preparation. Fine-tuning the adjustments generally includes adjustment of gradient volume, adjustment of flow rate, adjustment of equilibration volume, modification of fractionation, and modification of CIP routines. Scale up from 10- to 500-fold are routinely made; however, a stepwise approach is suggested to take into account unexpected nonlinearities particularly with reference to the column characteristics that may arise. One of the premier sources of support is obviously the column and media supplier such as Amersham, who are more than likely to walk you through the entire process of scale up. When projects of large dimension are installed, many suppliers would even offer to run your process

TABLE 8.2
Optimization Parameters in Chromatography and Its Effect on Process Parameters

Chromatographic	Process
Column length and diameter	Stability
Bead size	Working temperature
Flow rates	Viscosity
Sample capacity (volume/mass), conditioning, application	Concentration/dilution
Buffers and salts	Batch size
Gradient volumes and shape	Logistics of handling liquids and consumables
Regeneration/reequilibration	Cooperation between research/development and production

to ensure you are making the right selection. Chromatography media are one of the most expensive components of the entire process, and every effort should be made to make this as optimal as possible for long-term cost savings.

The primary objective of optimization is to reach the specified purity at the highest possible yield, at the lowest possible cost, and in the shortest possible time. There are two parallel activities: the optimization of each chromatographic step and the optimization of the process.

The method of optimization using process chromatography operates on a different principle than does analytical chromatography; in process chromatography the resolution is adjusted to increase sample loading (productivity) and increased yield through less peak cutting within a defined purity Rs; in analytical chromatography, resolution concerns the maximum number of peaks, identity, purity, and quantification. Similarly, in process chromatography the size of sample is as large as possible while the opposite holds true for analytical chromatography. The speed is measure in g/mL gel/h in process and in cycles/h in analytical chromatography. The optimization parameters related to chromatography and process are given in Table 8.2. Following is a detailed description of these parameters:

- *Bed height optimization* techniques depend on the required selectivity. For high selectivity techniques where efficiency is less important, chemistry is used to improve RS and adsorption techniques such as IEC, HIC, AC are used with typical bed height of 5 to 20 cm. In low selectivity techniques where efficiency is more important, isocratic techniques such as SEC are used with typical bed heights: 60 to 90 cm. Particle size is important; for purification, the bead size ranges from 1 to –90 mm and for polishing, 10 to 34 mm. Bead size greater than 90 mm causes fouling, pressure drop, flow rate, and higher costs. Flow rate adjustment requires equilibration, adsorption, wash, desorption, and regeneration consideration.
- Gradient optimization starts with a simple linear gradient wherein slopes and shapes are varied to improve Rs; in step gradients artifacts are often discovered.
- Sample loading optimization depends on the technique used. For adsorption techniques where very high selectivity or capture is desired, complete bed volume is used for sample binding. In adsorption chromatography is used for purification only first past of bed volume is used for sample binding; in isocratic techniques, the sample volume is limiting. Steps in the process inversely affect the yield regardless of the step yield proportion; therefore, keeping steps to a minimum is probably the most effective optimization for cost, yield, and productivity. Buffer systems are modified by setting a range of buffer conditions and avoiding expensive buffers, instead using the standard phosphate, acetate, or citrate buffer. Increases in temperature increase throughput and this is a good parameter to adjust if stability of target protein, media, and resultant interactions would allow.

- Gel filtration is optimized taking into account the matrix, selectivity, rigidity, chemical stability, bead size distribution, bed height, column packing, flow rate, sample volume, and viscosity.
- Ion exchange is optimized by binding pH and ionic strength, sample load (mass), flow rate (equilibration, adsorption, desorption, wash), gradient volume, and shape. The elution strength of different ions in anion exchange chromatography is: acetate < formate< chloride < bromide < sulfate < citrate; in cation exchange chromatography: lithium < sodium < ammonium < potassium < magnesium < calcium.
- Affinity chromatography has critical parameters that include the type of ligand and ligand density, binding conditions, dynamic capacity, and elution conditions. The binding of hIgG is increased due to coupling of the legend. The elution is often affected by denaturing conditions (low pH, chaotropic salts, urea, guanidine-HCL), in AF attempts should be made to immediately neutralize or remove eluting agents and remove aggregates simultaneously using gel filtration.

HIC optimization parameters include sample load, sample application, flow rate, gradient volume and shape, temperature dependence, and hydrophobicity of ligand and additives. Increased ligand density gives increased strength of interaction and increased capacity; increased temperature gives increased strength of hydrophobic interaction; however, one must be cognizant of temperature–dependent alteration of protein structure and that lower pH shows increased hydrophobic interaction. The productivity is improved by optimizing starting conditions like type of salt, concentration, and application mode, by optimizing the dynamic loading capacity, and by tuning the gradient, flow rate, and sample relationship to what is normally done for ion exchange chromatography.

9 Quality Assurance Systems

INTRODUCTION

The overarching philosophy articulated in both the current Good Manufacturing Practice (cGMP) regulations and in robust modern quality systems is that: *Quality should be built into the product, and testing alone cannot be relied on to ensure product quality.*

Several key concepts are critical for any discussion of modern quality systems. Every pharmaceutical product has established identity, strength, purity, and other quality characteristics designed to ensure the required levels of safety and effectiveness. *Quality by design* means designing and developing manufacturing processes *during the product development* stage to consistently ensure a predefined quality at the end of the manufacturing process. A quality system provides a sound framework for the transfer of process knowledge from development to the commercial manufacturing processes and for postdevelopment changes and optimization. Corrective and preventive action (CAPA) is a well-known cGMP regulatory concept that focuses on investigating and correcting discrepancies and attempting to prevent recurrence.

Change control is another well-known cGMP regulatory concept that focuses on managing change to prevent unintended consequences. The major implementation of change control in the cGMP regulations is through the assigned responsibilities of the quality control unit. Certain manufacturing changes (e.g., changes that alter specifications, a critical product attribute, or bioavailability) require regulatory filings and prior regulatory approval. A quality system also contains change control activities, including quality planning and control of revisions to specifications, process parameters, and procedures. In this guidance, *change* is discussed in terms of creating a regulatory environment that encourages change toward continuous improvement. This means a manufacturer is empowered to make changes based on the variability of materials used in manufacturing and optimization of the process from learning over time.

Many of the modern quality systems correlate very closely with the cGMP regulations. Current industry practice generally divides the responsibilities of the quality control unit (QCU), as defined in the cGMP regulations, between quality control (QC) and quality assurance (QA) functions.

- QC usually consists of testing of selected in-process materials and finished products to evaluate the performance of the manufacturing process and to ensure adherence to proper specifications and limits.
- QA primarily includes the review and approval of all procedures related to production and maintenance, and review of associated records, including auditing and performing trend analyses.

The concept of *quality unit* is consistent with modern quality systems in ensuring that the various operations associated with all systems are appropriately conducted, approved, and monitored. The cGMP regulations specifically assign the quality unit the authority to create, monitor, and implement the quality system. However, the quality unit is not meant to take on the responsibilities of other units of a manufacturer's organization, such as the responsibilities handled by manufacturing personnel, engineers, and development scientists.

Other cGMP-assigned responsibilities of the quality unit are consistent with a modern quality system approach:

- Ensuring that controls are implemented and completed satisfactorily during manufacturing operations;
- Ensuring that developed procedures and specifications are appropriate and followed, including those used by a firm under contract to the manufacturer;
- Approving or rejecting in-process materials and drug products — although such activities do not substitute for, or preclude, the daily responsibility of manufacturing personnel to build quality into the product;
- Reviewing production records and investigating any unexplained discrepancies.

Under a robust quality system, the manufacturing units and the quality unit can remain independent, but still be included in the total concept of producing quality products. In very small operations, a single individual can function as the quality unit. That person is still accountable for implementing all the controls and reviewing results of manufacture to ensure that product quality standards have been met.

Figure 9.1 shows the relationship among the six systems: the quality system and the five manufacturing systems. The quality system provides the foundation for the manufacturing systems that are linked and function within it. The quality systems model described in this guidance does not treat the five manufacturing systems as discrete entities, but instead integrates them into appropriate sections of the model. Those familiar with the six-system inspection approach will see organizational differences in this guidance; however, the interrelationship should be readily apparent. One of the important themes of the systems-based inspection compliance program is to be able to assess whether each of the systems is in a state of control. The quality system model presented in this guidance will also serve to help firms achieve the desired state of control. The model is organized into five major sections: management responsibilities; resources; manufacturing operations; evaluation activities; and management responsibilities.

Modern robust quality systems models call for management to play a key role in the design, implementation, and management of the quality system. For example, management is responsible for establishing the quality systems structure appropriate for the specific organization. Management has ultimate responsibility to provide the leadership needed for the successful functioning of the quality system.

Providing Leadership

In a robust, modern quality system, senior management demonstrates a commitment to developing and maintaining their quality system. Leadership is demonstrated by aligning quality system plans with the manufacturer's strategic plans to ensure that the quality system supports the manufacturer's mission and strategies. Senior managers set implementation priorities and develop action plans. Managers can provide support of the quality system by:

- Actively participating in system design, implementation, and monitoring, including system review;
- Advocating continual improvement of operations and the quality system;
- Committing necessary resources.

In a robust quality systems environment, managers should demonstrate strong and visible support for the quality system and ensure its global implementation throughout the organization (e.g., across multiple sites).

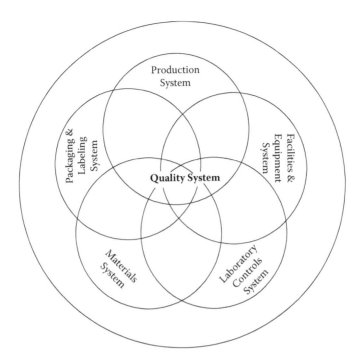

FIGURE 9.1 Six-way quality system. Guidance for Industry quality systems approach to pharmaceutical current good manufacturing practice regulations. (September 2004, available at http://www.fda.gov/cder/guidance/index.htm)

Managers should also encourage internal communication on quality issues at all levels in the organization. Communication should be ongoing among research and development, regulatory affairs, manufacturing, and quality unit personnel on issues that affect quality, with management included whenever appropriate.

STRUCTURING THE ORGANIZATION

When designing a robust quality system, management has the responsibility to determine the structure of the organization and ensure that assigned authorities and responsibilities support the production, quality, and management activities needed to produce quality products. Senior managers have the responsibility to ensure that the organization's structure is documented.

Managers have the responsibility to communicate employee roles, responsibilities, and authorities within the system and ensure that interactions are defined and understood.

An organization also has the responsibility to give the individual who is appointed to manage the quality system the authority to detect problems and effect solutions. Usually, a senior manager administers the quality system and can, thus, ensure that the organization receives prompt feedback on quality issues.

BUILDING QUALITY SYSTEM TO MEET REQUIREMENTS

Implementing a robust quality system can help ensure compliance with regulations related to safety, identity, strength, quality, and purity as long as the quality system addresses the minimum requirements of cGMP regulations as well as the needs of the manufacturer. Under the quality systems model, the agency recommends that senior managers ensure that the quality system they design and implement provides clear organizational guidance and facilitates systematic evaluation of issues.

For example, according to the model, when documenting a quality system, the following should be included:

- The scope of the quality system, including any outsourcing;
- The standard of quality that will be used;
- The manufacturer's policies to implement the quality systems criteria, and the supporting objectives;
- The procedures needed to establish and maintain the quality system.

It is recommended under a modern quality systems approach that a formal process be established to submit change requests to directives. It is also recommended that, when operating under a quality system, manufacturers develop and document record control procedures to complete, secure, protect, and archive records, including data that act as evidence of operational and quality system activities. This approach is consistent with the cGMP regulations, which require manufacturers to develop and document controls for specifications, plans, and procedures that direct operational and quality system activities and to ensure that these directives are accurate, appropriately reviewed and approved, and available for use.

ESTABLISHING POLICIES, OBJECTIVES, AND PLANS

Under a modern quality system, policies, objectives, and plans provide the means by which senior managers articulate their vision of quality to all levels of the organization. It is expected that under a quality system senior management would incorporate a strong commitment to quality into the organizational mission. Senior managers are expected to develop an organizational quality policy that aligns with this mission; commit to meeting requirements and improving the quality system; and propose objectives to fulfill the quality policy. Under a quality system, to make the policy relevant, it must be communicated to, and understood by, personnel and contractors (as applicable), and revised as needed.

Managers operating within a quality system are expected to define the quality objectives needed to implement the quality policy. Senior management is expected to ensure that the quality objectives are created at the top level of the organization (and other levels as needed) through a formal quality planning process. Objectives are typically aligned with the manufacturer's strategic plans. A quality system seeks to ensure that managers support the objectives with necessary resources and have measurable goals that are monitored regularly.

Under a quality system, managers would be expected to use quality planning to identify resources and define methods to achieve the quality objectives. It is recommended that quality plans be documented and communicated to personnel to ensure awareness of how their operational activities are aligned with strategic and quality goals.

REVIEWING THE SYSTEM

System review is a key component in any robust quality system to ensure its continuing suitability, adequacy, and effectiveness. Under a quality system, senior managers are expected to conduct reviews of the whole quality system according to a planned schedule. Such a review typically includes both an assessment of the product as well as customer needs (in this section, *customer* is defined as the recipient of the product and the product is the goods or services being provided). Under a quality system, the review should consider at least the following:

- The appropriateness of the quality policy and objectives;
- The results of audits and other assessments;

TABLE 9.1
21 CFR cGMP Regulations Related to Management Responsibilities

Quality System Element	Regulatory Citations
1. Leadership	—
2. Structure	Establish quality function: § 211.22 (a) (see definition § 210.3(b)(15))
	Notification: § 211.180(f)
3. Build QS	QU procedures: § 211.22(d)
	QU procedures, specifications: § 211.22(c), with reinforcement in: §§ 211.100(a), 211.160(a)
	QU control steps: § 211.22(a), with reinforcement in §§: 211.42(c), 211.84(a), 211.87, 211.101(c)(1), 211.110(c), 211.115(b), 211.142, 211.165(d), 211.192
	QU quality assurance; review/investigate: § 211.22(a), 211.100(a-b) 211.180(f), 211.192, 211.198(a)
	Record control: § 211.180(a-d), 211.180(c), 211.180(d), 211.180(e), 211.186, 211.192, 211.194, 211.198(b)
4. Establish policies, objectives, and plans	Procedures: § 211.22(c-d), 211.100(a)
5. System review	Record review: § 211.180(e), 211.192, 211.198(b)(2)

- Customer feedback, including complaints;
- The analysis of data trending results;
- The status of actions to prevent a potential problem or a recurrence;
- Any follow-up actions from previous management reviews;
- Any changes in business practices or environment that may affect the quality system (such as the volume or type of operations);
- Product characteristics meet the customer's needs.

When developing and implementing new quality systems, reviews should take place more frequently than when the system has matured. Outside of scheduled reviews, the quality system is typically included as a standing agenda item in general management meetings.

Review outcomes typically include:

- Improvements to the quality system and related quality processes;
- Improvements to manufacturing processes and products;
- Realignment of resources.

Under a quality system, the results of a management review should be recorded. Planned actions should be implemented using effective corrective and preventive action and change control procedures.

Table 9.1 shows how the cGMP regulations correlate to specific elements in the quality systems model for this section. Manufacturers should always refer to the specific regulations to ensure that they are complying with all regulations.

RESOURCES

Appropriate allocation of resources is key to creating a robust quality system and to complying with the cGMP regulations.

GENERAL ARRANGEMENTS

Under a robust quality system, there should be sufficient allocation of resources for quality system and operational activities. Under the model, senior management, or a designee, is responsible for providing adequate resources for the following:

- To supply and maintain the appropriate facilities and equipment to consistently manufacture a quality product;
- To acquire and receive materials suitable for their intended purpose;
- For processing the materials to produce the finished drug product;
- For laboratory analysis of the finished drug product, including collection, storage, and examination of in-process, stability, and reserve samples.

DEVELOP PERSONNEL

Under a quality system, senior management is expected to support a problem-solving and communicative organizational culture. Managers are expected to encourage communication by creating an environment that values employee suggestions and acts on suggestions for improvement. Management is also expected to develop cross-cutting groups to share ideas to improve procedures and processes.

In the quality system, it is recommended that personnel be qualified to do the operations that are assigned to them in accordance with the nature of, and potential risk to, quality presented by their operational activities. Under a quality system, managers are expected to define appropriate qualifications for each position to help ensure individuals are assigned appropriate responsibilities. Personnel should also understand the impact of their activities on the product and the customer (this quality systems parameter is also found in the cGMP regulations, which identify specific qualifications, i.e., education, training, and experience or any combination thereof).

Under a quality system, continued training is critical to ensure that the employees remain proficient in their operational functions and in their understanding of cGMP regulations. Typical quality systems training would address the policies, processes, procedures, and written instructions related to operational activities, the product/service, the quality system, and the desired work culture (e.g., team building, communication, change, behavior). Under a quality system (and the cGMP regulations), training is expected to focus on both the employees' specific job functions and the related cGMP regulatory requirements.

Under a quality system, managers are expected to establish training programs that include the following:

- Evaluation of training needs;
- Provision of training to satisfy these needs;
- Evaluation of effectiveness of training;
- Documentation of training or retraining.

When operating in a robust quality system environment, it is important that supervisory managers ensure that skills gained from training be incorporated into day-to-day performance.

FACILITIES AND EQUIPMENT

Under a quality system, the technical experts (e.g., engineers, development scientists), who have an understanding of pharmaceutical science, risk factors, and manufacturing processes related to the product, are responsible for specific facility and equipment requirements.

According to cGMP regulations, the QCU has the responsibility of reviewing and approving all initial design criteria and procedures pertaining to facilities and equipment and any subsequent

TABLE 9.2
21 CFR cGMP Regulations Related to Resources

Quality System Element	Regulatory Citation
1. General arrangements	—
2. Develop personnel	Qualifications: § 211.25(a)
	Staff number: § 211.25(c)
	Staff training: § 211.25(a-b)
3. Facilities and equipment	Buildings and facilities: §§ 211.22(b), 211.28(c), 211.42 – 211.58, 211.173
	Equipment: § 211.63 – 211.72, 211.105, 211.160(b)(4), 211.182
	Lab facilities: § 211.22(b)
4. Control outsourced operations	Consultants: § 211.34
	Outsourcing: § 211.22(a)

changes (see § 211.22(c)). FDA can, as resources permit, provide a preoperational review of manufacturing facilities.

According to the cGMP regulations, equipment must be qualified, calibrated, cleaned, and maintained to prevent contamination and mix-ups. Note that the cGMP regulations require a higher standard for calibration and maintenance than most generic quality system models. The cGMP regulations place as much emphasis on process equipment as on testing equipment, while most quality systems focus only on testing equipment.

CONTROL OUTSOURCED OPERATIONS

When outsourcing, a second party is hired under a contract to perform the operational processes that are part of a manufacturer's inherent responsibilities. For example, a manufacturer may hire another firm to package and label or perform cGMP regulation training. Quality systems call for contracts (quality agreements) that clearly describe the materials or service, quality specifications responsibilities, and communication mechanisms.

Under a quality system, the manufacturer ensures that the contract firm is qualified. The firm's personnel should be adequately trained and monitored for performance according to their quality system, and the contract firm's and contracting manufacturer's quality standards should not conflict. It is critical in a quality system to ensure that the contracting manufacturer's officers are familiar with the specific requirements of the contract. However, under the cGMP requirements, the QCU is responsible for approving or rejecting products or services provided under contract.

As Table 9.2 illustrates, the cGMP regulations are consistent with the elements of a quality system in many areas in this section. However, manufacturers should always refer to the specific regulations to ensure that they are complying with all regulations.

MANUFACTURING OPERATIONS

There is significant overlap between the elements of a quality system and the cGMP regulation requirements for manufacturing operations. It is important to emphasize again that FDA's enforcement programs and inspectional coverage remain based on the cGMP regulations.

DESIGN AND DEVELOP PRODUCT AND PROCESSES

In a modern quality systems manufacturing environment, the significant characteristics of the product being manufactured should be defined, from design to delivery, and control should be exercised over all changes. Quality and manufacturing processes and procedures — and changes to them — should be defined, approved, and controlled. It is important to establish responsibility for designing or changing products. Documenting associated processes will ensure that critical variables are identified.

This documentation includes:

- Resource and facility needs;
- Procedures to carry out the process;
- Identification of the process owner who will maintain and update the process as needed;
- Identification and control of critical variables;
- Quality control measures, necessary data collection, monitoring, and appropriate controls for the product and process;
- Any validation activities, including operating ranges and acceptance criteria;
- Effects on related process, functions, or personnel.

Management calls for managers to ensure that product specifications and process parameters are determined by the appropriate technical experts (e.g., engineers, development scientists). In the pharmaceutical environment, experts would have an understanding of pharmaceutical science, risk factors, and manufacturing processes as well as how variations in materials and processes can ultimately affect the finished product.

Monitoring Packaging and Labeling Processes

Packaging and labeling controls, critical stages in the pharmaceutical manufacturing process, are not specifically addressed in quality systems models. Therefore, the FDA recommends that manufacturers always refer to the packaging and labeling control regulations at 21 CFR 211 Subpart G.

In modern quality systems environments, when new or reengineered processes are developed, it is expected that they will be designed in a controlled manner. A design plan would include authorities and responsibilities; design and development stages; and appropriate review, verification, and validation. If different groups are involved in design and development, the model recommends that responsibilities of the different groups be documented to avoid omission of key duties and ensure that the groups communicate effectively. Plans should be updated when needed during the design process. Prior to implementation of processes (or shipment of a product), a robust quality system will ensure that the process and product will perform as intended. Change controls should be maintained throughout the design process.

Examining Inputs

In modern quality systems models, the term *input* refers to any material that goes into a final product, no matter whether the material is purchased by the manufacturer or produced by the manufacturer for the purpose of processing. *Materials* can include items such as components (e.g., ingredients, process water, and gas), containers, and closures. A robust quality system will ensure that all inputs to the manufacturing process are reliable because quality controls will have been established for the receipt, production, storage, and use of all inputs.

The quality systems model calls for the verification of the components and services provided by suppliers and contractors; however, the model offers a method for implementing verification that is different from those in the cGMP regulations.

The cGMP regulations require either testing or use of a certificate of analysis (CoA) plus an identity analysis. The preamble to cGMP states that reliability can be validated by conducting tests or examinations and comparing the results to the supplier's CoA. Sufficient initial tests must be done to establish reliability and to determine a schedule for periodic rechecking. As an essential element of purchasing controls, it is recommended that data for acceptance and rejection of materials be analyzed for information on supplier performance.

The quality systems approach also calls for the auditing of suppliers on a periodic basis. During the audit, the manufacturer can observe the testing or examinations conducted by the supplier to help determine the reliability of the supplier's CoA. An audit should also include a systematic examination of the supplier's quality system to ensure that reliability is maintained. The FDA recommends that a combination approach be used (i.e., verifying the suppliers' CoA through analysis and audits of the supplier). If full analytical testing is not done, the audit should cover the supplier's analysis; however, a specific identity test is still required.

Under a quality systems approach, there should be procedures to verify that materials are from approved sources (for application and licensed products, certain sources are specified in the submissions). Procedures should also be established to encompass the acceptance, use, or the rejection and disposition of materials produced by the facility (e.g., purified water). Systems that produce these in-house materials should be designed, maintained, qualified, and validated where appropriate to ensure the materials meet their acceptance criteria.

In addition, we recommend that changes to materials (e.g., specification, supplier, or materials handling) be implemented through a change control system (certain changes require review and approval by the quality control unit). It is also important to have a system in place to respond to changes in materials from suppliers so that necessary adjustments to the process can be made and unintended consequences prevented.

PERFORMING AND MONITORING OPERATIONS

The core purpose of implementing a quality systems approach is to enable a manufacturer to more efficiently and effectively perform and monitor operations. The goal of establishing, adhering to, measuring, and documenting specifications and process parameters is to objectively assess whether an operation is meeting its design (and product performance) objectives. In a robust quality system, production and process controls should be designed to ensure that the finished products have the identity, strength, quality, and purity they purport or are represented to possess.

In a modern quality system, a design concept established during product development typically matures into a commercial design after process experimentation and progressive modification. Areas of process weakness should be identified, and factors that are influential on critical quality attributes should receive increased scrutiny. The FDA recommends that scale-up studies be used to help demonstrate that a fundamentally sound *design* has been fully realized. A sufficiently robust manufacturing process should be in place prior to commercial production. With proper design and reliable mechanisms to transfer process knowledge from development to commercial production, a manufacturer should be able to validate the manufacturing process. In a quality system, process validation provides initial proof, through commercial batch manufacture, that the design of the process produces the intended product quality. Sufficient testing data will provide essential information on performance of the new process, as well as a mechanism for continuous improvement. Modern equipment with the potential for continuous monitoring and control can further enhance this knowledge base. Although initial commercial batches can provide evidence to support the validity and consistency of the process, the *entire life cycle* should be addressed by the establishment of continuous improvement mechanisms in the quality system. Thus, in accordance with the quality systems approach, process validation is not a one-time event, but an activity that continues.

As experience is gained in commercial production, opportunities for process improvements may become evident. cGMP regulations require the review and evaluation of records to determine the need for any change. These records contain data and information from production that provide insights into the product's state of control. Change control systems should provide for a dependable mechanism for prompt implementation of technically sound manufacturing improvements.

Under a quality system, written procedures are followed and deviations from them are justified and documented to ensure that the manufacturer can trace the history of the product, as appropriate, concerning personnel, materials, equipment, and chronology and that processes for product release are complete and recorded.

Both the cGMP regulations and quality systems models call for the monitoring of critical process parameters during production:

- Process steps should be verified using a validated computer system or a second person. Batch production records should be prepared contemporaneously with each phase of production. Although time limits can be established when they are important to the quality of the finished product, this does not preclude the ability to establish production controls based on in-process parameters that can be based on desired process endpoints measured using real-time testing or monitoring apparatus (e.g., blend until mixed versus blend for 10 minutes).
- Procedures should be in place to prevent objectionable microorganisms in a finished product that is not required to be sterile and to prevent microbial contamination of finished products purported to be sterile. Sterilization processes should be validated.

Pharmaceutical products must meet their specifications and manufacturing processes must consistently meet their parameters. Under a quality system, selected data are used to evaluate the quality of a process or product. In addition, data collection can provide a means to encourage and analyze potential suggestions for improvement. A quality systems approach calls for the manufacturer to develop procedures that monitor, measure, and analyze the operations (including analytical methods and/or statistical techniques). Knowledge continues to accumulate from development through the entire commercial life of the product. Significant unanticipated variables should be detected by a well-managed quality system and adjustments implemented. Procedures should be revisited as needed to refine operational design based on new knowledge. Process understanding increases with experience and helps identify the need for change toward continuous improvement. When implementing data collection procedures, consider the following:

- Are collection methods documented?
- When in the product life cycle will the data be collected?
- How and to whom will measurement and monitoring activities be assigned?
- When should analysis and evaluation (e.g., trending) of laboratory data be performed?
- What records are needed?

A modern quality system approach indicates that change control is warranted when data analysis or other information reveals an area needing improvement. Changes to an established process should be controlled and documented to ensure that desired attributes for the finished product will be met.

Change control with regard to pharmaceuticals is addressed in more detail in the cGMPs. When developing a process change, it is important to keep the process design and scientific knowledge of the product in mind. When major design issues are encountered through process experience, a firm may need to revisit the adequacy of the design of the manufacturing facility, the design of the manufacturing equipment, the design of the production and control procedures, or the design of laboratory controls. When implementing a change, determining its effect should be based on monitoring and evaluating those specific elements that may be affected based on understanding of the process. This allows the steps taken to implement a change and the effects of the change on the process to be considered systematically. Evaluating the effects of a change can entail additional tests or examinations of subsequent batches (e.g., additional in-process testing or additional stability studies).

The quality system elements identified in this guidance, if implemented, will help a manufacturer manage change and implement continuous improvement in manufacturing.

Under a quality system, procedures should be in place to ensure the accuracy of test results. Test results that are out of specification may be due to testing problems or manufacturing problems and should be investigated. Invalidation of test results should be scientifically and statistically sound and justified.

The U.S. FDA recommends that, upon the completion of manufacturing and to maintain quality, the manufacturer should consider shipment requirements to meet special handling needs (in the case of pharmaceuticals, one example might be refrigeration).

Under a quality system, trends should be continually identified and evaluated. One way of accomplishing this is the use of statistical process control. The information from trend analysis can be used to continually monitor quality, identify potential variances before they become problems, bolster data already collected for the annual review, and facilitate improvement throughout the product life cycle. Process capability assessment can serve as a basis for determining the need for changes that can result in process improvements and efficiency.

ADDRESSING NONCONFORMITIES

A key component in any quality system is handling nonconformities or deviations. The investigation, conclusion, and follow-up should be documented. To ensure that a product conforms to requirements and expectations, it is important to measure process and the product attributes (e.g., specified control parameters strength) as planned. Discrepancies may be detected during any stage of the process by an employee or during quality control activities. Not all discrepancies will result in product defects; however, it is important to document and handle them appropriately. A discrepancy investigation process is critical when a discrepancy is found that affects product quality.

In a quality system, it is critical to develop and document procedures to define responsibilities for halting and resuming operations, recording the nonconformity, investigating the discrepancy, and taking remedial action. The corrected product or process should also be reexamined for conformance and assessed for the significance of the nonconformity. If the nonconformity is significant, based on consequences to process efficiency, product quality, safety, and availability, it is important to evaluate how to prevent recurrence.

Under a quality system, if a product or process does not meet requirements and has not been released for use, it is essential to identify or segregate it so that it is not distributed to the customer by accident. Remedial action may include correcting the nonconformity; or, with proper authorization, allowing the product to proceed with proper authorization and the problem documented, or using the product for another application; or rejecting the product. If an individual product that does not meet requirements has been released, the product can be recalled. Customer complaints should be handled as discrepancies and be investigated.

Table 9.3 shows how the cGMP regulations correlate to specific elements in the quality systems model. Manufacturers should always refer to the specific regulations to ensure that they are complying with all regulations.

EVALUATION ACTIVITIES

As in the previous section, the elements of a quality system correlate closely with the requirements in the cGMP regulations.

ANALYZING DATA FOR TRENDS

Quality systems call for continually monitoring trends and improving systems. This can be achieved by monitoring data and information, identifying and resolving problems, and anticipating and preventing problems.

Quality systems procedures involve collecting data from monitoring, measurement, complaint handling, or other activities, and tracking this data over time, as appropriate. Analysis of data can

TABLE 9.3
21 CFR cGMP Regulations Related to Manufacturing Operations

Quality System Element	Regulatory Citation
1. Design and develop product and processes	Production: § 211.100(a)
2. Examine inputs	Materials: §§ 210.3(b), 211.80 – 211.94, 211.101, 211.122, 211.125
3. Perform and monitor operations	Production: §§ 211.100, 211.103, 211.110, 211.111, 211.113
	QC criteria: §§ 211.22(a-c), 211.115(b), 211.160(a), 211.165(d)
	QC checkpoints: §§ 211.22 (a), 211.84(a), 211.87, 211.110(c)
4. Address nonconformities	Discrepancy investigation: §§ 211.22(a), 211.115, 211.192, 211.198
	Recalls: 21 CFR Part 7

provide indications that controls are losing effectiveness. The information generated will be essential to achieving problem resolution or problem prevention.

Although the annual review required in the cGMP regulations call for review of representative batches on an annual basis, the quality systems approach calls for trending on a regular basis. Trending enables the detection of potential problems as early as possible to plan corrective and preventive actions. Another important concept of modern quality systems is the use of trending to examine processes as a whole; this is consistent with the annual review approach. These trending analyses can help focus internal audits.

CONDUCTING INTERNAL AUDIT

A quality systems approach calls for audits to be conducted at planned intervals to evaluate effective implementation and maintenance of the quality system and to determine if processes and products meet established parameters and specifications. As with other procedures, audit procedures should be developed and documented to ensure that the planned audit schedule takes into account the relative risks of the various quality system activities, the results of previous audits and corrective actions, and the need to audit the entire system at least annually. Quality systems recommend that procedures describe how auditors are trained in objective evidence gathering, their responsibilities, and auditing procedures. Procedures should also define auditing activities such as the scope and methodology of the audit, selection of auditors, and audit conduct (audit plans, opening meetings, interviews, closing meeting, and reports). It is critical to maintain records of audit findings and assign responsibility for follow-up to prevent problems from recurring.

The quality systems model calls for managers who are responsible for the areas audited to take timely action to resolve audit findings and ensure that follow-up actions are completed, verified, and recorded.

ASSESSING RISK

Effective decision making in a quality systems environment is based on an informed understanding of quality issues. Elements of risk should be considered relative to intended use, and in the case of pharmaceuticals, this includes patient safety and ensuring availability of medically necessary drug products. Management should assign priorities to activities or actions based on the consequences of action or inaction — otherwise known as *risk assessment*. It is important to engage appropriate parties in assessing the consequences. Such parties include customers, appropriate manufacturing personnel, and other stakeholders. Assessing consequences includes using the manufacturer's risk assessment model to address risks, developing a strategy by deciding which options to implement, taking actions to implement the strategy, and evaluating the results. Since risk assessment is a reiterative process, the assessment should be repeated if new information is developed that changes the need for, or nature of, risk management.

In a manufacturing quality systems environment, risk assessment is used as a tool in the development of product specifications and critical process parameters. Used in conjunction with process understanding, risk assessment helps manage and control change.

TAKING CORRECTIVE ACTIONS

Corrective action is a reactive tool for system improvement to ensure that significant problems do not recur. Both quality systems and the cGMP regulations emphasize corrective actions. A quality systems approach calls for procedures to be developed and documented to ensure that the need for action is evaluated relevant to the possible consequences, the root cause of the problem is investigated, possible actions are determined, a selected action is taken within a defined time frame, and the effectiveness of the action taken is evaluated. It is essential to maintain records of corrective actions taken.

It is essential to determine what actions are needed to prevent problem recurrence using information from sources such as:

- Nonconformance reports and rejections;
- Complaints;
- Internal and external audits;
- Data and risk analyses related to operations and quality system processes;
- Management review decisions.

TAKING PREVENTIVE ACTIONS

Being proactive is an essential tool in quality systems management. Tasks can include succession planning, training, capturing institutional knowledge, and planning for personnel, policy, and process changes. A preventive action procedure will help ensure that potential problems and root causes are identified, possible consequences assessed, and actions considered. The selected preventative action should be evaluated and recorded, and the system should be monitored for the effectiveness of the action. Problems can be anticipated and their occurrence prevented using information from reviews of data and risk analyses associated with operational and quality system processes, and by keeping abreast of changes in scientific and regulatory requirements.

PROMOTING IMPROVEMENT

The effectiveness and efficiency of the quality system can be improved through the quality activities described here. Management may choose to use other improvement activities as appropriate. It is critical that senior management be involved in the evaluation of this improvement process.

Table 9.4 shows how the cGMP regulations correlate to specific elements in the quality systems model presented in this section. Manufacturers should always refer to the specific regulations to ensure that they are complying with all regulations.

SUMMARY

Implementation of a *comprehensive quality systems model* for human and veterinary pharmaceutical products, including biological products, will facilitate compliance with 21 CFR parts 210 and 211. The central goal of a quality system is to ensure consistent production of safe and effective products and that these activities are sustainable. Quality professionals are aware that good intentions alone will not ensure good products. A robust quality system will promote process consistency by integrating effective knowledge-building mechanisms into daily operational decisions. Specifically, successful quality systems share the following characteristics, each of which have been discussed in detail above:

TABLE 9.4
21 CFR cGMP Regulations Related to Evaluation Activities

Quality System Element	Regulatory Citation
1. Analyze data for trends	Annual Review: § 211.180(e)
2. Conduct internal audits	Annual Review: § 211.180(e)
3. Risk assessment	—
4. Corrective action	Discrepancy investigation: § 211.22(a), 211.192
5. Preventive action	—
6. Promote improvement	—

- Science-based approaches;
- Decisions based on an understanding of the intended use of a product;
- Proper identification and control of areas of potential process weakness;
- Responsive deviation and investigation systems that lead to timely remediation;
- Sound methods for assessing risk;
- Well-defined processes and products, starting from development and extending through-out the product life cycle;
- Systems for careful analyses of product quality;
- Supportive management (philosophically and financially).

Both good manufacturing practice and good business practice require a robust quality system. When fully developed and effectively managed, a quality system will lead to consistent, predictable processes that ensure that pharmaceuticals are safe, effective, and available for the consumer.

IMPLEMENTING QUALITY ASSURANCE SYSTEMS

The quality assurance (QA) systems are established to ensure that every batch produced has similar characteristics. The quality systems plan described above lists the basic principles of ensuring quality. Implementation of these standards requires careful planning, often very early in the scheme of developing a biological process.

Whereas the role of in-process controls, standard operating procedures, and extensive documentation control is the key to good QA practices, the specific process requirements in recombinant manufacturing and the inherent variability of biological systems makes the QA system more complicated, and the need for stringent controls is evident in light of reported incidents in the use of products of biological products where the most common incidents involve either incomplete virus inactivation, endogenous viral contamination, adventitious viral contamination, or entry of other infectious agents such as prions. It is important to realize that the QA system is supposed to prevent manufacturing of out-of-specification product and not to prevent side effects or lack of efficacy if that is built into the process. For example, the most recent reporting of pure red cell aplasia (PRCA) in the use of epoietin formulation in Europe was not a QA issue but a design issue; when albumin was removed and replaced with polysorbate, there was an aggregation that could not be predicted, which resulted in several PRCA cases. Such incidences are less frequent than the issues related to products being out of specification. The regulatory guidelines from International Conference on Harmonisation (ICH), FDA, European Medicines Evaluation Agency (EMEA), and Japan are very detailed in how the specifications are to be laid out and the tolerance allowed for each test. However, the manufacturers inevitably develop their in-house specifications, limits, and QA procedures, which are generally more stringent; in some instances manufacturers add tests that are neither required nor reported to the regulatory agencies. This is one of strongest claims made by the innovator companies as they defend their position that there can never be a biogeneric product.

When new products are developed, whether generic or innovative, the planning for regulatory controls and compliance starts very early in the process; despite this well-established practice, most delays in the approval of drug products occur because of poor early planning relating to QA issues. Some of these issues are:

- Companies should arrange meetings with the FDA as early as possible; the Division of Therapeutic Proteins is now a well-defined section under FDA's Center for Drug Evaluation and Research (CDER) fully staffed to attend to all inquiries. The well-established system of filing for pre-IND conferences should be used extensively; otherwise the best place to contact is the Division of Therapeutic Proteins (DTP) Amy Rosenberg, M.D., Director, or Barry W. Cherney, Ph.D., Deputy Director, for monoclonal antibodies for *in vivo* use; cytokines, growth factors, enzymes, immunomodulators, and thrombolytics; proteins intended for therapeutic use that are extracted from animals or microorganisms, including recombinant versions of these products (except clotting factors) and other nonvaccine therapeutic immunotherapies. For all other products the contact point is CBER. You will most likely be speak to someone whose main concern regarding biogeneric products is their immunogenicity potential; be prepared to offer a protocol to compare your product to an innovator's product in its 3D and 4D structures.
- The time lines for the development of process should be made realistic; however, marketing pressures often cause the regulatory staff to squeeze the time lines. The same holds for adequate resources, both manpower and financial set aside to develop the chemistry, manufacturing, and control (CMC) sections. Greatest difficulties arise in securing and qualifying equipment. It is for this reason that I have repeatedly emphasized the need to outsource initial manufacturing and then later use the comparability protocol to move the process in-house.
- The problems related to product definition area readily solved in a generic situation, but when faced with a new product, the final product composition and definition often changes during development, making the regulatory filings more difficult and time consuming. However, the definition of product related to its immunogenicity potential remains; this will require using some sophisticated methods to ascertain that at least the 3D structure in the native state is comparable to the innovator's product or to the natural product as the case may be.
- The choice of cell line is critical; for example, growth hormone is produced using different types of cell lines; the choice of one over another will depend on a large number of factors, not necessarily the financial ones; the safety of the product and ease of production should be the prime considerations. Cell lines must be optimized and characterized in accordance with the ICH guidelines. The cells must come from certified traceable sources. This aspect was earlier alluded to by Professor Baralle in his Foreword to this volume. Developing cell line in-house should be a second choice to licensing a stabilized cell line; if one examines the overall cost of the project, this may turn out to be the best investment made.
- The process design for cGMP manufacturing should include robustness and scalability; though the FDA allows for process change through comparability protocols, these are expensive to run and should be highly discouraged; all factors should be studied prior to finalizing the process with as few changes made to it later. This is one reason why delays take place in kicking off the project; companies like BioMetics (Boston, MA) are well equipped to assist you in laying out the process flow, material balance, and appropriate sizing of all processes. Again, the aim should be to avoid any process changes later.

- The availability of raw materials can often be a major problem, such as when securing albumin from a reliable source; all materials should be manufactured under cGMP compliance. Fortunately, many companies with delivery points around the world are ready to supply material on a just–in–time (JIT) basis. In an earlier chapter, a list of suppliers was provided. To ensure steady supply, agreements should be made with these companies. Many of these companies have developed their own specification for raw materials, and it may be worthwhile to develop a process around these materials, specially when it comes to chromatography media, which may be interchangeable between vendors, but this switching is not recommended. Prior to selecting a vendor, insist on a CoA, Good Manufacturing Practices (GMP) compliance, and where applicable, access to their Drug Master File (DMF).
- In-process controls often prove inadequate when the process is scaled up; a small-scale process using a starter 3L fermenter has a different set of conditions that control the process than a 1000 L fermenter; more differences become apparent in downstream processing. In other words, in-process control does not scale up linearly.
- Ensure that the documentation is as comprehensive as possible. This is one area where you will find that most of initial time and money is invested; from IQ/OQ/PQ exercises to SOPs to VMP, etc., there is a new set of documentation to be created and revised several times very early in the process development stage.
- Analytical procedures should be adequately validated, the assays rugged, and sufficient testing included. This applies to both the in-process control systems as well as compliance to release specifications. Whereas many methods required are now well defined in pharmacopoeia, it is inevitable that additional methods will be required. As discussed above, the prime concern of the regulatory authorities is comparability regarding immunogenicity potential; one way to address this is through complete characterization of the drug substance as well as the drug product. This will require developing additional methods like CD, 3D, NMR, etc.; often validation of these methods is more difficult than the methods routinely described in pharmacopoeia.
- Parameters should be stated in intervals with a set point. Product specification and acceptance criteria should be well defined. Later in the chapter a discussion regarding factorial analysis will allude to selection of parameters, the need for a practical intervals, keeping in mind that larger variations occur at larger scale; for example, it is possible to keep the pH constant within an interval of 0.1 unit, but in a larger container, just the mixing inefficiencies can lead to greater pH variation.

VALIDATION MASTER PLAN

The U.S. FDA defines process validation as "establishing documented evidence which provides a high degree of assurance that a specific process will consistently produce a product meeting its pre-determined specifications and quality characteristics." The validation of pharmaceutical production is a general requirement of the cGMP for finished pharmaceuticals, 21 CFR 210 and 211. The validation procedure comprises production facility qualification and a process validation. Validation ensures that safe and efficacious products are manufactured, and this requires not just controlling the finished product but the manufacturing process itself. Process validation starts early; however, full validation is not required until Phase III cGMP manufacture.

The process validation program is comprised of several common elements; however, each product is unique and requires a dedicated listing of important elements of validation. The plan suggested here will be discussed under three categories:

- *Acceptance criteria* of raw materials and equipment,
- *Process rationale* and strategy,

- *A flow sheet,* defining parameter intervals, defining critical parameters, column cleaning, column life time, filter cleaning, filter life time, process performance qualification and removal of process and product related impurities.

The validation master plan (VMP) begins with the process development and is updated throughout the process. An appropriate VMP reduces the risk of missing essential components in the CMC section, while ensuring batch compliance.

PROCESS VALIDATION

Process validation is a major component of the VMP and includes such elements as:

- The process rationale, stating reasons why certain steps are chosen, is developed based on the type of target protein, the expression system used, and the specific demands to posttranslational modifications such as glycosylation, acylation, phosphorylation, or pegylation. The process strategy should include the considerations related to product safety, process robustness, scale up, cGMP manufacture, and economy. The strategy should allow VMP revisions as the process "changes" from a Phase I process to a mature Phase III process.
- Acceptance criteria for every analysis of in process materials, drug substance (DS), and drug product (DP).
- Identification of all analytical methods used, including plans for qualification and validation.
- Characterization of the cells used for propagation into cell cultures. The program comprises cell line history, substrate and raw material characterization, test for microbial agents, fungi, mycoplasma, viruses, and prions. The ICH guideline on cell characterization is usually followed.
- Identification of critical parameters for each unit operation. Statistical factorial design is used to identify critical parameters.
- Stability studies, both short term and long term, for the product and for intermediary products stored for a certain amount of time. Product stability under the given storage conditions must be ensured throughout the storage period.
- Process robustness testing results include specified parameter intervals, identification of critical parameters by statistical analysis, recoveries, yields, batch data, column and filter performances, columns and filter life times.
- Flow sheets describing every unit operation. A flow sheet showing all process unit operations with an indication of where critical raw materials or adventitious agents are entering the process and at which steps they are removed is required. This includes removal of host cell-, product-, and process-related impurities. All parameters derived from validation studies are listed in the flow sheet.
- Identification and clearance methods for impurities. Host cell–related impurities come from the host organism (e.g., endotoxins from *E. coli*, viruses from insect cells, animal cells or transgenic animals, host cell proteins, host cell DNA). Process steps, which are especially powerful in removing a specific impurity, should be identified and a clearance factor calculated, if possible. Process-related impurities are substrates and reagents required by the process (viruses, prions, chemical compounds, enzymes, leachable from chromatographic resins). Process steps, which are especially suitable for removing a specific impurity, should be identified and a clearance factor calculated, if possible. Product-related impurities are derivatives or isoforms of the target protein (e.g., di- and polymers, des-amido forms, oxidized forms, split products, scrambled forms, carbamylated forms). Product-related impurities are normally removed in the polishing step(s).

- Protocols for every validation study should be conducted; these include, statement of experimental objective, definition of what is to be qualified or validated, experimental plan, sampling plans, test plans with acceptance criteria to be met or established, description of statistical analyses to be applied.
- Parameter intervals should be established for every unit operation and include proven acceptable range, regulatory range, control range, and defined operating range.
- Identity, safety, process criticality, release procedures, and certificates of analysis must be addressed. ISO 9000-9004 standards are often used.
- References are made to:
  - analytical methods used: descriptions, method qualification, and validation;
  - pilot and manufacturing protocols and batch documentation;
  - relevant development documentation, direct or indirect (development report);
  - summary reports, unit operation descriptions, protocols and batch records;
  - stability reports, short and long term.
- Sampling and testing plans to include sampling for end of production test, in process control, quality control, target protein characterization, holding times, and stability studies.
- Specifications include the analytical test program for active pharmaceutical ingredient (API) and drug product (DP).
- Validation task reports include product development summary, lot summary report, process performance report, in-process control report, and validation protocol completion report.

VALIDATION STUDIES

Validation studies depend on the type of protein but mostly these comprise:

- Column lifetime is crucial and requires cleaning validation, sanitization, and test for leachables.
- Assessment of column performance. Critical parameters are determined by statistical methods (e.g., fractional factorial design is common practice).
- Filter lifetime requires cleaning validation, sanitization, and test for filter extractables.
- Process robustness requires manufacturing three to five continuous batches in small or pilot scale meeting specification accept criteria. The measurement of unit operation includes recoveries and total yield.
- Raw materials require identification of critical raw materials and identity, purity, suitability, and traceability are included.
- Removal of impurities comprises control of host cell-, process-, and product-related impurities.
- Virus validation requires assurance of virus removal from the target protein.

REGULATORY REQUIREMENTS

In regulatory filings, the requirement of validation studies depends on the phase of study:

- Phase I: Virus validation with one or two model viruses, sterility and mycoplasma tests, critical analytical methods, removal of impurities of biological origin, generic assays for HCP, DNA, and endotoxins; product impurity profile, API, and DP to meet specification accept criteria. Process validation is *not* required.
- Phase II: Critical analytical methods, others qualified; product impurity profile, API, and DP meet acceptance criteria. No virus validation studies and no specific process validation are required unless changes have been made.

- Phase III: Extensive virus validation, process validation on three or more consecutive batches, all analyses, specific assay for HCP, cleaning validation, and lifetime studies for chromatographic columns, clearance studies for removal of HCP, DNA, and specific impurities; product-related impurities characterized if present in amounts of $> 0.1\%$; API and DP to meet specification acceptance criteria; critical process parameters and operating ranges defined taking into account the worst scenarios.

RAW MATERIALS

All raw materials, biological and chemical, such as cell culture nutrients, serum components, and inorganic salts, detergents, antifoam agents, enzymes, reagents, organic compounds, organic solvents, cleaning agents, growth factors, and chromatographic media, etc., should be manufactured under cGMP; paying closer attention to such materials as chromatographic media where the supplier should certify its cGMP status. The qualification of raw materials is an ongoing process, starting during process development. It is recommended to draft the master plan prior to entering production of material for Phase I clinical studies, and to establish specifications and standard operation procedures for all material used. Critical materials should be identified and supplier data obtained. During Phase II production, the master plan is updated, critical raw material assays are in put place and the test of noncritical materials should be initiated. Stability assays should be established, where relevant. The basic quality concepts include assurance of the identity, purity, suitability, and traceability of all the raw materials used, meeting standards appropriate for their intended use. Raw materials must be quarantined, identified, and released by an authorized person, and their identity proven by specific assays (often available from the vendor). A CoA should be received for each lot of raw material. Each vendor must undergo a vendor qualification program (audit) such as described by the Parenteral Drug Association. Some raw materials such as chromatographic media require substantial testing before release for clinical production (a test period of 1 year or more should be expected). Some vendors have overcome this hurdle by providing regulatory support files for media to be used in biopharmaceutical processes.

EQUIPMENT

The equipment that comes in contact with the product must be of GMP grade, which simply means that it should be sanitizable with full provision for validating the cleaning process. Whereas this requirement applies at all stages of manufacturing, it is obviously more rigid during the downstream processing, the purification stages where any contamination from other batches or adventitious exposure should be minimized. The fermenter is a key piece of equipment and it is available in various arrangements, from laboratory scale autoclavable equipment to CIP large vessels (e.g., BioFlo from New Brunswick); there is a need to use the same vendor for different size fermenters as most of them will be scaleable and the vendor will be able to provide additional support as well. The same applies to cell disrupters (when used) and other such storage and centrifugation vessels.

The considerations in downstream processing are substantially more important and the choice of a column system should be made early in the process development; ideally, a manufacturer should source as many supplies from the same vendor as possible. In this regard companies such as Amersham (now GE) can be very helpful. For example, the BioProcess HPLC columns (Amersham) comprise a family of stainless steel, high-pressure chromatography columns with a wide range of bed heights and inner diameters. Their well-proven chromatographic design simplifies packing and ensures the speedy, reliable, and convenient process-scale purification of small biomolecules such as peptides. BioProcess HPLC columns (Figure 9.2) are particularly suitable for processes involving reversed phase chromatography (RPC) media. BioProcess HPLC columns comply with the technical performance demands placed on equipment operated at pressures up to 100 bar in industrial bioprocessing. In addition, they withstand temperatures up to 50°C, which

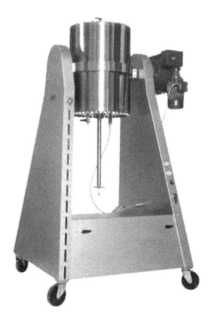

FIGURE 9.2 BioProcess HPLC column.

allows effective cleaning with warm water. Construction is in stainless steel AISI 316 L, and the sanitary design includes Quick connections. Sealing materials are resistant to organic solvents, and a leakage detection system is included.

The columns feature dynamic axial compression that uses solvent as the compression medium. In addition, dynamic axial piston pressure eliminates the formation of voids or channels in packed beds. A specially designed flow distribution system fitted at both the piston and the bottom of the column ensures a uniform distribution of the mobile phase across the whole bed. Figure 9.3 shows a schematic diagram of the general column construction. Filling the column is facilitated by the accessory slurry tank that both prepares the medium in slurry form and pumps it directly into the tube. Liquid is then pumped into the hydraulic chamber to move the adaptor up. For BioProcess HPLC columns, the working bed height extends up to 1.0 m. An automated packing set-up means that the medium can be packed in minutes with precise pressure regulation to prevent bead crushing. It also results in a homogeneous bed plus good contact with the distributor plate. Operation is further enhanced by low dead volumes, which promote excellent chromatographic performance as well as enabling effective cleaning-in-place (CIP).

The media and the column selected should be such that these simple systems can be deployed for CIP. The description above lists the various features of raw materials that are important to select as early as possible.

COST EFFICIENCY AND QUALITY MATTERS

Whereas the purpose of quality assurance is to ensure quality of a product, this must be accomplished at a reasonable cost as well. Fortunately, there is a parallel that can be drawn between simplicity and quality and thus the cost of achieving it. Improved planning in the manufacturing process also provides better efficiency. It should be noted that almost 70% of the cost of manufacturing is incurred in the downstream, purification stage, so the main concern is the life of the column and its reusability. Here are some considerations:

- Combining inclusion bodies from different batches can be allowed since the process at this stage is yielding a crude preparation; the inclusion bodies can be kept frozen for a

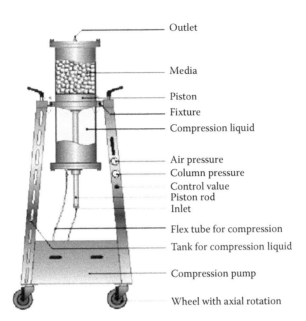

Outlet

Media

Piston

Fixture

Compression liquid

Air pressure
Column pressure
Control value
Piston rod
Inlet

Flex tube for compression

Tank for compression liquid

Compression pump

Wheel with axial rotation

FIGURE 9.3 Schematic flow in column construction.

long time and then taken out to process specific size batches. This allows use of smaller fermenters, yet provides for large-scale downstream processing. It is noteworthy that the scale up of fermenters is a nonlinear process in terms of cost of installation. Installing a 500 L fermenter may require highly specialized facility compared to what is required for a 30 L fermenter.

- In a typical chromatographic unit operation the column is washed in one to several volumes of a specific wash buffer intended to remove impurities. If the process is run in campaigns to improve cost, storage of the column(s) is an integrated part of the procedure requiring defining storage time and conditions. It should be kept in mind that even the use of strong cleaning agents does not guarantee total removal of impurities and thus the lifetime of a column used for campaign manufacturing should be cost-justified. Such studies are for economic reasons usually carried out in small-scale test columns operating under identical conditions except for the column diameter and load (prospective validation). Another approach is to correlate column performance with readily measurable attributes (e.g., recovery, clearance of specific impurities, back pressure, TOC) with specified acceptance criteria (concurrent validation). The advantage of the latter procedure is that it can be carried out in full scale during manufacture. However, demands for fast and reliable analytical methods and the risk of failed batches due to column failure should be taken into consideration.

- The cleaning procedure is obviously a very important part of the chromatographic unit operation. The lifetime of a column may be several hundred cycles and build up of impurities may severely affect the column performance (e.g., reduced capacity) and even result in leakage of tightly bound impurities into the product. Therefore, critical factors such as type and concentration of cleaning agent, contact time, flow rate, and temperature should be investigated during process development. Typically analytical methods such as ELISA, HPLC, TOC, total protein, and visual inspection are used to measure the outcome. The final cleaning validation must be carried out in full scale. The cleaning procedure should also be tested (challenge studies) for its ability to sanitize the column with respect to microorganisms, fungi, and spores. Examples of sanitizing agents are NaOH or Hibitane (0.5%) in 20% ethanol, or 20% ethanol. A typical CIP protocol should be suitable for most applications using BioProcess HPLC columns (Amersham) is to circulate 1.5 column volumes of 20% acetic acid at a low flow rate (60 cm/h) for 15 min, upward flow; then reverse the flow for 15 min; repeat with 1.0 M NaOH; finally, slowly circulate 1.0 M NaOH in the column for a further 60 min.

- Virus validation is an integrated part of the program if the target protein has been expressed in insect cells, mammalian cells, or transgenic animals. The first virus validation study is carried out before or during manufacture for Phase I clinical material. Although column lifetime usually comprises a few cycles at this stage, the issue should be a part of the overall strategy. A more comprehensive virus validation study is carried out usually prior to Phase III manufacture. The ICH Guideline on Viral Safety states that: "over time and after repeated use, the ability of chromatographic columns and other devices used in the purification scheme to clear virus may vary." Thus a repeated virus validation study may be needed at the end of the column lifetime study.

- The integrity of the column bed needs to be measured to confirm the quality and consistency of the chromatographic operation. Commonly used measures are the number of theoretical plates (N), the height equivalent to theoretical plate (HETP), the tailing factor (T), and the asymmetry (As). A high HETP indicates inefficient column packing, while a low HETP indicates that the probe molecule is retained on the column. The typical range of As is from 0.8 to 1.4. Values lower than 0.8 indicate column over packing, packing a too high pressure, or bed cracking. A value over 1.4 indicates that the column is not packed tight enough, there are air pockets in column hardware void spaces, or poor injection technique.

ROBUSTNESS STUDIES AND FACTORIAL DESIGNS

Robustness is introduced by controlling each step, and this requires developing critical process parameters. In fermentation or cell culture and downstream processing the parameter intervals are identified; the operational parameters (factors) are linked to performance parameters (responses) by means of statistical methods. The identified lower and upper parameter limits help achieve uniformity in large-scale production where worse-case scenarios are tested to ascertain homogeneity. Given below are some of these parameters and their selection process:

- Upstream process:
  - Seed flask and fermentor culture is tested for pH, conductivity, and temperature, and the parameter tested is cell density.
  - Bioreactor is monitored, in addition to oxygen supply, nitrogen supply, nutrient supply, dissolved oxygen, aeration rate, agitation rate, pCO_2, methanol concentration, ethanol concentration, holding time. Measured parameter tested is cell density in addition to viability, respiration quotient, biomass, cell number, target protein concentration.
- Centrifugation is monitored by pH conductivity, temperature, rotations per minute, g-force, time, holding time. The tested parameters are recovery and volume of supernatant.
- Filtration is monitored by pH, conductivity, temperature, inlet flow velocity, cross flow velocity, filtrate flux, retentate flux, recirculation rate, back pressure, inlet pressure, outlet pressure, holding time, load. The tested parameters are transmembrane pressure, volume of filtrate, volume of retentate, protein concentration, protein stability, amount of process-related impurities, bioburden, yield.
- Precipitation is monitored by pH, conductivity, temperature, protein concentration, holding time. The tested parameter is recovery.

- Chromatography conditions are monitored by pH, conductivity, load, linear flow, temperature, bed height, column diameter, holding time. The tested parameters are back pressure, recovery, protein concentration, protein stability, amount of process-related impurities, ultraviolet profile, selectivity, resolution.

Robustness studies are conducted using a fractional factorial design wherein variables are tested at two levels, usually a low and a high value, to allow statistical variance analysis. The process takes several well-defined steps:

- Identifying the goals of the unit operation or process: The purpose and expected outcome (e.g., recovery, protein stability, impurity profile) of the unit operation are defined in terms of minimally acceptable performance.
- Choosing operational parameters. The number of variables to investigate is often large; however, this can be reduced by excluding extremely well-controlled parameters (e.g., narrow range parameters) or parameters not expected to interact or influence the process outcome. On the other hand, parameters with strong process impact need investigation. Also, some parameter interactions can be predicted, e.g., interaction of pH and conductivity in ion exchange chromatography.
- Defining ranges. Parameter ranges are difficult to define in early stages; however, narrow ranges can jeopardize large-scale operations, e.g., adjusting pH in large volume tanks to a narrow range is more difficult than in liter flasks, requiring a broader range. Broader validated ranges add to robustness and allow for optimization. An acceptable range developed earlier is narrowed down to control range or operating range. The limits are used to create worst and best case scenarios and are within two to three standard deviations.
- Defining responses. Responses are unit operation/process outputs that measure performance against the predetermined goals, e.g., specific biological activity, recovery, target protein stability, and content of specific impurities (e.g., DNA, endotoxins, viruses). Operational parameters are associated to specific responses in the process control (in process analytical control).
- Designing the experiment. In many cases, it is sufficient to consider the factors affecting the production process at two levels. For example, the temperature for a fermentation process may either be set a little higher or a little lower, the amount of solvent in a chromatographic eluant can either be slightly increased or decreased, etc. The experimenter would like to determine whether any of these changes affects the results of the production process.

The most intuitive approach to study those factors would be to vary the factors of interest in a full factorial design, that is, to try all possible combinations of settings. This would work fine, except that the number of necessary runs in the experiment (observations) will increase geometrically. For example, if you want to study seven factors, the necessary number of runs in the experiment would be $2**7 = 128$. To study 10 factors you would need $2**10 = 1,024$ runs in the experiment. Because each run may require time-consuming and costly setting and resetting of machinery, it is often not feasible to require that many different production runs for the experiment. In these conditions, *fractional factorials* are used that "sacrifice" interaction effects so that main effects may still be computed correctly. In general, it will successively "use" the highest-order interactions to generate new factors. For example, consider the following design that includes 11 factors but requires only 16 runs (observations).

Design: 2**(11 – 7), Resolution III

Run	A	B	C	D	E	F	G	H	I	J	K
1	1	1	1	1	1	1	1	1	1	1	1
2	1	1	1	-1	1	-1	-1	-1	-1	1	1
3	1	1	-1	1	-1	-1	-1	1	-1	1	-1
4	1	1	-1	-1	-1	1	1	-1	1	1	-1
5	1	-1	1	1	-1	-1	1	-1	-1	-1	1
6	1	-1	1	-1	-1	1	-1	1	1	-1	1
7	1	-1	-1	1	1	1	-1	-1	1	-1	-1
8	1	-1	-1	-1	1	-1	1	1	-1	-1	-1
9	-1	1	1	1	-1	1	-1	-1	-1	-1	-1
10	-1	1	1	-1	-1	-1	1	1	1	-1	-1
11	-1	1	-1	1	1	-1	1	-1	1	-1	1
12	-1	1	-1	-1	1	1	-1	1	-1	-1	1
13	-1	-1	1	1	1	-1	-1	1	1	1	-1
14	-1	-1	1	-1	1	1	1	-1	-1	1	-1
15	-1	-1	-1	1	-1	1	1	1	-1	1	1
16	-1	-1	-1	-1	-1	-1	-1	-1	1	1	1

The design displayed above should be interpreted as follows. Each column contains +1s or −1s to indicate the setting of the respective factor (high or low, respectively). So, for example, in the first run of the experiment, set all factors *A* through *K* to the plus setting (e.g., a little higher than before); in the second run, set factors *A, B,* and *C* to the positive setting, factor *D* to the negative setting, and so on. Note that there are numerous options provided to display (and save) the design using notation other than ±1 to denote factor settings. For example, you may use actual values of factors (e.g., *9 C* and *100C*) or text labels (*Low* temperature, *High* temperature). Because many other things may change from production run to production run, it is always a good practice to randomize the order in which the systematic runs of the designs are performed. The design above is described as a 2**(11 − 7) design of *resolution* III (three). This means that you study overall *k = 11* factors (the first number in parentheses); however, *p = 7* of those factors (the second number in parentheses) were generated from the interactions of a full 2**[(11 − 7) = 4] factorial design. As a result, the design does not give full *resolution*; that is, there are certain interaction effects that are confounded with (identical to) other effects. In general, a design of resolution *R* is one where no *l*-way interactions are confounded with any other interaction of order less than *R-l*. In the current example, *R* is equal to 3. Here, no *l* = 1 level interactions (i.e., main effects) are confounded with any other interaction of order less than *R-l* = 3 − 1 = 2. Thus, main effects in this design are confounded with two-way interactions; and consequently, all higher-order interactions are equally confounded. If you had included 64 runs, and generated a 2**(11 − 5) design, the resultant resolution would have been *R = IV* (four). This will lead to the conclusion that no *l* = 1-way interaction (main effect) is confounded with any other interaction of order less than *R-l* = 4 − 1 = 3. In this design then, main effects are not confounded with two-way interactions, but only with three-way interactions. Regarding the two-way interactions, no *l* = 2-way interaction is confounded with any other interaction of order less than *R-l* = 4 − 2 = 2. Thus, the two-way interactions in that design are confounded with each other. One way in which a resolution III design can be enhanced and turned into a resolution IV design is via *foldover.* For example, for a 7-factor design in 8 runs, the following holds:

Design: 2**(7–4) design

Run	A	B	C	D	E	F	G
1	1	1	1	1	1	1	1
2	1	1	-1	1	-1	-1	-1
3	1	-1	1	-1	1	-1	-1
4	1	-1	-1	-1	-1	1	1
5	-1	1	1	-1	-1	1	-1
6	-1	1	-1	-1	1	-1	1
7	-1	-1	1	1	-1	-1	1
8	-1	-1	-1	1	1	1	-1

This is a resolution III design, that is, the two-way interactions will be confounded with the main effects. A typical design would test pH (7.5 to 8.5), conductivity (15 to 20 mS/cm), temperature (18° to 25°C), flow (100 to 130 cm/h), load (10 to 15 mg/mL); the responses measured could be recovery, DNA content, and target protein stability. When critical parameters have been identified, further factorial studies link different unit operations, providing information on the entire process. This type of experimental design can be used to show process robustness during process validation at Phase III manufacture.

This design can be turned into a resolution IV design via the *foldover* (enhance resolution) option. The foldover method copies the entire design and appends it to the end, reversing all signs:

Design: 2**(7–4) design (+Foldover)								
Run	A	B	C	D	E	F	G	New: H
1	1	1	1	1	1	1	1	1
2	1	1	-1	1	-1	-1	-1	1
3	1	-1	1	-1	1	-1	-1	1
4	1	-1	-1	-1	-1	1	1	1
5	-1	1	1	-1	-1	1	-1	1
6	-1	1	-1	-1	1	-1	1	1
7	-1	-1	1	1	-1	-1	1	1
8	-1	-1	-1	1	1	1	-1	1
9	-1	-1	-1	-1	-1	-1	-1	-1
10	-1	-1	1	-1	1	1	1	-1
11	-1	1	-1	1	-1	1	1	-1
12	-1	1	1	1	1	-1	-1	-1
13	1	-1	-1	1	1	-1	1	-1
14	1	-1	1	1	-1	1	-1	-1
15	1	1	-1	-1	1	1	-1	-1
16	1	1	1	-1	-1	-1	1	-1

Thus, the standard run number 1 was *-1, -1, -1, 1, 1, 1, -1*; the new run number 9 (the first run of the "folded-over" portion) has all signs reversed: *1, 1, 1, -1, -1, -1, 1*. In addition to enhancing the resolution of the design, we also have gained an eighth factor (factor *H*), which contains all +1s for the first eight runs and −1s for the folded-over portion of the new design. Note that the resultant design is actually a 2**(8–4) design of resolution IV.

To summarize, whenever it is desired to include fewer observations (runs) in the experiment than would be required by the full factorial 2**k design, there is a "sacrifice" interaction effect, and that assigns them to the levels of factors. The resulting design is no longer a full factorial but a *fractional* factorial. The 2**(k–p) designs are the "workhorse" of industrial experiments. The impact of a large number of factors on the production process can simultaneously be assessed with relative efficiency (i.e., with few experimental runs). The logic of these types of experiments is straightforward (each factor has only two settings). The simplicity of these designs is also their major flaw. As mentioned before, underlying the use of two-level factors is the belief that the resultant changes in the dependent variable are basically *linear* in nature. This is often not the case, and many variables are related to quality characteristics in a nonlinear fashion. Often there is a *curvature* in the relationship between the factors in the design and the dependent variable can be detected if the design includes center point runs, but one cannot fit explicit nonlinear (e.g., quadratic) models with 2**(k-p) designs (however, central composite designs will do exactly that). Another problem of fractional designs is the implicit assumption that higher-order interactions do not matter; but sometimes they do, for example, when some other factors are set to a particular level, temperature may be *negatively* related to protein structure through changes in dielectric value. Again, in fractional factorial designs, higher-order interactions (greater than two-way) particularly will escape detection.

STATISTICAL ANALYSIS PRESENTATION

Frequency diagrams indicate the distribution of all outputs. Pareto plots estimate the relative strength of each variable and interaction. Analysis of variance (ANOVA) determines the statistical significance of the effects.

VIRUS VALIDATION

Virus safety evaluation requires selecting virus-free cell lines, testing unprocessed bulk, assessing the capacity of the downstream process to remove or clear viruses, and finally testing the drug substance and the drug product to ensure absence of contaminating viruses.

TESTING REQUIREMENTS

Viruses are introduced into the cell bank by several routes such as derivation of cell lines from infected animals, use of viruses to establish the cell line, use of contaminated reagents (e.g., animal serum), and contaminants during handling of cells. The testing plan involves:

- Extensive screening for both endogenous and nonendogenous viral contamination is performed on the master cell bank (MCB).
- Less extensive testing of working cell bank (WCB).
- It is not necessary to assay for presence of the noninfectious virus particles in the purified bulk if cell lines (e.g., Chinese hamster ovary [CHO] cells), which have been extensively characterized, have been used to express the protein and if adequate clearance has been demonstrated.
- Cells at the limit of *in vitro* cell age are evaluated for those endogenous viruses that may not have been detected in the MCB and WCB.
- Substrate testing is required to eliminate viral sources in the feeding during fermentation. (See WHO requirements for the use of *in vitro* substrates for the production of biologicals and the ICH guidelines Q5A, B, and D.)
- Serum and trypsin should be free of infectious viruses.
- Testing should be done using cell cultures to test monolayer cultures. polymerase chain reaction (PCR) technology can be used (seek regulatory guidance on this first). Tests for adventitious viruses in continuous cell line cultures used for expression of recombinant proteins should include inoculation onto monolayer cultures of the same species and tissue type such as that used for production, cultures of human diploid cell line, and cultures of another cell line from different species.
- Testing of viruses is also performed in animals and eggs for pathogen viruses not able to grow in cell cultures (e.g., suckling mice, adult mice, guinea pigs, fertilized eggs).
- Test for retroviruses, endogenous viruses, or viral nucleic acid include infective assays, transmission electron microscopy (TEM), and reverse transcriptase (Rtase) of cells cultured up to or beyond *in vitro* cell age.
- Induction studies are generally not very useful. Testing for specific viruses is done for murine cell lines using mouse, rat, and hamster antibody production (MAP, RAP, HAP) tests.
- *In vivo* testing for lymphocytic chorimeningitis virus is required. Human cell lines are screened for human viral pathogens (Epstein-Barr virus, cytomegalovirus, human retroviruses, hepatitis B and C, viruses with appropriate *in vitro* techniques). PCR technology may be useful in specific virus testing.
- Transgenic animals used for the production of biotechnological products should be kept according to good agricultural practices (GAP) and tested for viruses as described above.

The primary harvest material (milk) from animals is an equivalent stage of manufacture to unprocessed bulk harvest from a bioreactor.

- Adventitious agent contamination is tested at the end of the cell culture in the unprocessed bulk (if multiple harvest pools are prepared at different times, the culture should be tested at the time of the collection of each pool).

INACTIVATION AND REMOVAL

The validation of the virus removal involves evaluation of the cell substrates, raw materials used, virus inactivation/removal, and test of final product. Generally, a retrovirus or adventitious virus contamination raises serious questions about product safety. Even when viruses are not present, the presence of virus-like particles (VLPs) is often demonstrated by electron microscopy and the overall reduction should take into account the VLPs even though these may not point to an infective contamination. Similarly, when viruses of unknown origin are present, this should always be a matter of grave concern because there is no assay available to test what is totally unexpected; only preventive measures including extensive testing of the producer cells for specific viruses and testing for adventitious virus at a number of stages during fermentation can work.

The assessment of viral clearance or inactivation requires process evaluation using: viruses that are identical, a virus from the same genus or family, a virus closely related to the known or suspected virus, and nonspecific viruses. The process quantitatively estimates the overall level of relevant virus reduction obtained in the process (of viruses known to be present). It is not necessary to evaluate every unit of operation of the downstream process if adequate clearance has been demonstrated in selected steps by deliberate addition of virus to the unit operation application sample. Because of the complexity of carrying out viral clearance studies and the fact that log reduction factors of one do not contribute to the overall clearance factor, focus is on a few but efficient unit operations for virus removal (typically two to three in a downstream process). It may be difficult to assess the excess clearance (clearance measured minus risk measured), but this should be a central part of the effort to reduce the risk from viral contamination. Also, it is not recommended to perform the virus spiking experiments in the cGMP facility.

When scaling up to large-scale manufacturing, it is acceptable to perform the virus validation studies in small-scale studies (with scalable equipment), preferably around the capture and intermediary steps to avoid any potential virus burden at the polishing step. Steps that are likely to clear a virus should be individually assessed with sufficient virus present for adequate assessment. Chromatographic columns and filter devices used repeatedly should be validated with respect to cleaning in place and performance. Down-scale factors of 100 to 1000 can be achieved. Studies are best conducted under fractional factorial designs, as described above.

In virus activation studies, samples are taken at different time intervals, and an inactivation curve is constructed including at least one time point less than the minimum exposure time. The methods of testing meet all requirements of test method validation, and large variation in response seen is similar to what is observed in biological assays. As a result, the need for objective statistical evaluation has been emphasized by the FDA in the "Points to Consider," by the EMEA in the "Notes for Guidance," in the ICH Guidelines, and otherwise in the literature. The two main *in vitro* assay methods used in quantitative virus clearance studies are the plaque formation assay and the cytopathic assay. Both assays have been validated and they are routinely used to determine virus titers. The ICH Harmonised Tripartite Guideline, Q5A, step 4 further describes details of assays.

Examples of useful model viruses used as an unknown source of infection are SV40, human polio virus 1, animal parvovirus, a parainfluenza virus or influenza virus, Sindbis virus, RNA viruses, and murine retroviruses.

The downstream processing provides clearance of virus when using mammalian cell culture or components of biologic origin; the efficacy of these processes is verified much like the sterility testing that is done for bacterial contamination, and thus a statistical sample of the lot can be tested in accordance with sterility testing protocols. The effect of virus clearance is determined by spiking experiments for the respective unit operations. Virus distribution is monitored and balanced for the individual intermediates of such an operation: the virus titer of the load is measured and compared to the (residual) virus titer of the product containing fraction after processing, e.g., the flow-through or eluate of a chromatographic process or the permeate of a filtration process. The reduction factor of a unit operation is calculated upon the volume of the process fluids, and the virus titers measure for the load and the product-containing fraction after processing. The reduction factor is typically expressed in log 10 units, the "individual reduction factor" R_i for each unit of operation. The overall reduction factor for a virus within the entire purification process is the cumulation of the individual reduction factors. However, the cumulation of virus clearance can only be claimed for process steps, which represent different physicochemical measures. Based on cell assay variability, which is measured in a logarithmic scale, a logarithmic reduction factor in the order of 1, i.e., a 90% reduction in titer, is considered to be not significant for virus clearance. To set a numerical figure for the virus burden of a cell culture fluid at the time of harvest, electron microscopy is applied for counting viral particles in a distinctive volume. However, this approach raises additional questions: How representative can a few mLs of sample be for a few hundred l to several thousand l scale of cell culture fermentation? Furthermore, the cells in culture are grown to densities between 10^6 to 10^7/mL; the number of cells investigated by EM is reduced by several logs and is about 10^3/mL. The identification of virus particles and their differentiation from particulate matter due to the preparation procedure require extensive experience, and a confirmation of the viral nature is impossible. Examples are artifacts, which are originated from sample preparation, e.g., high speed centrifugation of cell culture supernatant; the pellets derived from centrifugation typically harbor complex aggregates, which often conceal those details necessary to identify virus structures.

ANALYTICAL METHOD VALIDATION

QA systems ensure that the analytical procedures are reliable and suitable for the intended use. The extent of validation depends on the stage of development; in the early phases, the methods are evolving and the main interest is in testing for efficacy and toxicity; however, prior to manufacturing clinical test batches, the methods must be fully validated. The elements of validation include specificity, linearity, range, accuracy, precision, detection limit, quantification limit, robustness, and system suitability testing. These requirements are identical to those used for any other testing method used as part of CMC preparation; details can be found elsewhere. For example, the validation of analytical procedures is described in the ICH harmonized tripartite guideline Q2B (http://www.ich.org/MediaServer.jser?@_ID=418&@_TYPE=MULTIMEDIA&@_TEMPLATE= 616&@_MODE=GLB). Revalidation may be necessary if the manufacturing process is changed, if the drug product composition is changed, or if the analytical method is changed. The degree of revalidation required depends on the nature of changes. An analytical validation plan is a description of how the validation will be carried out and is a part of the master validation plan. A formal report on analytical method description, including sample preparation instructions, raw material and equipment list, method description, data collection procedure, results, data interpretation, should be provided. A formal validation protocol, including specific sample and control replicate analysis sequences, validation characteristics, method of data analysis and reporting, working values for system suitability, assay performance requirements, assay limitations, and reference standard identification, should be provided.

10 Quality Control Systems

INTRODUCTION

Testing of therapeutic proteins follows similar methods and protocols as used for chemically derived or small molecule products; this includes the in-process testing as discussed under quality assurance issues. An example of required quality control (QC) tests would be given in a monograph such as the one included for interferon and erythropoietin in the European Pharmacopoeia (EP) or British Pharmacopoeia (BP). This would be release testing; testing is also a part of a comprehensive QC program that monitors various parameters and responses, definition of critical parameters, in-process control of intermediary compounds, and tests of drug substance and drug product. In its usual description, the quality control comprises in-process control, control of drug substance/product, and a description of analytical methods used to characterize intermediary and final products.

The most common in-process tests include measures for pH, conductivity, total protein, and redox potential. The drug substance/product testing follows the International Conference on Harmonisation (ICH) guidelines in which the product is characterized with respect to identity, biological activity, immunoreactivity, purity, and quantity comparing data with specified acceptance criteria. Where a compendium monograph exists, such as in the case of interferon, erythropoietin, growth hormone, or insulin, the testing on a final product and the concentrate is accordingly performed. The methods used are validated (and verified where there exists a compendium method) and appropriate documentation is created to support this.

IN-PROCESS CONTROLS

For biological products, safety is considered a larger issue than in the case of chemical products; impurities in the system are of lesser concern in chemical system than in biological systems as they can alter the three-dimensional structure of protein affecting its immunogenicity; so, while the levels of impurities may be well below what is considered unsafe or even undetectable, they can adversely affect the product. As a result, the product quality is inevitably linked to the process design, process robustness, process compliance with current Good Manufacturing Practice (cGMP), and extensive QC programs including product specifications, process specifications, in-process control, drug substance and drug product testing, regulatory policies, and scientific understanding. In-process controls apply to control of raw materials, control of process variables, analytical testing of intermediary compounds, end of production test after termination of cell culture, etc. In addition, in-process controls are included to control quality by monitoring of process parameters and responses. This requires complete characterization of the process where the parameters and their action limits are well defined. This is accomplished in the early stages of process development and scale up in the manufacturing of Phase I and Phase II clinical supplies and finalized with completion of process validation during manufacture of Phase III material including regulatory ranges and operating ranges. Retrospective validation, though routinely used in pharmaceutical manufacturing, may not be sufficient to ensure that all essential parameters have been optimized to monitor in-line, on-line, or at-line processes during manufacture.

The goal of PAT (Process Analytical Techniques of the FDA) is to understand and control the manufacturing process, which is consistent with our current drug quality system: *quality cannot be tested into products; it should be built-in or should be by design.* Process analytical technology is a system for designing, analyzing, and controlling manufacturing through timely measurements (i.e., during processing) of critical quality and performance attributes of raw and in-process materials and processes with the goal of ensuring final product quality. It is important to note that the term *analytical* in PAT is viewed broadly to include chemical, physical, microbiological, mathematical, and risk analysis conducted in an integrated manner. There are many standard and new tools available that enable scientific, risk-managed pharmaceutical development, manufacture, and quality assurance. These tools, when used within a system, can provide effective and efficient means for acquiring information to facilitate process understanding, develop risk-mitigation strategies, achieve continuous improvement, and share information and knowledge. In the PAT framework, these tools can be categorized as:

- Multivariate data acquisition and analysis tools;
- Modern process analyzers or process analytical chemistry tools;
- Process and endpoint monitoring and control tools;
- Continuous improvement and knowledge management tools.

An appropriate combination of some, or all, of these tools may be applicable to a single-unit operation, or to an entire manufacturing process and its quality assurance. A desired goal of the PAT framework is to design and develop processes that can consistently ensure a predefined quality at the end of the manufacturing process. Such procedures would be consistent with the basic tenet of quality by design and could reduce risks to quality and regulatory concerns while improving efficiency. Gains in quality, safety, or efficiency will vary depending on the product and are likely to come from:

- Reducing production cycle times by using on-, in-, or at-line measurements and controls.
- Preventing rejects, scrap, and reprocessing.
- Considering the possibility of real-time release.
- Increasing automation to improve operator safety and reduce human error.
- Facilitating continuous processing to improve efficiency and manage variability:
  - Using small-scale equipment (to eliminate certain scale-up issues) and dedicated manufacturing facilities.
  - Improving energy and material use and increasing capacity.

A combination of increased automation and real-time analysis reduces human error, facilitates continuous processing, and shortens process time.

Parameters

The biological manufacturing processes are clearly divided into distinct unit operations, normally comprising a single technical procedure (e.g., filtration) in which a sample is treated according to a protocol resulting in an output pool, precipitate, supernatant, filtrate (e.g., sample procedure output). The sample and procedure parameters can be controlled, but the output is difficult to control because of a large number of parameters that control the upstream and downstream operations. In typical upstream processes, parameters like pH, redox potential, and dissolved oxygen affect cell growth and stability; temperature, agitation rate, and flow rates affect cell growth, redox potential, and metabolic activity, which is further controlled by the supply of glucose and glutamine. Similarly, the parameters of importance in the downstream process and how they affect the outcome include:

- Back pressure affects protein aggregates or other high-molecular increase pressure (should be kept constant).
- Conductivity affects stability, binding to chromatographic media, viscosity, turbidity, and holding times.

- Filtration inlet pressure affects flux, fouling, and cross-flow velocity.
- Filtration outlet pressure affects flux, fouling, and cross-flow velocity.
- Holding time affects stability and solubility.
- Linear flow affects protein binding ability in chromatographic media.
- Load affects capacity of chromatographic media (adjust accordingly).
- pH affects stability, precipitation reactions, formulation of des-amido forms, -elimination, racemization, disulfide bond and cleavage, binding to chromatographic media, solubility, and holding times.
- Protein concentration affects stability, solubility, viscosity, turbidity, and holding times.
- Rexod potential affects stability of inter- and intramolecular disulfide bonds, formation of oxidized forms, and holding times.
- Temperature affects stability, solubility, formation of protein derivatives, enzymatic activity of proteolytic enzymes, reaction kinetics, and holding times.
- Transmembrane pressure affects filtrate flow, flux, and fouling.
- Turbidity affects ability to pass filters and chromatographic media.
- Viscosity affects ability to pass filters and chromatographic media.

Because of complex composition of the sample, it is frequently difficult to fully characterize the sample, a prerequisite to operation control since the procedure applied can have unpredictable responses such as cell density, cell viability, specific production rate, ammonia concentration, expression level, specific amino acid concentration, NADH/NADPH ratio, and lactate dehydrogenase activity in the upstream and yield, retention time, UV-profile, protein stability, and biological activity in the downstream processes.

The parameters are stated in terms of intervals and not set points to allow for adjustments particularly in large-scale operations, defining lower and upper limits allows for statistical multivariate data analysis and allows for process optimization without process redesign. The specified range intervals in regulatory documents are further refined with internal action limits, which are a proven acceptable range (PAR) based on small-scale experiments, to comply with the worst-case scenarios as dictated by the U.S. FDA. The statistical methods applied to validating the interval ranges are arrived at using factorial designs as described in the chapter on quality assurance.

The intermediate products are tested analytically and extensively in the process development stages to obviate such testing during manufacturing operations. Typical in-process control analyses are tests for microbial agents, fungi, mycoplasmas, viruses, endotoxins, 1D-SDS, HP-IEC, HP-RPC, HP-SEC, and ELISA. Given below are details on some of these tests and their limitations.

Parameters are often monitored using a continuous probe system such as observed in the many automated controls offered in a modern fermenter. An unusual situation arises in the monitoring of biological manufacturing where the properties of the medium monitored change with time; for example, the pH change may be accompanied by a change in temperature, ionic strength, other solute strengths, and redox potential; the pH probes therefore should be validated to take into account all of these factors. This type of work will likely be conducted as part of a PAT exercise; however, it will be impossible to select all pertinent factors ahead of the completion of the process development, requiring revalidation of the probes. Another problem arises in the stability and robustness of the probe itself. In many instances the solutions probed can alter the probe because of chemical or biological reactions and thus a shelf-life of each probe must be predetermined. Other aspects that must be examined include the common factors in the measurement of parameters. For example, pH measurements are affected by the ionic strength of the solution and the temperature (which should be the same as during calibration). When measuring redox potential it is often impossible to obtain stable measurements. Instead, the potential will shift toward more negative values (e.g., biological systems) because of the slow exchange of electrons with the platinum electrode, as the redox center is often shielded by protein. A rapid measurement can be achieved by adding a redox mediator capable of making rapid exchanges of electrons with the electrode. In practice, a mediator is chosen having E_{m7} (the midpoint redox potential at pH 7.0) close to the estimated redox potential of the solution at a given pH (the above E_m values can be used at a different pH considering pH (2-10) ~ -400 mV or approximately –50 mV per increase in pH unit). The volume of the mediator must be small compared to the volume of the solution. Good results are often obtained with a mediator volume of a few drops of a 0.05% solution to 100 mL of test solution. It is common practice to perform redox titration in both oxidative and reductive sequences, vary the concentration of mediators in 10 to 6 to 10 to 3 range, and use mediators in the range of Em ($\pm$ 60 mV) to the redox couple being measured.

As is well known for the pKs of the pH buffers, the E region of greatest resistance is close to the redox Em value of the mediator. Because of temperature fluctuations in the process, one must ensure that all redox potential measurements include a temperature reference. Special precautions must be taken regarding the influence of oxygen, for example, by use of an oxygen-free protective gas like nitrogen.

TOTAL PROTEIN

In testing protein content, sensitivity is not an issue and the method chosen is a matter of convenience, sample, amount, purity, interfering compounds, sensitivity, accuracy, and assay time. The chromogenic assays are used for a fast evaluation of protein content in crude samples, but may later be exchanged with quantitative methods, such as Kjeldahl. The UV-spectrometry assay is preferably used in purified samples where a high content of target protein and amino acid analysis is typically used for quantification of the drug substance reference standards. It may be a useful strategy to use two different methods for determination of total protein and compare the results.

The methods of choice are:

- The bicinchinonic acid assay (BCA) is a copper based spectrophotometric assay often preferred to the biuret or Lowry assay due to its simplicity and ruggedness toward many buffer components. The accuracy is good, but protein-to-protein differences in reactivity can occur. Major interfering agents are strong acids, ammonium sulfate, and lipids.
- The copper-based biuret assay is among the oldest of the total protein assays offering low sensitivity (1 to 10 mg/mL) and is still used frequently in more concentrated solutions. The major interfering agents are ammonium salts.
- The Bradford assay uses the ability of the Coomassie brilliant blue G-250 dye to bind to peptides and proteins. Upon binding the dye undergoes a color shift from 465 to 595 nm. This assay can be used in dilute solutions.
- The Lowry assay and its modifications (Hartree-Lowry) are enhancements of the biuret reaction making use of the Folin-Ciocalteau reagent. The color reaction is time dependent and protein-to-protein variations may occur. The accuracy is good. Numerous buffer components can interfere with the assay (e.g., strong acids, ammonium sulfate).
- The Kjeldahl assay is a quantitative method for nitrogen determination in crude samples. The method is based on the fact that nearly all proteins contain approximately 16.5% nitrogen by weight, which gives a conversion factor between nitrogen and protein content of approximately 6. The sample must be free of interfering nitrogen containing compounds.
- UV-spectrometry measures the absorbance at 277 to 280 nm (tyrosine and tryptophan), which is an indirect measure of the protein concentration. In protein mixtures an average extinction coefficient must be used, and the method is consequently semiquantitative if not used relative to a quantitative method such as Kjeldahl. Major interfering agents are detergents, nucleic acids, particulates, and lipid droplets.

The accuracy of the assay depends on the validity of the standard curve and thereby the quality of the standard solution used (stability, purity, protein). In addition the buffers used for the standard curve must reflect the buffer of the sample to be analyzed. Interfering compounds should preferably be identified and the signal from blank samples monitored. Time of reaction is of importance for some assays (e.g., Lowry), and test samples must be treated accordingly. Common practice is to prepare a minimum of 5 standard points in duplicate or triplicate across a five- to 10-fold range of concentration. It is important to realize that good performance in calibration with single, fairly pure proteins does not necessarily translate into reliable performance with real samples. Samples are generally dialyzed, desalted, or precipitated with trichloroacetic acid (TCA) prior to analysis to remove interfering compounds where suspected; for example, nucleic acids are precipitated with polyethyleneimines (PEI).

SPECIFICATIONS

Specifications comprise a list of tests, references to analytical procedures, and appropriate criteria, which are numerical limits, ranges, or other criteria for the test described to establish the set of criteria to which a drug substance or drug product or an intermediary compound should conform to; this conformity of batch data to specification test accept-criteria is an important part of the batch quality control release (certificate of analysis, COA).

The specifications are developed in the early part of process and product development (process design, scale up, non-GMP manufacture, and cGMP manufacture for clinical Phase I and II) wherein the active drug is fully characterized for its physiochemical properties, biological activity, immunochemical properties, purity, and quantity. The acceptance criteria are related to the analysis method chosen and established as early as possible; however, throughout the development process, these specifications change, partly as a result of scale up and partly as a result of a better understanding of the relevance of the parameters to activity including the identification of product and process impurities. Examples of the ICH recommendations of characterization parameters include appearance (color, clarity), identity (amino acid composition, amino acid sequence, CD, DSC, EPR, MS, IE focusing, isoform pattern, native electrophoresis, NIR, NMR, peptide map, 2D electrophoresis, X-ray diffraction), biological activity (animal assays, cell assays, receptor assays, as applicable), immunochemical properties (antigen binding assays), purity (capillary electrophoresis, ELISA-HCP, HP-IEC, HP-RPC, HP-SEC, LAL test, PCR), quantitative amino acid analysis (Kjeldahl analysis, UV absorbance), sterility, pH, osmolality, etc.

Identity of the active product is established using tests for primary, secondary, and tertiary structures, posttranslational modifications, and physiochemical properties of the drug substance/product. These tests include determining molecular weight, isoform pattern, extinction coefficient, electrophoretic patterns, liquid chromatography patterns, and spectroscopic profiles. The structural characterization program often includes amino acid sequence, amino acid composition, terminal amino acid sequence, peptide map, sulfhydryl group(s) and disulfide bridges, X-ray diffraction, NMR analysis, and carbohydrate structure. The biological activity is tested using animal, cell, receptor, ligand, and biochemical assays and may be used to determine the biological activity of the product. Potency (expressed in units) is the quantitative measure of biological activity. When possible, the biological activity should be compared to that of the natural product.

Additional tests required for therapeutic proteins include tests for potential to induce immunogenicity, which is difficult to assess, and the only real test of the immunogenicity potential is ascertained once the drug goes into actual use where millions of doses are administered over a longer period of time to provide the only correct evaluation of immunogenicity. Early studies can only identify significant hypersensitivity and allergic reactions. However, assays that like binding to antibodies are becoming increasingly accepted and the FDA has been emphasizing development of highly sensitive assays to detect antibodies at below nanogram levels. The immunogenicity potential becomes more relevant when the molecules are modified from their natural state, like pegylation, wherein unexpected immunogenic responses can be expected.

Impurities in biological products can be adventitious agents, process, and product impurities. Virus infection risk is a lesser concern if a bacterial expression system has been used, but presence of scrambled forms of the target protein arising from the *in vitro* folding could be an issue. Therefore, protein purity should not be related to a few analytical methods, but rather be analyzed on the basis of the expression system used, the process design, and the derivatives of the target protein arising as a consequence of upstream and downstream processing.

Impurity identification and quantitation are more important for biological products because even small concentrations of impurities can significantly alter the protein structure, though they themselves may not be harmful. The host-related impurities arrive from the construction of the recombinant organism, from eventual infections of the cell, and from compounds coexpressed with the target protein or from cells undergoing apoptosis and lysis. Examples of host-related impurities are endotoxins, viruses, prions, nucleic acids, host cell lipids, proteins, and proteolytic enzymes. The process-related impurities encompass those derived from the manufacturing process (upstream, downstream, and formulation). Examples of process-related impurities are bacteria, yeast, fungi, mycoplasmas, viruses, prions, endotoxins, raw materials, and cell culture substrates. This category also includes adventitious agents not intentionally used in the process such as mycoplasma infections of the cell culture. The product-related impurities are target product derivatives such as des-amido forms, oxidized forms, scrambled forms, glycosylated forms, cleaved forms, carbamylated forms, acylated forms, and polymeric forms. These forms may be physically and chemically closely related to the target protein and may also exhibit full or partial biological activity. Especially the polymeric forms may be immunogenic. In a regulatory sense some of these derivatives are not regarded as impurities if they have similar properties (activity, efficacy, safety) as the desired product.

Quantity is usually measured as the amount of total protein present in the sample of highly purified recombinant products. Quantitative methods such as amino acid analysis, Kjeldahl, or UV-absorbance are used for quantity determination. In less pure products immunogenic assays (e.g., ELISA) may be used to determine the quantity of the active drug.

IDENTITY

An important part of the overall characterization program for a recombinant-derived protein is the identity tests confirming molecular weight, isoelectric point, primary structure, secondary structure, tertiary structure, quaternary structure, possible posttranslational modifications, liquid chromatography patterns, and biomolecular interactions. Identity is generally a qualitative measure of the physical and chemical target protein properties favoring specificity over sensitivity.

Protein structure and function are closely related. Even minor deviations in the three-dimensional conformation or in the posttranslational modifications (e.g., glycosylation, phosphorylation, or acylation pattern) may result in altered biological activity or in an adverse immunogenic/allergic response.

During the drug development phase extensive characterization programs are exerted on reference materials (often of the drug substance level) in order to confirm the chemical and physical properties of the protein and to compare the recombinant product with it natural counterpart, if possible. Only a minority of the identity tests will be used for batch release.

The standard methods for determination of molecular weight (MW) are Electrospray MS, MALDI TOF, HP-SEC, and ultrafiltration. The MW can be determined if the sedimentation coefficient is known. Various ultrafiltration sedimentation velocity measurements (sedimentation velocity, difference sedimentation, and sedimentation equilibrium) are used to gain information on shape and conformation. This is a useful check of homogeneity. Scanning transmission electron microscopy is used to determine the molecular weight of large particles.

The isoelectric point (pI) is the pH level where the protein has no net charge. The standard methods for determination of pI are IEF in polyacrylamide gels and CE-IEF. The separation principle is based on charge heterogeneity caused by differences in amino acid residue charges. It is common practice to include a sample of the natural protein, if possible. The pI may also be determined by means of 2D-electrophoresis, where molecules are separated according to pI and MW.

The primary structure provides information on the amino acid sequence of the protein. For most proteins a primary structure analysis comprises N-terminal sequencing by Edman degradation, C-terminal analysis, and peptide mapping followed by HP-RPC purification and subsequent determination of the MW of the fragment by mass spectroscopy. Peptides and smaller proteins may be sequenced by means of Edman degradation only. The amino acid sequence is often supported by total amino acid analysis, comparison of the cloned gene sequence, and the molecular weight determination. Comparative fingerprints between the natural and the recombinant protein are also used to confirm primary structure identity.

The secondary structure provides information on disulfide bond arrangement, -helix, and -sheet content. The standard methods for determination of disulfide arrangements are peptide mapping by HP-RPC or SDS-PAGE. Structural information is obtained by means of fluorescence, far UV circular dichroism, Raman scattering, and infrared absorption using FTIR. The spectroscopic methods are very powerful when used for comparison analysis with the natural counterpart. The confirmation of correct disulfide linkage is usually carried out on appropriate enzymatic or chemical digests of the target protein followed by HP-RPC purification of the fragments and subsequent mass analysis using ESI-MS or MALDI-TOF. The analysis may be challenged by close neighboring cystinyl residues, making it difficult to cleave the protein at least once between successive cys residues. Cleavage techniques must take the possibility of disulfide bond interchange into consideration at pH above 7, where some proteolytic enzymes have their optimum. Scrambling is catalyzed by presence of free cystinyl residues or free cystine, but these can be blocked before digestion.

The tertiary structure is the three-dimensional structure of the molecule. The standard methods for tertiary structure determination are NMR (in solution), X-ray diffraction using crystals at high atomic resolution (< 3Å), and near UV circular dicroism. The latter method is very powerful for comparison analysis with the natural counterpart.

The quaternary structure of a protein results from interaction between individual polypeptide chains to yield larger aggregates. The individual chains are often referred to as subunits. The standard methods for determination of quaternary structure are HP-SEC, Raman scattering, and light scattering, useful for determination of large macromolecular assemblies and scanning transmission electron microscopy for determination of molecular weight of large particles.

Posttranslational modifications are chemical modifications of side groups (e.g., oxidation of Met, de-amidation of Asn of Gln), phosphorylation, glycosylation, fatty acid acylation, farnesylation, sialic acid capping, N-methylation, and acetylation. Typical standard methods for the detection of posttranslational modifications are HP-RPC, HP-IEC, or mass spectroscopy. In mass spectroscopy, the MW of the molecule can be determined with high accuracy and precision (better than 0.01%). This performance is normally sufficient to identify modifications such as missing residues or additional groups. Peptide mapping, using specific enzymes and subsequent HP-RPC purification of the fragments prior to MW detection, is also used for example for determination of glycosylation patterns. Heterologous glycosylated products are often identified by their isoelectric focusing slab gel pattern or more rarely by 2D-electrophoresis. A thorough carbohydrate structural analysis may include glycosylation site(s), carbohydrate chain structure, the oligosaccharide pattern, and the content of neutral sugars, amino sugars, and sialic acids.

The extinction coefficient can be determined from a known protein quantity (protein concentration) and the absorbance at 277 to 280 nm.

In chromatography evaluation, the target protein retention time using HP-IEC or HP-RPC can be used as an identity marker. For biomolecular interaction analysis, the method uses surface plasmon resonance to detect biomolecular interactions.

BIOLOGICAL ACTIVITY

The biological activity describes the ability or capacity of the drug substance to achieve a defined biological effect. Examples of procedures used to measure the biological activity include animal-based biological assays, cell culture-based biological assays, biochemical assays, and ligand and receptor binding assays. A biologic assay may be replaced by physicochemical tests provided sufficient information and correlation between the bioassay and the said tests can be given and there exists a well-established manufacturing history (ICH Harmonized Tripartite Guideline. Specifications: Test Procedures and Acceptance Criteria for Biotechnological Products (Q6B) on March 10, 1999). In some cases, the specific biological activity may provide additional useful information.

PURITY

Protein purity has been historically linked to the specific biological activity in terms of units of biological activity per mass unit of the product. The purest product was that of the highest specific biological activity. In contrast to drugs based on small molecules, which could be controlled on the drug product level, protein-based pharmaceuticals were closely linked to the process itself due to the complexity of the active pharmaceutical ingredient and the lack of proper characterization of the final product. With the introduction of recombinant technology and modern analytical methods, a much better drug substance/product characterization became possible resulting in the well-characterized protein concept and the widespread use of comparability studies. The importance of a stronger focus on presence of adventitious agents and specific impurities was also recognized, as the presence of even minor amounts of toxic, immunogenic, or adventitious compounds proved to have severe side effects. Unless otherwise specified, the acceptable level of impurities depends on the nature of the drug product and the dose.

ENDOTOXINS

Endotoxins come from gram-negative bacteria (e.g., *E. coli*), if it is used as the expression system. Presence of endotoxins indicates bacterial contamination in raw materials, columns, water, and buffers. Endotoxins bind strongly to anion exchange media even at high ionic strength and thus HIC and cation exchange chromatography (CEC) are used for their removal provided the target protein binds to the matrix. Binding of the target protein to cation exchange also allows effective endotoxin clearance. SEC can remove endotoxins provided the differences in molecular weight between the endotoxins and the protein are sufficient. However, SEC may be an unpredictable method, since endotoxins range in size from subunits of 10 to 20 kDa in the presence of detergents to vesicles of 0.1 Pm in diameter in the presence of divalent cations. In the absence of significant levels of divalent cations and surface-active agents, they dissociate into micelles of 300 to 1000 kDa.

Traditional inactivation methods (clean-in-place [CIP]) against endotoxins include acid hydrolysis, base hydrolysis, oxidation, alkylation, and heat and ionizing radiation. To ensure complete removal from chromatographic columns, the use of NaOH is recommended (the concentration depends on the matrix used). Endotoxins are destroyed by exposure to NaOH or peracetic acid, but are not affected by ethanol.

NUCLEIC ACIDS

Nucleic acid contamination comes from host cell DNA/RNA or retroviral RNA. Molecules with more than 150 to 200 base pairs will behave as flexible coils in size exclusion chromatography, while molecules up to 18 base pairs behave as globular proteins. In between the rigid rod structure should be expected. Their presence results in increased viscosity of the solution. Circular DNA is often super-coiled and will elute as a molecule of smaller size. Preventive action nucleic acid free biopharmaceutical products are obtained by using nucleases (e.g., Benzonase) or by minimizing release of nucleic acids from the host cell organism. Anion exchange chromatography has been shown to be effective in binding the highly charged nucleic acids at ionic strength at which most proteins elute. Due to the negative net charge and hydrophilic character binding of the target protein to a cation exchanger, hydrophobic interaction or affinity matrix may reduce the nucleic acid content.

DNA binds to hydroxyapatite at low to moderate phosphate concentrations. Precipitation of nucleic acids with polyethyleneimine or magnesium chloride has been reported. Use of 1 M NaOH is recommended (make sure that equipment, filters, and chromatographic media are not affected by NaOH) for CIP. Nucleic acids are detected by monitoring absorption of light at 260 nm. The residual content in drug substance (DS) or drug product (DP) is usually measured by PCR or amplification techniques. The maximum allowable content of nucleic acid per dose has been under continuous evaluation since the initially proposed content of 10 pg per dose was suggested by FDA's Center for Biologics Evaluation and Research (CBER). The World Health Organization (WHO) has stated that 100 pg per dose is acceptable. CBER now states that "Lot-to-lot testing for DNA content in biological products produced in cell lines should be performed and lot release limits established that reflect a level of purity that can be achieved reasonably and consistent."

Host Cell Proteins

Host cell proteins come from the host organism and constitute a major purification problem due to variability structure and surface properties. The amount released into the culture medium depends on the expression system used, the culture conditions, and whether or not the cells are disrupted in order to extract intracellular expressed target protein. Notice that "foreign" cellular proteins can be introduced by means of recombinant derived raw materials (e.g., enzymes) used in the downstream process. The range of preventive actions include use of expression systems with direct expression of the target protein to the culture medium, gentle handling of intact cells, and purification procedures such as chromatography, filtration, precipitation, and crystallization. If milk from transgenic animals is used as the product source, presence of the animal equivalent to the target protein should be of concern (as it might copurify with the target protein). Protein impurities should be considered on a case-by-case basis and be relegated to process validation rather than final product testing. Due to molecular diversity no specific purification method can be recommended, as the separation depends on the difference in affinity (selectivity) between HCP and the target protein for chosen chromatographic media and operating conditions. Use of a combination of different chromatographic principles is recommended. Most proteins will be removed (CIP) by means of 0.1 to 1 M NaOH (make sure that equipment, filters, and chromatographic media are not affected by NaOH). Several analytical methods have been used to monitor HCP including SDS-PAGE, 2D-electrophoresis, Western blot (WB), and immunoassays. SDS-PAGE separates molecules according to the molecular weight of the protein. The method, which is semiquantitative, has a sensitivity of 100 pg/band (silver staining). Two-dimensional electrophoresis (IEF in combination with SDS-PAGE) provides the most powerful separation of protein mixtures. The method, which is semiquantitative, provides the widest window of the methods used with a sensitivity of 100 pg/spot. The WB method provides information of immunological identity. The sensitivity is 0.1 to 1 ng/band and the method is qualitative. Immunoassays are widely used for HCP analysis in drug substances and drug products. The method depends on the nature and quality of antibodies used and not all proteins (regardless of quantity) are detected. The method, which is semiquantitative, provides the highest sensitivity (< 0.1ng/mL). Two types of assays have been used to detect HCPs: generic and specific assays. In generic assays, the host cell proteins typical for a given expression system are detected. If the assays are based on competently produced antibodies raised against cell lysates, the quality may be adequate or better than those produced by individual companies. Generic assays are typically used during process development, as process-specific assays by definition are not available before the process has been locked. However, it is recommended also to use generic HCP assays for lot release for several reasons. First, the protein patterns are highly conserved between strains, and second, a generic HCP assay will be a very strong tool for detection of variations in the process, which could lead to a different impurity profile. Process-specific assays are directed against host cell proteins copurifying with the target protein. The assays are typically developed by purifying the cell lysate without target protein, using the exact process used for the licensed product. By definition, the process-specific assay cannot be developed before the process is locked. The assay, which typically takes from 1 to 2 years to develop, may thus be a time-delaying factor. The process-specific assays provide a much narrower window than do generic assays and their value as a lot-release test has recently been challenged because these assays most probably will fail to detect atypical HCP contaminants. There are some significant differences between WB technology and immunoassays. In WB the denaturation and solubilization steps can destroy some native epitopes, while the immunoassay technology relies on reaction with the native protein. The immunoassay technology provides an objective result, while the WB depends on a subjective interpretation. Finally, the sensitivity of immunoassays is generally higher than for WB assays. None of the methods mentioned are quantitative. They are at best semiquantitative. Even the commonly used HCP immunoassay lack the linear accuracy applied to single analyte immunoassays due to variance in relative affinities between antibodies and HCP antigens and HCP concentrations. Instead assay results are correlated with clinical conditions and to process control. The amount of HCP to be accepted depends on the antigenicity of the copurifying proteins. Recognizing the complexity of the task and the inability of quantitative measurements it is not possible to state a general acceptable level.

VIRUSES

Virus contamination comes from the host cell, the culture medium, and infections during manufacture. The host cell may contain a genomic virus or virus vectors used to transform the cell line. The type of viral genome or vector depends on the cell line history. Continuous cell lines are extensively characterized, but chronic or latent viruses may be present. The retroviruses associated with continuous cell lines are noninfectious, but oncogenic. Epstein-Barr virus or Sendai virus is often used for cell transformations. Contaminants such as BVDV, IBR, reovirus, PI-3, bovine leukemia virus, and bovine polyoma virus should be expected from serum-supplemented media. Virus control is executed on several levels. The cell line history reveals all information on the origin and identity of the cell line and the host genome vectors used to establish the cell line. The master cell bank (MCB) is extensively characterized using viral identity tests, *in vitro* tests, and *in vivo* tests to ensure freedom of adventitious viruses. The end of production test of the cell culture is carried out to ensure that the cells are free of viruses. Viruses are brought into the process from the environment either because of contaminated equipment, infected raw materials, water, or because of nonsterile handling procedures. Working in closed systems and avoidance of raw materials of animal origin will help reduce the risk of infection. Strict control of equipment cleaning and sanitization procedures during processing will also help reduce contamination risk. Removal viruses may be inactivated by heat, radiation, chemical compound, or low pH, or removed by chromatography or filtration techniques. Due to molecular diversity no specific chromatographic purification method can be recommended, and virus reduction factors must be determined for selected unit operations. Nano-filtration is a very efficient virus removal step, often resulting in logarithmic reduction factors of 5 to 8. A commonly used reagent for cleaning of chromatographic media is 0.1 to 1 M NaOH. Viruses can be destroyed successfully with peracetic acid (make sure that equipment, filters, and chromatographic media are not affected by NaOH or peracetic acid). A variety of purity analyses are available: mono-layer cultures, test for pathogen viruses not able to grow in cell cultures in both animals and eggs, test for retroviruses, endogenous viruses, or viral nucleic acid, and test for selected viruses using mouse, rat, and hamster antibody production. It is necessary to document utilization of adequate virus removal and inactivation strategies to ensure the exclusion of contaminating viruses. Different modes of action should ensure overlapping and complementary levels of protection. The purification process is validated with respect to virus removal and inactivation. The final product is rarely tested if continuous mammalian cell lines have been used as an expression system.

Prions

Prions come from transmissible spongiform encephalopathies (TSE), including scrapie in sheep and goats, chronic wasting disease in mule deer and elk, bovine spongiform encephalopathy (BSE) in cattle, and Kuru and Creutzfeldt-Jakob disease (CJD) in humans. The disease-causing agents (prions) replicate in infected individuals generally without evidence of infection detectable by available diagnostic tests applicable *in vivo*. The major source of contamination of a recombinant product is the use of animal-derived raw materials, which could harbor bovine prions (BSE agent). Currently, there are no assays that are sensitive or specific enough to test raw materials or sources, and the only reliable prevention is to include barriers, such as avoidance of animal or human raw materials (e.g., trypsin, serum, transferin, bovine/human serum albumin, protein supplements, peptones). However, this is not always possible (e.g., in the propagation of cells for the establishment of cell banks), and inactivation and removal procedures during downstream processing become of interest. Milk is unlikely to present any risk of prion contamination. Filtration has proven efficient in the removal of prion particles. Thus, size exclusion partitioning of abnormal prion particles using normal flow filtration or tangential flow filtration resulted in significant reduction of the infectious agent. The most effective inactivation methods include chloride dioxide, glutaraldehyde, 4 M guanidium thiocyanate, sodium dichloroisocyanurate, sodium metaperiodate, 6 M urea, and autoclaving at 121 qC for 15 min, of which several will not be suited if the target protein is present. Biological assays such as *in vivo* infection of susceptible animals are time consuming (months to years). They will not be of practical use in the test of biopharmaceutical products. The best semiquantitative biochemical assays include WB, capillary immunoelectrophoresis, conformation-dependent immunoassay, and dissociation-enhanced, time-resolved fluoimmunoassay. The infectious dose is not known. Accept criteria must be decided on a case-by-case basis.

Proteolytic Enzymes

Proteolytic enzymes are released to the medium because of cell death, mechanical stress, or induced cell lysis. Their presence should be expected during fermentation and initial downstream unit operations. Measures are taken to work fast at low temperatures and to avoid working near the pH optimum of the enzyme. The most rewarding strategy is to prevent proteolysis during fermentation either by use of mutant strains or by optimizing the conditions toward minimum enzymatic activity. Most enzymes of the vacuoles and lysozomes will be minimally active at slightly alkaline pH (7 to 9), a pH interval strongly recommended for extraction of proteins expressed in bacteria. Proteins are probably more resistant toward proteolytic attacks in their native state and stabilizing factors (e.g., cofactor, correct parameter interval, cosolvent) should always be considered optimized. Use of protein inhibitors is not recommended for safety reasons. Proteolytic enzymes are typically removed during the capture and intermediary purification steps and they rarely copurify with the target protein throughout the downstream process. Despite the variety of enzymes present in the cell cytosol, proteolytic enzymes rarely constitute a problem in final products. Selective removal (e.g., affinity chromatography) of specific enzymes should be considered. Most proteins will be removed by means of 0.1 to 1 M NaOH (make sure that equipment, filters, and chromatographic media are not affected by NaOH). Suited analytical methods for early control are SDS-PAGE and WB. Purified preparations may be analyzed by means of HP-IEC, HP-RPC, MS, and peptide mapping. Ascertain that the degradation observed is not a function of the analytical assay. Enzyme inhibitors can be used for prevention of enzymatic activity in analytical assays.

Lipids

Lipids (lipoproteins, triglycerides, phospholipids, cholesterol) are brought to the medium by cell lysis. If transgenic animals are used, the protein is expressed into the milk containing up to 4% fat. Lipids can be removed from the feedstock by centrifugation, specific adsorption to hydrophobic compounds such as Hyflow by precipitation with Dextran sulfate, by binding to anion exchangers, or by affinity chromatography, allowing for specific binding of the target protein. Lipids will bind to hydrophobic media and surfaces. Lipids are retarded (two to three column volumes) by adsorption to Sephadex. Milk fat is usually removed by centrifugation. Lipids are removed by means of NaOH or organic solvents (make sure that equipment, filters, and chromatographic media are not affected by NaOH or organic solvents).

MICROBIAL AGENTS

Microbial agents and fungi come from infection of the bioreactor during cell culture. Other sources are contaminated water, buffers, raw materials, chromatographic columns, and equipment. Fermentation and cell culture bioreactors are prone to microbial infections. As the use of antibiotics in large-scale operations should be avoided, strict demands to the design of bioreactors and handling procedures are the key measures to avoid microbial infections. Testing for microorganisms at the end of production ensures that no infections have taken place during culture. The nature of samples and buffers used during downstream processing makes these excellent growth substrates for microorganisms. For that reason water quality control, sterile filtration of buffers prior to use, sterile filtration of intermediary products, and effective cleaning and sanitization procedures are key elements of the downstream operations. Filtration should be through 0.22 μm filters. Bacterial spores are typically removed by means of 0.1 Pm filters. Cleaning with 60 to 70% v/v ethanol is a commonly used disinfectant against microbial agents; often 20% v/v ethanol is used as a storage solution for chromatographic resins, but the solution has no sporicidal effect, while 0.1 to 1.0 M NaOH is widely used to kill microorganisms. Peracetic acid has both bacterial and sporicidal effects. Viable cells can be identified by spread out of the cell suspension or sample solution on agar plates.

MYCOPLASMA

Mycoplasmas have for long been recognized as a contaminant of continuous cell cultures caused by an infection of the cell line or bioreactor. Working in closed systems under GMP will reduce the risk of infection. The end of production test includes screening for mycoplasmas. Mycoplasmas are extremely sensitive to osmotic shock and pH extremes and should not constitute a problem in downstream processing provided sanitization and CIP procedures are carried out according to GMP. Mycoplasmas are resistant to most antibiotics. Frequent testing (at every passage) is recommended. The cell culture is discarded upon infection. Cleaning with 0.1 to 1 M NaOH will inactivate mycoplasmas. Mycoplasmas are difficult to detect, the only reliable way of demonstrating infection is by agar plating, fluorescent dying of DNA, or by PCR. Recently, a selective biochemical test that exploits the activity of certain mycoplasma enzymes has been made commercially available.

RAW MATERIALS

Raw materials are themselves considered impurities, which should be removed from the final product. Raw materials include cell culture substrates, enzymes, reagents, amino acids, peptides, proteins, chromatographic media, inhibitors, and antibiotics. Raw materials should not be of animal origin due to the potential virus and prion infection risk. Raw materials are intentionally introduced in the process. The basic quality concepts include assurance of the identity, purity, suitability, and traceability of all the raw materials used in the manufacturing process. The quality of the raw materials used should meet standards appropriate for their intended use. Quality requirements for raw materials are met somewhat differently in production of clinical batches (process evolution) and manufacturing of licensed product. Special attention should be paid to raw materials of animal or human origin. They should, as a general rule, be avoided. Chromatographic media must be supplied with a regulatory support file. Specific analytical assays may be required in order to detect residual amounts of critical raw materials in the final product. Critical reagents such as toxic compounds, enzymes, detergents, and stabilizers must be accounted for and their removal validated. Large amounts of hydrophobic reagents may affect hydrophobic interaction chromatography. DS or DP should be tested for residual content by specific assays. Detection-specific assays are required. Be aware of ligand leakage from chromatographic media and be prepared for setting up specific assay for their detection (ELISA or total organic carbon).

Des-Amido Forms

Des-amido forms are target protein derivatives in which one or several of the glutaminyl or asparagyl amino acid residues are converted to the corresponding acids (glutamyl and asparagyl). The deamidation reaction is slow at pH 3 to 5, at low temperatures, and at low conductivity. Deamidated forms are removed by HP-IEC and HP-RPC. Des-amido forms are detected by analytical HP-IEC, HP-RPC, native PAGE, IEF, MS, or CE. The content accepted depends on the nature of the drug product and the dose.

Oxidized Forms

Oxidized forms are target protein derivatives in which one or several Met, Cys, His, Trp, or Tyr residues have been oxidized. The oxidation of cystinyl residues results in formation of a disulfide bond (cystinyl residue). The oxidation reaction is slow at low pH and low temperature. Formation of disulfide bonds will take place above 0 mV. Oxidized forms are removed by HP-IEC and HP-RPC. Disulfide aggregates can be removed by size exclusion chromatography (SEC). Oxidized forms are detected by analytical HP-IEC, HP-RPC, native PAGE, IEF, MS, or CE. The content accepted depends on the nature of the drug product and the dose.

Carbamylated Forms

Carbamylated forms are target protein derivatives in which one or several primary amino, sulfhydryl, carboxyl, phenolic hydroxyl, imidazole, and phosphate groups react with cyanate to form a derivative. The blocking may change the pI of the protein. Cyanate is formed spontaneously in urea solutions, which is the primary source. The formation is slow at low temperatures, but it is nevertheless strongly recommended to purify the urea solution by means of mixed ion exchangers before use. Carbamylated forms are removed by HP-IEC and HP-RPC and detected by analytical HP-IEC, HP-RPC, native PAGE, IEF, MS, or CE. The content accepted depends on the nature of the drug product and the dose.

Aggregates

Aggregates are target protein derivatives in which two or more molecules are linked together either by covalent interdisulfide bonds or by hydrophobic interaction. Target protein aggregates are formed as a result of hydrophobic intermolecular reactions or because of intermolecular disulfide bond formation under oxidizing conditions. Aggregates are very often antigenic, resulting in formation of target protein antibodies. Proteins exposed to even mildly denaturing conditions may partially unfold, resulting in exposure of hydrophobic residues to the aqueous-solvent favoring aggregation. The aggregation process is assumed to be controlled by the initial dimerization step in a second-order reaction. Consequently, high protein concentrations will increase the aggregation rate. Intermolecular disulfide bond formation between cystinyl residues takes place at alkaline pH under oxidizing conditions. Proteins with reactive free thiol groups should be purified under reducing conditions (typically 1 to 10 mM reducing agent) in the presence of EDTA. Even proteins with disulfide bonds may participate in intermolecular disulfide bond reactions due to disulfide bond shuffling at neutral and alkaline pH. The aggregation reaction based on intermolecular disulfide bond formation is prevented at pH < 6 and under reducing conditions. The hydrophobic aggregation reaction strongly depends on the hydrophobicity of the molecule. Preventive actions are to keep the protein in its native conformation during processing in order to avoid unfolding and exposure of hydrophobic sites. Hydrophobic proteins (e.g., certain membrane proteins) may be kept soluble by addition of specific cosolvents (e.g., detergents). Aggregates may be removed by filtration or SEC. Disulfide-based aggregates can be detected by nonreducing (no boiling of sample) 1D-SDS, HP-SEC, MS, or CE. Hydrophobic aggregates may be detected by HP-SEC. The content accepted depends on the nature of the drug product and the dose.

Scrambled Forms

Scrambled forms are target protein molecules with a disulfide bond pattern different from that of the native molecule. Scrambled forms are typically formed during *in vitro* folding of proteins, but disulfide bond shuffling at neutral pH or above also occurs. This requires studies on control of protein stability during downstream processing. The formation of scrambled forms is closely linked to the folding procedure. The best preventive action is to optimize the procedure. As the folding reaction is protein specific, no general rules can be given. Scrambled forms are removed by HP-IEC and HP-RPC and detected by analytical HP-IEC, HP-RPC, CE, or peptide mapping. The content accepted depends on the nature of the drug product and the dose.

Cleaved Forms

Cleaved forms are typically used for target protein derivatives with almost identical molecular weight (± a few hundred Daltons), where a peptide bond is cleaved, resulting in loss of a N- or C-terminal site or where an internal peptide bond is cleaved, while at the same time the resulting fragments are kept together by means of disulfide bonds. Gentle handling of cells, low temperatures, and working in pH intervals where enzymatic activity is low reduces proteolysis. The use of enzyme inhibitors is not recommended for safety reasons. Removal of proteolytic enzymes during capture prevents formation of cleaved forms as well. Cleaved forms are removed by HP-IEC and HP-RPC and detected by analytical HP-IEC, HP-RPC, native PAGE, IEF, MS, peptide mapping, or CE.

Glycosylated Forms

Glycosylated forms appear in the yeast, insect cell, mammalian cell, transgenic animal, and plant expression systems. The glycosylation pattern is a consequence of the molecular biology and the fermentation conditions. Unwanted glycoforms are removed by HP-IEC or HP-RPC methods. Glycosylated forms are detected by analytical HP-IEC, HP-RPC, native PAGE, IEF, MS, peptide mapping, or CE.

Quantity

The quantity of target protein is determined as the total peptide/protein content in a given sample, excluding any inactive derivatives such as des-amido forms, oxidized forms, or polymeric forms. High performance chromatographic methods are used to quantitate both the target protein as well as its derivatives using UV-detection and determination of peak areas. If the extinction coefficient is not known (e.g., analogues), amino acid or Kjeldahl analysis is used as a primary reference method. Bioassays are often replaced with quantity determination partly because of the usual high costs associated with biological assays and partly because of the much higher accuracy of quantitative assays. The subject is of great interest to regulatory authorities as the principal goal of biogeneric manufacturers is to reduce the cost of product, and much work has been done to create surrogate tests for target proteins. The commonly used quantity methods are amino acid analysis, Kjeldahl analysis, ultraviolet spectrometry, and high-performance chromatographic procedures.

Amino Acid Analysis

Amino acid analysis (AAA) involves hydrolysis of peptides and proteins into free amino acids followed by derivatization and separation (or vice-versa) of the amino acid derivatives. The method is in principle independent of protein shape, charge, hydrophobicity, or molecular weight because the peptide/protein is fully degraded. Protein hydrolysis is commonly accomplished by acid hydrolysis of the peptide bonds under vacuum and heat, typically at 110 to 165°C for 1 to 24 hours. Only 16 of the common 20 amino acids are usually measured by this technique, as Cys, Trp, Ser, and Tyr are degraded during acid hydrolysis. Eight amino acid residues are well recovered (Asp, Glu, Asn, Gln, Ala, Leu, Lys, and Gly) and they are commonly used for protein quantitation. The sample must be highly purified; an ideal sample would contain from 1 to 10 nmol protein in a volume of 10 to 100 Pl water or very low concentration of defined buffer. If interfering compounds are present, dialysis of the sample prior to analysis is recommended. In the precolumn method, the hydrolysis is followed by derivatization of the free amino acids with reagents such as phenylisothiocyanate (PITC), o-phthalaldehyde (OPA), or Fmoc-chloride before the chromatographic separation (e.g., HP-RPC-C18). In the postcolumn method, the hydrolysis is followed by chromatographic separation (HP-IEC) of the free amino acids, which are then mixed with ninhydrin at approximately 135°C. The reaction forms a blue derivative detectable at 570 nm. The preferred postcolumn method is the more precise of the two, but is less sensitive (picomolar quantities). It is strongly recommended to establish an internal standard such as norvaline or norleucine in order to minimize the variability of the assay and to provide an additional parameter in the event of method problems. Hydrolysis and analysis of a protein standard (e.g., bovine serum albumin available from the National institutes of Standards and Technology: http://www.nist.gov) should be compared to predefined suitability requirements and acceptance criteria. Theoretically, the yield of just one well-recovered amino acid in a protein sample can be used for quantitation. However, using an average of several stable residues is preferred to ensure accurate and precise measurements. The amount of protein can be correlated to the absorbance at maximum wavelength (typically 280 nm) with the purpose of determination of the extension coefficient and protein concentrations in solution. A comparative study between amino acid analysis, Kjeldahl analysis, and UV determination of protein content in good correlation was found for proteins in the range 6 to 22 kDa. For larger proteins such as immunoglobulins (150 kDa) amino acid analysis may underestimate the total protein concentration (evaluation of amino acid analysis as reference method to quantitative highly purified proteins). The AAA technology also provides support to primary structure studies (amino acid composition), identification of odd or modified residues, and identification of proteins by way of computer database searches. This method should be the primary method for measuring the protein content. The range of sensitivity is about 1 pmol of each amino acid.

Amino Acid Sequencing

Amino acid sequencing is divided into N-terminal and C-terminal sequencing. Amino terminal (N-terminal) sequence analysis is based on the modification of the unmodified N-terminal amino group of the peptide/protein with phenylisothiocyanate (PITC) followed by acid cleavage of the peptide bond releasing the phenylthiohydantoin (PTH) derivative of the amino acid. A new amino group of the next amino acid is now available to react with PITC and the protein sequencing will thus take place in a cyclic manner (Edman degradation). The resulting PTH-amino acid derivative is thereafter analyzed on a PTH amino acid analyzer based on HP-RPC separation technology. The cyclic reaction is not 100% effective and in practice from 20 to 40 amino acid residues can be sequenced by the method described in the low picomol range. Entire sequences may be obtained by cleavage of the protein with specific proteases such as trypsin, V8 protease, or chymotrypsin followed by HP-RPC separation, MALDI mass spectroscopy (MALDI-MS), and Edman sequencing of the peptides separated. Carboxy-terminal (C-terminal) sequence analysis is used for confirmation of the C-terminal part of the peptide or protein. Typically, the peptide/protein is digested with enzymes such as carboxypeptidase A, P, or Y, which are exopeptidases removing one amino acid residue at a time from the C-terminus of the peptide/protein. The enzymes have different specificity and mixtures may be used. After digestion, the released amino acids are removed from the residual peptide/protein and analyzed by amino acid analysis. The reaction is followed over time allowing for determination of relative amounts released. Recently an automated procedure has been introduced consisting of two principal reaction events. First, the D-carboxylic acid group of the C-terminal amino acid residue is activated with trifluoroacetic acid (TFA) and coupled with diphenyl phosphoroisothiocyanatidate (DPP-ITC) in the presence of pyridine. The resulting peptide/protein thiohydantoin is then cleaved with potassium trimethylsilanolate to release the thiohydantoin amino acid from the now shortened peptide/protein. The thiohydantoin derivative is identified by RP-HPC analysis at 269 nm. The method is currently able to provide three to five cycles of sequence information. The range of sensitivity is from 10 to 20 pmol of protein.

BICINCHONINIC ASSAY

The bicinchoninic assay is a modification of the biuret assay. Bicinchoninic acid (BCA) sodium salt is a stable water-soluble compound capable of forming an intense purple complex with cuprous (Cu) ions under alkaline conditions. The maximum absorbance is at 562 nm. The end product is stable for hours and the assay is not affected by detergents and denaturing agents such as urea. This, combined with the simplicity of the assay (only one reagent), makes the BCA assay very attractive compared with the Lowry and biuret assays. Compounds interfering with the assay are: EDTA, sucrose (> 10 mM), glucose (> 10 mM), glycine (1 M), ammonium sulfate (> 5%), sodium acetate (2 M), sodium phosphate (> 1 M), and reducing mercapto reagents. Samples containing lipids show high absorbencies. The sensitivity range is from 0.2 to 1 mg/mL. The sample may be treated with trichloroacetic acid (TCA) or deoxycholate-trichloroacetic acid in order to precipitate the protein before analysis, as most proteins are almost quantitatively precipitated even from dilute solutions. The TCA precipitate should be dissolved in base or appropriate buffer prior to analysis. Samples may also be dialyzed against a suited buffer in order to remove substances interfering with the assay. Desalting is also recommended, but a loss of protein in the range from 10 to 15% should be expected. The BCA assay is typically used during development for in-process control.

BIURET ASSAY

The biuret assay is based on polypeptide chelation of cupric ion in strong alkaline solution. The reaction of the peptide bond with copper sulfate reduces copper, resulting in a color shift (deep purple) to 540 nm. Although the assay is less susceptible to chemical interference than other copper-based assays, Tris, glycerol, glucose, ammonium sulfate, sulfhydryl compounds, and sodium phosphate containing buffers may interfere with the assay. Samples should contain from 1 to 10 mg/mL of protein. The sample is diluted about fivefold upon addition of reagent to give a concentration of 0.2 to 2 mg/mL final assay volume.

The biuret assay is relatively independent on the protein standard of choice, as the reaction chemistry is based on polypeptide structure and not on the composition of the amino acid residue side chains. The sensitivity range is from 0.5 to 10 mg/mL, making the assay the least sensitive among the colorimetric assays. The sample may be treated with TCA or deoxycholate-trichloro-acetic acid in order to precipitate the protein before analysis, as most proteins are almost quantitatively precipitated even from dilute solutions. The TCA precipitate should be dissolved in base or appropriate buffer prior to analysis. Samples may also be dialyzed against a suited buffer in order to remove substances interfering with the assay. Desalting is also recommended, but a loss of protein in the range from 10 to 15% should be expected.

Bradford Assay

The semiquantitative assay is based on the dye Coomassie brilliant blue G-250, which undergoes a shift from 465 nm to 595 nm when binding to peptide bonds under acidic conditions. The binding of the dye to protein is a very rapid process (approximately 2 min) and the protein-dye complex remains dispersed in solution for up to an hour. Some variability in response between different proteins should be expected. The protein is irreversibly denatured by the reaction. The assay is relatively insensitive to most commonly used buffer components. However, detergents such as SDS and Triton X-100 interfere with the assay, although small amounts of detergent may be eliminated by the use of proper control. By comparison of four different methods (Kjeldahl, biuret, Lowry, and Bradford) an underestimated protein content by a factor of two was observed relative to the other assays. The reliability of the Coomassie dye binding assay should therefore be verified case-by-case. The sensitivity is about 25 Pg/mL. The sample may be treated with TCA or deoxycholate-trichloroacetic acid in order to precipitate the protein before analysis, as most proteins are almost quantitatively precipitated even from dilute solutions. The TCA precipitate should be dissolved in base or appropriate buffer prior to analysis. Samples may also be dialyzed against a suited buffer in order to remove substances interfering with the assay. Desalting is also recommended, but a loss of protein in the range from 10 to 15% should be expected.

Capillary Electrophoresis

The basic principle of capillary electrophoresis (CE) is to apply high voltage to a fused silica capillary filled with an appropriate electrolyte and with both ends dipped in the same solution. The separation occurs due to the combination of electrophoretic migration and electro-osmotic flow. The fused silica capillary column may be derivatized or filled with different types of material (polyacrylamide, agarose) or filled with ampholyte solutions allowing for separation according to iso-electric points. CE can be viewed as a combination of traditional electrophoresis and HP-RPC, offering rapid, precise, and highly efficient analysis of complex mixtures (amino acids, peptides, DNA). Protein analysis is difficult to carry out. Proteins bind to uncoated columns and each protein tends to have its own set of optimal separation parameters (pI, stability, solubility, hydrophobicity) not easily transferred to other proteins. However, the before mentioned separation techniques, based on charge alone (IEF-CE), molecular weight (CE in the presence of SDS), or by means of derivatized columns, have made CE a reliable technique for characterization of recombinant proteins as demonstrated in the separation of human growth hormone and insulin molecular forms. CE offers several separation modes. Capillary zone electrophoresis (CZE) is based on the differences in the electrophoretic mobility of sample ions that migrate with a linear velocity proportional to their charge-mass ratio. SDS is often used to form a protein-SDS complex allowing for separation according to molecular radius. Micellar electrokinetic capillary electrophoresis (MECC) is based on a separation of molecules (according to hydrophobicity) between an aqueous phase and a micellar pseudo-stationary phase comprising a surfactant in an amount above its critical micellar concentration. Capillary isoelectric focusing (CIEF) is based on separation according to isoelectric focusing using a background electrolyte to establish the pH gradient. Charged molecules will migrate to their isoelectric point. Capillary isotachophoresis (CITP) is based on sample separation at constant velocity.

The sample is applied between two solutions of different ionic mobilities with an electrolyte that is more mobile than any sample ion and a terminating electrolyte that is least mobile. The peak capacity is in the range of 18 peaks per minute (compared to HP-RPC of 3 peaks per minute). Unlike conventional electrophoresis, the method is highly efficient with small sample requirements. The CE methods are quantitative. Small sample sizes are required (from 1 to 10 Pl).

HIGH PERFORMANCE ION EXCHANGE CHROMATOGRAPHY

Analytical high performance liquid chromatography offers a high level of resolution and precision, making the technology available for identity, purity and quantity determinations. High performance ion exchange chromatography (HP-IEC) is based on highly specific analytical columns comprising monodispersed particles with a diameter of 5 to 10 Pm, separating proteins according to their electrical charge. The resolution may be comparable to that of high performance reversed phase chromatography (HP-RPC) and the technology will apply to almost all types of globular proteins. The HP-IEC is used for detection of target protein-related compounds (e.g., des-amido forms, oxidized forms, scrambled forms, cleaved forms), which may be present in amounts from 1 ppt and upward. The resulting UV-diagram provides an impurity profile within the relatively narrow window offered by the technology, but it should be kept in mind that not all impurities are detected by this or similar methods. Impurities present in 0.1% or higher should be fully characterized no later than Phase III of manufacture. HP-IEC offers two separation modes: CEC and anion exchange chromatography (AEC). In CEC positively charged biomolecules typically are retained due to interaction with negatively charged groups (e.g., sulfonic acid) on the surface of the chromatographic resin. The buffer pH must favor a net charge of the biomolecule lower than pI in order to maintain separation. CEC primarily retains biomolecules by the interaction with histidine, lysine, and arginine (pKa about 6.5, 10, and 12 respectively). In AEC negatively charged biomolecules typically are retained due to interaction with positively charged groups (e.g., quaternary amine) on the surface of the chromatographic resin. The buffer pH must favor a net charge of the biomolecule higher than pI in order to maintain separation. AEC primarily retains biomolecules by the interaction with aspartic or glutamic acid side chains (pKa about 4.4). The separation is affected by temperature (due to structural changes of the protein molecule), presence of displacer ions such as Na and Cl, presence of denaturing agents, presence of organic solvents, and hydrophobic interactions with the resin. HP-IEC is used for in-process control analysis of target protein identity (retention time), quantity (peak area), and purity (215nm or 280 nm profile). The method is also used for drug substance/product impurity profiles and determination of quantity.

HIGH PERFORMANCE REVERSED PHASE CHROMATOGRAPHY

Analytical high performance liquid chromatography offers a high level of resolution and precision, making the technology available for identity, purity, and quantity determinations. HP-RPC is based on highly specific analytical columns comprising monodispersed particles with a diameter of 5 to 10 Pm, separating proteins according to their hydrophobicity. The high resolution methodology is restricted to analysis of hydrophilic or semihydrophobic proteins of a molecular weight of 3000 to 100,000. Retention of molecules of interest can be controlled by manipulating the properties of the mobile phase, and separation of molecules with only small differences in hydrophobicity can be performed. The HP-RPC is used for detection of target protein-related compounds (e.g., des-amido forms, oxidized forms, scrambled forms, cleaved forms), which may be present in amounts from 1 part per thousand (ppt) and upward. The resulting UV diagram is said to provide an impurity profile within the relatively narrow window offered by the technology, but it should be kept in mind that not all impurities are detected by this or similar methods. Impurities present in 0.1% or higher should be fully characterized no later than Phase III of manufacture. HP-RPC is used for in-process control analysis of target protein identity (retention time), quantity (peak area), and purity (215 nm or 280 nm profile). The method is also used for drug substance/product impurity profiles and determination of quantity.

HIGH PERFORMANCE SIZE EXCLUSION CHROMATOGRAPHY

High performance size exclusion chromatography (HP-SEC) is based on highly specific analytical columns comprising uniform particles of a given diameter depending on the molecular weight of the target protein. The principal feature of SEC is its gentle noninteraction with the sample, enabling high retention of biological activity, while separating multimers that are not easily distinguished by other chromatographic methods.

The resolution is less than for HP-IEC and HP-RPC techniques. The technology applies for almost all types of globular proteins. HP-SEC can be coupled directly to electrospray ionization (ESI) and mass spectrometry (MS) by means of ammonium formate buffer (typically 50 mM), making direct determination of molecular weights possible.

HP-SEC is used for detection of di- and polymeric target protein content in the drug substance/product. It is a purity analysis.

ISOELECTRIC FOCUSING

Isoelectric focusing (IEF) is one of the electrophoretic methods comprising SDS-PAGE, native electrophoresis, IEF, 2D-electrophoresis, and capillary electrophoresis. One-dimensional SDS-PAGE offers separation of proteins according to their molecular weight. Samples run under denaturing, but nonreducing conditions, will detect the presence of other molecular species and of disulfide intermolecular di- and polymers. Samples run under denaturing and reducing conditions will detect monomeric compounds. Notice that in the latter procedure, it is common practice to boil the sample in the denaturing and reducing buffer before application. The boiling procedure must not be used if information of aggregates is required (denaturing but non-reducing conditions). Native electrophoresis separates proteins according to charge, molecular weight, shape, and other factors (samples are typically applied under conditions maintaining the tertiary structure). IEF separates proteins according to the isoelectric point (samples may be applied under native or denaturing conditions). The method offers very high resolution and is often used to provide information of presence of closely related derivatives (e.g., des-amido forms) or presence of glycosylated derivatives of the target protein. Two-dimensional electrophoresis separates proteins according to the proteins isoelectric point (first dimension) and its molecular weight (second dimension). The method is a combination of IEF and SDS-PAGE. The resulting coordinate (pI, Mw) provides a unique identification of the protein.

Differences in posttranslational modifications (e.g., phosphorylation) will often result in separate spots (slightly different pI and Mw). CE offers similar separation technologies, which can be used as a purity analysis. In IEF the movement of the protein through the gel matrix is modulated by a pH gradient created by soluble ampholytes, which are small organic molecules with various isoelectric points and buffering capacities. The pH-gradient is produced when the soluble ampholyte migrate in the gel matrix until they reach their isoelectric points. Stable pH gradients are difficult to establish outside the range 3.0 to 8.0 and nonequilibrium conditions are required.

Commercial carrier ampholyte mixtures comprise hundreds of individual polymeric species with pIs spanning a specific pH range. When a voltage is applied across a carrier ampholyte mixture, the carrier ampholytes with the lowest pI (and the most negative charge) move toward the anode, and the carrier ampholytes with the highest pI (and the most positive charge) move toward the cathode. The other carrier ampholytes align themselves between the extremes, according to their pIs, and buffer their environment to the corresponding pH. The result is a continuous pH gradient. An attractive alternative to soluble ampholytes is the use of immobilized pH gradient gels (IPG), where buffering side chains are covalently incorporated into the acrylamide matrix. The pH gradient is stabilized by an electric field allowing the proteins to migrate until they reach their isoelectric point, where the protein has no net charge. Because reproducible linear gradients with a slope as low as 0.01 pH units/cm can separate proteins with pI differences of 0.001 pH units, the resolution possible with immobilized pH gradient gels is 10 to 100 times greater than that obtained with carrier ampholyte–based IEF. IEF can be run in either a native or a denaturing mode.

Native IEF is the more convenient option, as precast native IEF gels are available in a variety of pH gradient ranges. This method is also preferred when native protein is required, as when activity staining is to be employed. The use of native IEF, however, is often limited by the fact that many proteins are not soluble at low ionic strength or have low solubility close to their isoelectric point. In these cases, denaturing IEF is employed. Urea is the denaturant of choice, as this uncharged compound can dissolve many proteins not otherwise soluble under IEF conditions. Detergents and reducing agents are often used in conjunction with urea for more-complete unfolding and solubilization. Urea is not stable in aqueous solution, so precast IEF gels are not manufactured with urea. Dried precast gels are a convenient alternative; they have been cast, rinsed, and dried and can be rehydrated with urea, carrier ampholytes, and other additives before use. Samples are typically dialyzed against buffer containing a nonionic detergent (e.g., TX-100), urea, a reducing agent (DTT or 2-ME), and ampholytes before electrophoresis. Multisubunit proteins dissociate and each polypeptide migrates as a single species, according to its mass and charge. Specific isoelectric focusing standards are included in the electrophoretic run. The standards have a range of isoelectric points and will carry a net positive, negative, or zero charge depending on the pH of the system.

The IEF slab gel method is very powerful and even closely related derivatives such as phosphorylated or glycosylated forms are detected. The method is primarily used for identification of glycosylation patterns (protein microheterogeneity) and for determination of product-related impurities (des-amido forms, oxidized forms, scrambled forms, blocked amino groups). However, the method is semiquantitative only, at its best, and one must be very careful about method validation, if the method is used for purity purposes.

The IEF tube gel method is typically used for the first dimension of 2D-electrophoresis run. Coomassie blue and silver staining are the two most common staining methods used for band detection on slab gels. Coomassie staining has a sensitivity of 0.05 to 0.5 pg protein per band. Silver staining is about 10 to 100 times more sensitive, enabling detection of 1 to 5 ng of protein per band. IEF is used as a target protein identity method according to the pI of the molecule. The powerful resolution of closely related derivatives makes the method suited for pattern recognition of, for example, glycosylated forms. One should in general be careful to use electrophoretic methods as purity analyses due to difficulties in quantifying the method.

KJELDAHL ANALYSIS

The Kjeldahl analysis is used for quantitative determination of the nitrogen content in protein samples. In the Kjeldahl analysis, nitrogen is converted to ammonium sulfate by digestion of the protein in a mixture of concentrated sulfuric acid, copper sulfate (to raise the boiling point), and a catalyst (typically copper II, Mercury II, or selenium salts) under high temperature. Sample nitrogen is converted to ammonium sulfate by this procedure. Ammonia is released by a change in pH to alkaline conditions (addition of NaOH), and steam distillation is followed by a titration to determine the quantity of ammonia released. To account for potential environmental contaminants, a reagent blank without protein is run. An ammonium sulfate reference can be used as a standard to ensure assay accuracy.

An alternate method is the Nessler assay in which hydrogen peroxide is used to accelerate the oxidation of nitrogen to ammonium sulfate. After digestion, the Nessler reagent (mercury and potassium chloride in sodium hydroxide) is added to produce a colored complex. Both methods exploit the observation that nearly all proteins contain approximately 16.5% nitrogen by weight. Multiplication of the weight of nitrogen determined by a factor of 6 should provide a valid benchmark measure of the weight of protein. The methods are not as sensitive as the other methods described. However, the accuracy is high, and the indirect determination of the nitrogen content may be one of the most reliable methods for determination of total protein in crude samples. This type of assay does not demonstrate the protein-to-protein variation of colorimetric methods. Note that mg amounts are required for analysis. Also, make sure that the sample does not contain nonprotein nitrogen-based compounds such as tris and amino acids; precision can be decreased due to loss of ammonia by leakage or adsorption.

The Kjeldahl analysis quantitatively determines the total amount of protein present in a sample. The method is typically used for total protein determination in crude samples.

LIMULUS AMEBOCYTE LYSATE ASSAY

The Limulus amebocyte lysate (LAL) test is used to detect endotoxins. Pyrogens are a group of chemically diverse substances that cause fever and shock in severe cases. The most important pyrogenic substances in pharmaceutical industry are bacterial endotoxins. There are two methods of detection: the pyrogen test, which is based upon the measurement of body temperature of rabbits before and after injection of the specimen, and the LAL test, which is based upon the clotting reaction of an enzyme complex of cells of the horseshoe crab together with bacterial endotoxins (*in vitro* test).

Although the LAL test is widely used, a total replacement of the Pyrogen test still is not possible since on the one hand the LAL test will only detect bacterial endotoxins and on the other hand not all specimens can be tested with the LAL test because of interference with the test. LAL is the aqueous extract obtained after the lysis of the blood cells from the horseshoe crab, *Limulus polyphemus*. This extract contains blood proteins, causing clotting of the crab's blood when exposed to lipopolysaccharides (LPS) from gram-negative bacteria (e.g., *E. coli*). Presence of LPS located within the cell wall, also named endotoxins, is an indicator of bacterial contamination in water, buffers, chromatographic columns, and raw materials. There are currently three LAL methods in use: the gel clot test, the turbidimetric test, and the chromogenic test method. All methods allow for reading after a fixed time interval (end-point tests). The turbidimetric and the chromogenic test methods can also be read continuously (kinetic tests).

The gel clot test is the simplest and most widely used form. A mixture of test sample and LAL reagent is mixed in a test tube and incubated for a given time interval (typically 1 h at 37°C) and then read for presence or absence of a firm gel clot. The turbidimetric test is a spectrophotometric method based on the optical density (at 340 or 405 nm). End point tests do not require very many data points, while kinetic assays will require a computer for data handling. Optical density values must be collected without disturbing the integrity of the coagulation matrix formed. It is therefore advisable to use optical readers where the samples are fixed. The chromogenic test is a spectrophotometric method based on measurement of the optical density of the leaving group (e.g., para-nitroaniline).

For most chromogenic assays, turbidity develops along with the increase in color intensity. It is advisable to fix the samples in the optical reader in order not to disturb the coagulin matrix formed. The kinetic assays make use of the time period after mixing sample and LAL reagent in which the optical density increases. The differences in the rate of increase in optical density are a function of the endotoxin concentration: the rates of increase in optical density increase with increasing concentration of endotoxin. The endotoxin concentration is calculated from a standard curve constructed by linear regression of the log of the onset time, on the log of the endotoxin concentration. The absolute coefficient of correlation recommended by FDA is 0.980.

One of the most important aspects of LAL test is that the test is in accordance with the latest demand of the European Pharmacopoeia Commission for the replacement of the animal-based tests in favor of alternative methods where possible. The USP endotoxin reference standard has a defined potency of 10,000 EU per vial. It must be demonstrated that the sample does not inhibit or enhance the LAL reaction. It is used as an in-process control procedure, typically during development, and as a purity test of the drug substance/product.

LOWRY ASSAY

The Lowry assay is a colorimetric method based on cupric ions and the Folin-Ciocalteau reagent for phenolic groups. The phosphomolybdate-phosphotungstate salts are reduced to produce a maximum absorbance at 750 nm. Little variation between different proteins is observed by this method, making it very useful for protein mixtures. The color reaction is light sensitive and can vary from protein to protein. The protein is irreversibly denatured. Numerous buffer components can interfere with the Lowry assay including potassium ions, magnesium ions, EDTA, GuCl, Triton X-100, SDS, Brij 35, tris (> 0.1 M), ammonium sulfate, sodium acetate (> 1 M), sodium phosphate (> 1 M), thiol reagents, and carbohydrates. The two-step nature of the Lowry assay, the instability of the reagent in alkaline solutions, and the different compounds interfering make it a complex and cumbersome assay to use. The Hartree version of the Lowry assay makes use of three reagents instead of five. The method is less laborious than the original method, and it maintains the sensitivity of the original. The sensitivity range is from 0.01 to 1 mg/mL. The sample is treated with trichloroacetic acid (TCA) or deoxycholate-trichloroacetic acid in order to precipitate the protein before analysis, as most proteins are almost quantitatively precipitated even from dilute solutions. The TCA precipitate should be dissolved in base or appropriate buffer prior to analysis. Samples may also be dialyzed against a suited buffer in order to remove substances interfering with the assay. Desalting is also recommended, but a loss of protein in the range from 10 to 15% should be expected. Note that most of the interfering substances can be removed by precipitating the protein with deoxycholate-trichloroacetic acid prior to running the assay; color development reaches a maximum in 20 to 30 min; lipids can be removed by chloroform extraction; the reaction is pH dependent, and it is important to keep pH in the range from 10 to 10.5. The Lowry assay is typically used during development for in-process control of total protein, preferentially in crude samples.

NATIVE ELECTROPHORESIS

Native electrophoresis is one of the electrophoretic methods comprising SDS-PAGE, native electrophoresis, IEF, 2D-electrophoresis, and capillary electrophoresis. One-dimensional SDS-PAGE offers separation of proteins according to their molecular weight. Samples run under denaturing, but nonreducing, conditions will provide information of presence of other molecular species and of disulfide intermolecular di- and polymers. Samples run under denaturing and reducing conditions will provide information on monomeric compounds. Notice that in the latter procedure, it is common practice to boil the sample in the denaturing and reducing buffer before application. The boiling procedure must not be used if information of aggregates is required (denaturing but nonreducing conditions).

SDS-PAGE

SDS-PAGE is one of the electrophoretic methods comprising SDS-PAGE, native electrophoresis, IEF, 2D-electrophoresis, and capillary electrophoresis. One-dimensional SDS-PAGE offers separation of proteins according to their molecular weight. Samples run under denaturing, but nonreducing, conditions will provide information of presence of other molecular species and of disulfide intermolecular di- and polymers. Samples run under denaturing and reducing conditions will provide information on monomeric compounds. Notice that in the latter procedure, it is common practice to boil the sample in the denaturing and reducing buffer before application. The boiling procedure must not be used if information of aggregates is required (denaturing but nonreducing conditions).

SDS is an anionic detergent that denatures proteins by wrapping the hydrophobic tail around the polypeptide backbone. For almost all proteins, SDS binds at a ratio of approximately 1.4 g SDS of protein, thus conferring a net negative charge to the polypeptide in proportion to its length. The SDS also disrupts hydrogen bonds, blocks hydrophobic interactions, and substantially unfolds the protein molecules, minimizing differences in molecular form by eliminating the tertiary and secondary structures. DTT is a reducing agent, and 50 to 100 mM of DTT will cleave protein disulfide bonds, and in the presence of SDS the protein will unfold. Standard proteins of known molecular weight are included in the electrophoretic run. Coomassie blue and silver staining are the two most common staining methods used for band detection on slab gels. Coomassie staining has a sensitivity of 0.05 to 0.5 pg protein per band. Silver staining is about 10 to 100 times more sensitive, enabling detection of 1 to 5 ng of protein per band. SDS-PAGE is used as a target protein identity method (separation according to molecular weight). The method may also be used under nonreducing conditions to evaluate the pattern of di- and polymeric target protein impurities. One should in general be careful to use electrophoretic methods as purity analyses due to difficulties in quantifying the method.

Native electrophoresis separates proteins according to charge, molecular weight, shape, and other factors (samples are typically applied under conditions maintaining the tertiary structure). IEF separates proteins according to the isoelectric point (samples may be applied under native or denaturing conditions). The method offers very high resolution and is often used to provide information of presence of closely related derivatives (e.g., des-amido forms) or presence of glycosylated derivatives of the target protein. Two-dimensional electrophoresis separates proteins according to the protein's isoelectric point (first dimension) and its molecular weight (second dimension). The method is a combination of IEF and SDS-PAGE. The resulting coordinate (pI, Mw) provides a unique identification of the protein. Differences in posttranslational modifications (e.g., phosphorylation) will often result in separate spots (slightly different pI and Mw).

CE offers similar separation technologies. The CE methods can be used as a purity analysis. SDS-PAGE under denaturing (and reducing) conditions separates proteins according to the molecular size as they move through the gel toward the anode (positively charged electrode). The system comprises a large pore stacking gel (in which the sample is loaded) and a running gel (in which the proteins are separated). Because of the high resolution obtainable with discontinuous buffer systems, the SDS discontinuous system is usually used. In the discontinuous system, protein mobility, a quantitative measure of the migration rate of a charged species in an electric field, is intermediate between the mobility of the buffer ion of the same charge (usually negative) in the stacking gel (leading ion) and the mobility of the buffer ion in the upper tank (trailing ion). When electrophoresis is started, the ions and the proteins begin migrating into the stacking gel. The proteins concentrate in a very thin zone, called the stack, between the leading ion and the trailing ion. The proteins continue to migrate in the stack until they reach the separating gel. At that point, due to a pH or an ion change, the proteins become the trailing ion and "unstuck" as they separate on the gel. Although a continuous system is slightly easier to set up than a discontinuous system and tends to have fewer sample precipitation and aggregation problems, much greater resolution can be obtained with a discontinuous system. Only minimal concentration of the sample takes place with continuous gels, and proteins form zones nearly as broad as the height of the original samples in the sample wells, resulting in much lower resolution. Other buffer systems can be used, for example the Tris™-tricine system for resolution of polypeptides in the size range below Mr 10,000. The sample may be treated in different ways according to the type of information the electrophoresis should reveal in the presence of SDS and no boiling (separation according to size — disulfide bonds are intact and aggregates with intermolecular disulfide bonds will separate from the monomer) or in the presence of SDS and a reducing agent (50 to 100 mM DTT) and boiling (only monomers will appear).

2D-Electrophoresis

Two-dimensional electrophoresis is one of the electrophoretic methods comprising SDS-PAGE, native electrophoresis, IEF, and capillary electrophoresis. One-dimensional SDS-PAGE offers separation of proteins according to their molecular weight. Samples run under denaturing, but nonreducing conditions, will provide information on the presence of other molecular species and of disulfide intermolecular di- and polymers. Samples run under denaturing and reducing conditions will provide information on monomeric compounds. Notice that in the latter procedure, it is common practice to boil the sample in the denaturing and reducing buffer before application. The boiling procedure must not be used if information of aggregates is required (denaturing but nonreducing conditions).

Native electrophoresis separates proteins according to charge, molecular weight, shape, and other factors (samples are typically applied under conditions maintaining the tertiary structure). IEF separates proteins according to the isoelectric point (samples may be applied under native or denaturing conditions). The method offers very high resolution and is often used to provide information of presence of closely related derivatives (e.g., des-amido forms) or presence of glycosylated derivatives of the target protein. Two-dimensional electrophoresis separates proteins according to the proteins isoelectric point (first dimension) and its molecular weight (second dimension). The method is a combination of IEF and SDS-PAGE. The resulting coordinate (pI,Mw) provides a unique identification of the protein. Differences in posttranslational modifications (e.g., phosphorylation) will often result in separate spots (slightly different pI and Mw). CE offers similar separation technologies.

The CE methods can be used as a purity analysis. Two-dimensional electrophoresis is a combination of isoelectric focusing (first dimension) and SDS-electrophoresis (second dimension), revealing information about a protein's charge and molecular coordinates (pI,Mw). It is very unlikely that two different proteins will have identical pI and Mw, making 2D-electrophoresis a very powerful protein identification technique. Further, 2D-electrophoresis offers unique separation and identification even of complex protein mixtures, making comparability analyses possible. From 1000 to 2000 well-resolved spots can be expected, when sensitive detection methods are used. There are, however, some restrictions to the methods usability, as proteins normally are reduced and denatured prior to IEF electrophoresis in the first dimension. One should therefore be careful to interpret the results obtained correctly, as pI and Mw may not be that of the native protein. Further, even when extreme care is taken in producing first and second dimension gels, some gel-related variability among gel casts occurs. The comments related to IEF and SDS electrophoresis will apply for 2D-electrophoresis as well. The method will apply for determination of target molecule pI and Mw, purity analysis with respect to target molecule derivatives, identity of post-translational forms, and as a method for determination of host cell protein patterns supporting immunoassay methods. However, the method is semiquantitative only, at its best, and one must be very careful about method validation. A specific feature of the method is diagonal gel electrophoresis for investigation of subunit composition of multisubunit proteins containing interchain disulfide bonds. Very basic proteins must be analyzed by nonequilibrium pH gradient electrophoresis, one-dimension method. Instead of applying the sample to the basic end of the gel, it is applied to the acidic end. In order to prevent the proteins from running to the end of the gel, short run times are used before an equilibrium state is reached.

Coomassie blue and silver staining are the two most common staining methods used for band detection on slab gels. Coomassie staining has a sensitivity of 0.05 to 0.5 pg protein per band. Silver staining is about 10 to 100 times more sensitive, enabling detection of 1 to 5 ng of protein per band. Two-dimensional electrophoresis is used as a target protein identity method (separation according to molecular weight and pI). One should in general be careful to use electrophoretic methods as purity analyses due to difficulties in quantifying the method.

UV Absorbance

The method is based on the absorbance of tyrosine, tryptophan, and phenylalanine residues at 275 to 280 nm (ultraviolet region). Phenylalanine is only weakly absorbing and is usually neglected for most purposes. The protein structure is not affected by the method, making on-line measurement a possibility. Pigments, organic cofactors, and phenolic compounds interfere with the assay. The protein concentration measurement is based on Beer's law: $280 = E \times C \times L = H \times C \times L/Mw$; where OD is the optical density at 280 nm, E is the absorptivity (nm × ml)/(mg × cm); C is the protein concentration in mg/ml; L is the light pathway (cm); H is the molar extinction coefficient;

Mw is the molecular weight (g/mol). The curve is normally linear between an OD of 0.05 and 0.8. It is common practice to use an extinction coefficient of 1 for protein mixtures, accepting the great variability in the extinction 1% coefficient between different proteins. Weight absorbance coefficients, *E* (gram dry protein per 100 ml) range between 3 and 30 optical density at 280 nm units for most proteins. The sensitivity range is from 0.05 to 1.0 mg/mL. Note that presence of nucleic acids in the sample will interfere with the absorbance, and the extinction coefficient of a protein is pH dependent. The UV absorbance method is used for determination of total protein in semi- and purified samples. The assay may be used as an on-line in-process control method for determination of total protein in intermediary samples and in the drug substance/product.

11 Regulatory Affairs

The regulatory filing of biological products is made in accordance with the rules established by the regulatory agencies as shown below. These rules are being revised worldwide to accommodate filings of generic biological products, particularly therapeutic proteins. Most of the current chatter about the therapeutic proteins revolves around their regulatory status.

U.S. Food and Drug Administration (FDA): (http://www.fda.gov) On October 1, 2003, FDA transferred certain product oversight responsibilities from the Center for Biologics Evaluation and Research (CBER) to the Center for Drug Evaluation and Research (CDER). This consolidation provides greater opportunities to further develop and coordinate scientific and regulatory activities between CBER and CDER, leading to a more efficient, effective, and consistent review program for human drugs and biological drugs. FDA believes that as more drug and biological products are developed for a broader range of illnesses, such interaction is necessary for both efficient and consistent agency action. Under the new structure, the biologic products transferred to CDER will continue to be regulated as licensed biological drugs. The therapeutic biological products now under CDER's review include:

* Monoclonal antibodies for *in vivo* use;
* Cytokines, growth factors, enzymes, immunomodulators, and thrombolytics;
* Proteins intended for therapeutic use that are extracted from animals or microorganisms, including recombinant versions of these products (except clotting factors);
* Other nonvaccine therapeutic immunotherapies.

The Investigational New Drug (IND) filings and filings of the Biological License Application (BLA) for therapeutic proteins are now received at CDER and not at CBER (http://www.fda.gov/cder/biologics/default.htm). Even though the therapeutic proteins mentioned above have been moved to CDER, the requirement for filing BLA continues. In the past, the approved biological products were not listed in the Orange Book (the FDA's listing of generic equivalent products) as there was no generic equivalent, so the information was not readily available on these products. Now a new listing method at FDA (http://www.accessdata.fda.gov/scripts/cder/drugsatfda/index.cfm) shows a listing of all approved products. The U.S. FDA has not yet developed a mechanism to accept generic applications for biological products. The EMEA has released guidelines for "biosimilar" products (EMEA/CHMP/49348/05, CRMP/437/04), and concept papers (CHMP/146710/2004, CHMP/146701/2004, CHMP/146489/2004, and CHMP/146664/2004).

Sandoz has filed generic biological applications for growth hormone at both EMEA and FDA but at both of these agencies the review process has been held back and the matter is in the courts. To begin the process of developing guidelines for biogeneric products, the FDA had held a public workshop, "Scientific Considerations Related to Developing Follow-On Protein Products," on September 14–15, 2004. It was open for comments until November 12, 2004. The presentation made at this public hearing reveals the many hurdles that the biogeneric manufacturer is likely to face and these can be read at: http://www.fda.gov/cder/meeting/followOn/followOnPresentations.htm.

In 1984, Congress created a mechanism for the approval of generic chemistry-based drugs in the Hatch-Waxman amendments to the federal Food, Drug, and Cosmetics Act. Under Hatch-

Waxman, once a drug reaches the end of its patent life, a competitor can get approval to market the same product using much of the first manufacturer's formulas and testing data. Without making the investment in drug discovery and clinical testing, generic manufacturers can offer their products at a much lower price than the company that did the original research. When a generic competitor enters the pharmaceutical market, prices for an already existing drug typically fall 70%. Biotech analysts say the price differential will be less for biological drugs because of the complexities of manufacturing protein-based drugs. Up until now most biotech companies believed their drugs, spawned by recombinant technology that evolved in the 1970s and 1980s, would remain free of generic competition because no similar pathway existed for abbreviated approvals. In the U.S., most biotech drugs have been approved for market under the Public Health Service Act (PHSA), which was used to regulate vaccines and serums in the early 1900s. When bioengineered products began to come through the approval process, they fell under a different center in the FDA than did chemical-based drugs, which had been governed by the Food, Drug, and Cosmetics Act and later, Hatch-Waxman. In June, those centers merged to streamline administration, but the move provided FDA with an opportunity to examine its policy on generics. The FDA's current review began with insulin and human growth hormone, because those products are easier to characterize than the more complex biotech drugs; also, they had always been regulated under the drug laws and not the PHSA.

Some relevant documents at FDA include:

- Guidance for Industry: Monoclonal Antibodies Used as Reagents in Drug Manufacturing (March 29, 2001);
- Guidance for Industry: Content and Format of Chemistry, Manufacturing and Controls Information and Establishment Description Information for a Biological *In vitro* Diagnostic Product (March 8, 1999)
- Points to Consider in the Manufacture and Testing of Monoclonal Antibody Products for Human Use (February 28, 1997);
- Guidance for Industry for the Submission of Chemistry, Manufacturing, and Controls Information for a Therapeutic Recombinant DNA-Derived Product or a Monoclonal Antibody Product for *In vivo* Use (August 1996)
- 21 CFR 120: *Hazard Analysis and Critical Control Point Systems*
- 21 CFR 210: Current Good Manufacturing Practice (cGMP) in Manufacturing, Processing, Packing, or Holding of Drugs, General
- 21 CFR 211: Current GMP for Finished Pharmaceuticals
- 21 CFR 610: General Biological Products Standards
- 21 CFR 809: *In vitro* Diagnostic Products for Human Use
- Draft Guidance for Industry: Drug Substance — Chemistry, Manufacturing, and Controls Information (January 6, 2004)
- Draft Guidance for Industry: Comparability Protocols — Protein Drug Products and Biological Products: Chemistry, Manufacturing, and Controls Information (September 3, 2003)
- Draft Guidance for Industry: Sterile Drug Products Produced by Aseptic Processing — Current Good Manufacturing Practice (September 3, 2003)
- Draft Guidance for Industry: Comparability Protocols — Chemistry, Manufacturing, and Controls Information (February 20, 2003)
- Draft Guidance for Industry: Drug Product — Chemistry, Manufacturing, and Controls Information (January 28, 2003)
- Draft Guidance for Industry: Preventive Measures to Reduce the Possible Risk of Transmission of Creutzfeldt-Jakob Disease (CJD) and Variant Creutzfeldt-Jakob Disease (vCJD) by Human Cells, Tissues, and Cellular and Tissue-Based Products (HCT/Ps) (June 14, 2002)

- Draft Guidance for Industry: Biological Product Deviation Reporting for Licensed Manufacturers of Biological Products Other than Blood and Blood Components (August 10, 2001)
- Guidance for Industry: Content and Format of Chemistry, Manufacturing and Controls Information and Establishment Description Information for a Biological *In vitro* Diagnostic Product (March 8, 1999)
- Guidance for Industry: Content and Format of Chemistry, Manufacturing and Controls Information and Establishment Description Information for a Vaccine or Related Product (January 5, 1999)
- FDA Guidance Concerning Demonstration of Comparability of Human Biological Products, Including Therapeutic Biotechnology-Derived Products (April 1996)
- FDA Guidance Document Concerning Use of Pilot Manufacturing Facilities for the Development and Manufacturing of Biological Products
- Draft Points to Consider in the Characterization of Cell Lines Used to Produce Biologicals (July 12, 1993)
- Supplement to the Points to Consider in the Production and Testing of New Drugs and Biologics Produced by Recombinant DNA Technology: Nucleic Acid Characterization and Genetic Stability (April 6, 1992)
- Guideline on General Principles of Process Validation (May 1987)
- Points to Consider in the Production and Testing of New Drugs and Biologicals Produced by Recombinant DNA Technology (April 10, 1985).

European Medicines Evaluation Agency (EMEA): (http://www.emea.eu.int/) On October 25, 2004, the EU accepted BioPartner's interferon alpha as the first "biosimilar" filing. If approved, the "biosimilar" could be on the market as early as next year. BioPartner's filing represents the first occasion that the EMEA has accepted an application for a biosimilar drug for review. This development comes shortly after the U.S. government turned down an application to market Omnitrop/Omnitrope (somatropin), a generic version of recombinant human growth hormone developed by Sandoz, citing problems in establishing an appropriate regulatory route for "biogeneric" products. In 2004 the European Parliament approved new pharmaceutical legislation that, among other things, set out a legal framework for the registration of so-called biosimilars, biological therapies that are therapeutically the same as existing, approved biological products. Sandoz had also filed for approval with the European Medicines Evaluation Agency for Omnitrop, but was unable to progress the application. Documents of interest at EMEA include:

- 3AB4A: Production and Quality Control of Monoclonal Antibodies
- 3AB8A: Virus Validation Studies — The Design, Contribution and Interpretation of Studies Validating the Inactivation and Removal of Viruses
- 3AB9A: *Validation of Virus Removal/Inactivation Procedures — Choice of Viruses* Regulation No. 1946/2003 of the European Parliament and of the Council of 15 July 2003 on Transboundary Movements of Genetically Modified Organisms
- 21/04/02 EudraLex Volume 4: Medicinal Products for Human and Veterinary Use — Good Manufacturing Practices
- 2000/608/EC: Commission Decision of 27 September 2000 Concerning the Guidance Notes for Risk Assessment Outlined in Annex III of Directive 90/219/EEC on the Contained Use of Genetically Modified Microorganisms (notified under document number C(2000) 2736)
- Commission Directive 91/356/EEC, of 13 June 1991, Laying Down the Principles and Guidelines of Good Manufacturing Practice for Medicinal Products for Human Use
- Council Directive 90/219/EEC of 23 April 1990 on the Contained Use of Genetically Modified Microorganisms

- 3AB1A: Production and Quality Control of Medicinal Products Derived by Recombinant DNA Technology
- 3AB2A: Quality of Biotechnological Products — Analysis of the Expression Construct in Cells Used for Production of R-DNA Derived Protein Products
- 3AB3A: Production and Quality Control of Cytokine Products Derived by Biotechnological Process
- 3AB6A: Gene Therapy Product Quality Aspects in the Production of Vectors and Genetically Modified Somatic Cells
- 3AB10A: Minimizing the Risk of Transmitting Agents Causing Spongiform Encephalopathy via Medicinal Products
- 3AB14A: Harmonization of Requirements for Influenza Vaccines

Japanese Ministry of Health and Welfare (MHW): (http://www.nihs.go.jp) Japanese health authorities mainly follow the ICH guidelines.

World Health Organization (WHO): (http://www.who.int/biologicals/) WHO provides International Biological Reference Preparations, which serve as reference sources of defined biological activity expressed in an internationally agreed unit. These preparations are the basis of a uniform reporting system, helping physicians and scientists involved in patient care, regulatory authorities, and manufacturing settings to communicate in a common language for designating the activity or potency of biological preparations used in prophylaxis or therapy and ensuring the reliability of *in vitro* biological diagnostic procedures used for diagnosis of diseases and treatment monitoring. The concept of using well-characterized preparations as references against which batches of biological products are assessed remains fundamental to ensuring the quality of biological products as well as the consistency of production and is essential for establishment of appropriate clinical dosing. These preparations are generally intended for use in the characterization of the activity of secondary reference preparations (regional, national or in-house working standards). The National Institute of Biological Standards and Control (http://www.nibsc.ac.uk/) is an international laboratory of WHO that supplies standards. The World Health Organization (www.who.int) has published a general guide to Good Manufacturing Practices for Pharmaceutical Products (Technical Report Series No. 823, Geneva, 1992), which is a good place to start when looking for regulatory guidance.

International Conference on Harmonization (ICH): (http://www.ich.org) There are currently no official guidelines for the development of recombinant products. However, the rationale and views expressed by the International Conference on Harmonisation of Technical Requirements for Registration of Pharmaceuticals for Human Use (ICH) on licensed products are relevant. ICH is a project that brings together the regulatory authorities of Europe, Japan, and the U.S. and experts from the pharmaceutical industry in the three regions to discuss scientific and technical aspects of product registration. The purpose is to make recommendations on ways to achieve greater harmonization in the interpretation and application of technical guidelines and requirements for product registration in order to reduce or obviate the need to duplicate the testing carried out during the research and development of new medicines. The ICH quality web page is available at http://www.ich.org/TxtServer.jser?@_ID=476&@_TYPE=HTML&@_TEMPLATE=616 and should be consulted for all aspects of biogeneric product filing. Some of the most relevant documents include:

- ICH Harmonized Tripartite Guideline Q5B, Analysis of the Expression Construct in Cells Used for Production of r-DNA Derived Protein Products, Step 4 (http://www.ich.org/ich5q.html)
- ICH Harmonized Tripartite Guideline Q5D, Derivation and Characterization of Cell Substrates Used for Production of Biotechnological/Biological Products, Step 4 (http://www.ich.org/ich5q.html)
- ICH Guidance on Viral Safety Evaluation of Biotechnology Products Derived from Cell Lines of Human or Animal Origin (September 24, 1998), ICH Draft Guidance: Q5E

Comparability of Biotechnological/Biological Products Subject to Changes in Their Manufacturing Process (March 29, 2004)

- ICH Guidance: Q7A Good Manufacturing Practice Guide for Active Pharmaceutical Ingredients (September 25, 2001)
- ICH Guidance on Quality of Biotechnological/Biological Products: Derivation and Characterization of Cell Substrates Used for Production of Biotechnological/Biological Products (September 21, 1998)
- ICH Final Guideline on Quality of Biotechnical Products: Analysis of the Expression Construct in Cells Used for the Production of r-DNA Derived Protein Products (February 1996)

REGULATORY ISSUES

Regulatory issues are mostly related to product safety, which is ensured not only by product control but also in use of established and extensively tested cell banks, process robustness, well-characterized raw materials, and in-process control procedures generally decided on a case-by-case basis. The newest guidelines of the FDA related to PAT (see Chapter 9 on Quality Assurance Systems) go into great detail on how to ensure process robustness. The risks related directly to the use of recombinant technique relate either to contamination or immunogenicity, over and above the risks of manufacturing, that are common and well defined in the cGMP guidelines. The contamination results from viruses and other transmissible agents, cellular DNA, and host cell proteins (e.g., growth factors). The potential introduction of adventitious agents such as fungi, bacteria, viruses, and prions in cell culture media is of major concern and has prompted constant improvements in media and raw materials used. Thus raw materials possessing high contamination risk (e.g., hydrolysates and peptones produced from animals or by means of animal-derived enzymes) should be avoided. The use of antibiotics is discouraged, but when used, the selection markers are selected with care (e.g., kanamycin). Content of endotoxins (gram negative bacteria), nucleic acids, host cell proteins, and correct N-terminal in the drug substance/product are of major regulatory concern. These topics are adequately covered in Chapter 10 on Quality Control Systems.

One of the most important components of regulatory scrutiny is the master cell bank (MCB) and a thorough cell line characterization is required. The testing of the cell substrate is the first part of the biosafety program carried out for each biopharmaceutical drug substance/product used in clinical trials. For example, mammalian cell line characterization would typically include:

- Rodent retrovirus assays including RT, mus Dunni, XC, S+L–, and ERV
- Human pathogens including HIV-I & II, HBV, HCV, HAV, HSV-I, HSV-2, HSV-6, HTLV-I, HTLV-II, and CMV
- Primate pathogens including SIV, STLV, foamy agent, and SMRV
- Mycoplasma testing
- *In vivo* and *in vitro* adventitious agents testing
- Karyology and isoenzymes
- Electron microscopy.

STERILITY

Further issues are end of production tests, test of raw materials, and quality control analyses of drug substance and drug product (the latter are rarely tested for viruses if produced in continuous cell lines). The potential risks associated with the use of microbial or metazoan expression systems are partly related to contaminants from the cells and partly from raw materials used to propagate the cells. Cell-related impurities are nucleic acids and host cell proteins. Metazoan cells may be infected with viruses or other transmissible agents and they may produce growth-promoting proteins. Insect cells that have been introduced as the baculoviral vector do not infect mammals, but the transfected insect cell line cannot be considered completely free of contaminating viruses (e.g., Flaviviridae), and it is strongly advised to set up test programs similar to those of metazoan cells. It should be mentioned that mycoplasma infections might constitute a greater problem than previously anticipated. The extensive characterization of the MCB does to some point overcome the concerns of using serum and perhaps other raw materials of animal origin. It is strongly advised not to use raw materials of animal origin at any point after MCB characterization as safety could be compromised by such an act.

The downstream process is required to be fully validated for regulatory submissions. Some of the documents that may be required to establish the validation include:

- Batch records (downstream part)
- Development report (downstream part)
- In-process control analytical method descriptions including typical data
- Laboratory notebooks
- List of raw materials used
- Protocol for validation
- Strategy and rationale report for the downstream part
- Summary reports
- Unit operation description.

PURITY CONTROL PROGRAMS

Purity of target protein is the most important consideration in supporting a regulatory filing. The analytical program is product specific and the rationale of the suggested program is to analyze the drug substance extensively in the early phases to ensure safety and prevent unintended process redesign later on. It is highly recommended that the biogeneric product manufacturer discuss the regulatory analytical procedures with the official authorities as early as possible; however, in those instances where compendial monographs exist, the choice of analytical methodology is well established. The manufacturers, however, must still demonstrate its plan for purity control. The purity control program depends on the expression system and the intended use of the material produced. In a typical microbial expression system, identity and biological activity are required for all four phases of development: preclinical, Phase I, Phase II, and Phase III; immunogenicity is not required at the preclinical level but must be evaluated at all other stages. Similarly, all tests related to purity are required at all levels, except viruses and prions. Virus clearance is performed prior to Phase I and is not repeated until prior to Phase III unless the process is changed in a way that invalidates the preclinical study.

The prion test program is yet unclear. Virus and prions testing is required in Phase I and Phase III when using insect cell, mammalian cells, and transgenic animal expression The tests for impurity that are required include host cell proteins, DNA, endotoxins, bioburden, cosolvents, leachable (if affinity chromatography has been used or if a new polymeric matrix has been introduced) components, and the impurity profile (impurities exceeding 0.1% should normally be fully characterized prior to Phase III clinical studies). If the impurity comprises less than 0.5% it is suggested to suspend the characterization program until Phase III. Transgenic animals may coexpress the equivalent animal protein. Its removal must be documented by means of specific test procedures. The target protein requires quantification at all stages, but the toxicity is evaluated only at the preclinical stages. When preparing a regulatory filing for the biogeneric product, many of these analyses may be redundant, and it is recommended that the regulatory authorities be consulted within the early phase of development.

TABLE 11.1
The Four Levels of Effects of Antibodies on the Clinical Outcome in the Use of Recombinant Products

Clinical Concern	Clinical Outcome
Safety	Neutralize endogenous counterpart with unique function causing deficiency syndrome; hypersensitivity reactions
Efficacy	Inhibition or enhancement of product efficacy
Pharmacokinetics	Changes in dosing level due to PK changes
None	Despite generation of antibodies, no discernible impact

IMMUNOCHEMICAL PROPERTIES

Immunogenicity is the ability of therapeutic protein products to elicit immune responses; antibodies are the most frequent measure of immune response to soluble protein products.

Cell-mediated immune responses to proteins may be critically important to generation of antibodies. The T-cell dependent antibody responses are generally required for antibodies to proteins or generally required for class switching to IgG and affinity maturation. T-cells and B-cells are activated by different segments of the same protein. The clinical concerns for antibodies to therapeutic proteins fall into several categories, as shown in Table 11.1.

Several recent case examples need to be reviewed to understand the potential and extent of the immunogenicity potential.

- PEG-MGDF: The biologically unique function of MGDF/TPO is its megakaryocyte/platelet growth and development potential. Literature reports that its neutralizing antibody caused thrombocytopenia in healthy platelet donors (4%) and oncology patients (0.5%). This illustrates the effect of immune status on host. Furthermore, in healthy donors, tolerance was easily broken (2 to 3 doses) in some cases and TCP developed in all animal models tested, including nonhuman primate-using species specific product; however, antibody was present in some patients prior to treatment.
- Erythropoietin: The neutralizing antibody to erythropoietin induces PRCA and approximately 300 cases have occurred from 1997 to 2003. Incidentally, nearly all cases are related to use of Eprex brand of erythropoietin and nearly all cases developed following packaging changes (prefilled syringes), formulation changes (delete HSA), and shift in route of administration (to SC from IV). These cases turned out not to be an isolated group, but clearly part of a more pervasive problem. By December 2003, a total of 262 cases had been reported.

It is possible to break immunologic tolerance to endogenous proteins because mammals are not fully tolerant to endogenous proteins and this forms the basis for autoimmune diseases such as autoimmune thyroiditis, MS, RA, etc. as well as the basis for regulation of inflammatory cytokines and fail-safe mechanism for potent growth factors (Epo, TPO, G-CSF). As a result, the immune response can abort efficacy of life-saving or life-enhancing protein therapeutics to glucocerebrosidase in Gaucher's disease, where most patients tolerize with continued treatment, and in a small percentage high titer antibodies persist and neutralize activity, to Factor VIII in hemophilia A where approximately 30% develop "inhibitors" or neutralizing antibody, to alpha-glucosidase in Pompe's disease, and to mAbs in treatment of autoimmune disease.

As a result, regulatory agencies like the FDA assess the risk of immune responses to therapeutic proteins by estimating the likelihood of development of an immune response as learned from known-product and patient-risk factors; potential clinical sequelae resulting from generation of immune response from understanding of biological function and redundancy of protein; alternative products for indication if available; and ability to terminate immune response. Predicting immunogenicity is a difficult task and factors such as evaluation, if it is derivation, self or foreign, product-specific attributes, patient/immune system–specific attributes, and the results of animal immunogenicity testing are important. Immunogenicity is expected from proteins of foreign origin as it would neutralize the product and produce hypersensitivity; in the case of immunogen created by the body itself, there is a potential for immunogenicity that would neutralize endogenous protein and produce severe deficiency syndrome. The product-specific factors of importance are: molecular structure, aggregation, novel epitope(s) spreading, degradation, oxidation/deamidation, and glycosylation.

The important factors to assess the potential of a product to raise an immune response include product-specific factors and patient-specific factors that impact decisions regarding testing. Aggregation remains one of the most important factors. It is important to remember that there can be covalently bonded aggregates, which may be measured by standard means in current use, and there can be noncovalently bonded aggregates resulting from hydrophobic or weaker ionic interactions, which are difficult to quantitate using standard techniques. Covalent aggregates are mostly affected by the molecular structure, while noncovalent aggregates are a result of formulation effects. Recently, greater understanding has developed about the role of aggregation in inducing immunogenicity. The presence of aggregates precludes tolerance in naive immune systems, and the product changes associated with enhanced immunogenicity (oxidation, degradation) are associated with protein aggregation. For example, tolerance to interferon alpha breaks when aggregates are formed at room temperature storage; IL-2 exists as microaggregates (average size 27 mols) and is highly immunogenic, resulting in antibody development in 47 to 74% of instances; in a study on mAb, the elimination of aggregates eliminated immunogenicity.

The methods to detect aggregation include those that disrupt noncovalent or weak aggregates and include SDS-Polyacrylamide gel electrophoresis, capillary electrophoresis, and size exclusion HPLC. Methods that better detect weak aggregates include analytical ultracentrifugation, field flow fractionation, and atomic force microscopy. The problem of aggregate formation requires studies using sensitive methods to quantitate product aggregation for covalently bonded and weak aggregates. The effects of product aggregates in *in vitro* and *in vivo* systems should be assessed to understand what level of aggregates can break tolerance. And obviously, the processing steps should be designed to minimize product aggregation.

The product-specific factors also include the inherent immunomodulatory activity. An example of immune suppression would be anti-CD4 mAb CTLA4-Ig and of immunostimulatory, GM-CSF; Flt-3L; CpG oligos. The formulation factors are also product-specific factors that may arise from novel epitope formation with protein adducts, patient/immune system factors. Immune competency is more likely to generate a response than immune compromise. The route of administration takes its importance in the following hierarchy: SC/ID > IM > IV. The dose and frequency of administration also play an important role; for example, it was demonstrated that frequent intravenous dosing of Factor VIII resulted in generating therapeutic counterpart of endogenous, leading to tolerance.

The usefulness of animal immunogenicity testing depends on homology of human to animal protein. For example, studies with TPO and PEG-MGDF precisely predicted immunogenicity results in humans; however, it is not generally useful if homology is low as a result of xenogeneic responses. Other uses of animal models include deliberate provocation of immunity to assess effects of neutralization of endogenous product; the use of knock out animals may predict effect of loss of endogenous product due to antibody neutralization.

The risk of immunogenicity is determined by analysis of factors critical for generation of immune responses, how they apply to the product in question, and the clinical consequences of such responses. For products that are critical components of therapy for life-threatening or debilitating diseases, sensitive immunogenicity assays should be in place at the earliest stages of product development. This should include evaluation of the manufacturing changes (formulation, specification, virus or adventitious agent removal/inactivation, establishment of MCB) on immunogenicity.

Examples of formulation changes that have demonstrated impact on aggregation-related effects include the observation that addition of sucrose to buffer eliminated aggregation in mAb products, in the case of Eprex, removal of human serum albumin increased immunogenicity while removal of human serum albumin from interferon alpha reduced immunogenicity; heat denaturation during virus/adventitious agent removal increased product aggregation in the case of urokinase; shear force from product filtration increased product aggregation and so did low pH as shown in the case of interferon alpha; renaturation or refolding induced protein aggregation and in some instances protein overexpression can theoretically lead to aggregation; even such changes as storage commodity have shown an impact on aggregation. The syringe material may affect hydrophobic interaction and thus aggregation of product. Additionally, in one instance leaching from the syringe gasket activated metalloprotease-product truncation or leaching from syringe barrel caused product oxidation regaling in aggregation. There are reported incidences where prefilled syringes stored at home storage condition alter immunogenicity of photo and heat labile molecules like erythropoietin; even mechanical agitation would induce or disrupt structure for most proteins.

Testing for immunogenicity for high-risk manufacturing changes can take many routes; the most important being upfront testing, but it is generally insufficiently powered to detect relatively rare events, i.e., < 1/1000; this leaves postmarketing adverse event assessment, passive AE surveillance programs, epidemiological studies, and postmarketing commitments for active data collection as the only viable choices. Requirement for further *in vivo* testing depends on the product, the manufacturing change, and results of extended comparability assessment including comprehensive aggregate analysis.

As elaborated earlier, one of the most important concerns of the regulatory authorities is the immunogenic potential of generic proteins. During recent considerations by the FDA, this has been the prime concern, over and above all other considerations. The first generation of protein drugs was based on tissue extracts from animals (e.g., bovine insulin, porcine insulin) or from human extracts (pituitary glands). The foreign origin and the lack of purity of these earlier preparations often resulted in immune responses in patients. With the introduction of the recombinant technology, it was hoped that the near identity with the human "natural" protein and better purification procedures would reduce the problem due to immunological tolerance of "self" proteins. Although replacement of the animal protein with the human species' protein reduced the problem, it still persisted, and it was learned that the incidence of immunogenicity does not necessarily correlate with the sequence homology to the human protein. Interestingly, it has been observed that the target protein may induce an immune response even in individuals not being deficient in the protein, but merely produces an insufficient amount. Furthermore, individuals with no predisposition to autoimmunity often produce antibodies against the target protein. Even minor amounts of protein impurities may raise an antigenic response (the limit for presence of bovine proinsulin in bovine insulin preparations can be 1 ppm), making it mandatory to use well-designed, robust, and controlled downstream processes to produce the product and to use validated host cell protein assays to detect for content of HCP in the drug substance/product. Apparently modern process technologies and designs cope well with the challenge, resulting in a reduction of immunogenic responses due to host cell proteins. Product-derived impurities such as target protein aggregates may also be antigenic, making protein stability during processing and storage a central safety issue.

The target protein may be immunogenic for several reasons:

- It has a different amino acid sequence from the human protein equivalent
- It has an incorrect three-dimensional structure
- It has incorrect posttranslational modifications
- It is aggregated
- It is chemically modified

- It is administered together with an adjuvant
- The protein is administered in large amounts
- The protein is delivered by a method raising an immune response.

An immune response should be expected if there is a sequence difference between the target protein and the human equivalent. However, an indication of the complexity of immunogenicity is illustrated by a lack of antibody response in patients having received animal proteins even after years of use. Further, administration of deaggregated nonself proteins without adjuvants has induced immunological tolerance. Foreign proteins may also be of bacterial or plant origin, for example, introduced as impurities. In some diseases the patient lacks the human protein (e.g., hemophilia patients carrying a homozygous deletion), and the recombinant human protein must be considered foreign. Human protein analogues comprise a specific class of proteins having high homology with the native protein. These products predominantly induce immune responses in patients who lack immune tolerance because of an innate insufficiency of the native gene.

Incorrect native structure is often associated with scrambled forms resulting from *in vitro* folding of proteins expressed in *E. coli*. Posttranslational modifications (e.g., glycoproteins) not resembling those of the natural product may also be immunogenic. It is a common observation that several different forms are expressed and copurified resulting in a mixed product. A consistent pattern at IEF or peptide mapping should be provided to demonstrate identity between batches.

Protein aggregates have been shown repeatedly to cause immunogenicity in patients. The immune response is usually weak and is generally observed after long-term treatment. The clinical consequence is usually minor and loss of efficacy can be compensated for by increased doses. In rare cases the antibody neutralizes the native protein with severe biological consequences. Formation of protein aggregates is a function of upstream processing, downstream processing, formulation, and storage conditions, making protein stability a key issue not only in process design but also in broader aspect. It should be noted that animals rendered fully tolerant to monomeric proteins will not mount an immune response when challenged with an aggregated version of the protein. Chemically modified forms such des-amido and oxidized forms may also be antigenic. Interestingly, chemically modified analogues (e.g., pegylated products) have been introduced with the purpose of altering the protein half-life and the immune reactive response. The effect on the immune system is still unclear. Administration of self proteins to patients can break immunological tolerance due to the presence of adjuvants such a lipopolysaccharides. Administration of the protein in large amounts may induce an immunogenic response. The route of administration also influences the local inflammatory response or induction of antibodies in patients.

The formation of antibodies may have several, sometimes severe consequences for the patient. Those cases with the most serious adverse events have been those instances where antibodies raised against product cross-react with endogenous proteins as seen with inhibition of endogenous thrombopoietin and subsequent development of autoimmune thrombocytopenia. Examples of therapeutic proteins resulting in antibody formation in patients are streptokinase, staphylokinase, bovine adenosine deaminase, calcitonin, trichosanthin, gonadotropin, erythropoietin, interleukin 2, TNF receptor 2-Ig, and Denileukin diftitox. Other clinical consequences are hypersensitivity reactions including fever, nausea, chills, and allergic reactions. Immediate hypersensitivity responses that cause anaphylactic or anaphylactoid responses are of major concern.

Better process design, control of protein stability, generation of soluble nonaggregated native proteins, high purification factors of immunogenic substances, avoidance of contaminating adjuvants, and better formulations are examples of process-related preventive actions. The impact of the process, also on long-term product stability, should be taken into consideration throughout the drug development program.

Covalent binding with polymers such as polyethylene glycol (e.g., in PEG-Intron) and dextran may reduce the antigenicity and immunogenicity of proteins. The effect of proteins, which are homologous with human proteins, is unclear as exemplified in the serious clinical consequences observed with pegylated TNF- treatment. Sequence modifications, especially where T-cell epitopes have been removed or changed, are in the form of interesting modifications meant to reduce the immune response.

The ability to predict immunogenicity is the key issue at most regulatory authorities. The approaches include bioinformatics, screening for T-cell epitopes, detection of antibiotics, the use of animal models, and ultimately, the response in patients. Bioinformatics approaches are based on identification of super motifs present across different MHC alleles or to identify "promiscuous" epitopes capable of binding different MHC alleles regardless of "super type" family. Algorithms allow for the construction of a matrix of all possible amino acid side chain effects for a single MHC binding motif. The screening of T-cell epitopes relies on the induction of T-cell activity from cells derived from previously exposed subjects or the identification of priming T-cell epitopes using a dendritic cell-based assay — the i-mune assay. The detection of antibodies is a common methodology to confirm an immune response in patients. Typical immunoassays are ELISA (direct binding and competitive ELISA), ELISA in combination with bioassays and surface plasmon resonance (BIAcore technology), electrochemiluminescence (ECL), SDS-PAGE, and Western blot technology. However, it should be noticed that the antibody level might be too low for detection in some of the assays mentioned (lack of sensitivity).

The goals of antibody testing include detecting all antibodies capable of binding to the target protein, identifying all antibodies of clinical relevance, determining whether the antibodies can neutralize the drug's biological effect, characterizing the antibodies of relevance, and assessing the impact of antibodies on the therapeutic protein program. The animal models have in general not been able to predict the immunogenicity of recombinant biopharmaceuticals in humans, the main issue being that the administration of a human protein into an animal species is likely to be immunogenic. In addition, the said biopharmaceutical cannot be expected to be biologically active, which can affect the immunogenicity. The use of transgenic animals is a promising technology as shown for interferon-α studies in human interferon-α transgenic mice.

Since therapeutic proteins can provoke life-threatening autoimmune responses, regulatory agencies will expect, prior to licensure, detailed clinical evaluation of the potential for immunogenicity. CBER (and now CDER) considers immune responses to biological therapeutic agents in a hierarchy, structured by clinical effects. The greatest concern regards immediate hypersensitivity responses that cause anaphylactic or anaphylactoid responses. Also the presence of neutralizing antibodies is of major concern as seen in patients exhibiting pure red blood cell aplasia and immune-mediated thrombocytopenia after treatment with recombinant erythropoietin and thrombopoietin. Of importance, but posing less threat, is generation of binding antibodies, which can diminish product efficacy. The Concerted EU Action started in 1993 with the purpose of coordinating research on the immunogenicity of biopharmaceuticals is an important learning exercise.

Immunochemical properties are described in the ICH Harmonized Tripartite Guideline. Specifications: Test Procedures and Acceptance Criteria for Biotechnological Products (Q6B) (March 10, 1999), for example, see http://www.ich.org/TxtServer.jser?@_ID=476&@_TYPE= HTML&@_TEMPLATE=616 and in Pre-clinical Safety Evaluation of Biotechnology Derived Pharmaceuticals, ICH topic S6, see http://www.ich.org/TxtServer.jser?@_ID=501&@_TYPE= HTML&@_TEMPLATE=616.

PROTEIN DEGRADATION

Proteolysis is a selective, highly regulated process that plays an important role in cellular physiology. *E. coli* contains a large number of proteases that are localized in the cytoplasm, the periplasm, and the inner and outer membranes. These proteolytic enzymes participate in a host of metabolic activities, including the selective removal of abnormal proteins. Protein damage or alteration may result from a variety of conditions, such as incomplete polypeptides, mutations caused by amino acid substitutions, excessive synthesis of subunits from multimeric complexes, posttranslational damage through oxidation or free-radical attack, and genetic engineering. Such abnormal proteins are efficiently removed by the bacterial proteolytic machine. To date, the mechanisms of protein degradation are incompletely understood, and it is unlikely that all proteolytic pathways or enzymes operating in *E. coli* have been identified. For example, a new protease associated with the outer membrane was recently discovered and a fascinating new mechanism for the degradation of abnormal proteins in *E. coli* has just been uncovered. Nevertheless, the intense scientific interest in this area has generated new tools and strategies for minimizing the degradation of heterologous proteins in *E. coli*.

Although the precise structural features that impart lability to proteins are not known, some determinants of protein instability have been elucidated. In a series of systematic studies, Varshavsky and colleagues formulated the "N-end rule" that relates the metabolic stability of a protein to its amino-terminal residue. Thus, in *E. coli*, N-terminal Arg, Lys, Leu, Phe, Tyr, and Trp conferred 2-min half-lives on a test protein, whereas all the other amino acids except proline conferred more than 10-h half-lives on the same protein. As discussed above (see the section on cytoplasmic expression), amino acids with small side chains in the second position of the polypeptide facilitate the methionine aminopeptidase catalyzed removal of the N-terminal methionine. Therefore, these studies suggest that Leu in the second position would probably be exposed by the removal of the methionine residue and would destabilize the protein.

The second determinant of protein instability is a specific internal lysine residue located near the amino terminus. This residue is the acceptor of a multiubiquitin chain that facilitates protein degradation by a ubiquitin-dependent protease in eukaryotes. Interestingly, in a multisubunit protein, the two determinants can be located on different subunits and still target the protein for processing.

Another correlation between amino acid content and protein instability is presented in the PEST hypothesis. On the basis of statistical analysis of eukaryotic proteins that have short half-lives, it was proposed that proteins are destabilized by regions enriched in Pro, Glu, Ser, and Thr, flanked by certain amino acid residues. Phosphorylation of these PEST domains leads to increased calcium binding, which in turn facilitates the destruction of the protein by calcium-dependent proteases. It was suggested that PEST-rich proteins may be produced efficiently in *E. coli*, which apparently lacks the PEST proteolytic system.

Strategies for minimizing proteolysis of recombinant proteins include protein targeting to the periplasm or the culture medium, the use of protease-deficient host strains, growth of the host cells at low temperature, construction of N- or C-terminal fusion proteins, tandem fusion of multiple copies of the target gene, coexpression of molecular chaperones, coexpression of the T4 *pin* gene, replacement of specific amino acid residues to eliminate protease cleavage sites, modification of the hydrophobicity of the target protein, and optimization of fermentation conditions.

Although the variety of approaches for protein stabilization attests to the ingenuity of the investigators, the usefulness of some of the above methods may be limited, depending on the intended use of the recombinant protein. Thus, for example, the presence of fusion moieties on the target protein may interfere with functional or structural properties or therapeutic applications of the product. The engineering of enzymatic or chemical cleavage sites for the subsequent removal of the fusion partners is a complex process that involves numerous considerations: the accessibility of the cleavage sites to enzyme digestion; the purity, specificity, and cost of the commercially available enzymes; the authenticity of the N- or C-termini upon enzymatic digestion; the possible modification of the target protein upon chemical treatment, and so forth. For the large-scale production of fusion proteins, some of these difficulties are amplified. Similarly, the fusion of multiple copies of the target gene to create multidomain polypeptides requires the subsequent conversion to monomeric protein units by cyanogen bromide cleavage. In this case, the target protein must not contain internal methionine residues and must be able to withstand harsh reaction conditions. Moreover, a limited extent of amino acid side chain modification may occur, and the toxicity of cyanogen bromide presents a significant issue for large-scale cleavage reactions. Similarly, the rational modification of a protein sequence requires extensive structural information that may not be available. Molecular chaperones have been used successfully to stabilize specific proteins, but this approach remains a hit-or-miss affair.

The cytoplasm of *E. coli* contains a greater number of proteases than does the periplasm. Therefore, proteins located in the periplasm are less likely to be degraded. For example, proinsulin localized to the periplasm was 10-fold more stable that when produced in the cytoplasm. However, proteolytic activity in the periplasm is substantial. Secretion into the culture medium would provide a better alternative in terms of protein stability. Unfortunately, the technology for secretion of proteins from *E. coli* into the culture medium is still in its infancy. A major catalyst of protein degradation in bacteria is the induction of heat shock proteins in response to a variety of stress conditions, such as the thermal induction of gene expression or the accumulation of abnormal or heterologous proteins in the cytoplasm. Under these conditions, the production of the *lon* gene product, protease La, and other proteases is enhanced. This problem is minimized by the use of host strains deficient in the *rpoH* (*htpR*) locus. The *rpoH* gene encodes the RNA polymerase subunit, which regulates several proteolytic activities in *E. coli*. Hosts that carry the *rpoH* mutation have been patented and have been demonstrated to dramatically increase the production of foreign proteins in *E. coli*. Strain SG21173, which is deficient in proteases La and Clp and the *rpoH* locus, is particularly effective in protein production. A large number of protease-deficient hosts exist, including some that are deficient in all known protease loci that affect the stability of secreted proteins.

Before leaving this section, it is worth repeating a caveat on the use of protease-deficient strains: proteolysis may be an effect rather than a cause of folding problems, serving as a disposal system to remove misfolded and aggregated material. Therefore, it is possible that the absence of proteases will result in increased toxicity to the host as a result of the accumulation of abnormal proteins.

Like other small molecules, protein drugs are subject to demonstration of stability (providing a predetermined minimum potency) to the time of use and in addition, a safety profile since the degradation products of protein drugs can be immunogenic, compared to small molecules where the concern is mainly creation of toxic molecules. The stability studies for therapeutic proteins are conducted at three levels: preformulation, formulation development, and formal GMP studies. The preformulation studies determine basic stability properties of bulk protein or peptide and the accelerated studies at this stage are primarily intended to establish stability indicating assays and other analytic methods. The formulation development studies are intended for the candidate formulation and encompass large studies that evaluate the effects of excipients, container/closure systems, and where lyophilized, a study of myriad factors that can alter the characteristics of products. The data generated in the formulation development studies are used to select final formulation and to design the studies that follow: formal GMP studies. The formal stability studies are used to support clinical use, IND, and then all the way through a Biological License Application (submitted to CDER; effective June 2003, therapeutic proteins are now handled by CDER). When preparing supplies for clinical use, it is important to know that there is no need to demonstrate shelf-life for the commercial dosage form and only stability demonstration is required during the testing phase, such as 6 months; many manufacturers use frozen product to ensure adequate stability; this may create a logistics problem of ensuring that the clinical sites can store the produce frozen. Obviously, products that can be adversely affected by freezing will not be subject to this method of reducing the clinical startup time. Also, at this stage of initial clinical testing under an IND, the test methods need not be fully validated or have demonstrated robustness; as long as reproducibility and repeatability is demonstrated, this should be acceptable to FDA. The formal GMP studies monitor commercial lots, and clear ICH guidelines are available to follow the protocols of these studies in ICH Stability Guidelines for Biologics, Federal Register July 10, 1996, Volume 61, No. 133, p 36466-36469.

STABILITY CONSIDERATIONS

Commercial viability of recombinant production processes depends on the final product yield; this is a particularly more significant issue as biogeneric manufacturers will bring their line of products to be sold at a lower price than the innovator's products; thus, the issue of yield becomes more important. A primary cause of poor yield is neither the quality of the gene construct nor the nature of molecule but the degradation of the product during the manufacturing process. Protein degradation therefore becomes a key factor that must be thoroughly understood, and steps must taken to minimize this degradation step wherever possible. This chapter deals with this significant issue and makes suggestions on how to avoid the degradation of proteins in the downstream processing.

PROTEOLYSIS

In contrast to the cellular environment, where enzymatic degradation of proteins is highly controlled, extra cellular protease is the cause of uncontrolled protein degradation. The result of the proteolytic attack may vary from complete hydrolysis, single breaks within the peptide chain, or loss of a few N- or C-terminal amino acid residues. Besides losing the product, presence of truncated forms may seriously challenge the purification design.

Proteolytic enzymes are released to the medium because of cell death, mechanical stress, or induced cell lysis. Their presence should be expected during fermentation and initial downstream unit operations. Most enzymes of the vacuoles and lysozomes will be minimally active at slightly alkaline pH (7 to 9), a pH interval strongly recommended for extraction of proteins expressed in bacteria.

Proteins are probably more resistant toward proteolytic attacks in their native state, and stabilizing factors (e.g., cofactor, correct parameter interval, cosolvent) should always be considered optimized. Use of protein inhibitors is not recommended for safety reasons. The primary mechanism of proteolysis is the enzymatic hydrolysis of the peptide bond. The indicators of this reaction taking place in the system include loss of product or poor yield, lack of expected activity, changes in specific activity, change in molecular weight, high background staining in 1D SDS electrophoresis, smeared bands and many lower Mw bands of poor resolution, bands that may disappear, and discrepancies in Mw. The actions to prevent proteolysis are listed in Table 11.2.

TABLE 11.2
Factors and Their Control to Prevent Proteolysis

Factor	Comment
pH	There is no specific pH range in which all enzymes are considered inactive; at slightly alkaline pH the nonspecific enzymes of the vacuoles and lysozomes will be minimally active. Use strong buffers for extraction to prevent unintended shift in pH as a result of cell disruption. Some yeast enzymes are least active in the pH range 4 to 5, but active in the pH range 7 to 9. Phosphate may exhibit a stabilizing effect on proteins.
Temperature	Low temperature decreases the proteolytic activity. It is recommended to store harvest at 4 to 8°C or frozen.
Time	Enzymatic protein degradation is a function of time. Lengthy procedures and long storage times should be avoided during harvest, capture, and initial purification steps.
Conductivity	Noncritical
Redox potential	Reducing and oxidizing conditions may alter the disulfide bridge arrangement and state of free cysteine residues thus influencing the protein secondary and tertiary structures.
Cosolvents	Presence of other proteins in excess (e.g., albumin) will reduce the proteolytic damage. Cosolvents such as glycerol or dimethylsulfoxide may have a stabilizing effect, but will probably be too expensive for large-scale operations.
Low Mw compounds	Substrates, substrate analogues, and cofactors can help stabilize the protein. Potential proteinase activators (e.g., divalent metal ions) should be excluded from the extraction buffer.
Techniques	Careful cell disruption and specific extraction procedures may lower the enzymatic cleavage.
Denaturation	The proteolytic enzymes lose their biological activity upon denaturation. However, some enzymes are stable under mild denaturing conditions, leading to increased activity if the target protein is partly denatured under the same conditions.

TABLE 11.3
Factors and Their Control to Prevent Deamidation

Factor	Comment
pH	Deamidation should be expected above pH 5. The optimal working range in which to avoid deamidation is probably between 3.0 and 5.0.
Temperature	The deamidation rate increases with increasing temperature.
Time	The deamidation rate is a function of time. Presence of des-amido forms is a marker for drug product stability and shelf life.
Conductivity	The ionic strength of the solution should be kept low. At high ionic strength the deamidation reaction can be fast even at neutral pH.
Redox potential	Nonessential parameter.
Cosolvents	In general the buffer species and the buffer strength will influence the rate of deamidation. High solvent dielectrics favor deamidation.
	In model peptides the protein stability was higher in Tris buffer than in phosphate buffer.

The use of enzyme inhibitors is not recommended as they are harmful to human beings. Ascertain that the degradation observed is not a function of the analytical assay. Enzyme inhibitors can be used for prevention of enzymatic activity in analytical assays. Mild denaturation may accelerate enzymatic digestion. Selective removal (e.g., affinity chromatography) of specific enzymes should be considered, too.

DEAMIDATION

Two amino acid residues are involved in the deamidation reaction: asparagyl and glutamyl. The conversion to the corresponding carboxylic acid residues results in a shift in net charge of the protein at pH above the pKa. As the deamidation may influence the biological activity and the stability of the molecule, the maximal content of des-amido formed in bulk materials and in biopharmaceutical preparations is constantly being debated. The list of proteins undergoing deamidation is comprehensive and includes well-known proteins such as insulin, human growth hormone, and cytochrome C.

Asparagyl residues tend to be more susceptible to deamidation that glutamyl residues. Further, the deamidation reaction is strongly sequence-specific in model peptides with the half-life of the –Asn-Pro– sequence being 100-fold greater than that of –Asn-Gly. To some extent these observations can also be used on proteins taking the structural steric factors and nearby amino acid residues into consideration.

At pH above 5, deamidation of asparagyl or glutamyl occurs via a relatively slow intermediate succinimide formation. The succinimidyl derivative is rapidly hydrolyzed at either the α- or β-carbonyl group to generate a mixture of normal- and iso-residues. Under strongly acidic conditions asparagyl or glutamyl residues are hydrolyzed to the corresponding carboxyl residue. The indicators of deamidation include extra bands in electrophoresis and extra peaks in chromatographic recordings. Table 11.3 lists preventive actions against deamidation.

OXIDATION

The amino acid residues histidyl, methionyl, cystinyl, tryptophanyl, and tyrosinyl are potential oxidation sites at neutral or slightly alkaline conditions. Oxidation of the said residues often results in loss of immunological or biological activity. The list of proteins that have been oxidized is comprehensive and includes biopharmaceutical products such as albumin, growth hormone, glucagons, interleukin-1, and interleukin 2. In many cases, the immunological or biological activity was only partially lost. In general, oxidation of methionyl to methionyl sulfoxide does not affect protein

TABLE 11.4
Factors and Their Control to Prevent Oxidation

Factor	Comment
pH	The oxidation rate is assumed low at slightly acidic pH.
Temperature	Working at low temperatures decreases the rate of oxidation.
Time	The oxidation reaction is a function of time.
Conductivity	No data available.
Redox potential	Disulfide bond formation will take place at a redox potential above 0 mV. A high redox potential indicates presence of oxidizing agents.
Cosolvents	Avoid oxidizing agents and protect against light. Addition of chelating agents (EDTA, citric acid, thioglycolic acid), antioxidants (BHT, BHA, propyl gallate, Vitamin E), or reducing agents (Cys, DTT, methionine, ascorbic acid, sodium sulfite, thioglycolic acid, thioglycerol) may reduce oxidation.

antigenicity, probably because the conformational structure of the oxidized protein is close to the native structure. On the other hand, oxidation of a single amino acid residue often causes changes in the biological activity, and all efforts should be taken to minimize oxidation reactions.

The mechanism of oxidation involves methionyl residues that are converted to methionyl sulfoxide residues under mild oxidizing conditions. The most reactive residues are those exposed to the solvent, while those residues buried within the hydrophobic regions are fairly inert to oxidation (e.g., methionine residues in myoglobin and trypsin). Methionyl residues are susceptible to auto oxidation, chemical oxidation, and photo oxidation.

The cystinyl residues are easily oxidized and the reaction is usually accelerated at alkaline pH, where the thiol group is deprotonated. Under mild oxidizing conditions the reactions are oxidation of cystinyl residues to sulfenic/sulfonic acid (alkaline conditions), cystinyl residues to dehydroalanyl residues (alkaline conditions), or cystinyl to cystine residues (neutral to alkaline conditions). In the absence of a thiol reagent or a nearby thiol, the cysteine may instead oxidize to sulfenic acid.

The oxidation reaction is strongly catalyzed by divalent metal ions (e.g., copper). The indicators of oxidation include extra bands in gel electrophoresis and extra peaks in chromatographic recordings. Preventive actions against oxidation are listed in Table 11.4.

The degradation rate is often governed by trace amounts of peroxides, divalent metal ions, light, and base and free radicals. There are three classes of anti-oxidants:

- Phenolic compounds: BHT, BHA, propyl gallate, vitamin E
- Reducing agents: Cysteine, DTT, methionine, ascorbic acid, sodium sulfite, thioglycolic acid, thioglycerol
- Chelating agents: EDTA, citric acid, and thioglycolic acid.

CARBAMYLATION

Cyanate is able to react with amino, sulfhydryl, carboxyl, phenolic hydroxyl, imidazole, and phosphate groups in proteins according to the general scheme, RXH + HNCO = RXCONH$_2$. Cyanate is easily soluble in water. Most reactions have a pH optimum around 7. Acidic pH should be avoided as acidic conditions are ideal for modifications of carboxyl groups. For the same reason reactions with cyanate should not be terminated with acid. At high concentrations cyanate may react with itself to form cyanuric acid and cyamelide and it is recommended to work at concentrations about 0.2 M. Cyanate reacts rapidly with amino groups. At neutral pH and below the α-amino group can be expected to react about 100 times faster than the α-amino group. The resulting carbamoylamino groups are stable even in dilute NaOH. Typical reaction conditions are 3 mg/mL protein, 0.1 M cyanate at pH 8, 25°C for 1 h. Cyanate also reacts even more rapidly with sulfhydryl groups than amino groups resulting in the formation of S-carbamylcysteine residues. Since cyanate reacts rapidly with sulfhydryl groups, labile disulfide bonds may be ruptured. The resulting carbamylmercaptans decompose readily to free mercaptan and cyanate at alkaline pH. Consequently, cyanate can be used as reversible blocking agent for –SH groups. At acidic pH cyanate reacts with carboxylic groups under formation of a mixed anhydride, which can react with many nucleophiles (e.g., formation of amides). The reaction can be avoided entirely at pH 7 to 8. Aliphatic hydroxyl is resistant to carbamylation even at high cyanate concentrations at low pH. However, the reactive hydroxyl groups of chymotrypsin and other proteases react with cyanate to give urethans. Phenolic hydroxyl groups react more readily than aliphatic groups in a reversible reaction that is quite analogous to the one that occurs with –SH groups.

Cyanate present in aqueous urea solutions reacts with the free amino and sulfhydryl groups of proteins. Urea is often tacitly assumed to be a reagent, which alters the structure of the protein and may be used to keep target proteins in their monomeric form during purification. However, at pH 6 and above urea hydrolyzes under formation of cyanate leads to carbamylation reactive groups in proteins.

The equilibrium $(NH_2)_2CO = NH_4CNO$ between an undissociated urea and dissociated cyanate in aqueous urea solutions is the main course of unintended carbamylation of primary amino groups in proteins. As the protein concentration normally is from 0.1 to 30 mg/mL corresponding to the μM range, a considerable part of the protein mass is expected to undergo carbamylation under these conditions. Thus, the exposure of ribonuclease to cyanate in aqueous solution leads to a considerable loss of enzymatic activity. Formation of cyanate is prevented by storage of neutral urea solutions at 4°C or by buffering the solution at pH 4.7. Thus, acidification of urea solutions just before use will decompose any cyanate present. Cyanate can be removed from urea solutions by mixed ion exchange chromatography. The method of Salinas describes a sensitive and specific method for quantitative estimation of carbamylation in proteins (see Bibliography).

β-Elimination

The β-elimination reaction is caused by the abstraction of a β-hydrogen from cystinyl, seryl, and threonyl residues under alkaline conditions. The cystinyl residue decomposes as a result of β-elimination under formation of HS⁻ and free sulfur thus affecting the redox potential of the solution. Several studies indicate that the rate of reaction is proportional to the hydroxide ion concentration and pH should consequently be kept low (use dilute NaOH solutions to adjust pH preferably below 0.1M NaOH). In alkaline solutions the abstraction of β-hydrogen from cystinyl, seryl, and threonyl residues result in formation of a carbanion. Depending on the nature of the side-chain, the carbanion can rearrange to form an unsaturated derivative (dehydroalanine or β-methyl-dehydroalanine) or add a proton to give the L- and D-amino acid residues (racemization). The derivatives formed are reactive with a number of nucleophilic protein groups. The reaction is independent of the primary structure of the protein. The indicators of β-elimination include degradation of the protein, cleavage of disulfide bridges, and smell of sulfur. Preventive actions against β-elimination are listed in Table 11.5.

Racemization

All amino acid residues except glycine are subject to racemization at alkaline pH, resulting in formation of the D-enantiomers of the residue. Racemization is inevitably associated with conformational changes and thereby loss of function. The racemization of proteins has been described in several reports. The initial step of the reaction is abstraction of the β-hydrogen by hydroxide ions. Uptake of a proton will result in either the L- or D-amino acid residue. The carbanion formed may also undergo β-elimination. At pH 5 to 12 Asn, Asp, Gln, and Glu may modify via a succinimidyl intermediate resulting in both the D- and L-derivatives. The indicators of racemization include

TABLE 11.5
Factors and Their Control to Prevent β-Elimination

Factor	Comment
pH	pH should be kept below 10. Do not use NaOH solutions above 0.1 M to adjust pH.
Temperature	High temperature even at pH 4 to 8 results in β-elimination.
Time	The β-elimination reaction is a function of time.
Conductivity	Increased ionic strength increases the rate of β-elimination.
Redox potential	Cystinyl rich proteins may decompose under formation of HS^-, which will lower the redox potential of the solution. Reduction of disulfide bonds may result.
Cosolvents	Removal of divalent metal ions with EDTA.

TABLE 11.6
Factors and Their Control to Prevent Racemization

Factor	Comment
pH	High pH will favor abstraction of the β-hydrogen under formation of a carbanion. pH should be kept below 10 and use of NaOH in concentration above 0.1 M should be avoided when adjusting pH.
Temperature	The temperature should be kept low.
Time	The reaction is a function of time.
Conductivity	No data are available.
Redox potential	No data are available.
Cosolvents	No data are available.

change of protein structure and loss of biological activity. The change in optical rotation correlates with the rate of racemization. The amino acid residues undergo racemization at different rates. Preventive actions against racemization are listed in Table 11.6.

CYSTINYL RESIDUES

The reactive site of the cystinyl residue is the thiol group, which is deprotonated at alkaline pH (pKa around 8.5). The residue is under oxidizing conditions (and neutral to alkaline pH) and able to react with a similar residue under formation of a disulfide bond. Many proteins are stabilized by intramolecular disulfide bonds (e.g., insulin, growth hormone, IGF-1), but intermolecular bonds may also result from the reaction under formation of aggregates. In order to avoid unintended disulfide bond formation/cleavage, the redox potential of the solution must be monitored and controlled. In practice, aqueous buffers contain μ-molar amounts of dissolved oxygen, ensuring a redox potential of 200 to 600 mV, which is sufficient to maintain the intramolecular disulfide bonds. Proteins with free cysteines may prefer slightly reducing conditions, which can be obtained by addition of μ-molar amounts of reducing agent (e.g., cystine or DTT). The number of proteins containing both — SH groups and disulfide bonds — is relatively small (e.g., albumin, β-lactoglobulin). In many cases the disulfide bond stabilization is essential for maintaining the biological activity. Ribonuclease, for example, loses almost all activity when the four disulfide bonds are reduced. The mechanism of reaction involves cystinyl and cystinyl residues in the disulfide bond formation by oxidation or reduction, conversion of a cystinyl residue to a cystinyl residue, and a sulfenic/sulfonic acid residue at alkaline pH and decomposition to a dehydroalanine residue at alkaline pH (-elimination reaction). Disulfide bond formation is often catalyzed by the presence of a mercapto reagent (e.g., DTT, cystine) in mM concentrations (typically 1 to 10 mM). Controlled disulfide bond formation has gained much attention in the biopharmaceutical industry in connection

TABLE 11.7
Factors and Their Control to Prevent Cystinyl Residue Loss

Factor	Comment
pH	Minimum reactivity should be expected in the pH range 3 to 7. The reactivity of the –SH group is at maximum above the pKa (8.5), where the group is deprotonated. In strongly acidic media the reaction is expected to take place via a sulfenium cation by an electrofil displacement.
Protein concentration	The intramolecular disulfide bond formation is a first order reaction and thus independent of protein concentration. Intermolecular reactions via the cystinyl residue may be affected by the protein concentration (aggregation). The aggregation rate is favored by high protein concentration.
Temperature	The temperature should be kept low (4 to 20°C) especially at pH above 9.5.
Time	The reaction is a function of time.
Conductivity	No data available.
Redox potential	Reducing conditions favor free cystinyl residues. Oxidizing conditions favor disulfide bonds. The redox potential is a function of pH (60 mV/pH unit).
Cosolvents	Cystine (nonanimal origin) is recommended as a reducing agent for large-scale operations. Divalent metal ions should be removed by EDTA.

with *in vitro* folding of proteins expressed in *E. coli*. Presence of divalent metal ions (typically Cu^{++}) may result in oxidation of cystinyl residues by an ill-defined reaction mechanism. Cleavage of the disulfide bond is initiated by an attack on a sulfur atom by a nucleophile reagent (HS^-, RS^-, CN^-, SO_3^{--}, OH^-). The reaction, which takes place at neutral to alkaline pH, consists of two steps with a formation of a mixed disulfide as the intermediary step. The indicators of cystinyl residues include intermolecular disulfide bond formation resulting in aggregation, under reducing conditions the disulfide bonds destabilize, resulting in conversion of cystinyl to cystinyl residues (*in vitro* refolding may be the only solution to reestablish the correct disulfide bonds), presence of scrambled and structural altered forms, and smell of sulfur. Be careful when adjusting pH with high concentrations of NaOH. Locally high pH may facilitate β-elimination. Preventive actions against cystinyl residue loss are listed in Table 11.7.

HYDROLYSIS

The peptide bond is not undergoing significant hydrolysis in the pH interval (3 to 9.5) usually used in industrial downstream processing. However, in dilute acid, where the carboxyl group of aspartyl residues is not dissociated, the peptide bond is cleaved 100 times faster than other peptide bonds and especially the –Asp-Pro- sequence is prone for degradation. The guanidinium group of arginine is hydrolyzed by OH⁻ to give ornithine and possibly some citrulline, depending on the nature of the protein. The mechanism of hydrolysis includes hydrolysis of the peptide bond, hydrolysis of the amide group of Asn and Gln, and hydrolysis of the guanidine group from Arg residues, resulting in the formation of ornithine residues (hydroxide ion catalyzed). The indicators of hydrolysis include formation of split products and formation of a split product of identical molecular weight (the peptide fragments are linked via disulfide bonds). Actions to prevent hydrolysis are summarized in Table 11.8.

DENATURATION

The native protein molecule loses its tertiary structure upon denaturation, resulting in a population of partially unfolded molecules. In practice the denaturation process will lead to a mixture of more or less unfolded molecules comprising residual secondary structure elements (helix, β-sheet, β-turn, cis-trans isomery around the prolinyl residue). A population of random coil molecules should not be expected even under strong denaturing and reducing conditions. Upon denaturation the inner

TABLE 11.8

Factors and Their Control to Prevent Hydrolysis

Factor	Comment
pH	The Asp-peptide bonds are prone to degradation at acidic pH.
	Deamidation of Asn and Gln at pH above 5. Arg is converted to ornithine by OH⁻ in a concentration-dependent manner
Temperature	The deamidation rate increases with increasing temperature.
Time	The degradation reactions are a function of time.
Conductivity	The ionic strength of the solution should be kept low in order to prevent deamidation. At high ionic strength the deamidation reaction can be fast even at neutral pH.
Redox potential	No data available.
Cosolvents	No data available.

hydrophobic core of the protein molecule is exposed to the hydrophilic environment (solvent water) often resulting in (irreversible) aggregation of the target protein. The cooperativity of the denaturation process results in an abrupt transition from the native to the unfolded state within a narrow range of pH, temperature, ionic strength, and denaturant concentration, meaning that protein denaturation may come quickly and unexpectedly. As globular proteins are only marginally stable in aqueous solutions, parameter interactions should be well understood and described using for example factorial design experiments. Proteins with disulfide bonds may undergo unfolding under reducing conditions, where the covalent bond is cleaved.

A denatured protein may be brought back to its native form by *in vitro* folding. The folding process is often slow and yields can be poor. As each protein is unique, the *in vitro* folding conditions must be determined case by case, often using specific cosolvents as additives. An example is the group of proteins where disulfide bonds must be reestablished as part of the renaturation process.

Hydrogen bonds and intramolecular interactions (electrostatic, van der Waals) are stabilizing the native structure of the protein in a cooperative manner. Upon denaturation, the cooperative effect is lost, resulting in unfolding of the molecule and exposure of the inner hydrophobic core to the hydrophilic aqueous environment. For small globular proteins denaturation it is an almost all-or-none process approximated rather well by the two-stage transition. Thermodynamically, the denaturation process can be observed by an increase of molar heat capacity and a rapid enthalpy increase with increasing temperature. The primary structure (amino acid sequence) is not affected by denaturation. The indicators of denaturation include loss of structure and loss of biological activity and aggregation. Prevention methods for denaturation are given in Table 11.9.

AGGREGATION

Protein aggregation is a major problem in the purification and formulation of protein biopharmaceuticals. Two types of intermolecular reactions dominate: aggregation resulting from hydrophobic interactions and aggregation stemming from intermolecular disulfide bond formation between cystinyl residues.

Proteins exposed to even mildly denaturing conditions may partially unfold, resulting in exposure of hydrophobic residues to the aqueous solvent favoring aggregation. The aggregation process is assumed to be controlled by the initial dimerization step in a second-order reaction. Consequently, high protein concentrations will increase the aggregation rate.

Intermolecular disulfide bond formation between cystinyl residues takes place at alkaline pH under oxidizing conditions. Proteins with reactive free thiol groups should be purified under reducing conditions (typically 1 to 10 mM reducing agent) in the presence of EDTA. Even proteins

TABLE 11.9
Factors and Their Control to Prevent Denaturation

Factor	Comment
pH	Loss of tertiary structure should be expected at pH above 9.5. Proteins tend to be most stable near the isoelectric point.
Temperature	The unfolding process is a function of temperature. Many proteins have optimal stability in the temperature range 10 to 30°C. Loss of structure should be expected both at low temperatures (cold denaturation) and at elevated temperatures. The reason that many protein biopharmaceuticals are stored at low temperatures is to minimize chemical degradation (e.g., deamidation).
Time	The denaturation reaction can be very fast.
Conductivity	No data available.
Redox potential	Cleavage of disulfide bonds should be expected under reducing conditions. A redox potential below 100 mV is considered unstable for some proteins (e.g., insulin). Not all proteins will undergo conformational changes upon reduction of the disulfide bond(s).
Cosolvents	Sucrose, mannose, glucose, glycine, alanine, glutamine, and ammonium sulfate are examples of compounds acting as protein stabilizers (weak or no binding to the protein surface).
	Magnesium sulfate, guanidinium sulfate, sodium chloride, and other weakly interacting salts will exhibit an effect depending on protein charge and concentration.
	Polyethylene glycol (PEG) and 2-methyl-2,4-pentanediol (MPD) act as stabilizers due to steric exclusion and repulsion from charged groups. Both PEG and MPD may destabilize the protein under certain circumstances, where binding is favored over exclusion.
	Cosolvents such as urea or guanidinium chloride, which binds strongly to the protein surface, are strong denaturants).

with disulfide bonds may participate in intermolecular disulfide bond reactions due to disulfide bond shuffling at neutral and alkaline pH.

Expression of proteins in *E. coli* often results in the formation of insoluble aggregates called inclusion bodies, probably comprising fully or partially unfolded protein. Inclusion bodies are brought to their monomeric form by extraction with a denaturant (e.g., 8 M urea) under reducing conditions (e.g., 0.1 M cysteine).

The mechanism of reaction is primarily hydrophobic interaction or interaction via disulfide formation. Exposure of hydrophobic residues to the surface of the molecule leads to disorganization of the surrounding water molecules, thus increasing the entropy of the system. In order to avoid the change of the hydration shell structure, the protein molecules are forced to aggregate. The aggregation reaction can be very fast and will, in severe cases, lead to formation of insoluble polymers. The dominant mechanism is presumably specific interaction of certain conformations of intermediates rather than nonspecific coaggregation. Proteins comprising free thiol groups may form intermolecular disulfide bonds, leading to aggregation of the protein. The reaction takes place at alkaline pH (presence of $-S^-$) under oxidizing conditions. Indicators of aggregation include loss of structure and biological activity, turbid solution, presence of fibrils in the solution, precipitation, and formation of gels. Formation of inclusion bodies in *E. coli* is an example of *in vivo* protein aggregates. Hydrophobic protein aggregates will often dissolve at high pH (> 11). Intermolecular disulfide aggregates may dissolve under reducing conditions (presence of DTT, cystine, or the like). Prevention strategies for aggregation are listed in Table 11.10.

PRECIPITATION

Protein precipitates are aggregates large enough to be visible. However, in practice aggregates not visible by the naked eye may result in severe problems as filters and chromatographic columns can be blocked.

TABLE 11.10
Factors and Their Control to Prevent Aggregation

Factor	Comment
pH	High pH should be avoided in order to prevent protein unfolding. Some proteins do change conformation as a function of pH and certain pH intervals should be avoided. PH < 7 will protect the protein from intermolecular disulfide bond formation.
Temperature	The unfolding process is a function of temperature. Many proteins have optimal stability in the temperature range 10 to 30°C. Loss of structure should be expected both at low temperatures (cold denaturation) and at elevated temperatures.
Protein concentration	Low protein concentrations should be favored.
Time	The aggregation reaction can be very fast.
Conductivity	No data available.
Redox potential	Oxidizing conditions results in formation of disulfide bonds and intermolecular interactions should be expected. Reducing conditions will prevent intermolecular disulfide bond formation.
Cosolvents	Denaturing or destabilizing agents (e.g., urea, certain alcohols, organic solvents) should be used with care. Detergents may prevent aggregation, but they often bind strongly to the protein.

Protein precipitation is typically observed at high ionic strength, in the presence of organic solvents, or close to the isoelectric point, where solubility is low due to the zero net charge of the protein. Presence of precipitates is not always easily observed. Typical markers are presence of large, often white particles or flocculates, a turboid appearance, fibrils, or increased viscosity.

Unintended precipitation can be difficult to predict as the effect depends on a combination of the distribution of hydrophilic and hydrophobic residues on the proteins surface, the pH, ionic strength, protein concentration, temperature, and composition of the aqueous phase. A perfectly clear solution may gradually become turbid during application to a chromatographic column, resulting in column blocking.

The mechanism of precipitation involves salting out, iso-precipitation, or the presence of polar solvents. In most cases high salt concentrations will lead to precipitation of the protein. The process is largely dependent on the hydrophobicity of the protein, and the optimal salts are those favoring dehydration of the nonpolar regions without binding to the protein. At zero net charge of the protein, the electrostatic repulsion between the molecules is minimal. Therefore, proteins tend to precipitate near the pI of the molecule. Addition of nonpolar organic solvents reduces the water activity. The organic solvent reducing the hydrophobic attraction will displace the water molecules around hydrophobic areas. The principal forces leading to precipitation are, therefore, likely to be electrostatic forces and dipolar van der Waals forces. The indicators of precipitation include cloudy solution and precipitation of solid material (the precipitates often appear white). The Hofmeister series provides the impact of various cations and anions:

Cations:

$$NH_4^+ > K^+ > Na^+ > Li^+ > Mg^{++} > Ca^{++} > Gdn^+$$

Anions:

$$SO_4^{--} > HPO_4^{--} > CH_3COO^- > Cl^- > NO_3^- > SCN^-$$

The ions to the left in the series exert a stabilizing effect on proteins. The ions to the right may bind to the protein surface and thereby destabilize the protein. The effect of the ions is additive. Ammonium sulfate is a stabilizing salt often used for precipitation of proteins (2 to 3 M solution). Gdn-sulfate is a stabilizing salt, while Gdn-chloride is a strong denaturant.

TABLE 11.11
Factors and Their Control to Prevent Precipitation

Factor	Comment
pH	The protein solubility is minimal near the iso-electric point.
	A change in pH may affect the redox potential of the solution, the protein solubility, and the protein stability.
Temperature	High temperature increases the conformational flexibility and organic solvents may more easily penetrate the internal structure of the protein.
Protein concentration	Low protein concentration will protect the protein from precipitation; concentrations below 0.1 mg/mL may be necessary to avoid precipitation.
Time	Precipitation is a function of time. Always determine the holding time for a given sample to ensure precipitates are not formed during storage.
Conductivity	High ionic strength normally results in protein precipitation. Keep the salt concentration low to moderate, but at the same time, be aware of the "salting in" effect. Ions such as NH_4^+ do stabilize the protein upon precipitation.
Cosolvents	Typical protein precipitation agents are salts (e.g., ammonium sulfate), polyethylene glycols (e.g., PEG 20000), polyelectrolytes (e.g., carboxymethyl cellulose), and organic solvents (e.g., acetone).

Precipitation is commonly used as a purification tool in downstream processing, as the biological activity is rarely affected by this procedure (organic solvents may result in denaturation). Iso-precipitation becomes more effective by adding alcohols or polyalcohols to the solvent. pH adjustment may result in unintended iso-precipitation of the protein. Passing the iso-electric point does not affect the biological activity or stability of the protein (in most cases), and the protein will normally enter into solution again 2 to 3 pH units from the pI. Precipitates may form hours after the protein solution has been prepared or adjusted. The precipitates are not always visible. Because the particles may result in blocking of filters and chromatographic columns, unintended precipitation in application samples constitutes a great problem in downstream processing. Table 11.11 lists the preventive measures for precipitation.

DOCUMENTATION

Regulatory filings often comprise truck-loads of documentation. This documentation is supposed to support technology transfer from research over to manufacturing of material for clinical trials. Although the major part of the development information and data gathered is not a part of the material submitted to regulatory authorities, it was a natural choice to use the structure of the Common Technical Document, ICH, section 3.2. A comprehensive regulatory filing will include documents related to authentication (sponsor's identification), the identification of the project (including the identification of the staff and facility participating), general characteristics of the protein, and the description of manufacturing and testing facilities (see The Common Technical Document, ICH Section 3.2.S. [NTA 2B, CTD module 3, July 2001]).

The control of materials (reagents, enzymes, substrates, solvents, catalysts, etc.) used in the process must be described in detail. It is common practice to establish a list of raw materials prior to the up-scaling program. The required information about the raw materials includes:

- Raw material name
- Manufacturer
- Lot number
- Batch number

- Raw material description
- Raw material accept criteria
- Analytical test methods
- Stability of the raw material
- Release procedure(s)
- Regulatory support files for chromatographic media
- Reference to EP and USP
- Where in the process is the raw material used
- Clearance control of adventitious agents
- Control of source and starting materials of biologic origin
- Source, history, and generation of cell substrate
- Cell banking system, characterization and testing.

The process is presented in the form a flow sheet, which is a rather detailed overview of the downstream process preferably using diagrams and boxes that identify: unit operations in sequential order; unit operation number; protocol reference; where in the process the raw material is introduced; where the raw material is removed; parameter intervals of each unit operation; critical parameters; buffer composition and description; chromatographic media used; and filters and membranes used. The details about this arrangement are available in the ICH CTD (www.nihs.go.jp/dig/ich/m4index-e.html; section 3.2.S. [NTA 2B, CTD module 3, July 2001]).

The rationale and strategy report is a final document describing the rationale and strategy behind the drug development program and process design. The report should be written at the initiation of the experimental process development work. The laboratory notebook is a written record of the laboratory work performed. It is a final document.

The laboratory notebooks are part of a suggested process development documentation system comprising the rationale and strategy report, the laboratory notebooks, the summary reports, the unit operation reports, the unit operation protocols and the development report. Specific rules regarding keeping records in laboratory books should be observed.

A summary report describes a study related to the process development, the development of an analytical method, or other specific development issues that need to be addressed during drug substance development. Usually, the summary report is a short and concise final document that summarizes the results from a development study shortly after the study has been performed. Typical examples are: reports describing a factorial design experiment, a unit operation optimization, chemical modifications of the protein, semisynthesis, and technical investigations.

The unit operation document describes the development work related to a given unit operation. The aim is to collect all information of relevance in one document, giving easy access to overview the rationale of the unit operation protocol. The report is a final document providing a status at the time of tech transfer from development to pilot.

The unit operation protocol is a live document describing the state of art of the unit operation. The combined collections of unit operation protocols comprise the manufacturing procedure of the drug substance batches produced.

The development report is the overall development document summarizing the drug development program.

All of these reports are part of a suggested process development documentation system comprising the rationale and strategy report, the laboratory notebooks, the summary reports, the unit operation reports, the unit operation protocols, and the development report.

A structural characterization report describes the analytical method used to characterize the structure of the drug substance. The structural characterization reports are part of the suggested drug substance quality control program comprising quality control and characterization methods.

The report on control of drug substance suggests the content of an analytical method report. The report will develop from a method description over qualification to a fully validated report.

The reference material is an internal standard used as a working standard during development and early phase production for clinical trials. The reference material precedes the reference standard normally established during production for Phase III clinical material.

12 Intellectual Property Issues

The Congress shall have Power ...To promote the Progress of Science and useful Arts, by securing for limited Times to Authors and Inventors the exclusive Right to their respective Writings and Discoveries.

— The U.S. Constitution

Everything that can be invented has been invented.

— Charles H. Duell, U.S. Patent Office Director, telling President McKinley to abolish the office in 1899. [Note: Until 1836 the U.S. Patent and Trademark Office had issued 9,957 patents; from 1837 to November 2004, it issued over 6.8 million patents.]

The development of new pharmaceutical or biotechnology derived products undergoes a lengthy and expensive cycle, which is adequately described elsewhere in this book. Given the cost of development now hovering around the billion dollar mark for each new drug, amortized over all other molecules racing, the only way to protect this investment is to create intellectual property claims to not only the active molecule but where possible, each and every step of its production, processing, and testing. Almost 4% of the development cost is spent on filing and prosecuting patents.

Typically, the research-based pharmaceutical companies spend about 15 to 20% of their total sales revenue on developing new drugs, as compared with less than 4% for the industry overall; the cost of patent protection ranges between 1 to 3% of the R&D expenditure. Successful patenting, patent protection, and exploitation of expired patents involve a complex interaction among scientists and lawyers. Generally, the development teams should have a basic understanding of the patenting process to be able to make the best use of legal expertise in the field; the more complex the field is, the more input from scientists becomes valuable. In this chapter, I describe the fundamentals of patenting that I consider important enough for scientists, administrators, and marketing personnel to understand well.

PATENTING SYSTEMS AND STRATEGIES

A patent is a grant by the state of exclusive rights for a limited time in respect of a new and useful invention; rights to prevent others from making or selling the invention (see later on making vis-à-vis the Food and Drug Administration) in a limited territory as defined by the patent issuing authority. It is not necessarily a right to practice an invention by the inventor. The word "patent" means "open," from the word, "letter patent," meaning an announcement to all that the inventor has been awarded rights to the invention. Open here means without having to break any seal as was the custom in the decrees issued by the sovereign governments and royalties. Note that "letters patent" are not restricted to inventions as even today these are issued to appoint judges in the U.K. Historically, patents were issued on elaborate stationary, and they still are to some extent. The point about the rights to exercise an invention vis-à-vis prevent others from practicing needs further elaboration. The new chemical entity patent for sildenafil citrate expired in March 2003; the use and composition patents listed for sildenafil citrate in the Orange Book (Food and Drug Administration) extend to 2012 and 2019; 17 U.S. patents issued to Pfizer on the various aspects of sildenafil citrate; a total of 44 patents making claims for sildenafil citrate including its use in Tourette's syndrome to its chewing gum formulations that require chewing the gum for not less than two minutes, etc.

The example of erythropoietin demonstrates how the patent laws can create great difficulties for biogeneric offering. For example, the following issued claims exemplify the numerous ways in which patent protection relating to a protein may be obtained.

U.S. Patent No. 5,621,080: An isolated erythropoietin glycoprotein having the *in vivo* biological activity of causing bone marrow cells to increase production of reticulocytes and red blood cells, wherein said erythropoietin glycoprotein comprises the mature erythropoietin amino acid sequence of FIG. 6 and has glycosylation which differs from that of human urinary erythropoietin.

U.S. Patent No. 6,048,971: A secretable mutant human erythropoietin protein having an amino acid residue which differs from the amino acid residue present in the corresponding position in wild type human erythropoietin, the amino acid residue of said wild type erythropoietin selected from the group consisting of: amino acid residue 103, amino acid residue 104, and amino acid residue 108.

U.S. Patent No. 5,955,422: A pharmaceutical composition comprising a therapeutically effective amount of human erythropoietin and a pharmaceutically acceptable diluent, adjuvant, or carrier, wherein said erythropoietin is purified from mammalian cells grown in culture.

U.S. Patent No. 4,703,008: A purified and isolated DNA sequence encoding erythropoietin, said DNA sequence selected from the group consisting of: a. the DNA sequences set out in FIGS. 5 and 6 or their complementary strands; and b. DNA sequences which hybridize under stringent conditions to the DNA sequences defined in (a). & 4. A prokaryotic or eukaryotic host cell transformed or transfected with a DNA sequence according to claim [1] in a manner allowing the host cell to express erythropoietin.

U.S. Patent No. 5,618,698: A process for the preparation of an *in vivo* biologically active erythropoietin product comprising the steps of growing, under suitable nutrient conditions, host cells transformed or transfected with an isolated DNA sequence selected from the group consisting of (1) the DNA sequences set out in FIGS. 5 and 6, (2) the protein coding sequences set out in FIGS. 5 and 6, and (3) DNA sequences which hybridize under stringent conditions to the DNA sequences defined in (1) and (2) or their complementary strands; and isolating said erythropoietin product therefrom.

U.S. Patent No. 5,641,670: A homologously recombinant cell having incorporated therein a new transcription unit, wherein the new transcription unit comprises an exogenous regulatory sequence, an exogenous exon and a splice-donor site, operatively linked to the second exon of an endogenous gene, wherein the homologously recombinant cell comprises said exogenous exon in addition to exons present in said endogenous gene.

The homologously recombinant cell of claim [1] wherein the endogenous gene encodes a protein selected from the group consisting of erythropoietin, calcitonin, growth hormone, insulin, insulinotropin, insulin-like growth factors, parathyroid hormone, beta-interferon, gamma-interferon, nerve growth factors, FSH-beta, TGF-beta, tumor necrosis factor, glucagon, bone growth factor-2, bone growth factor-7, TSH-beta, interleukin 1, interleukin 2, interleukin 3, interleukin 6, interleukin 11, interleukin 12, CSF-granulocyte, CSF-macrophage, CSF-granulocyte/macrophage, immunoglobulins, catalytic antibodies, protein kinase C, glucocerebrosidase, superoxide dismutase, tissue plasminogen activator, urokinase, antithrombin III, DNAse, alpha-galactosidase, tyrosine hydroxylase, blood clotting factor V, blood clotting factor VII, blood clotting factor VIII, blood clotting factor IX, blood clotting factor X, blood clotting factor XIII, apolipoprotein E, apolipoprotein A-I, globins, low density lipoprotein receptor, IL-2 receptor, IL-2 antagonists, alpha-1 antitrypsin, immune response modifiers, and soluble CD4.

U.S. Patent No. 6,048,524: A method of expressing erythropoietin in a mammal, comprising the steps of:

obtaining a source of primary cells from a mammal;

transfecting primary cells obtained in (a) with a DNA construct comprising exogenous DNA encoding erythropoietin and additional DNA sequences sufficient for expression of the exogenous DNA in the primary cells, thereby producing transfected primary cells which express the exogenous DNA encoding erythropoietin;

culturing a transfected primary cell produced in (b), which expresses the exogenous DNA encoding erythropoietin, under conditions appropriate for propagating the transfected primary cell which expresses the exogenous DNA encoding erythropoietin, thereby producing a clonal cell strain of transfected secondary cells from the transfected primary cell;

culturing the clonal cell strain of transfected secondary cells produced in (c) under conditions appropriate for and sufficient time for the clonal cell strain of transfected secondary cells to undergo a sufficient number of doublings to provide a sufficient number of transfected secondary cells to produce erythropoietin; and

introducing transfected secondary cells produced in (d) into a mammal of the same species as the mammal from which the primary cells were obtained in sufficient number to express erythropoietin in the mammal.

U.S. Patent No. 4,397,840: A method for the preparation of an erythropoietin product having no inhibitory effect against erythropoiesis which comprises the steps of:

adsorbing a crude erythropoietin product obtained from the urine of healthy human on to a weakly basic anion exchanger from a neutral or weakly acidic aqueous solution in the presence of an inorganic neutral salt in a concentration in the range from 0.1 to 0.2 mole per liter, and

eluting the thus adsorbed erythropoietin product with an aqueous eluant solution containing an inorganic neutral salt in a concentration in the range from 0.5 to 0.7 moles per liter.

U.S. Patent No. 4,667,016: A process for the efficient recovery of erythropoietin from a fluid, said process comprising the following steps in sequence: subjecting the fluid to ion exchange chromatographic separation at about pH 7.0, thereby to selectively bind erythropoietin in said sample to a cationic resin; stabilizing materials bound to said resin against degradation by acid activated proteases; selectively eluting bound contaminant materials having a pKa greater than that of erythropoietin by treatment with aqueous acid at a pH of from about 4.0 to 6.0; and selectively eluting erythropoietin by treatment with an aqueous salt at a pH of about 7.0; and isolating erythropoietin-containing eluent fractions.

U.S. Patent No. 6,001,800: A method for preparing spray dried recombinant human erythropoietin (rhEPO), comprising:

Providing an aqueous solution of rhEPO having a concentration within the range of about 20 mg/ml to about 100 mg/ml;

Atomizing said solution into a spray;

Drying said spray with hot drying air in order to evaporate the water from the spray to form a dried rhEPO; and

Separating dried rhEPO from the drying air to provide biologically active spray dried rhEPO.

U.S. Patent No. 5,629,175: A method for producing a mammalian peptide which comprises: growing tobacco plant cells containing an integrated sequence comprising, a first expression cassette having the direction of transcription (1) a transcriptional and translational initiation region functional in said plant cells, (2) a structural gene coding for said mammalian peptide, and (3) a termination region, whereby said structural gene is expressed to produce said mammalian peptide.

U.S. Patent No. 5,780,709: A method to increase water stress resistance or tolerance in a monocot plant, comprising: introducing into cells of a monocot plant an expression cassette comprising a preselected DNA segment comprising an mtlD gene, operably linked to a promoter function in the monocot plant cells to yield transformed monocot plant cells; and b) regenerating a differentiated fertile plant from said transformed cells, where in the mtlD gene is expressed in the cells of the plant so as to render the transformed monocot plant substantially tolerant or resistant to reduction in water availability that inhibits the growth of an untransformed monocot plant.

THE PATENT LAWS

It is noteworthy that patents are awarded for things or "*res*," which must have some use; there need not be any rationale provided why and an invention works, obviously it must meet all statutory requirements to be eligible for patenting (see below). The patent laws are extremely complex, often inexplicably irrational and in almost all instances questionable in their enforcement.

The following definitions and terms are commonly used in describing patent laws:

- Invention: An invention is the conception of a new and useful article, machine, composition, or process.
- Patent Application: A document describing an invention in detail, which is to be submitted to a patent office with the aim of obtaining a patent on the invention.
- Patent: Right of ownership granted by the government to a person that gives the owner the right to exclude others from making, selling, or using the claimed invention.
- Reduction to Practice: An in-depth description of how the invention works, described in concrete terms.
- Prior Art: The existing or publicly available knowledge available before the date of an invention or more than one year prior to the first patent application date.
- Utility: This is the most common type of patent. It includes inventions that operate in a new and useful manner.
- Design: The emphasis of this type of patent is on the design of the invention, not on its functionality. What is important with this type of patent is the invention's unique ornamental and aesthetic properties.
- Plant: This type of patent includes new varieties of asexually reproduced plants.
- Actual Reduction to Practice: Constructing the machine or article, synthesizing the composition, or performing the method and testing sufficiently to demonstrate that the invention works for its intended purpose. Testing is *not* required if one of ordinary skill in the art would recognize that it will work.
- Constructive Reduction to Practice: Filing a U.S. patent application — in compliance with the first paragraph of §112.
- Diligence: Working on reducing the invention either into practice or considering it abandoned.

The patenting of inventions is a complex process that has historically been confused, particularly by the inventors who may not be practitioners of patent law. For example:

- Patents are valuable only if they can be used to protect a profit stream by excluding others from making, using, or selling whatever is covered by the patent's claims.
- Having a patent does not mean that the invention works as verified by the government; it is left for the licensors to evaluate. It is suspected that as many as 10% of all issued patents are invalid for being nonfunctional as claimed.
- You cannot get a Provisional Patent, there is nothing like this. You can file a Provisional Patent Application for a small fee that allows you 12 months to file a regular application

while protecting your priority. A Provisional Application is not "just describing the idea," it is a complete application except the required claim(s). You may not change anything in the text when you file the regular application if you want to take priority advantage.

- You cannot get a patent for an idea or mere suggestion. Patents are granted to people who (claim to) "invent or discover any new and useful process, machine, manufacture, or composition of matter, or any new and useful improvement thereof" to quote the essence of the U.S. statute governing patents. Complete and enabling disclosure is also required.

- A patent can be enforceable from the time it issues until it expires, not necessarily 20 years. New rules provide some guarantee that the enforceable term of a utility patent will be at least 17 years and that some royalties may be collectable when a patent is published before it issues. Design patents are good for only 14 years and only cover the ornamental appearance of the item and not its structure or functionality.

- A patent does not give the owner the exclusive right to make, use, and sell his or her invention; it gives its owner the right to *exclude* others from making, using, and selling exactly what is covered by his or her patent claims. A holder of a prior patent with broader claims may prevent the inventor whose patent has narrower claims from using the inventor's own patent. A patent right is exclusory only.

- A U.S. patent is enforceable only in the U.S. It can be used to stop others from importing what the patent covers into the U.S., but people in other countries are free to make, use, and sell the invention anywhere else in the world that the inventor does not also have a patent. This is the reason why one must consider filing a Patent Cooperative Treaty and follow it up with either individual state filings or consortium filing such as the European Patent Office.

- A patent does not protect an invention because only a patent in conjunction with a legal opinion of infringement will give the owner(s) of the patent the right to sue in a civil case against the alleged infringer. The U.S. government does not enforce patents (however, the Customs Service can help block infringing imports), and infringement of a patent is not a crime. The responsibility, and all expenses, for enforcing the rights granted by a patent (and securing Customs Service help) lie with the patent owner(s).

- Filing for a patent is not the only way to protect an invention. When properly used, the U.S. Patent and Trademark Office Disclosure Document Program ($10), Non-Disclosure Agreements (Free), and Provisional Applications for Patent ($80) along with maintaining good records and diligent pursuit can keep your patenting rights intact until you do file.

- A patent attorney or agent is not needed to file your patent; an inventor may choose to go pro se (on his own). However, given the complexity of the law, advice from professionals always proves invaluable.

TYPES OF PATENT LAWS

There are two types of patent laws: the world laws and the U.S. laws. The U.S. Congress had many options in enacting laws in accordance with the Constitution; it chose to include many unique features not found in the laws of other countries. For example, the laws in the U.S. give the inventor the recognition, and the U.S. is the only country where the patent applications must be filed by the inventor and not by an assignee such as the inventor's employer. It is for this reason that correct designation of inventorship plays such an important role in U.S. patenting, whereas in most other countries it has little or no effect on patent validity, although it may be important for other reasons such as compensation for employee inventors. This issue is of particular importance in the pharmaceutical industry where a team of researchers often works on the same invention, often members of this team move to other companies, and at times they are not available or cooperative in the filing of a patent for an invention. The U.S. patent law goes into fine detail on how to handle all of these situations.

The U.S. law further distinguishes from the world law by establishing the precedence between two patent applications claiming the same invention on the simple basis that the first to invent has priority contrary to the rest of the world where the party who files first has the precedence. This creates significant legal issues often leading to lengthy and cumbersome "interference practice," in the prosecution of patent applications establishing when the invention was made vis-à-vis when it was filed. Not only is the date of filing important, the date when a "workable" model was conceived, the period when the inventor did not "diligently" follow the development, the dates when the inventor began working again, whether this renewed interest was in response to knowledge that someone else may be working on the same invention, along with a host of other related factors exemplify the complexity of legal proceedings in the practice of patent law, particularly in the U.S.

The U.S. laws assert that there is no requirement of a working model to declare that an invention has been made; it can be a mental process wherein all essential elements of invention are present. One of the most interesting recent court decision on this issue pertained to the legal battle between Amgen and Chugai. Chugai filed prior to Amgen but Amgen could show completion of invention prior to Chugai's date of invention; Amgen won and made billions. Legal cases like this establish interpretation of the laws — the so-called patent case law history.

The development of U.S. patent law has been strongly influenced by decisions of the courts, particularly of the U.S. Supreme Court. For example, the question of "how much invention is needed to support a patent" was resolved by the U.S. Supreme Court. It was said that it is clearly wrong that patents should be granted for improvements so minor that any competent mechanic or chemist could make them as a matter of course, for this would restrict all the normal day-to-day work of the workshop or laboratory. On the other hand, it was also ascertained to be wrong that patents should be granted only for outstanding inventions that revolutionize society. Many inventions are ingenious and at least potentially useful without being world shattering, and one great merit of the patent system is that the value of the patent grant is left to be determined by market forces. It is not as if the state, in granting a patent, guarantees to the patentee that he or she will profit by it; by and large a patent for a poor invention will not be very valuable. The extreme position that only outstanding inventions should be patentable was nevertheless adopted by the Supreme Court in 1941, when Justice William Douglas condemned the grant of patents for "gadgets" as being superfluous. The Cornell University Library provides an excellent resource on patent law.

Of great importance to the pharmaceutical industry is the Drug Price Competition and Patent Restoration Act of 1984, commonly known as the Hatch–Waxman Act, which provided for extensions of patent term for human drugs, food additives, and medical devices the commercialization of which had been delayed by regulatory procedures (in the Food and Drug Administration), and at the same time made registration easier for competitors when patent protection had expired. It also provided that testing for regulatory approval involving a patented drug did not amount to patent infringement. (Amendments to this act and the Greater Access to Affordable Pharmaceuticals Act [HR-2491] are pending in the U.S. Congress.) Several legislative changes to the U.S. patent law have been made since, but the most important was certainly the Uruguay Round Amendments Act (URAA) of 1995, which made changes necessary in order to bring U.S. law into line with the TRIPS agreement (Trade Related Intellectual Property).

ANATOMY OF A PATENT

A published patent (they are published every Tuesday in the U.S.) is a legal document, not unlike the deed for a real property that describes its boundaries. Each section of printed information on the patent has a special meaning; whereas it is most useful for the attorneys, scientists also have much to gain by understanding the anatomy of a patent; it can teach them how to design their searches and how to interpret the findings of an invention. Figure 12.1 shows the front page of a typical patent. Listed here are explanations to various parts of a patent.

PATENTABILITY

There are three principal requirements for an invention to be patented as set out in the European Patent Convention: (1) That the invention must be new; (2) That it must involve an inventive step; and (3) That it must be capable of industrial application. The same three requirements are met in one form or another in the U.S., Japan, and indeed in practically every country that has a patent system at all. Some countries and conventions exclude certain inventions, but these exclusions may be forbidden under TRIPs.

First Requirement: Novelty

A patent issued for what is already known would deprive the public of its use, and it is thus not permitted. In fact, the very reason a patent is awarded is to encourage new technology to come forth. Though the concept of novelty is rather basic in the human mind, its interpretations are not. Absolute novelty, as applied by European Patent Commission, requires that an invention is new if it is not part of the "state of the art," with state of the art being defined as everything that was available to the public by written or oral publication, use, or any other way in any country in the world, before the priority date of the invention. The law, particularly the U.S. law, goes into great detail in describing what is considered "prior art." This is exemplified by a situation where a later patent application is rendered invalid by written publication anywhere in the world but by use of the invention only in the home country; that is, prior use in a foreign country would not invalidate it if there was no written description. Under the absolute novelty system, which is now the law in the U.K. and under the European Patent Commission, prior use of an invention anywhere in the world would invalidate a British or European patent application if that use made the invention available to the public. The situation is clear if the invention is a machine, a gadget, or a chemical compound or composition that can be analyzed and reproduced by the skilled person "without undue burden." In this case, sale makes the invention available to the public, and it is immaterial whether in fact anyone did investigate the workings of the machine or analyze the compound or even whether or not anyone would have any motivation for doing so. However, the use, or even the widespread sale to the public, of a complex mixture that cannot be precisely analyzed may not be held to make the invention it represents available to the public. A special situation is that of so-called selection inventions, in which an earlier publication discloses a broad class and the invention is or is not characterized by a narrower subclass. This situation may occur in mechanical inventions in which the class is a group of structural elements, one of which is selected as being particularly useful. More usually, however, selection inventions are found in the field of chemistry, where a narrow group of compounds is selected from a known broad group. So long as no members of the narrow subgroup are specifically disclosed in the publication, it is generally considered, at least in the U.K., the U.S., and the European Patent Office, that the compounds are novel, even though they may have been described in general terms. The narrow subgroup of compounds will, however, be patentable only if it has some nonobvious advantage over the other members of the broad class, that is, if there is an inventive step in choosing that particular subgroup from all those generally disclosed.

An important question in considering novelty an inventive step is the position of earlier patent applications that were not published at the priority date of a later application. Unpublished patent applications are not available to the public; and on this basis one would expect that they should not be considered as part of the state of the art. On the other hand, it has been a principle of patent law from the earliest times that not more than one patent should be granted for the same invention, since, if this were not the rule, licensees could be forced to pay twice over to obtain the same rights, and the term of patent protection for one invention could be extended beyond the statutory period.

In the European Patent Office, an earlier unpublished European application is prior art against a later one, so long as it is not withdrawn before publication and to the extent that it validly designates the same countries. This means that the earlier application may be effective in respect to some states designated in the later application, but not against others. Unpublished European patent applications designating the U.K. can be prior art against a later British national application, and an earlier unpublished British application is prior art against a granted European patent (U.K.) under British law. In the European Patent Office, however, earlier unpublished national applications are not considered as prior art against European applications.

Although under the whole-contents approach the earlier unpublished application is considered to be part of the state of the art, this applies only to considerations of pure novelty and not to the question of whether there is an inventive step. The existence of an earlier unpublished application can destroy the novelty of an invention, but it cannot be used to argue that the invention is obvious. This possibility means that under the Patents Act 1977 lack of novelty and obviousness must be clearly distinguished from each other. In early reported cases in England this was often not the case, and many patents were found invalid for lack of novelty or "anticipation," whereas the real reason was lack of an inventive step. Nowadays the term "anticipation" is normally used to mean lack of novelty, and it is considered to occur when a piece of prior art (that is, a publication or use which was part of the state of the art before the priority date of the patent application in question) either is or describes something that would be an infringement of one or more of the claims in the application. That is, the test for anticipation is essentially the same as the test for infringement, and it is met in the case of a written publication if the publication clearly describes something having every feature of the claim or gives instructions to do something that if carried out would give something falling within the scope of the claim. Thus a claim to a chemical compound may be anticipated by a description of a process if carrying out the process will inevitably give that compound, even if the compound itself was not described. However, anticipation requires "more than a signpost upon the road to the patentee's invention ... the prior inventor must be clearly shown to have planted his flag at the precise destination" (1972, RPC.457 *General Tire and Rubber Co. v. The Firestone Tire and Rubber Co.*).

Japan also has a system in which earlier unpublished Japanese applications are part of the state of the art, but with the difference that earlier unpublished applications of the same applicant are

---

(12) **United States Patent**
　　　Niazi

US006447820B1

(10) **Patent No.:**　　**US 6,447,820 B1**
(45) **Date of Patent:**　　**Sep. 10, 2002**

(54) **PHARMACEUTICAL COMPOSITION FOR THE PREVENTION AND TREATMENT OF SCAR TISSUE**

(76) Inventor: Sarfaraz K Niazi, 20 Riverside Dr., Deerfield, IL (US) 60015

(*) Notice: Subject to any disclaimer, the term of this patent is extended or adjusted under 35 U.S.C. 154(b) by 0 days.

(21) Appl. No.: 09/681,137

(22) Filed: Jan. 22, 2001

(51) Int. Cl.^{7} A61K 35/78; A61K 9/00; A61K 9/50; A01N 25/00

(52) U.S. Cl. 424/767; 424/400; 424/502; 424/725; 514/946; 514/947

(58) Field of Search 424/400, 502, 424/725, 767; 514/946, 947

(56) **References Cited**
U.S. PATENT DOCUMENTS
5,405,608 A * 4/1995 Xu 424/195.1

6,126,950 A * 10/2000 Bindra et al. 424/401

OTHER PUBLICATIONS

Johnson, T. CRC Ethnobotany Desk Reference, 1999, CRC Press LLC, p. 568.*

*cited by examiner

Primary Examiner—Leon B. Lankford, Jr.
Assistant Examiner—Kailash C. Srivastava
(74) *Attorney, Agent, or Firm*—Welsh & Katz, Ltd.

(57)　　　　**ABSTRACT**

The disclosed is a treatment of existing and prevention of new skin scars in humans and animals using a topical application containing alcoholic extracts of *Cortex Phellodendri* and *Opuntia ficus indica* in a specific combination.

5 Claims, No Drawings

FIGURE 12.1 See caption, facing page.

excluded. In the U.S., a pending patent application of an earlier date is *a priori* prior art against a later application, unless the later applicant can show that he or she had an invention date earlier than the date of filing of the earlier application. If it is prior art, it can be applied to attack both novelty and the inventive step.

A disclosure formed by combining two documents is not novelty destroying, although it may be relevant to the question of the inventive step. Indeed it is not even permissible in the European

---

FIGURE 12.1 A typical patent front page. (10) Patent Number: The number assigned to the issued patent is the best place to branch out your search, particularly the patent numbers quoted in the front page of the patent that serve as a related reference.

(12) Publication type and inventor's family or surname.

(45) Date of Patent: The date the patent was issued (always on a Tuesday) is when it becomes effective; however, know that the date when the application was published under the new rules determines if the inventors of an issued patent are eligible to claim royalties to a marketed invention if it reads on the patent claims. This date also tells you the period of exclusivity remaining in the patent.

(54) Title: Patent title describes the broadest area of invention description; it is often misleading but very useful in determining the broadest classification of the invention. Most often the title is chosen for (the) express purpose of making a random search difficult to reveal the content of a patent.

(76) Inventor: Inventor's name and address can be a very useful lead if you want to know your competitor; the same inventor often files a series of patents on an invention; this information also helps track down reissues and reexamined patents. Given under the inventor information is a notice with an asterisk indicating patent term extension or reduction granted during prosecution delays by either the U.S. Patent and Trademark Office or the applicant. Almost invariably this entry would include any additional patent term extensions granted based on regulatory delays in the approval of a health care product, which can be found in the Official Gazette or through other searches as shown below.

(21) Application No.: The Application Number assigned to a patent application can be useful in tracking down its publication prior to issuance of patent to compare if there were any changes made in the application during prosecution (something you may get through the file wrapper as well).

(22) Patent Filing Date: The date the application was filed with the Patent and Trademark Office is a critical date for §102e prior art reference; this date also tells you about how long your competitors have been working on this project; since the patent wrapper (all correspondence between the U.S. Patent and Trademark Office and the inventor or whoever is prosecuting the patent) is public information, you may want to request the wrapper, particularly if there was a long delay between the filing and issuance of patent — meaning there was some admission by the filer, which may be of use to you in establishing the patentability of your invention).

(51) International Classification: This is an important field as it allows you to do comparable international searches (more on it later); notice that there is a conversion of classification available between the U.S. and the International System.

(52) U.S. Classification: Class and subclass information, the categories that the U.S. Patent and Trademark Office uses to classify or sort the various types of inventions. These numbers mean a lot for any patentability search.

(58) Field of Search: This indicates the class or subclasses searched for the purpose of determining patentability.

(56) Reference Cited: During the prosecution, the examiner may bring several references (patents and publications) that formed the basis of defining the scope of invention; given here are the patent number and class/subclass of patents that were brought up during prosecution; most likely, you would also want to see the full text of these patents. Other publications are also cited here. It is further indicated whether these references were brought up by the examiner (marked with an asterisk). Combined with the information in the file wrapper, these references provide the most significant data on evaluating the proposed invention. The names of examiner and primary examiner are also given here; chances are if your invention is similar you will see correspondence from the same examiner or primary examiner.

(74) Attorney, Agent or Firm: Identification of who did the prosecuting can be important if you want to track down what other patents were prosecuted by the same attorney, agent, or firm. If no name is listed here or the category is not listed, this patent was filed as a pro se patent.

(57) Abstract: This is usually one concise paragraph summarizing the invention in plain English (no legalese or technical jargon is preferred here). Since this appears on the front page of the issued patent, it is the most frequently referenced section of a patent. This is one of the most craftily written pieces of language in the patent; as you prepare patent searches, you will learn how to read between lines in an abstract.

Drawings: Drawings of the invention from different perspectives; also disclosed here is the number of drawings and claims in the patent. If there are no drawings reported, you may not want to switch to patent image (unless there are chemical structures or other graphic information). The text format of a patent is more suitable for cutting and pasting in your search document; the patent image is in a noneditable *.tiff format.

Background of the Invention: This section discusses any previous inventions related to the patented invention — prior art, in legal terms. Since you are allowed to incorporate other patents by reference, you may also include this material in your own application if it suits the purpose as well. A recent patent with an extensive background section provides a wealth of information and saves great effort on the part of the filer. Read it carefully as it may disclose information that may later be used by the patent examiner as §103e information.

Summary of the Invention: This is a discussion of the invention that captures its essential functions and features; this must be read first before reading the background section.

Brief Description of Drawings: A one-sentence description of each drawing figure is useful in ascertaining whether you want to switch to an image of the patent. It is noteworthy that the U.S. Patent and Trademark Office website allows searching of patents from 1790 through 1975 only by Patent Number and Current U.S. Classification; later patents are searchable by text entries. Online patent images were made available recently.

Detailed Description: This section is generally an in-depth discussion of the various aspects of the claimed invention. Detailed references to drawings are made in this section; here you see exactly what is invented.

Claims: Analogous to the boundaries of a real estate described in a deed, the claims layout the legal scope of the patent, going down from the broadest claim to the narrowest claim. This section determines if your invention infringes on a patent (reads onto claims). This section also provides you with the vocabulary you may want to use for your own invention. Often searches are made of the claims section only to determine patentability.

Patent Office to attack novelty by combining two embodiments described in the same document, unless the document itself indicates that they should be combined. Nevertheless, the prior art document must be interpreted in the light of the common general knowledge of the skilled worker in the relevant field as at the date of publication of the document. Needless to say, there is a gray area between what is clearly common general knowledge (for example, something in a standard reference book used by everyone in the field) and what is simply another publication, and there have been many decisions on this point both in the U.K. courts and in the European Patent Office.

Conception is the formation in the mind of the inventor of a definite and permanent idea of the complete and operative invention as it is thereafter to be applied in practice. An invention date is the date when diligence began and leads to reduction to practice. Section §104 prohibited evidence outside of the U.S. prior to December 8, 1993, except for filing of a Patent Cooperative Treaty or foreign application or acts domiciled in the U.S. but serving outside of U.S. on government business. After December 8, 1993, but prior to January 1, 1996, North American Free Trade Agreement countries were included and on or after January 1, 1996, all countries of WTO were included. If there were events prior to these dates, they are taken to the dates the privileges became available. This is important for overcoming 102(a) rejections.

The U.S. Patent law goes into great detail in describing various events that can be novelty defeating as described in 35 USC §102.

Section §102 events include:

- Novelty defeating events occurring prior to invention: 102(a), (e), and (g): AGE
- Time barring events occurring more than fixed time (e.g., 1 yr) prior to United States filing date: 102(b) and (d): ABSOLUTE TIME BAR
- Miscellaneous: 102(c) and (f): OTHERS.

Section §102(a) events include:

Events by OTHERS; public knowledge and use only in United States or patented or printed publication anywhere in the world — all prior to date of invention. By definition, the inventor himself cannot trigger a 102(a) event. Applicant's own publication is not but if someone else describes applicant's invention without learning anything from the applicant then it is a 102(a) event if it happened prior to date of invention.

"Knowledge" means the claimed invention must have been publicly known to a sufficiently large segment of the public, the size depending on the number of persons skilled in the art who have such knowledge — the more likely it is then for the invention to be in public knowledge.

"Use by others" means in use before the date of invention and by more than one person and the use must have been accessible to the public without deliberate attempt to keep the use secret, although it need not be "visible" to the public — a hidden device.

"Printed publication" is a reference only for what it discloses and enables (it cannot be a passing remark); the effective date of publication is when the document is indexed or cataloged in a library or disseminated by mail — the test being if one of ordinary skill would have had access to the document with reasonable diligence to locate it. The number of copies distributed, whether recipients constitute a significant portion of those interested in the subject matter, and whether the disclosure was an oral paper only at a conference, determines "Publication" status. It need not be in a classic printed form — the key is public accessibility, even if stored in a remote location in a remote library, even if no one read the document in the library. Electronic publication such as online databases or Internet resources are "printed publication" if accessible.

"Patent" is a reference to the date it becomes enforceable, but if it is kept secret (as in some countries) then it is the date it becomes sufficiently accessible to the public; if patent is published before its rights are exercisable, the date is when it becomes exercisable, not the date of publication.

The published patent is treated as "printed publication" not a patent until such time. The patented subject matter includes, in addition to claimed subject matter, subject matter disclosed in the specification that is covered by the claims: unclaimed species are covered by a genus claim. Specification that relates to the subject matter is also "patented" matter. The disclosure need not be enabling, quite unlike the requirements for a "printed publication."

Priority can be claimed to avoid 102(a) rejection based on earlier foreign, continuation, provisional, or nonprovisional filing for any claim (establishing its effective filing date) in the later U.S. application if the earlier application provides §112 ¶1 support, it is filed within one year (or 6 month for design) of the earlier application, and it makes a claim to priority.

§102(b): Events by ANYONE (including inventor); public use and on sale only in United States or patented or printed publication anywhere in the world, more than 1 year before filing date — the earliest United States filing date of application; also called "the critical date." If anniversary date of the critical date falls on a weekend or a federal holiday in the DC, the application may be filed on the next business day to avoid statutory bar. §102(b) is a statutory time bar — it cannot be removed or antedated regardless of date of invention or who was responsible.

A §102(b) event anticipates a claim if and only if all elements and limitations recited in the claim (under application) are present in the subject matter of the event, i.e., if the claim reads on the subject matter of the event.

A single public use of the claimed invention by a single person is sufficient for this bar. Hidden from sight but public uses are sufficient. Intentionally concealing (making it available on a restricted basis and confidentiality obligation) is not public use. Misappropriated use is still a public use. Experimental use is not public use (where it is necessary to demonstrate the workability and where the profit was incidental to the experimental use). Experimentation must be the primary purpose (control by the inventor, confidentiality agreements, record of performance and progress report kept, necessity of public testing, length of test period, whether payments were made, changes made as a result of use). Product acceptance by the market is *not* experimental use.

On sale bar applies when offered for sale in the U.S. and the invention was "ready for patenting," reduced to actual practice, or the inventor had prepared drawings or other descriptions of the invention sufficient to enable a person skilled in the art to practice the invention. The product sold need not be on hand or in physical existence. The sale offer can be made by anyone (inventor, assignee, or a third party). Published abstracts may qualify for on sale rejection if they identify the product's vendor, contain information useful for potential buyers (contact, price, warranties, etc.), along with date of product release or installation before the critical date. Note it can also be a §102/§103 bar as well (obviousness based on sale activity). A sale can be: conditional, secret (phone or discrete), without profits, an offer from the U.S. to an offeree abroad or vice versa, an offer originating but not received prior to critical date, an offer that never reaches, a rejected offer, not consummated, single sale, sale between two related entities not controlled by each other, or even sale made without the inventor's consent or in violation of any confidentiality agreement. Incidental sale to experimental use is *not* a sale even if it yields a profit provided the primary purpose was experimental study (see above for conditions); assignment of rights is not an "on sale" event, the "*res*" of invention must be sold.

Patents on the date of their availability become §102(b) bar. A foreign filing within 12 month of a §102 event and then filing for a U.S. patent within one year of the foreign filing does not remove §102(b) bar — it must be filed in the U.S. within 12 months either as provisional or nonprovisional. Foreign priority does not remove this bar, the U.S. priority does. A continuation application is governed by its ancestral filing date and thus it can avoid §102(b) bar.

§102 (c): Events by INVENTOR — abandonment of invention, expressed, implied, by action or by inaction. Unreasonable delays in filing the United States patent, developing invention, coupled with other evidence such as spurring into activity if someone else has commercialized or about to commercialize the product of invention. Delay alone is not sufficient to demonstrate abandonment. Disclosing but not claiming a distinct embodiment; can be overcome by filing another application claiming the disclosed embodiment within one year of the issue date of the patent or filing a broadening reissue application within two years of the patent. Abandoned invention may be recaptured by proceeding diligently to obtain a United States patent prior to another's invention of the same subject.

§102(d): Events by INVENTOR or AFFILIATE (as allowed in foreign filings) — filing abroad more than 1 year (six months for design) before United States filing date and patent must issue before United States filing date (unlike §102(a) and (b), the date of patent is the date rights attach even if the patent is kept secret. The same invention must be involved but not necessarily claimed in the United States application; a different aspect of the invention might be claimed.

§102(e): The default date of invention of a pending application is its filing date (constructive reduction to practice) unless otherwise proven. Events by OTHERS; published application in United States or in English if Patent Cooperative Treaty and designating United States or an issued United States patent filed before the date of invention of application in question. Note: the only date the United States Patent and Trademark Office has for a pending application is the filing date of application (constructive reduction to practice), which must then be challenged through affidavits if contested if rejection is based on §102(e). "Another" means an inventive entity different from the application's inventive entity. An inventive entity is different if not ALL inventors are the same. Rule 132 declaration can be used to establish this. §102(e)(2)[A]. A United States patent to "another" stemming from a domestic application (not a Patent Cooperative Treaty filing designating United States) has the effective date as a reference as of its United States filing date (with claim extending to its provisional or continuation application if applicable) as a prior art reference but NOT its foreign priority date, where applicable, against a pending United States application. On the contrary, the pending United States application against which the reference is used CAN use its foreign priority date as a SHIELD provided the reference's United States filing date is later than the foreign filing date of the application. This is applicable even if the reference has a foreign filing date prior to the foreign filing date of the application since the foreign filing date of the reference is immaterial. However, if the reference has domestic priority date prior to the applicant's foreign priority date then the foreign priority date of applicant cannot be used to overcome §102(e)(2)[A] rejection. §102(e)(2)[B]. A United States patent to "another" stemming from a national stage-Patent Cooperative Treaty application has the priority date depending on the filing dates of the pending applications against which it is used. If the application under examination was filed: for a pending United Sates Patent and Trademark Office application filed prior to November 29, 2000, and NOT voluntarily published, the priority date of the United States patent as a reference is the date when the Patent Cooperative Treaty application for this reference patent entered the national stage in the United States. For a pending United States Patent and Trademark Office application filed before November 29, 2000, and published voluntarily, the United States patent stemming from a national stage-Patent Cooperative Treaty filing has no effect on this application. [Meaning that the United States patent reference has no effective filing date. It does not exist.] For a pending United States Patent and Trademark Office application filed on or after November 29, 2000, the United States patent stemming from a national stage-Patent Cooperative Treaty filing has no effect on this application. [Meaning that the United States patent reference has no effective filing date. It does not exist.] §102(e)(1)[A]. Published domestic United States Patent Application is an anticipatory reference as of its filing date, even if it were subsequently abandoned. The §102(e) reference must contain an enabling disclosure relative to the application claim against which it is applied; an issued United States patent has a statutory presumption of validity, a published application does not. If the reference is not enabling, it cannot be a §102 event but can still be a §103 event. §102(e)(1)[B]. Published Patent Cooperative Treaty patent application (by WIPO or by United States Patent and Trademark Office — entering national stage) is a reference as of the Patent Cooperative Treaty filing date if it did designate United States and was published by WIPO in English. The United States Patent and Trademark Office-published national stage is a reference as of its Patent Cooperative Treaty filing date but only if the Patent Cooperative Treaty application was published by

WIPO in English. If a Patent Cooperative Treaty application does meet these requirements, it can be a §102(a) or (b) event but not §102(e).

§102(f): The inventor is the one who conceives the invention, not derives it from someone else — disclosed by someone else or getting the idea from someone else.

§102(g): §102(g)(2). A patent bar arises if the invention was made in this country by another inventor who did not abandon, suppress or conceal it. An interference proceeding or an *ex parte* examination decides and thus §102(g) becomes applicable ONLY after these evaluations. Five conditions apply: the invention must have been made, i.e., reduced to practice, in this country (§104 — invention in foreign countries does not apply), by another, before the applicant's date of invention and that the other did not abandon, suppress or conceal it. Reasonable diligence is a major key to these decisions. §102(g)(1). Applies only in an interference proceeding to establish than the invention was made within the limits of §104 — North American Free Trade Agreement country after December 7, 1993 or WTO country after December 31, 1996. Other conditions of abandoning, suppressing and concealing apply as above. Countries outside North American Free Trade Agreement or WTO are not considered regardless of date of activity in those countries. Even in North American Free Trade Agreement and WTO countries the latest date of activity is the date given above when they entered the jurisdiction; all prior dates are shifted to these dates. §102 Special Forms: Abandoned Applications: If an issued patent refers to an abandoned application, the content of that application become evidence of public-knowledge [§102(a)]. If an issued application expressly incorporates the disclosure of an abandoned application by reference, then the contents become part of the disclosure effective as of the patent's filing date under §102(e)(2). Material cancelled from an application is not part of the patent for the purposes of §102(e)(2), however the prosecution history becomes available to the public as of the issue date of the patent and becomes §102(a) event. Incipient §102(e) references: Unpublished applications cannot be cited as prior art under §102(e), however, claims in a later-filed application may be provisionally rejected over an earlier application under §102(e) if the two applications have a common inventor or assignee. Oral testimony alone, without at least some documentary corroboration, is generally insufficient to prove invalidity. SIRs (Statutory invention registration) examined in compliance with §112, ¶1 are treated the same as a patent for §102(e)(2) purpose — defensive purpose. The Doctrine of Forfeiture states that a commercial, purposely hidden use of a process or a machine by an applicant (but not by a third party) more than one year before the filing date of the application, coupled with a sale of the res precludes the application from obtaining a patent.

Second Requirement: Inventive Step

The question of whether something for which a patent is applied for involves an inventive step is one that is intrinsically much more difficult, since to some extent judgment of what is or is not obvious must be a subjective matter. Because the question is such a contentious one, there have been a great many patent cases in which obviousness has been at issue, and a great many judges have tried at various times to define what is meant by "obviousness," or to pose questions such as "is the solution one which would have occurred to everyone of ordinary intelligence and acquaintance with the subject matter who gave his mind to the problem" or, more bluntly, was it "so easy that any fool could do it"? Thus the person to whom the invention must be nonobvious if it is to be patentable is "the person skilled in the art"; a competent worker but without imagination or inventive capability. In the days when the great majority of patents were for relatively simple mechanical devices, it was common to describe the person skilled in the art as an "ordinary workman." This is no longer appropriate in view of the increasing technical sophistication of industry. For chemical patents the person skilled in the art may normally be considered as the average qualified industrial chemist, and for complex inventions such as in the field of biotechnology, the "person skilled in the art" may be considered to be a team of highly qualified scientists. When attacking a patent, it behooves to bring in a witness who is an ordinary worker rather than a nobel laureate, whose testimony will be challenged and likely thrown out as he is expected to know more than what would be known by "a person of ordinary skills."

The inventive step need not be a giant stride nor a result of any planned research; there is also no need to demonstrate a flash of genius in the process. An oft-asked question is that if this were obvious why didn't anyone else come up with this invention before? The answer to that is that this is that person. The patent examiners are also warned not to look at the invention in hindsight, as this may appear too obvious but only in the light of the art available at the time of invention; this is particularly true of fields of invention that are fast-growing.

The European Patent Office applies a "problem and solution approach" to the inventive step. The invention must attempt to solve a technical problem, a slightly better objective method than what U.S. Patent and Trademark Office practices. Anything in the state of the art, other than unpublished earlier patent applications, may be taken into account. It was not allowed to use different publications, reconstructing the invention by taking a piece from one and a piece from another, unless for example one document directly referred to the other. The documents can be combined together in considering obviousness if a man skilled in the art would naturally consider them in association; thus it may be enough if they simply relate to the same technical field. The jurisprudence of the European Patent Office is similar; it is permissible to combine documents in assessing the inventive step only if it would have been obvious for the skilled person to do so at the time of filing. In the U.S. it is allowed to combine any number of prior art documents including earlier filed applications.

The issue of obviousness is dealt with under 35 USC §103 of the U.S. Patent Law §103(a). If the difference between the claimed invention and the prior art are such that the invention *as a whole* would have been obvious *at the time of invention* to a person having ordinary skill in the art to which said subject matter pertains, a patent will not be granted. The manner in which the invention is made does not negate patentability (for example an invention made by someone not familiar with the field of invention or making an accidental invention). The famous *Graham v. John Deere* case decided that fundamental inquiry invokes the scope and content of the prior art, the difference between the prior art and the claims at issue, the level of ordinary skill in the pertinent art, secondary considerations, i.e., objective indicia of unobviousness. These measures may include: commercial success, long felt but unresolved needs, failure of others, etc., recognition of problem, failure to resolve problem, competitors' prompt copying, licensing of patent to industry, teaching away, unexpected results, disbelief, and incredulity.

Prima facie obviousness is the level of showing that the Patent and Trademark Office must make in order to shift to the applicant the burden of going forward with production of evidence or arguments tending to prove nonobviousness. The examiner, on the basis of prior art, proposes a combination that would be possible for one of ordinary skills to make. To protect the applicant:

- Hindsight is impermissible.
- Examiner must step back before invention.
- Knowledge of applicant's disclosure put aside.
- Only the facts gleaned from the prior art may be used.

The examiner bears the initial burden of supporting prima facie conclusion; otherwise the applicant has no obligation to submit evidence of unobviousness. Once so produced, the burden shifts to the applicant to submit additional evidence, e.g., commercial success, unexpected results, etc. The prima facie requirements state that there must be some suggestion or motivation, either in the references themselves or in the knowledge generally available to one of ordinary skill in the art, to modify the references or to combine reference teachings. Prima facie does not hold if it is shown that:

- Teachings can be modified or combined.
- Prior art does not suggest the desirability of combination.
- One of ordinary skill is merely capable of combining the teachings.

- Modifications or combinations destroy the intended function.
- There is a change in the principle of operation of the prior art.
- Modification or combination of prior art teaches away from such modification or combination.
- Applicant's invention is the discovery of problem or the source of problem.

There must be a reasonable, not absolute, expectation or predictability of success of the proposed modification or combination of the prior art at the time of invention was made, not when the examiner does evaluate it. The prior art reference(s) must teach or suggest *all* the claim limitations. This includes indefinite limitations (not meeting §112, ¶2) and limitations unsupported by the specification in the application. (Thus there may be rejection on §112 basis but not §103 in these situations.) Unclaimed features are not germane to the obviousness determination. The prior art must be "analogous" to invention — either in the field of invention or reasonably pertinent to it. Only the teachings of prior art must be combinable. It is not necessary that the specific structure be physically combinable; prima facie obviousness is not negated for business reasons not to combine; the issue is technologic combination. Prior art need not suggest the same advantage or results as the invention; motivation to modify or combine the prior art may be stimulated by a purpose different from that of the claimed invention, or the solution of a problem different from that solved by the claimed invention. Routine manipulative steps cannot be prima facie obvious when the claimed material it uses or produces is patentable, i.e., where either the starting or the ending material is patentable.

§102 (e), (f), and (g) Events as §103 Prior Art: Prior art under §102(e), (f), and (g) may be modified or combined to establish obviousness, except when the subject matter of prior art and the invention claimed in the application under examination were, at the time the claimed invention was made (not when it was filed), owned by the same person or subject to an obligation of assignment to the same person. With respect to §102(e), §103(c) is effective as of November 29, 1999 (AIPA). Rejections on §102(e)/§103 can be obviated using an affidavit if the ownership is same by an affidavit for an application filed after November 29, 1999. For applications filed prior to this date, a continuation application may be filed to take advantage of this ruling change. Whereas references in §103 are as of the date of invention, an exception arises when using a §102(e) event are applied, wherein the prior art is applied as of the date of the filing of the application vis-à-vis the filing date of the reference.

Admission as Prior Art Under §103: If an applicant admits a reference as prior art it cannot be reversed in a traversal; admissions include labeling drawings are prior art and any written admission during prosecution in addition to whatever has been submitted in the specification. A Jepsen claim however is rebuttable.

Third Requirement: Be Patentable

The third basic requirement of patentability is that the invention should be capable of industrial application, broadly defined, and includes making or using the invention in any kind of industry, including agriculture. Methods of medical treatment or diagnosis performed on the human or animal body are defined as being incapable of industrial application, although substances invented for use in such methods are patentable.

There are certain specific exceptions to patentability, which apply whether or not the invention is capable of industrial application. Artistic works and aesthetic creations are not patentable and are generally not industrially applicable either; but scientific theories and mathematical methods, the presentation of information, business methods, and computer programs are also unpatentable, although they may very well be applied in industry.

Animal and plant varieties are not patentable in countries adhering to the European Patent Commission, although in the U.S. plants may be protected either by normal utility patents or by special plant patents for plant varieties. In the U.K. and certain other European countries new plant varieties, although not patentable, can be protected by plant breeders' rights granted under the UPOV (International Union for the Protection of New Varieties of Plants) convention. Transgenic plants and animals are in principle patentable only if they do not constitute a variety raising a difficult and uncertain situation. A further exception applies to offensive, immoral, or antisocial inventions, it need not just be an article prohibited by the law; if it is abhorrent to society, it is unpatentable, though it may be legal. A portable nuclear device would be such an example. Also excluded are inventions contrary to well-established natural laws, for example, a perpetual motion machine, though European Patent Commission does not spell it out like this.

According to the U.S. laws, patentable inventions are defined as any new and useful process, machine, manufacture, or composition of matter, or any new and useful improvement thereof. The requirement that the invention be useful is rather stronger than the European Patent Commission requirement that it be capable of industrial application, and is more like the old British utility requirement.

PATENTABILITY AND TECHNICAL INFORMATION SEARCH

Before a patent application is filed, a thorough search of the subject matter is conducted to unearth prior art; this is, however, also an excellent means for scientists to learn about the state of science as well. Though many scientists remain skeptical about the correctness of information vis-à-vis refereed publications, there is no doubt that much time can be saved in conducting research if a thorough analysis of the invention and related inventions is made by the scientists. With the availability of Internet, it has now become routine for the scientists to present the most comprehensive analysis of the state of art prior to beginning the process of patenting. This search does not replace the search conducted by the patent attorneys.

PATENT OFFICE RESOURCE

The patent offices worldwide have opened their databases to the public; there is no better place to start the search for patentability than with these free databases; please know that the same databases are packaged by other vendors that provide additional services and literature search. The U.S. Patent and Trademark Office (http://www.uspto.gov) has created one of the world's largest electronic databases that includes every patent issued; recently, published applications are also available in the database. Scientists are strongly urged to develop strong skills on interacting with the database study of the U.S. Patent and Trademark Office. The search at U.S. Patent and Trademark Office can be most beneficial if the scientist learns how to use the patent classification system. (Tutorials are available at the U.S. Patent and Trademark Office website; alternately, please consult, *Filing Patents Online: A Professional Guide* by Sarfaraz K. Niazi, CRC Press, 2002.)

The U.S. Patent Office Classification 435 includes the following subcategories related to therapeutic proteins.

Class 435: Chemistry: Molecular Biology and Microbiology — provides for methods of purifying, propagating, or attenuating a microorganism; e.g., a virus, bacteria, etc., except for propagating a microorganism in an animal for the purpose of producing an antibody containing sera. Class 435 provides for methods of propagating animal organs, tissues, or cells; e.g., blood, sperm, etc., and culture media therefore. Class 435 is the generic home for processes of: (1) analyzing or testing which involve a fermentation step or (2) qualitative or quantitative testing for fermentability, or fermentative power.

435. Chemistry: Molecular Biology and Microbiology — see appropriate subclasses: for processes in which a material containing an enzyme or microorganism is used to perform a qualitative or quantitative measurement or test; for compositions or test strips for either of the stated processes; for the processes of making such compositions or test strips; for processes of using microorganisms or enzymes to synthesize a chemical product; for processes of treating a material with microorganisms or enzymes; to separate, liberate, or purify a preexisting substance or to destroy hazardous or toxic waste; for

processes of propagating microorganisms; for processes of genetically altering a microorganism; for processes of tissue, organ, blood, sperm, or microbial maintenance; for processes of malting or mashing; for microorganisms, per se, and subcellular parts thereof; for recombinant vectors and their preparation; for enzymes, per se, compositions containing enzymes not otherwise provided for and processes of preparing and purifying enzymes; for compositions for microbial propagation; for apparatus for any of the processes of the class; for composting apparatus; and subclasses 4+ for *in vitro* processes in which there is a direct or indirect, qualitative or quantitative, measurement or test, by or of a material which contains an enzyme or microorganism (for the purposes of Class 435, microorganism includes bacteria, actinomycetales, cyanobacteria [unicellular algae], fungi, protozoa, animal cells, plant cells, and virus). Class 424 definition contains controlling statements on the class lines.

93.2 Genetically modified microorganism, cell, or virus (e.g., transformed, fused, hybrid, etc.) — This subclass is indented under subclass 93.1. Subject matter involving a microorganism, cell, or virus that (a) is a product of recombination, transformation, or transfection with a vector or a foreign or exogenous gene or (b) is a product of homologous recombination if it is directed rather than spontaneous or (c) is a product of fused or hybrid cell formation. (1) Note. Examples of subject matter included in this and the indented subclass are compositions containing microorganisms, cells, or viruses resulting from (a) a process in which the cellular matter of two or more fusing partners is combined, producing a cell that initially contains the genes of both fusing partners or (b) a process in which a cell is treated with an immortalizing agent, which results in a cell that proliferates in long-term culture or (c) a process involving recombinant DNA methodology. (2) Note. Excluded from this subclass are products of unidentified or noninduced mutations; products of microbial conjugation wherein specific genetic material is not identified and controlled; and products of natural, spontaneous, or arbitrary conjugation or recombination events. These products are not considered genetically modified for this subclass and therefore will be classified as unmodified microorganisms, cells, or viruses.

93.21: Eukaryotic cell — This subclass is indented under subclass 93.2. Subject matter involving an eukaryotic cell, such as an animal cell, plant cell, fungus, protozoa, or higher algae that has been genetically modified. (1) Note. An eukaryotic cell has a nucleus defined by a nuclear membrane wherein the nucleus contains chromosomes that comprise the genome of the cell.

93.3: Intentional mixture of two or more microorganisms, cells, or viruses of different genera: This subclass is indented under subclass 93.1. Subject matter involving a mixture consisting of two or more different microbial, cellular, or viral genera. (1) Note. A mixture of *E. coli* and *Pseudomonas* or a mixture of *Aspergillus* and *Bacillus* would be considered proper for this subclass, while a mixture of *Bacillus cereus* and *Bacillus brevis* would be classified under Bacillus rather than in this subclass since they are both in the genus, *Bacillus*. (2) Note. Rumen, intestinal, vaginal, etc., microflora mixtures are mixtures appropriate for this subclass unless mixture constituents are disclosed and are found to be contrary to the subclass definition.

133.1: Structurally modified antibody, immunoglobulin, or fragment thereof (e.g., chimeric, humanized, CDR-grafted, mutated, etc.) — This subclass is indented under subclass 130.1. Subject matter involving an antibody, immunoglobulin, or fragment thereof that is purposely altered with respect to its amino acid sequence or glycosylation, or with respect to its composition of heavy and light chains or immunoglobulin regions or domains, as compared with that found in nature; or wherein the antibody, immunoglobulin, or fragment thereof is part of a larger, synthetic protein. (1) Note. Structurally modified antibodies may be made by chemical alteration or recombination of existing antibodies, or by various cloning techniques involving recombinant DNA or hybridoma technology. (2) Note. Structurally modified antibodies may be chimeric (i.e., comprising amino acid sequences derived from two or more nonidentical immunoglobulin molecules, such as interspecies combinations, etc.). (3) Note. Structurally modified antibodies may have domain deletions or substitutions (e.g., deletions of particular constant-region domains or substitutions of constant-region domains from other classes of immunoglobulins). (4) Note. Structurally modified antibodies may have deletions of particular glycosylated amino acids, or may have their glycosylation otherwise altered, which may alter their function. (5) Note. While expression of cloned antibody genes in cells of species other than from which they originated may result in altered glycosylation of the product, compared with that found in nature, this subclass and indented subclasses are not meant to encompass such antibodies or fragments thereof unless such cloning is a deliberate attempt to alter their glycosylation. However, such antibodies or fragments thereof may still be classified here or in indented subclasses if they are structurally modified in other ways (e.g., if they are single chain, etc.). (6) Note. It is suggested that the patents of this subclass and indented subclasses be cross-referenced to the appropriate subclass(es) that provide for the binding specificities of these antibodies, if disclosed.

141.1: Monoclonal antibody or fragment thereof (i.e., produced by any cloning technology): — This subclass is indented under subclass 130.1. Subject matter involving an antibody or fragment thereof produced by a clone of cells or cell line, which clone of cells or cell line is derived from a single antibody-producing cell or antibody-fragment-producing cell, wherein said antibody or fragment thereof is identical to all other antibodies or fragments thereof produced by that clone of cells or cell line. (1) Note. This and the indented subclasses provide for bioaffecting and body-treating compositions of antibodies or fragments thereof as well as bioaffecting and body-treating methods of using said compositions, said antibodies, or said fragments, which antibodies or antibody fragments are produced by any cloning technology that yields identical molecules (e.g., hybridoma technology, recombinant DNA technology, etc.). (2) Note. Monoclonal antibodies, per se, are considered compounds and are provided for elsewhere. See the search notes below. (3) Note. Monoclonal antibodies are sometimes termed monoclonal receptors or immunological binding partners.

1.49 and 1.53, for methods of using radiolabeled monoclonal antibodies or compositions thereof for bioaffecting or body-treating purposes and said compositions, per se.

9.1+ for methods of using monoclonal antibodies or compositions thereof for *in vivo* testing or diagnosis and said compositions, per se.

178.1+ for bioaffecting or body-treating methods of using monoclonal antibodies or fragments thereof that are conjugated to or complexed with nonimmunoglobulin material; bioaffecting or body-treating methods of using compositions of monoclonal antibodies or fragments thereof, which monoclonal antibodies or fragments thereof are conjugated to or complexed with nonimmunoglobulin material; and said compositions, per se.

199.1: Recombinant virus encoding one or more heterologous proteins or fragments thereof: This subclass is indented under subclass 184.1. Subject matter involving a virus into whose genome is integrated one or more nucleic acid sequences encoding one or more heterologous proteins or fragments thereof. (1) Note. A heterologous protein is one derived from another species (e.g., another viral species). (2) Note. Such genetically modified viruses may be used as multivalent vaccines.

200.1: Recombinant or stably transformed bacterium encoding one or more heterologous proteins or fragments thereof — This subclass is indented under subclass 184.1. Subject matter involving a bacterium into whose genome is integrated one or more nucleic acid sequences encoding one or more heterologous proteins or fragments thereof; or involving a bacterium that carries stable, replicative plasmids that include one or more nucleic acid sequences encoding one or more heterologous proteins or fragments thereof. (1) Note. A heterologous protein is one derived from another species (e.g., another bacterial species). (2) Note. Such genetically modified bacteria may be used as multivalent vaccines.

201.1: Combination of viral and bacterial antigens (e.g., multivalent viral and bacterial vaccine, etc.) — This subclass is indented under subclass 184.1. Subject matter involving a combination of viral and bacterial antigens, such as that found in a multivalent viral and bacterial vaccine.

202.1: Combination of antigens from multiple viral species (e.g., multivalent viral vaccine, etc.) — This subclass is indented under subclass 184.1. Subject matter involving a combination of antigens from multiple viral species, such as that found in a multivalent viral vaccine. (1) Note. A combination of antigens from multiple variants of the same viral species should be classified with that viral species.

203.1: Combination of antigens from multiple bacterial species (e.g., multivalent bacterial vaccine, etc.) — This subclass is indented under subclass 184.1. Subject matter involving a combination of antigens from multiple bacterial species, such as that found in a multivalent bacterial vaccine. (1) Note. A combination of antigens from multiple variants of the same bacterial species should be classified with that bacterial species.

801: Involving Antibody or Fragment Thereof Produced by Recombinant DNA Technology — This subclass is indented under the class definition. Subject matter involving an antibody or fragment thereof produced by recombinant DNA technology.

A search under CCL/"435/69.1" yields 8898 patents, including the earliest patents wherein insulin was produced by genetically modified fungi from the University of Minnesota and the two classic patents from Stanford and Columbia.

Second to the U.S. Patent Office, the largest database is accessed through the European Patent Office, where one should conduct a similar classification search as suggested above for the U.S. Patent and Trademark Office (http://ep.espacenet.com).

The World Intellectual Property Organization (http://ipdl.wipo.int/) offers many useful features including complete details of the Patent Cooperative Treaty and its gazette.

The Canadian Patent Office can be reached at http://patents1. ic.gc.ca/srch_bool-e.html.

INTERNET SEARCH ENGINES

Though intended for the lay public, the use of Internet search engines can reveal remarkable information, particularly as it pertains to prior art. The following sites are recommended:

http://www.searchenginecolossus.com/
http://www.searchengineguide.com/
www.google.com/
www.lycos.com/
www.yahoo.com/
www.altavista.com/
www.alltheweb.com/
www.webcrawler.com/
www.excite.com/
www.infoseek.com/
www.msn.com/
www.infospace.com/

INFORMATION PORTALS

Listed here is a guide to information portals available on the Internet.

http://lcweb.loc.gov The Library of Congress is the best place to start as it is the world's largest library.
http://www.firstgov.gov/ Gateway to all government information.
http://spireproject.com/ A guide to what is coming online.
http://scout.cs.wisc.edu/ The Scout Report is one of the Internet's longest-running weekly publications, offering a selection of new and newly discovered online resources.
http://infomine.ucr.edu/Main.html A University of California Library service on what is available on the Internet in the sciences.

http://www.ipl.org/ref/RR/Internet Public Library. An annotated collection of high quality Internet resources for their usefulness in providing accurate, factual information on a particular topic or topics.

http://www.invent.org/ A highly artistic website on the patenting process with much support for independent inventors.

http://www.access.gpo.gov/getcfr.html This page describes the HTML coding necessary to link directly to documents contained in the Code of Federal Regulations (CFR) databases resident on GPO's WAIS servers.

http://vlib.org/ The WWW Virtual Library.

http://www.invent1.org/ Minnesota Inventors Congress; inventor resources and the oldest convention center.

http://www.uww.edu/business/innovate/innovate.htm; http://www.innovationcentre.ca The Canadian Innovation Center.

http://www.sul.stanford.edu/depts/swain/patent/pattop.html. Selected Resources for Patents, Inventions, and Technology Transfer selected by Stanford University.

http://www.bl.uk/ The 150 million volume British Library is a good source; search here with the key word "patent."

http://www.rand.org/radius The most comprehensive listing of federally funded research projects, free to federal employees.

http://www.knowledgeexpress.com/ Knowledge Express provides business development and competitive intelligence resources — including intellectual property, technology transfer, and corporate partnering opportunities — to organizations involved with science/technology research and new inventions.

http://searchlight.cdlib.org/cgi-bin/searchlight Publicly available databases and other resources.

http://productnews.com New product information on thousands of products weekly.

http://www.techexpo.com Aimed at manufacturers and inventors.

http://www.pubcrawler.ie/ Health and medical information

http://medlineplus.gov/National Library of Medicine consumer site on health.

http://clinicaltrials.gov/ Information on all U.S. clinical trials under way and you can branch out to learn about how to do clinical trials.

http://www.pubmedcentral.nih.gov/ A major archive of free online life sciences journals.

http://highwire.stanford.edu/lists/freeart.dtl Free online journals in science, technology, and medicine.

http://www.healthfinder.gov/ Reliable health information from government agencies.

http://www.cdc.gov/ The Centers for Disease Control.

http://www.fda.gov Food and Drug Administration regulations.

http://www.nal.usda.gov/fnic/ USDA food and nutrient information center.

http://www.mdtmag.com Medical design technology for devices.

http://www.medscape.com/ Medical information from WebMD.

http://bmn.com Biomedical information portal.

http://www.intelihealth.com Consumer healthcare information from Harvard.

http://www.bmj.com *British Medical Journal*; prestige medical issues.

http://www.devicelink.com/ Medical devices.

http://www.ornl.gov/hgmis/ The human genome project.

TECHNICAL DATABASES

National Institutes of Health (http://www.ncbi.nlm.nih.gov/PubMed) offers over 12 million research papers mainly in the biomedical sciences that are available through the National Library of Medicine. This free database allows downloads of abstract in an ASCII format for direct placement into programs like Word to develop a comprehensive bibliography.

Derwent (http://www.derwent.com) is one of the most widely used databases, from which the U.S. Patent and Trademark Office examiners benefit as well.

Dialog (http://www.dialog.com) is another large database that allows you to search without having to register an account; you pay as you go along using your credit card. You cannot do this if you are searching for trademarks.

Delphion (formerly IBM Intellectual Property database) (http://www.delphion.com/) allows for more in-depth search of patents as well as access to many consolidated databases. It is a low cost solution.

American Chemical Society offers its large database (http://stneasy.cas.org/html/english/login1.html). This is one of the premier scientific databases from where you will be able to get original papers faxed to you if you need them urgently.

Nerac (http://www.nerac.com) also offers numerous online databases.

PATENT SEARCH AND IP SERVICES

Patent Café (http://www.patentcafe.com) is a hangout for patent product vendors.

Investor's Digest (http:/www.inventorsdigest.com/) has many resources for inventors. It is a very active site.

MIT has provided an elaborate and detailed website for invention development; worth a detailed look (http://web.mit.edu/invent/).

PATENT COPIES, SEARCH FACILITIES

Micropatent (http://www.1790.com/0/patentweb9809.html) has perhaps the most comprehensive service available, very reasonable cost, and an easy website to navigate. It is highly recommended.

Questel (http://www.questel.orbit.com/)

Faxpat (http://www.faxpat.com)

Patentec (http://www.patentec.com)

Lexis-Nexus (http://www.lexis-nexis.com)

Mayall (http://www.mayallj.freeserve.co.uk/)

COMPONENTS OF A PATENT APPLICATION

A patent specification (not specifications) is a legal document that ends up getting published as the patent, if allowed. Great care and detail go into writing this document in defining the scope of invention, deciding what is claimed, and wording the claims (which are part of specification) such that they can withstand challenges.

Deciding on what is "invented" is the job of the research scientist, but the decision to patent is made in light of prior art; for example, if there is a discovery of a new group of chemicals, the breadth of group should be ascertained in light of the prior art available and obviously what can be reasonably predicted regarding the structure of chemicals and the ability to synthesize representative chemicals, if not all. Where a completely new molecular structure has been invented, a broad scope, including all kinds of derivatives of the basic structure that the inventor thinks may be useful, is possible. It is surprising what scientists who are sure of the novelty of a structure, composition, or application find out when a thorough search is made of the possible prior art. It is worth realizing that with the availability of databases in electronic format, the Internet, and generally faster access to remote publications (even brochures for promotion in remote countries), what a thorough search would reveal; know that the patent examiners have access to these same channels of information and then some. I have been humbled more than once on what the patent examiner dug out. So, scientists are advised not to jump the gun in making very broad claims until so advised by the patent attorneys after conducting a thorough patent search. Obviously, the scope is narrowed down gradually as more and more prior art emerges. The goal is not to narrow it down to a point where it loses its commercial importance. The scope of protection, which it is commercially important to achieve, varies from one field to another. In extreme situations it is sufficient to have a scope that includes a singular compound, if that is what the company wishes to market. The strength in this approach comes from the regulatory control of pharmaceutical products. Once a company received marketing authorization from the Food and Drug Administration, at great expense, imitators would like only to reproduce the invention, which they cannot do through the course of patent term and any other extensions granted by the Food and Drug Administration. So, while there may be other molecules, perhaps better ones, available, imitators are unlikely to invest in their development since they are unprotected and there is no guarantee that the Food and Drug Administration will approve them. So, in the field of new drug development, a single chemical entity does have substantial value. This is not the case in other industries where regulatory costs are not involved, such as in the chemical industry.

Once a decision is made about what is invented, how much to claim, and what specifically to claim, the process of drafting specification begins. One method is to draft the main claim, defining the scope of the invention in the form of the statement of invention, which is the heart of the patent specification, then the rest of the specification will be drafted, along with the rest of the claims.

Specification begins with a title. Newcomers to the field of patenting would be amazed or perhaps amused at the choice of patent titles and even the language used to describe an invention. Historically, inventors kept the titles vague to keep the searchers (who then did manual searches) from finding out about their inventions. Today, as most patent offices have gone electronic, this is no longer an issue, nevertheless the practice continues.

Patent applications have fixed formats that often vary between patent offices but nevertheless require a similar information submission: a background, a summary, a detail of invention, etc. The patent application must be comprehensive to demonstrate novelty and the inventive step in light of prior art; it should be understood that the purpose is not to fool the patent examiner into allowance but to protect the invention from competitors who will challenge it, should it be worth anything. A full disclosure is required to keep the infringers out as the chance of their success in knocking out a patent goes down. Additional statements are included defining the features of the invention for use as a basis for specific claims. For example, stating that: "In one aspect the invention provides …," "In another aspect the invention provides …," "The above defined widgets are new and form part of the invention." Attorneys have their preferences and standard statements that fill the specification write up quickly.

After the statements of invention, there is a description of indication of what are the preferred parts of the scope, and one or more formulae may be given defining narrower subgeneric scopes. This section fulfills the requirement of adequacy of description. The specification must also describe how the invention is to be carried out, an essential part of a patent application. This is a critical stage in deciding how and what to disclose. As discussed earlier, often at this stage a decision may be made not to file for a patent application for the disclosure will inevitably cause the invention to escape from the hands of inventors, and if there were no certain ways to determine infringement, this would make patenting useless. It is also not a smart move to be deceptive when it comes to describing how the invention works; many a patent applications have been declared invalid after the companies have made significant investment in marketing the invention because a competitor was able to demonstrate that the inventors hid certain critical facts. It must be understood that the disclosure need not be for a commercial model of invention and thus need not include many fine details generally required for a large-scale production of the invention, such as in-process specifi-cations, certain handling conditions, the grade of excipients used, etc., which may be material to produce a product fit for a particular purpose, such as human consumption. As long as the competitor can manufacture the article, not necessary for commercial production, using the details provided, the requirement of sufficiency of disclosure is met. This becomes more important in the discovery of new chemical entities where chemical synthesis can be described adequately, but not necessarily for the grade of material required; for example, the impurity profile of an NCE (New Chemical Entity: Food and Drug Administration) is critical for the purpose of an NDA (New Drug Application: Food and Drug Administration); manufacturers often are able to produce a product that would meet Food and Drug Administration's requirement for quality, yet not report this method in the patent, which would allow the competitor to manufacture the product with impurities only. The reason the companies are able to get away with this trick is that the patent claims a chemical compound, not necessarily what would be suitable for ingestion by humans. Obviously, if the molecule turns out to be a blockbuster, many will imitate the process and may challenge the patent; case law on this aspect is silent. It is well known, as a result, once an NCE comes to the end of its patent cycle, new sources of API are developed with greater difficulty than what would be anticipated from the disclosures in the patent.

Next comes an indication of what the invention is useful for, a part of the specification usually called the utility statement. Whereas in the case of mechanical inventions it is often obvious, it requires explanation for chemical inventions along with any peculiar or particular advantages. It is important to know that there is no requirement to explain how and why the invention works; thus, it is best not to offer any hypothesis about the invention. However, if a theory must be given, one should leave room for a change of mind later, for example, by wording such as "while we do not intend to be bound to any particular theory, it is believed that …" In a chemical case a number of examples are given with detailed instructions for the preparation of at least one of the compounds within the scope, and for the use of the compounds.

After this comes the heart of patent, the claims. There is no limitation on how many claims are made; however, redundant and superfluous claims are frowned upon by the examiners and should be avoided. It is important to know that all dependent claims are narrower in scope and written exclusively for the purpose of protecting the invention, or any part of it, should the broader claim or claims be knocked out in court proceedings.

Other parts of a patent application such as priority dates, affidavit requirements, assignment, or appointment of attorney or agents is best left to patent practitioners and the company legal department to worry about; however, there may be some interaction with the inventor in filling out certification documents. The filing of an application is followed by numerous communications and office actions from the patent office, the responses to which are drafted in full consultation with the scientists and their approval for accuracy of information and its interpretation. A word of caution is needed here. In the U.S., there is a clause of "estoppel," under which admissions made in the specification or in responses to office action about what is actually taught by the prior art may be binding upon the applicant. A wrong statement about accepting an article as prior art may be reversed later. Court proceedings will have the entire text of correspondence available for examination, and the "file wrapper" becomes part of the patent. The safest rule is to admit nothing and say as little about the prior art as possible. Of course, all relevant prior art known to the applicant or his or her attorney must be brought to the attention of the U.S. Patent and Trademark Office, but this does not mean that it has to be mentioned in the specification.

There must be at least one claim in each patent application. Claims define the scope of subject matter for which protection is sought. A competitor does not infringe and cannot be stopped unless he or she makes, sells, offers for sale, imports, or does something falling within the scope of at least one claim of the granted patent, in order words, if the infringing object "reads onto claim," then it is an infringement. How claims are interpreted keeps the courts filled with opportunities to create case laws. Claims are always read in light of the published specification and thus the issue of prior art comes up again; had there been a mistake in allowing a claim in the light of prior art, the claim will be thrown out and in some cases the entire patent rendered invalid.

All claims fall into one of two broad categories: they claim either a product (a mechanical device, a machine, a composition of matter, etc.) or a process (a method of making, using, or testing something). For chemical patents, this may include the chemical per se as a useful intermediate, as a composition in a pharmaceutical product, be a specific form (optical isomer, crystal form, etc.), or for use direct use. The process claims would include process of synthesis, isolation, or purification as the case may be; the methods of use may be the first or a subsequent use as a method of medical treatment or diagnosis or testing and analysis methods.

4.1 DRAWING(S) (§ 113)

When necessary, most likely in mechanical or electrical and some chemical applications. Filing date not assigned if drawings not provided at the OIPE level of evaluation; examiner may require drawings but filing date not affected; drawings MUST show all of the claimed elements; drawings may be added later by amendment if already described in the specification or claim as originally filed; no need for manufacturing drawings (such as tolerances or in-process controls).

4.3 SPECIFICATION (§112 ¶1)

The written description, the manner and process of making and using, in such full, clear, concise, and exact terms as to enable any personal skilled (with ordinary skills) in the art to which it pertains, or with which it is most nearly connected, to make and use the invention and setting forth the best mode contemplated by the inventor for carrying out his invention. There are three requirements of disclosure:

4.4 DESCRIPTION:

- Must described what is claimed clearly.
- Focus is on the claimed invention only.
- Scope commensurate with scope of claim(s): disclosure of a single species may or may not support a generic claim.
- Critical or essential element MUST be recited in claims.
- The vantage point is one of ordinary skill in the art.
- The inventor may be his/her own lexicographer); spell out but not befuddle, not use in a contrary manner to what is commonly acceptable.
- Theory need not be set forth; if theory is wrong, the error is not fatal (unless theory is claimed invention).
- Manner of invention is not important (how the invention was made).

4.5 ENABLEMENT:

- To one of ordinary skills to make and use.
- Without undue experimentation.
- Not necessarily for commercial production.
- This requirement different from §101 requirement of being useful.
- Claim not reciting essential matter may be rejected for lack of enablement or failing to claim the subject matter applicant regards as the invention.
- Publications after filing date may not be used to support enablement but may be used to defeat enablement (such as by examiner).
- Scope of enablement must be commensurate with scope of claim(s).
- Amount of disclosure required depends on the state of the art and predictability — the more is known and the greater is the predictability, the less the disclosure is required.

4.6 BEST MODE:

- What inventor considers best mode, not what anyone or everyone else considers and not what is objectively best.
- At the time the application is filed; need not and cannot be updated by amendment (as it will be considered new matter) even in a division or continuation but can be updated in CIP if it pertains to a new claim made.
- Must be disclosed though not necessarily identified as such; embodiment disclosed is automatically considered as the best mode; several embodiments may be disclosed without identifying which one is the best.

4.7 PARAGRAPH 1 35 USC §112 REQUIREMENT:

Description, enablement and best mode for each claim as filed or else it renders claims invalid if contested. Mythical person is one of ordinary skills in the art not a layperson. Need to disclose what is considered as required knowledge of one of ordinary skill. Any one or more of can satisfy each of these three requirements: specification, drawing(s) and claims as originally filed. Unclaimed inventions need not satisfy this requirement.

4.8 PARAGRAPH 2 35 USC §112 REQUIREMENT: PARTS OF A CLAIM

- Preamble sets for the invention's technical environment and class (composition, process or apparatus, etc.: A method of ......, Apparatus for ......, A composition ......). It is not limiting if it only merely states the purpose of the invention; however if it breathes life and meaning into the claim (such as if it is essential to tell what is claimed of if the body of claim refers to it as antecedent support) it can become limiting.
- Transitional phrase connects the body of the claim to preamble: comprising, consisting of, consisting essentially of, etc. Three types: open-ended: comprising, including, containing, characterized by, etc.; closed: consisting of, also composed of, having, being etc., some of these can be interpreted differently; partially closed: consisting essentially of ... wherein it allows only those additional elements that do not affect the basic and novel characteristics of invention. No synergism. The applicant has burden of proof to show that additional elements in prior art would materially change the characteristics of the invention. If ABCD is known and ABC is claimed; absence of D must be demonstrated to affect materially the invention.
- Body is a list of elements such as ingredients of a composition, components of the apparatus; all elements must be interconnected. (There must a reason why a component is recited; not just to list it.).

4.9.0 READING A CLAIM

Claim reading onto prior art is to prove validity of claim, a device or process to indicate infringement or own specification satisfies §112 ¶1 requirements. Claim does not read on prior art with elements ABCD if the claim is ABC and closed (consisting of) but it reads if the transitional phrase is open such as "comprising" and may or may not read if it is "consisting essentially of."

4.10.0 PUNCTUATION OF CLAIM

One sentence, comma after preamble; colon after transitional; each element gets own paragraph; semicolon at the end of each paragraph; "and" between last two elements. More than one period means more than one sentence and thus an indefinite claim (¶2 §112).

4.11. DEFINITENESS OF CLAIM

- Without proper antecedent basis a claim is rendered indefinite. "A" or "an" introduces an element for the first time except in a means-plus-function format. "Said" or "the" refers back to previously introduced elements or limitations or refer to inherent properties (not required to be recited for antecedent purpose; example, "the surface of said element" when "surface" is not defined earlier).
- Inferential claiming where interconnectivity of elements is not certain — does not tell if the element is part of combination or not.

4.12 NARROWING OF CLAIM

Narrowed by adding an element or limitation to a previously recited element; narrow claim can be dependent or independent. Adding a step narrows method claims. Adding an element to a closed (such as Markush Group) claim broadens not narrows claim.

4.13 DEPENDENT CLAIMS (§112 ¶3 ¶4)

- Claim can be dependent or independent; a dependent claim incorporates by reference all the limitations of the claims to which it refers and is always narrower; must depend from a preceding claim not a following claim (numbering of claims is readjusted during prosecution).
- "Further comprising" or "further including" used to narrow a claim by adding another element or step.
- Claimed narrowed by further defining an element or the relationship between elements. Transitional element "wherein" used to add limitation. Narrowing can be both adding an element and further defining their relationship.
- Defining a step further narrows method claim.

4.14 MULTIPLE DEPENDENT CLAIMS (§112 ¶5)

- A claim referring to more than one previously set forth claim but only in the alternative ("or") and narrows the claim from which it depends.
- Cannot serve as a basis for another multiple dependent claim; may refer to other dependent claim and a dependent claim may depend from a multiple dependent claim.
- Incorporates by reference all the limitations of the particular claim in relationship to which it is being considered (individually and not collectively).
- It takes place of writing several dependent claims — in its spirit.
- A flat special fee is charged at the time of filing application if multiple dependent claim or claims are included.

4.15 DOMINANT-SUBSERVIENT CLAIMS

Dominant (Subcombination or genus)-Combination (Subservient-species). Need two members (species) to have genus, which is illustrated by the selection of species; genus is an inherent commonality among embodiments (species).

4.16 MEANS-PLUS-FUNCTION CLAUSES §112 ¶6

Claim defining an element by its function not what it is. Means for performing a function. Interpreted by the literal function recited and corresponding structure or materials described in specification and equivalents thereof. Does not cover all structures for performing the recited function. A claim reciting only a single means-plus-function clause without any other element is impressible. Must have the phrase, "means for," which then must be modified by functional language but not modified by the recitation of structure sufficient to accomplish the specific function. If specification does not adequately disclose the structure corresponding to the "means" claimed the claims fails to comply with paragraph 2 requirement for "particularly pointing out and distinctly claiming" the invention. If disclosure is implicit (for those skilled in the art), an amendment may be required or stated on record what structure performs the function. Equivalents: examiner must explain rationale; prior art must perform, not excluded by explicit definition in the specification for an equivalent, prior art supported by:

- Identical function, substantially same way, substantially same results.
- Art-recognized interchangeability.
- Insubstantial differences.
- Structural equivalency.

4.17 Process Claims

A method for making a product, comprising the steps of ...; a method of using a specified or known material, comprising the steps of ...; recitation of at least one step required and a single step method claim is proper.

4.18 Step-Plus-Function Clauses

- Functional method claims reciting a particular result but not the specified act — i.e., techniques used to achieve results — adjusting pH, raising temperature, reducing friction, etc.
- No recital of acts in support required.
- Typically introduced by words like "whereby," "so that" or "for."
- Addition of a functional description alone is not sufficient to differentiate claim—rejected under §102.
- Functional language without recitation of structure, which performs the function, may render the claim broader (rather than narrower) and rejected under §112 ¶1.

4.19 Ranges

Commonly used for temperature, pressure, time and dimensional limitations. "Up to" means from zero to the top limit; "at least" means not less than (does not set upper limit, which must be fully disclosed in specification); specification must support eventual ranges. A dependent claim cannot broaden the range. Range within range is indefinite in a claim but acceptable in specification.

4.20 Negative Limitations

Permissible if boundaries set forth definitely, such as free of an impurity or a particular element or incapable of performing a certain function. Absence of structures cannot be claimed: holes, channels, etc. as structural elements.

4.21 Relative and Exemplary Terminology

Imprecise language may satisfy definiteness requirement (for one of ordinary skill). "So dimensioned" or "so spaced" can be definite if it is as accurate as the subject would permit; "about" is clear and flexible but rendered indefinite if specification or prior art does not provide indication about the dimensions anticipated. "Essentially," "substantially," "effective amount" are definite if one of ordinary skills would understand. Exemplary terminology is always indefinite: such as, or like material, similar — all rejected.

4.22 MARKUSH GROUP

Closed form. Two forms: wherein P is a material selected from a group consisting of A, B, C, and D; or wherein P is A, B, C or D. Members must belong to a recognized class, possess properties in common as disclosed in specification and these properties mainly responsible for their function or the grouping is clear from their nature or the prior art that all members possess the property.

Adding members broadens claim. Prior art with one of the members anticipates the claim.

4.23 MARKUSH ALTERNATES

"Or" terminology if choices are related: one or several pieces; made entirely or part of; red, blue or white. If unrelated choices, the use of "or" will lead to indefinite interpretation. "Optionally" if definite if there are no ambiguities in the scope of claim as a result of choices offered.

4.24 JEPSON-TYPE CLAIMS — IMPROVEMENT CLAIMS

Preamble defines what is conventional; transitional phrase, "wherein the improvement comprises"; body builds on preamble; can add element or modify element in preamble. Preamble is limiting.

4.25 MIXED-CLASS CLAIMS

Mixed elements are improper: methods claims should have no structural elements; apparatus claims should have no step elements. Limitations can be mixed, such as method step may include a structural limitation and an apparatus may include a process limitation.

4.26 PRODUCT-BY-PROCESS CLAIMS

A product claim that defines the claimed product in terms of the process by which it is made: A product made by the process comprising of steps .... Patentability based on product itself and NOT on method of production. If the product is same (as prior art) using another process does not make it patentable. If examiner shows that product appears to be the same or similar the burden shifts to applicant; United States Patent and Trademark Office bears lesser burden of proof in making out a case of prima facie obviousness. One step method claims acceptable but claims where body consists of single "means" elements are not acceptable.

PATENT TERM ADJUSTMENT

The U.S. Congress passed legislation known as the Hatch–Waxman Act in 1984 that weakened patent law for pharmaceuticals, making it easier for generic copies to enter the market based on the innovator's safety and effectiveness data. Under the Act, pharmaceutical research companies lost nearly all of their rights to defend their unexpired patents before generic copies enter the market. Patent holders can sue to defend their unexpired patents *only* when a generic drug manufacturer submits a filing to the Food and Drug Administration seeking to bring the generic copy to market. The Act also created a 30-month stay procedure to allow patent holders the opportunity to obtain a court ruling on whether the generic copy infringes their patent. Thirty-month stays do not extend patents — they are triggered *before* the patent expires and provide a period of time during which patent infringement cases can be resolved.

Patent lawsuits based on the Act are rare because generally challenges to patents on prescription medicines are rare. Food and Drug Administration reports that of 8259 generic applications filed between 1984 and 2001, only 6% raised a patent issue, the necessary condition for patent litigation. According to the Federal Trade Commission, more than one quarter of patent challenges studied did not result in a lawsuit by the innovator company. Since enactment of the law, generic company share of prescription medicine use has increased from 19% of prescription units in 1984 to 50% today.

The average effective patent life for prescription medicines under the Hatch–Waxman Act is 11 to 12 years, compared to an average of 18.5 years for other products.

Effective August 18, 2003, the Food and Drug Administration has revising its regulations to:

- Permit only one 30-month stay in the approval process for a generic drug pending resolution of patent litigation. Past regulations acquiesced to the delayed launch of generic versions beyond 30 months when there were multiple, consecutive patent challenges that were made against the launch of the generic versions, even if the challenges were frivolous.
- Clarify the types of patents that may be listed in the "Orange Book," which is the Food and Drug Administration's official register of approved pharmaceutical products that provides notice to generic drug makers of name brand patent rights. Patents may no longer be listed that cover drug packaging or other minor matters not related to effectiveness. Patents are to be listed that pertain to active ingredients, drug formulations/compositions, and approved uses of a drug. A more detailed, signed attestation will be required to accompany a patent submission. False statements in the attestation can lead to criminal charges.
- Allow, for patents that are granted after the drug application is filed, the brand name drug maker 30 days to list the patent(s) from the grant date.
- Require the generic drug maker, when seeking approval for a generic, to certify to the Food and Drug Administration that either (1) there are no Orange Book listed patents for the name brand drug or (2) the patent(s) has (have) expired or (3) will expire by the time approval is sought or (4) the listed patent(s) is (are) invalid or will not be infringed. If the latter, notice of the certification is given to the patent owner and to the brand name drug maker with an explanation as to why the patent(s) is (are) invalid or not infringed. If the patent owner does not bring a patent infringement suit against the generic drug maker within 45 days, the Food and Drug Administration may approve the generic version. Otherwise, the approval process is stayed for the shorter of 30 months or the date when a court concludes the patent(s) is (are) either invalid or not infringed.
- Require generic manufacturers to demonstrate to the Food and Drug Administration that their generic drug is therapeutically equivalent to an approved brand name drug. That is, equivalence in terms of safety, strength, quality, purity, performance, intended use, and other characteristics.
- Review drug applications for generics more quickly. The Food and Drug Administration is hiring 40 generic drugs experts to expedite the approval process and to institute targeted research to expand the range of generic drugs available to consumers.
- Improve the review process for generic drugs by instituting internal reforms. The reforms include making early communications with generic drug manufacturers who submit applications and guiding generic manufacturers in preparing and submitting quality, complete applications.

The recent decision in the U.S. patent infringement case *Madey v. Duke* is very important to academic researchers as well as the industry. Duke University had challenged the general assumption that academic research using a patented device or method cannot constitute infringement. The subject matter was a laser device that had originally been developed and patented by Duke University. When the inventor left the University to pursue commercial applications for the laser,

Duke University continued to use their model for research purposes. Duke claimed that it was entitled to continue using the laser for noncommercial purposes under the experimental use exception in U.S. patent law. However, the court held that Duke University's use of the laser "unmistakably" furthered its commercial goals, including facilitating the education of students. The court further held that research using the laser had helped the University to obtain research grants. The equivalent provision in English law is section 60(5)(b) of the Patents Act of 1977, which states that an act relating to the subject matter of a patent that is done for "experimental purposes" will not constitute infringement. The provision does not set out whether the exemption is available to those whose experimental purposes have a commercial element. There is no U.K. equivalent, however, of the U.S. exemption that permits the unauthorized use of a patented device or method by a person seeking Food and Drug Administration approval to market a new product. The exemption applies only while the application is pending but extends to the use of patented devices or drugs in clinical trials, their sale for use in trials, demonstrations at trade shows, and the reporting of clinical data to potential investors.

The U.S. Patent Office prescribes specific regulations regarding patent term adjustment:

- Application filed prior to June 8, 1995: 17 years from the date of issuance regardless of the length of prosecution.
- Application filed June 8, 1995–May 28, 2000 The Uruguay Round Agreements Act (URAA): 20 years from filing date but with up to 5 years extension for delays resulting from secrecy orders, interferences, or successful appearances.
- Application pending or patent in force on June 8, 1995: 17 years from issue date or the period between the issue date and the twentieth anniversary of the filing date, whichever is greater.
- Application filed on or after May 29, 2000, American Inventors Protection Act (AIPA) may be entitled to patent term adjustment (PTA) in a continuing application including Continued Prosecuting Application (CPA), Request for Continued Examination (RCE) filed after May 29, 2000, in an application filed before May 29, 2000, does *not* provide PTA eligibility; Patent Cooperative Treaty's eligibility depends on its filing date, not its national stage entry date [Patent Cooperative Treaty must be filed on or after May 29, 2000, to be eligible for PTA].
- PTA: termination date (twentieth anniversary from filing date) is extended by number of days Patent and Trademark Office delays minus the number of days applicant delays.

4.31 PATENT AND TRADEMARK OFFICE DELAYS: GUARANTEED ADJUSTMENT BASIS (GAB):

GAB1: Patent and Trademark Office failure to take certain actions within 14 months from filing date and 4 month from other events: Patent and Trademark Office must mail an examination notification (first Office action including Quayle action or notice of allowability, restriction requirement and request for information, but NOT OIPE notice of incompleteness of application or other such notices) to applicant within 14 months of filing date; Patent and Trademark Office must also respond within 4 month to applicant's reply to an office action or applicant's opening appeal brief; Patent and Trademark Office must act within 4 months of a BPAI or court decision where allowable claims remain in the application; Patent and Trademark Office must issue the patent within 4 months of date the issue fee is paid and all outstanding requirements are satisfied.

GAB2: Patent and Trademark Office delays due to interference, secrecy order or successful appellate review (where BPAI or court reverses determination of patentability of at least one claim [allowance by examiner after a remand from BPAI is not a final decision]. GAB2 were also the bases of PTA under URAA but for a maximum of 5 years, AIPA removes 5-year limit.

GAB3: Patent and Trademark Office fails to issue a patent within 3 years excluding time consumed in RCE, secrecy order, interference, or appellate review (whether successful or not), time consumed by applicant requested delays (e.g., suspension of action up to 6 months for "food and sufficient cause," up to 3-month delay request at time of filing RCE or CPA, up to 3-year deferral of examination requested by applicant. Filing an RCE for an application filed on or after May 29, 2000) cuts off any additional PTA due to failure to issue patent within 3 years but it does NOT eliminate PTA in GAB 1 and 2.

4.32 REQUIRED REDUCTION BASIS (RRB)

Applicant's delay for failure to engage in reasonable effort to conclude prosecution of the application is subtracted from GAB1-3: failure to reply within 3 months to any notice from the office making any rejected, objection, argument or other request [even though applicant pays for and received extension], days in excess of 3 months are deducted; reinstatement of deduction of up to 3 months can be made by applicant showing that "in spite of all due care, the applicant was unable to reply," due perhaps to testing to demonstrate unexpected results, death of applicant's sole practitioner or a natural disaster. [Do not confuse the 3 months concession with 3 months required to respond.] Additional RRBs are generated because of: suspension of action under Rule 1.103, deferral of issuance under Rule 1. 3114, abandonment or late payment of issue fee, petition to revise more than 2 months after notice of abandonment, conversion of provisional to nonprovisional, preliminary amendment within one month of office action that requires supplemental office action (i.e., a response is sent when an office action was to come within one month)*, inadvertent omission in reply to office action*, supplemental reply not requested by examiner*, submission filed after BPAI or court decision within one month of office action that requires supplemental office action*, submission filed after notice of allowance* and filing a continuing application to continue prosecution. Note that in instances marked with an asterisk (*) IDS submission will not create reduction if information is received from foreign patent office within the last 30 days (i.e., the applicant responds within 30 days of receiving such information.),

4.33 NOTIFICATION

Notification of PTA is first given in the notice of allowance assuming that the applicant WILL pay the fee within 3 months and that the patent will issue within 6.5 months of Notice of Allowance; applicant may request revision or correction of PTA before payment of issue fee by showing that failure to reply within 3 months occurred "in spite of all due care," for reinstatement (a three months maximum is available for this reinstatement), the applicant may also point to Patent and Trademark Office miscalculations; in either case (even if it were Patent and Trademark Office error) a fee is required. Final PTA is listed in the Issue Notification that comes about two weeks prior to issue of patent — this includes any corrections made; applicant may request Patent and Trademark Office reconsideration (with payment of fee) for until 30 days after patent issues; no third party challenge to PTA is permitted in the Patent and Trademark Office. If correction accepted, it is printed in Certificate of Corrected; if applicant dissatisfied, applicant may appeal to United States District Court for the DC within 180 days of patent grant.

Summary: Patent term begins the day of patent issuance; terminal disclaimer date ends patent term; failure to pay a post issuance maintenance fee ends patent term (notice: no such fee required for design and plant patents); term extension beyond statutory period only through private congressional legislation or by showing government agency delays (e.g., Food and Drug Administration); 20-yr term begins from the earliest ancestral application from which priority is claimed [does not include provisional application or a foreign application for term running purpose]; design applications excluded from URAA and AIPA as they have fixed 14 year term from issue.

FOOD AND DRUG ADMINISTRATION

A listing of drugs for which the patent term had been extended by the United States Food and Drug Administration is available at http://www.uspto.gov/web/offices/pac/dapp/opla/term/156.html.

The longest patent term extension given by the U.S. Food and Drug Administration to any drug belongs to U.S. Patent 3,737,433 (Trental) for 2,494 days.

The point in the development program at which a patent application is filed will vary somewhat from company to company, but will normally be at an early stage in the process, when the substance has been made and been shown to be active in early screening. For a patent with a nominal term of 20 years from filing the effective term during which the patentee has exclusive rights to a marketed product is only eight to 12 years. This explains the importance attached by the pharmaceutical industry to provisions to extend the patent term, whether directly, as in U.S. and Japan, or indirectly by way of the Supplementary Protection Certificates (SPC) in Europe, in order to compensate for this loss of effective patent term. It also explains the importance to the industry of the minimum 20-year term guaranteed by the TRIPS agreement. The SPC for medicinal and plant protection products by the U.K. Patent Office does not extend the entire scope of the patent on which it is based, but is limited to the product covered by the marketing authorization and for any medicinal use of the product that has been authorized before the expiry of the certificate. Thus sales of the product for nonmedicinal uses do not infringe, but the SPC would be infringed by sales of a medicinal product by a third party even if that party had a marketing authorization for a different indication. Apart from this, the SPC confers the same rights as the basic patent and is subject to the same limitations and obligations to allow existing licenses under the basic patent to continue under the SPC. The scope of protection given by a U.S. patent during the Hatch–Waxman extension period is essentially the same.

INVENTIONS OF INTEREST TO PHARMACEUTICAL SCIENTISTS

Chemical compounding per se, a main requirement of TRIPs, is a relatively recent development in many countries, even in Germany, Japan, the Netherlands, Switzerland, Scandinavian countries, Austria, Spain, Greece, with several countries still not awarding patents for chemicals per se, though they may recognize the process being patentable. Much of this changed on January 1, 2005, the WTO deadline when countries became required to adopt the TRIPs requirements. The process patents are notoriously difficult to write and defend. The strength emanates from whether it is a "product-by-process" or a pure process; or, whether in a given country the onus lies on the infringer to prove innocence (a requirement of TRIPs). A process method can have value if the options available for synthesis are limited, such as in the case of diazo coupling to produce azo dyes, but if a compound can be synthesize alternately, the patent becomes very weak indeed; in some instances, the process of patenting opens up the opportunity for others to "design around" a given patent, something that is widely practiced today as the chemical processes have become more sophisticated; the same applies to production of chemical through biotechnology.

Pharmaceutical compositions remain at the top of the list of inventions patented by pharmaceutical companies. It is important to design these patents such that the claims provide a range of components, beyond which the product will not be effective; however, such tight ranges are not necessary and often not allowed by the patent office or for reasons such as prior art. However, the fact that a product may have to be approved by the Food and Drug Administration makes such patents very valuable; meaning that a generic equivalent cannot be filed until the expiry of patents. Of great importance to pharmaceutical research is the Hatch-Waxman Act of 1984, which allows patent term extension; this is described in detail later.

This use of a new strain of microorganism, whether this is found in nature, selected from organisms produced by artificially induced random mutation, or transformed by recombinant DNA technology, often presents special problem of sufficient disclosure (a requirement), requiring depositing the strain in a bank, which can result in loss of control. As a result, many companies decide not to pursue a patent filing. The products of rDNA are getting easier to disclose sufficiently.

Patents have historically been denied for an invention of a method of treatment of the human or animal body by surgery or therapy or of diagnosis practiced on the human or animal body as it is not considered to be capable of industrial application. However, this does not prevent a compound for specific use from having a useful application. Novel compounds that have a pharmaceutical utility are patentable per se in all countries that have implemented TRIPs.

Prodrugs are compounds that breakdown into active drugs in the body, anywhere along the delivery path. If the discovery of prodrug is made after the active drug, this may be infringing on the patent of the active drug if there are no additional benefits in using the prodrug; for example, hetacillin, an acetone adduct of ampicillin, which quickly hydrolyzes into penicillin, would infringe a patent for ampicillin. As long as it was not known that hetacillin converts to ampicillin, use of hetacillin would not have infringed ampicillin patent.

A patent claiming "a novel cephalosporin, its salts and a pharmaceutically acceptable bioprecursors thereof" is making a very broad claim that may lack sufficiency of disclosure since it will require an undue amount of experimental work to determine whether or not a given compound could fall under the vague definition of "bioprecursor." It is nevertheless possible to draft allowable claims to drugs which literally cover prodrugs, e.g., one can claim "physiologically hydrolysable and acceptable esters" of alcohols or acids. The situation is different when a compound is patented as a drug and subsequently found to be only a precursor of the real active substance, the active metabolite. This should not affect the patentability of the substance; if a pharmacological result is obtained by administering the substance, it is immaterial by what process the result is obtained, the mechanism need not be determined to be a patentable invention. However, if claims to the first substance do not include the second, they cannot be construed to cover it indirectly. The active metabolite, if novel and inventive, can be patented separately, and then the question arises whether sales of the original drug substance infringe the patent claiming the active metabolite. A classic example is that of terfenadine and fexofenadine, the active metabolite of terfenadine. The U.S. Patent 6,558,931 concerns a method for preparing fexofenadine from terfenadine by a bioconversion process using *Absidia corymbifera* LCP 63-1800 or *Streptomyces platensis* NRRL 2364 strain. However, before this patent, Merrell Dow had patented fexofenadine as an attempt to obviously extend the life of terfenadine patent. When a generic competitor began to sell terfenadine, Merrell Dow contended infringement (effectively, contributory infringement) under the metabolite patent, meaning that since terfenadine converts to fexofenadine, administering terfenadine is like administering fexofenadine — an audacious attempt. To prevent this misuse of patent system in this case (*Merrell Dow v. Norton* [1996] RPC 76 (HL)), the U.K. House of Lords, the U.S. District Court, and in courts in Germany declared that the patent holds but there is no infringement — perhaps the most bizarre judgment ever rendered. The arguments that lead to this conclusion are interesting and worth examining here. Obviously, there is never an "inherent lack of novelty" in any invention so that patent could not be rendered invalid. It was suggested that fexofenadine was manufactured prior to Merrell Dow's knowledge about what is happening in the liver of patients taking terfenadine; however, they did not know this so this could not be a novelty-destroying event. However, though the disclosure of the terfenadine patent specification did not mention the active metabolite, it made available to the public the invention of the acid metabolite because it "enabled the public to work the invention by making the active metabolite in their livers," i.e., by taking terfenadine. Accordingly the patent was held invalid to the extent that it covered this way of making the claimed metabolite. For the patent to be valid, it should include a disclaimer to the substance when prepared by ingestion and metabolism of terfenadine. Obviously, Merrell Dow did not have any further interest in the patent after these decisions.

Generally, whatever is available in nature is not patentable; however, if the claimed product is different from what is found in the nature, it can be patented. For example, a purified or extracted form of a natural product can be patented wherein the "specification" section of patent application would include limits of purity, etc. For example, adrenal gland could not be patented but pure adrenaline from the gland was patented. A large number of patents have been granted covering newly isolated hormones, cytokines, and other substances occurring in the human body. Whereas all antibiotics are natural products, identification and purification of these molecules allow their patenting. Even when purity limitations are not known, the natural products can be patented provided they are described in the claim in such a way that it would not include or cover the product as it is found in nature. To test this, one needs to determine if the claim infringes on the natural product; if it does not, then in patent jargon, "the claim is not anticipated" and thus allowed. Remember that only a claim is read onto a product and not vice versa. Where the chemical structure of a natural product is discovered, this can be patented as a new chemical but this would exclude the product from nature and thus it does not provide any significant protection.

In the grand scheme of delivery new chemical entities, the pharmaceutical research relies heavily on novel techniques besides the classical method of synthesizing related structures based on known structure-activity relationship and testing them pharmacologically. Some of these techniques include the following:

- Rational drug design is based on the dependence of a great many biochemical processes on specific interaction of a receptor molecule with a corresponding ligand. This interaction requires exact three-dimensional configuration of the receptor and ligand molecules, which must fit closely together. By X-ray diffraction and other physical methods it is often possible to determine exact three-dimensional structures of even large protein molecules. Sophisticated computer modeling enables scientists to predict which molecules, existing or hypothetical, would mimic the effect of the natural ligand, or to block the receptor-ligand interaction, whichever is desired. Whereas the industry has invested large sums of money in this science, the results have not been very promising compared to other most traditional methodologies of drug discovery.
- Random screening of large number of chemicals used in other trades or industries or found in nature often turn up with excellent lead compounds. Plant extracts, soil samples, or fermentation broths from microorganisms are good examples. If activity is found, the active compound can be isolated and identified subsequently. This is indeed a long-shot strategy.
- Combinatorial chemistry involves simultaneous synthesis of hundreds or even thousands of different compounds by a combination of different starting materials, reaction steps, and reagents to produce a "library" of compounds that are screened using such methods as reactions on a solid surface, for example, a plastic bead, or "tagging" the bead in some way so as to identify the sequence of reactions and reagents to which the original compound on the bead was subjected, and hence the structure of the final compound on the bead. Patenting a library or groups within the library presents some interesting options and problems. Generic claims to a group of compounds may include compounds known in prior art and chances are many of the members of group may be inactive. The library may be claimed the way it was synthesized or tagged in testing, and the only way to overcome the utility question is to show that there is a use (or value) for these libraries; recently, an assertion was made that since this database can be sold, there is an inherent value in it and thus it is "useful" in generating income; case law has yet to validate this concept.

Patentable pharmaceutical compositions and modalities can be:

- Combination preparations comprising two or more known pharmaceutically active ingredients; whereas, it is easier to make such claims in chemical compositions (see above), pharmaceutical compositions are more difficult to patent in the U.S. as these may be easily rendered prima facie obvious unless the patentee can demonstrate some synergism or a definite additive effect, not just the sum effect which is anticipated. Unlike the combinations in the chemical industry, the pharmaceutical compositions must further pass the regulatory test; however, this does not obviate the patenting objections of usefulness and the patent office need not agree with the argument that if the Food and Drug Administration has approved a product, this proves its utility. Synergism between two drugs is difficult to prove in the absence of knowledge about what to predict otherwise if they were given separately. This would require long dose-response studies of individual components and in combination to prove synergism, if at all measurable. The costs of these studies in the experimental stage can be prohibitive. However, the inventor may exploit any advantageous and unpredictable results to support the inventive steps. For example, a patent issued to me is for reduction of side effects in the use of orlistat (a patent product of Roche); use of natural fibers results in a dramatic decrease in the rectal leakage of oil and a patent was granted. However, based on the arguments presented above, this invention cannot be exercised until the use patent on orlistat (Xenical; Roche) expires. This also demonstrates the basic concept of patenting — to prevent others from practicing — as Roche cannot use this invention but neither can the inventor because of the protection in place.

- New drug delivery systems or forms such as a new kind of tablet that gives a controlled rate of release of drug when swallowed can be patented. Here the inventive step lies not in the active drug but in other constituents that enable it to be administered in a particular way to achieve such effects as a sustained blood level. Other examples would include using adhesive patches to deliver drugs, bypassing the first pass phenomenon using buccal delivery, or nasal sprays for hormones like insulin.

- Compositions comprising a compound not previously used as a drug, together with any conventional pharmaceutical carrier or excipient. A routine claim for this type of invention would be, "a pharmaceutical composition comprising a compound of formula X in association with a pharmaceutically acceptable diluent or carrier," which would include all forms in which the compound could be administered, from a complex drug delivery system to a simple tablet or solution. Care must be exercised not to include claims that are not novel, for example, if the compound were reportedly used in a solution form then its claim in the same form will be inadmissible, regardless of the newly found application of composition.

- Compositions involving first-time use of a substance can be easily patented; however, if the compound is disclosed for another use, finding another (new) use does not allow patenting of the substance. The only solution then is to patent the substance in a pharmaceutical composition containing the active ingredient. These claims would not be limited to any specific pharmaceutical indication and would cover all delivery systems. An alternative approach would be to claim the use of the compound as a pharmaceutical or therapeutic agent provided the claims do not render it a medical treatment, which is not patentable. As an example, one way to claim it is to state: "an invention consisting of a substance or composition for use in a method of treatment of the human or animal body by surgery or therapy." Claims in the form "compounds of formula X for use as an active therapeutic substance" are allowable and cover all therapeutic uses of the substances and are not restricted to a specific indication that is disclosed. Know that the patent applies to the substance when packaged as a pharmaceutical preparation and does not apply to the bulk substance.

Second or later use of a new compound is exemplified by the patenting of sildenafil citrate for the treatment of male erectile dysfunction while it was already patented for use in the treatment of hypertension and also covered under a new chemical entity claim. There is no limitation to how many new uses can be invented for an existing moiety provided it is not "taught" or disclosed in prior art. In some instances, a contrary claim to what is "taught" in the literature forms enough basis for the inventive step. A patent on the use of apomorphine in alleviating male erectile dysfunction (which was in prior art) was allowed when the patentee claimed a sublingual dosage form that was otherwise listed as a "poor delivery system." Additional patents were secured by listing the range of plasma concentration to be obtained from the sublingual tablet composition.

Method treatment claims take the form: "[a] method of treating disease X by administering compound Y"; however, if this were written as "the use of compound Y in treating disease X," this will be a claim for medical treatment, which is not allowed under the assertion that a doctor must be free to treat patients as he or she sees fit, without having to worry about being sued for patent infringement. The British Patents Act provides that a claim to a pharmaceutical substance or composition is not infringed by a pharmacist making up an individual prescription written by a doctor or dentist. In the U.S., claims to medical treatment of humans have been allowed for a long time. A typical claim of this type relating to a new use of a pharmaceutical would read "[a] method of treatment of disease Y comprising the administration, to a human in need of such treatment, of an effective dose of compound X." Claims to surgical procedures are also patentable, and this caused controversy when a U.S. surgeon patented a new type of incision for eye operations, demanded royalty payment from hospitals carrying out this technique, and in 1993 sued a clinic in Vermont for patent infringement. Besides the fact that it made the AMA furious over the physician's behavior, this led to the introduction of a bill in the House of Representatives which, after undergoing a lot of political activity, resulted in a new subsection of the U.S. patent law, 35 USC 287(c), to exempt from infringement performance of a medical activity by a medical practitioner and a "related health care entity," for example the hospital where the doctor works. "Medical activity" does not include the use of patented drugs or equipment, nor patented uses of drugs, nor biotechnological processes, so that in practice only surgical procedures are protected from infringement suits. Other patenting agencies have yet to reciprocate with such specific declaration.

BIOTECHNOLOGY INVENTIONS

Biotechnology inventions generally fall into one of two classes:

- New compositions of matter related to newly discovered isolated genes or proteins or to pharmaceutical inventions based on those genes or proteins. One cannot patent a naturally occurring gene or protein as it exists in the body, but one can patent a gene or protein that has been isolated from the body and is useful in that form as a pharmaceutical drug, screening assay, or other application.
- Methods of treating patients with a given disease through the use of a particular gene or protein. Even if someone has a patent on a gene or protein, a second inventor can obtain a patent on a new use of that gene or protein, if the second inventor discovers a new use for the substance.

The world patent authorities give extreme importance to biotechnology related inventions. The *Manual of Patent Examination Procedures* used by the U.S. Patent examiners contains an entire chapter on biotechnology related inventions; a critical review of this document is highly recommended (http://www.uspto.gov/web/offices/pac/mpep/documents/2400.htm).

Biotechnology means the production of useful products by living microorganisms and includes such examples as production of ethanol from yeast cells or production of various industrial chemicals such as acetic acid and acetone by fermentation processes. The dairy industry represents the best example of biotechnology implementation. The first "biotechnology" patent was awarded to Louis Pasteur in 1873, claiming "yeast, free from organic germs of disease, as an article of manufacture." The antibiotics and the therapeutic proteins industry is based upon the isolation of products from selected strains of microorganisms or mammalian cells, natural or mutated, such as fermentation of cyclosporine and CHO-cell derived recombinant erythropoietin. The modern biotechnology, as distinct from the classical fermentation technology, began in the 1970s with the two basic techniques: recombinant DNA (rDNA) and hybridoma technology. The rDNA is also referred to as gene splicing or genetic engineering, where genetic material from an external source is inserted into a cell in such a way that it causes the production of a desired protein by the cell; in the hybridoma technology, different types of immune cell are fused together to form a hybrid cell line producing monoclonal antibodies. More recently, the techniques of genetic engineering have been applied to higher organisms to produce transgenic animals and plants, and even to humans (gene therapy), for example, to replace missing or defective genes coding for a protein required by the body, or to introduce genes into cancer cells, which will render them easier to kill. The early completion of the human genome project has allowed identification of genes that could make useful protein products, the implementation of gene therapy, the elucidation of disease mechanisms, designing of novel diagnosis tests, and better selection of drugs based on sensitivity to different molecules. A large number of new biotechnology related study tools have been developed, which are also patentable.

The patent law and practice have had serious difficulties in keeping up with the rapid scientific progress in this field, and issues such as inventive step, sufficiency of disclosure, and permissible breadth of claims have proved challenging. As a result, patent law has undergone significant changes to accommodate the inventions made in biotechnology. One question that arose was to define the "person of ordinary skills," as the science was new, the other was to define what is considered prior art and to resolve the argument that biotechnology products are natural products and not patentable.

Patentability of microorganisms generally involves the use of a new strain of microorganism to produce a new compound or to produce a known compound more efficiently (for example, in higher yield or purity). The new organism may be found in nature (for example, by screening of soil samples) or may have been produced in the laboratory by artificially induced random mutation or by more specific techniques such as genetic engineering or gene splicing. If the microorganism produces a novel product, such as a new antibiotic, of which the structure has been determined or which can be characterized by a "fingerprint claim," then the novel product may be claimed as a new chemical compound. If the end product is already known, the patentee may rely on the process protection, but this protection is weak and it would be preferable to patent the new microorganism itself as did Lilly for the production of human insulin and General Electric for the cleanup of oil spills.

Whereas the plant and animal varieties are excluded from protection, as are the biological processes for their production, the microbiological process or the product of such a process, including the microorganism, are not excluded. The TRIPs agreement makes it obligatory for all WTO members to grant patents for microorganisms. If the microorganism intended for patenting exists in nature, it will be necessary to claim it in the form of an isolated strain to avoid possible novelty objections. It must be remembered that the term "microorganism" is interpreted broadly to include not only bacteria and fungi but also viruses and animal and plant cells. The interpretation on patenting of microorganisms went through a total turnaround at the U.S. Patent and Trademark Office after the famous Chakrabarty case was decided by the Supreme Court (though by a narrow 5 to 4 majority) wherein General Electric claimed a bacteria useful in removing oil spills, which in itself was not a useful product, though it did have a useful property.

Patent disclosure requires complete description of invention to enable others to reproduce it. This is a relatively simple subject when it comes to chemicals or pharmaceutical compositions but it is almost impossible to define a strain of microorganism. This difficulty in adequately describing the invention has resulted in a worldwide requirement that the strain be deposited in a recognized culture collection. The designated centers will maintain the strain in a viable condition and make samples of it available to the public, when required. The deposit can be made at any time while the application is pending. The majority of developed countries have now adopted the solution of requiring deposit of strains, and the Budapest Treaty on International Recognition of the Deposit of Microorganisms for the Purpose of Patent Protection (1977), which came into force in 1980 and as of 2002 has been ratified by 56 countries; the European Patent Office provides a list of international depository authorities where a single deposit made will suffice for all signatory states. A redeposit of strain is required if it becomes nonviable on storage; a minimum storage period of 30 years from the original deposit is required. Whereas the depositories provide a means of fulfilling the most important requirement of patenting, the practice creates a serious problem associated with this type of disclosure. For example, if the patentee does not get the patent and the competitors get hold of the strain 18 month after the application is filed and published, when the strain becomes public, this will be like giving away highly proprietary information. It is important to differentiate this from the disclosure made for chemical or pharmaceutical inventions where adequate disclosure can be made. In the case of the deposited strain, the public has access to the "real" product that may have taken millions of dollars to create. This is of greater concern if the strain is mutated (genetically engineered) to produce specific molecules. Whereas the patent offices have modified rules requiring that deposits will be made available only to experts and not the competing parties, it is almost impossible to guarantee that the strain will not disseminate as it is very easy to do. After the fall of the Russian Empire, it was not difficult to locate vendors offering clandestine test tubes containing modified bacteria.

RECOMBINANT DNA TECHNOLOGY — THERAPEUTIC PROTEINS

The patents describing secretion of therapeutic compounds from biological cells number over 66,000 dating from 1976 in the U.S. Patent Office; one of earliest molecule for which such a patent exists is for urokinase (Nicol, U.S. Patent 3,930,944 January 6, 1976), wherein the addition of specified amounts of pronase to the production medium for urokinase using live cells increases the production of urokinase by 50 to 100%. The first patent (dating back to April 27, 1976) that uses recombinant technology is that of Peetermans (U.S. Patent 3,953,592): Live influenza virus vaccines and preparation thereof.

There are two basic types of patentable invention in the field of recombinant DNA technology. The first relates to techniques and methods that are generally applicable to the production of a wide range of gene products; the second relates to specific products, both the proteins and the DNA sequences coding for them. The complexity involved in patenting a product of recombinant technology requires some understanding of the history of technology development. The basic invention of gene-splicing techniques was made by Cohen at Stanford and Boyer at the University of California, and Stanford University filed patent applications to cover their invention, but because publication in a scientific journal had already taken place before filing, patents could be granted only in the U.S. (See above on 35 U.S. ¶ 102 bar events which allow 12 months to file patents after disclosure). The patent (U.S. Patent 4,237,2240) was issued in December 1980 and claimed a method of producing a protein by expression of a gene inserted into any unicellular host. This covered the great majority of all genetic engineering processes and, before expiring in December 1997, earned hundreds of millions of dollars in royalty payments for the two universities. Though not so broad, other key patents cover the purification process, novel vector systems (e.g., plasmids), or promoter systems to regulate inserted genes into high expression rates of product. Most of the early patents are now nearing expiry, including patents on drugs like human insulin, erythropoietin, and growth colony stimulating factor kicking off a race for biogeneric drugs with stakes into billions of dollars. Table 12.1 lists some key drug patent expiry in the recombinant field.

Another field of rDNA technology relates to the production of a specific protein product by a transformed microorganism. The structure (amino-acid sequence) may be known, or may have been isolated in pure state but whose structure is not yet elucidated, or a product known only by its activity in some impure mixture. In the last of these cases the product can be claimed per se as a new compound characterized by its structure (which will generally be known once the gene has been obtained and sequenced). The gene itself, or at least the cDNA coding for the protein, can also be claimed.

Where the product has been previously obtained in the pure state a per se claim is no longer possible, but the invention can still be claimed in a variety of ways, having the effect of covering the product whenever made by rDNA techniques. In the European Patent Office, for example, the

TABLE 12.1
Key Drug Patent Expiry in the Recombinant Field

Brand Name (Generic Name)	Marketing Company	Indication	2002 Sales ($, millions)	U.S. Patent Expiry
Rebetron Combination Therapy (Ribavirin and Interferon alfa-2b)	Schering-Plough	Chronic hepatitis C	1,361	2001
Ceredase (aglucerase)	Cenzyme	Gaucher disease	537	2001
Cerezyme (imiglucerase)	Cenzyme	Gaucher disease	537	2001
Humulin (human insulin)	Novo Nordisk	Diabetes	500	2002
Intron A (interferon alfa-2b)	Schering Plough	Leukemia; hepatitis B and C, melanoma; lymphoma	2,700	2002
Avonex (interferon beta-1a)	Biogen	Multiple sclerosis	1034	2003
Humatrope (somatropin)	Eli Lilly & Co.	Growth hormone deficiency	329	2003
Nutropin/Nutropin AQ (somatropin)	Genentech	Growth hormone deficiency	226	2003
Epogen (epoetin alpha)	Amgen	Anemia	2,300	2004
Procrit (epoetin alpha)	Johnson & Johnson	Anemia	4,283	2004
Geref (sermorelin)	Serono Laboratories	Growth hormone deficiency	0.07	2004
Synagis (palivizumab)	Abbott	Respiratory syncytial viral	480	2005
Activase (alteplase)	Genentech	Myocardial infarction, stroke, pulmonary embolism	180	2005
Protropin (somatrem)	Genentech	Growth hormone deficiency	2,100	2005
Neupogen (filgrastim)	Amgen	Neutropenia	1,400	2005
Albutein (human albumin)	Enzon	Shock and hemo-dialysis	4,509	2006

Source: IMS Health, ABN AMRO estimates and Food and Drug Administration Orange Book (patent expiry as quoted by Carl Peck, Center for Drug Development Science, Georgetown University at the Presentation on Principles of Clinical Pharmacology, NIH, 2003; updated sales figures from http://www.i-s-b.org/business/rec_sales.htm).

patentee could claim the isolated gene for the product, a vector containing the gene, the host cell transformed with the vector, the process for obtaining any of these, and finally the process for obtaining the end-product, which would be infringed by sale of the product obtained by that process. It may be possible to claim the unglycosylated protein per se even when the natural glycosylated form is known. In the U.K. it is possible to go further and claim for example "human tissue plasminogen activator as produced by recombinant DNA technology."

What constitutes an inventive step has changed rapidly in the field of biotechnology since the days of Cohen and Boyer. Genentech's European patent claiming a rDNA process for the preparation of known tPA, which was upheld by the Board of Appeal, albeit in restricted scope in the European Patent Office but turned down in England, stating that it was obviously desirable to create a recombinant form of a known protein. The U.S. Patent Office used to take the position that the gene coding for a protein of known amino acid sequence was prima facie obvious and unpatentable, but in 1993 the Court of Appeals for Federal Circuit (CAFC) held otherwise, considering that the redundancy of the genetic code meant that there were over 1036 distinct DNA sequences coding for the protein in question (insulin-like growth factor), and that the prior art may not suggest any particular one of these sequences. It is therefore now possible to patent a recombinant form of a known protein.

A claim to a recombinant product defined by one specific amino acid sequence is likely to give a scope of protection that is too narrow, since for any natural protein, there are some regions in which it is possible to change one or two amino acids without affecting the function of the protein, and other regions where any change in the exact amino acid sequence will alter or destroy the activity. Thus, although porcine and bovine insulin differ slightly from human insulin, they have essentially the same activity in humans. To solve this problem claims are drafted for proteins that have a certain degree of homology with the defined amino acid sequence, or that may have a certain number of possible amino acid deletions, additions, or substitutions (some of which have been so broad as to claim practically all possible proteins). However, such a claim must necessarily cover a large number of useless products in view of the fact that a change of one amino acid may cause complete loss of activity and is likely to be invalid for this reason. A better claim combines such possibility of structural variation with a requirement that the product must have a certain defined activity. Wishfully, the courts need to interpret a claim to a specific protein structure as covering also minor variations such as might be expected to occur in nature and do not alter the properties of the claimed product.

The claims to DNA sequences may be placed in four categories of increasing breadth:

- A "picture" claim to one specific DNA sequence;
- Including other DNA sequences coding for the same protein (genetic code redundancy);
- Including DNA sequences coding for modified proteins having the same function;
- Including DNA sequences coding for significantly modified proteins, some of which may not be functional, or including noncoding DNA sequences.

The first two comprise the majority of patents issued in the U.S. In the U.S., it is not only the literal wording of the claim granted by the U.S. Patent and Trademark Office that is important, but also the extent to which the courts will broaden the wording by application of the Doctrine of Equivalents. In the litigation between Genentech, Wellcome and Genetics Institute (GI) over the clot-dissolving drug tissue plasminogen activator (WA), Genetics Institute had developed a modification of tPA called FEIX, which had 15% fewer amino acids than did natural tPA, as well as several minor changes, and as a result stayed active in the blood 10 times longer than the natural product. Genentech's claims literally covered only the natural sequence and naturally occurring variants, but before the District Court a jury found infringement by equivalence. However, the CAFC reversed on appeal, "on the basis that there was no evidence that FEIX functioned in the same way as natural tPA."

The U.S. courts frequently find broad claims to proteins and DNA sequences to be invalid for lack of enabling disclosure. Thus for example in the litigation between Amgen and Chugai over erythropoietin (European Patent Office), a claim of category 3 above, claiming any purified and isolated DNA sequence "encoding a polypeptide having an amino acid sequence sufficiently duplicative of that of erythropoietin to allow possession of (biological properties of European Patent Office)," was held invalid for lack of an adequate disclosure of how to make other DNA species in this broad genus. However, the court made it clear that broad generic claims could be valid if they corresponded to a proper disclosure of the invention. A situation frequently arises where a patent application is written at an early stage of the work, when sufficient data are not available, yet based on the prior art and extrapolations, it is possible to guess how the results may turn out. In such cases, risk is taken and broad speculative claims are drafted, which may be allowed by the patent office. In the U.S., such claims, once granted, have at least until recently been very difficult to attack, but in the infringement litigation between the University of California and Eli Lilly, the CAFC dealt a serious blow to broad claiming. The University inventors had isolated and sequenced only the gene for rat insulin, and the patent claimed results for genes for all mammalian insulin, including human. The description was sufficient in that the reader would be able to isolate human insulin gene using the method described in the patent. But it did not meet the "written description" requirement of 35 USC ¶112 because the inventors did not make the human insulin gene and did not describe its structure. In the European Patent Office, it has been difficult to attack overbroad claims because the violation of Article 84 is not a ground of opposition, and for some time it was difficult to allege insufficiency of disclosure because of the Genentech case, which was interpreted to mean that a single working example establishes sufficiency for the entire scope, no matter how broad. Later cases now agree that the description has to be sufficient over the whole claimed scope. This situation exemplifies the dilemma a researcher and his company may face at the time of filing a patent; if you go too broad, you may be knocked out later; if you claim too narrow, you will soon have a competitor nevertheless.

For inventions in a rapidly moving field, it is often critical to file a patent application as early as possible so that the art appearing in the literature could not be used to invalidate the claims. This was shown in the U.K. in the case of *Biogen v.* Medeva, which illustrated the difficulty of upholding the validity of broad biotech claims. The patent claimed a rDNA molecule characterized by a DNA sequence for a polypeptide displaying HBV (hepatitis B virus) antigen specificity, and covered the genes for both core and surface antigen, although only one of these had been developed. In the European Patent Office the patent was opposed but the Board of Appeal ruled that it was sufficient disclosure as it enabled the user to make both core and surface antigens. The patent was upheld despite publication of methods during the prosecution of the patent that would have made the patent invalid had it not been filed earlier. Priority date (date when the claim is made) was also an issue in a case relating to a whooping cough vaccine, in which the inventor had discovered that a certain known protein was a protective antigen; however, by the time the European application was filed, it had been realized that the antigen that had been discovered was in fact a different protein and even though the patentee argued that both proteins could be manufactured by the described method, the application was turned down for lack of adequate disclosure compared to the breadth of claims.

MONOCLONAL ANTIBODY TECHNOLOGY

Biotechnology products are also derived from the workings of the immune system responsible for producing white blood cells, or lymphocytes. These cells originate as stem cells in the bone marrow, and then differentiate and mature either in the bone marrow to B-lymphocytes (B-cells), or in the thymus gland to T-lymphocytes (T cells). The main task of the B-cells is to produce antibodies in response to exposure to foreign substance through interaction on the surface receptors of B-cells. Upon activation, the activated B-cell undergoes rapid division and develops into a clone of identical plasma cells, all of which secrete antibody molecules, which have the same specificity to the antigen as did the original B-cell. The antibodies thus produced (immunoglobulins or Ig molecules) are complex proteins having the approximate shape of the letter Y with binding sites in its branches for a particular antigen. The antibodies react with antigen molecules and form a cross-linked insoluble structure, removing the antigen from circulation. Where the antigen is located on the surface of a foreign cell like a bacterium, the antibodies bind to the surface (opsonization), rendering the cell ready for destruction by macrophages or other components of the immune system.

Antibodies isolated from human blood, particularly in the form of immunoglobulin-G (IgG or gamma-globulin) have been used therapeutically for a long time such as to provide immunity against viral infections; the potency will depend on how recently the donor had experience the infection. Antibodies are also powerful tools in diagnosis of disease and also in identification of biological organisms. Recently, a test method has been developed to test for contamination with anthrax using an antigen-antibody reaction (http://www.osborn-scientific.com/); the pregnancy test kits routinely exploit this technique. Historically, antibodies were produced commercially from mice immunized with human T-cells; however, the antisera would contain a mixture even if pure antigen were used to immunize mice. Individual B-cell specific for a particular antigen isolated and cultured would provide a single antibody, but the normal B-cells cannot be kept alive in culture. It was discovered that myeloma, malignant tumors of the immune system, all derived from B-cells, sometimes producing large quantities of a single monoclonal antibody. Cloning of tumor cells thus represented an opportunity to produce monoclonal antibodies except the fact that in a natural myeloma, the antibody actually produced was a matter of chance. To overcome this problem, in 1975, Milstein and Kohler fused a malignant mouse myeloma cell with a normal B-cell from the spleen of a mouse to obtain a hybrid cell line, a hybridoma, which had the properties of both parent cells, producing antibody and growing in culture amounting to immortalization of B-cells. Choosing a myeloma that did not produce antibodies of its own, this technique will allow production of the antibody from the normal B-cell only. The technique was further refined by Kohler and Milstein using spleen cells from a mouse immunized with sheep erythrocytes (red blood cells); monoclonal antibodies (MAbs) against sheep erythrocytes were obtained. The importance of this work was only realized years later when MAbs against a desired antigen in a mouse or rat immunized with the antigen were obtained by recovering lymphocytes from the spleen of the animal and fusing them with cells from a suitable myeloma line to create individual hybridoma cells. Clones that produce the desired MAb may then be selected and the hybridoma line cultured to manufacture the MAb in commercial quantities.

Initial inventions could not characterize the sequence of the amino acid in the antibody molecules, and the hybridoma lines were deposited as part of patent application disclosure; later, as more refined methods became available, the sequencing of the antibodies was submitted in lieu of or in addition to cell line deposits. Characterization of amino acid sequencing of antibodies also allowed use of rDNA technologies to produce antibodies as well. The use of rDNA addressed another problem with the therapeutic use of monoclonal antibodies, where mouse proteins upon repeated administration reacted with the patient's immune system, reducing their effectiveness or even causing harmful allergic reaction. Antibodies produced by rDNA methods use chimeric MAbs in which the variable regions (the arms of the Y) remain murine but the constant regions (the base of the Y) are replaced with the constant regions of a human antibody. Another advancement in the technology came when there was replacement of all but the actual hypervariable regions, which give the specificity to give a humanized antibody.

More advances in technology allowed use of fragments of antibody genes to be expressed on the surface of a carrier, such as a bacteriophage enabling fragments coding for hypervariable regions of desired specificity for selection and incorporation into genes which can be expressed to give fully human monoclonal antibodies. This made the technology for the production of chimeric and humanized antibodies obsolete by the time the first of these products came on the market. The phage display technique can also be used to find large or small molecules that bind to a particular structure, for example, one corresponding to a receptor or its ligand. Antibodies having certain specificities are also used as catalysts by holding two reagent molecules together in the correct configuration for reaction to proceed.

Whereas the work of Cohen and Boyer (for rDNA technology) was patented only in the U.S. (as described above), the work of Kohler and Milstein could not be patented for merely lack of foresight. Many patents have been granted claiming MAbs directed to particular antigens, or classes of antigens in light of the case of Wistar Institute. Patent was at first denied in the U.K. to Wistar, which claimed broadly monoclonal antibodies to any viral antigens. It was allowed in the U.S. and Japan. Though several patents claim any MAbs to specific antigens (e.g. to alpha-interferon) or to certain groups of cells (e.g. certain groups of human T-cells), their validity is questionable. Once the general applicability of the hybridoma technique was recognized, it was argued that there was no longer any invention in producing MAbs to any previously known antigen, in the absence of special difficulties that had to be overcome. If the antigen was unknown at the time, the inventive step may not be an issue, but there are serious problems of sufficiency of disclosure given that fusion to produce hybridomas is a random process that is inherently nonreproducible, and that finding one MAb with a specific affinity does not necessarily make it any easier to find a second one.

In the case of Ortho before the European Patent Office Board of Appeal, the patent contained broad claims to antibodies reacting with certain human blood cells but not others, but there was only a single example, and it was shown not to fall within these claims. Not only were the broad claims invalid, a claim limited to the deposited hybridoma was also rejected since the written description did not correspond to what was deposited.

Where the new and useful individual MAbs have defined structure and the hybridoma deposited, patents can be obtained but only if they have some advantageous properties. The dilemma of depositing hybridoma (vis-à-vis a recombinant bacteria) is a moot point with the availability of sequencing of amino acids in antibodies.

ANTISENSE TECHNOLOGY

If a particular gene has a role in disease, and the genetic code of that gene is known, one could use this knowledge to stop that gene specifically. Genes are made of double-helical DNA. When a gene is turned on, the genetic code in that segment of DNA is copied out as a single strand of RNA, called messenger RNA. The messenger RNA is called a "sense" sequence because it can be translated into a string of amino acids to form a protein. The opposite strand in a DNA double helix (A opposite T, T opposite A, C opposite G, G opposite C) is called the "antisense" strand. The antisense coding sequence of a disease gene can be used to make short antisense DNAs to work as a drugs that binds to messenger RNAs from disease genes, so that the genetic code in the RNA cannot be read, stopping the production of the disease-causing protein.

Generally, a fragment of 20 bases length will be specific for one particular gene and, therefore, not interfere with the expression of other genes. Several difficulties arise in developing antisense drugs that range from the instability of single-stranded DNA *in vivo* to finding suitable delivery systems. The stability problem may be overcome by chemical modification of the backbone of the DNA chain, for example, replacing the phosphate groups with groups that are hydrolyzed less easily, and these modifications can be patented. The first antisense drug was approved in 1998: the first antisense therapeutic for treating CMV retinitis, Vitravene. In 2003, there were over 1500 patents making a claim for products related to antisense technology. The impact of biotechnology on antisense technology is expected to increase dramatically as the links between genetics, protein production, and disease are better understood. The application of antisense technology is not limited to human and veterinary medicine. It is also used to make biotechnology food products. For example, in agriculture, this technology was used to develop the Flavr Savr Tomato.

CELL THERAPY

A nontherapeutic use of monoclonal antibodies is in characterizing cells, particularly cells present in the blood, lymphatic system, and bone marrow for the cell-specific molecules carried on their surfaces. This is done by tagging monoclonal antibodies tagged with fluorescent molecules and differentiating and separating cells by the FACS (fluorescence activated cell sorting) technique. In this way, the development of the various types of blood cell (the hematopoietic system) can be traced back to a single type, the hematopoietic stem cell (HSC), which can give rise to all other types. Also, mesenchymal stem cells (MSCs) differentiating into all types of connective tissue such as cartilage, bone, and tendon can be isolated from bone marrow. These cells are patentable where claims are not made to cover the cells in their natural state in the human body. Such stem cells can have direct therapeutic uses, for example HSCs can be administered to cancer patients whose hematopoietic system has been damaged by chemotherapy or radiotherapy, and MSCs may be useful to regenerate cartilage damaged by injury or arthritis. Most likely these treatments would require harvesting cells from the patient, isolating them, expanding the culture, and infusing them back into patients. These cells may also be used in gene therapy (see below).

GENE THERAPY

Genes, which are carried on chromosomes, are the basic physical and functional units of heredity. Genes are specific sequences of bases that encode instructions on how to make proteins. Although genes get a lot of attention, it is the proteins that perform most life functions and even make up the majority of cellular structures. When genes are altered so that the encoded proteins are unable to carry out their normal functions, genetic disorders can result, such as hemophilia and cystic fibrosis.

Gene therapy is a technique for correcting defective genes responsible for disease development. Researchers may use one of several approaches for correcting faulty genes:

• A normal gene may be inserted into a nonspecific location within the genome to replace a nonfunctional gene. This approach is most common.
• An abnormal gene could be swapped for a normal gene through homologous recombination.
• The abnormal gene could be repaired through selective reverse mutation, which returns the gene to its normal function.
• The regulation (the degree to which a gene is turned on or off) of a particular gene could be altered.

In most gene therapy studies, a "normal" gene is inserted into the genome to replace an "abnormal," disease-causing gene. A carrier molecule called a vector must be used to deliver the therapeutic gene to the patient's target cells. Currently, the most common vector is a virus that has been genetically altered to carry normal human DNA. Viruses have evolved a way of encapsulating and delivering their genes to human cells in a pathogenic manner. Scientists have tried to take advantage of this capability and manipulate the virus genome to remove disease-causing genes and insert therapeutic genes. Target cells such as the patient's liver or lung cells are infected with the viral vector. The vector then unloads its genetic material, containing the therapeutic human gene, into the target cell. The generation of a functional protein product from the therapeutic gene restores the target cell to a normal state.

Besides virus-mediated gene-delivery systems, there are several nonviral options for gene delivery. The simplest method is the direct introduction of therapeutic DNA into target cells. This approach is limited in its application because it can be used only with certain tissues and requires large amounts of DNA.

Another nonviral approach involves the creation of an artificial lipid sphere with an aqueous core. This liposome, which carries the therapeutic DNA, is capable of passing the DNA through the target cell's membrane.

Therapeutic DNA also can get inside target cells by chemically linking the DNA to a molecule that will bind to special cell receptors. Once bound to these receptors, the therapeutic DNA constructs are engulfed by the cell membrane and passed into the interior of the target cell. This delivery system tends to be less effective than other options.

Researchers also are experimenting with introducing a 47th (artificial human) chromosome into target cells. This chromosome would exist autonomously alongside the standard 46 — not affecting their workings or causing any mutations. It would be a large vector capable of carrying substantial amounts of genetic code, and scientists anticipate that, because of its construction and autonomy, the body's immune systems would not attack it. A problem with this potential method is the difficulty in delivering such a large molecule to the nucleus of a target cell.

The Food and Drug Administration has not yet approved any human gene therapy product for sale. Current gene therapy is experimental and has not proven very successful in clinical trials. In January 2003, the Food and Drug Administration placed a temporary halt on all gene therapy trials using retroviral vectors in blood stem cells. Whereas the progress has been slow, it is anticipated that with greater advances in the technology there will eventually be a treatment found for diseases like cystic fibrosis, just to name one. There will definitely be many opportunities of patenting not just the products but also the methods to study gene therapy.

LIFE PATENTING

Techniques like microinjection can be used to introduce extraneous genetic material into a fertilized mammalian ovum, or insert the ovum into a pseudopregnant female, and obtain offspring in which the genetic material has become incorporated into the genome. By combining this process with classical breeding steps such as back-crossing it is possible to obtain a strain of animal that stably transmits the new gene to subsequent generations, which will display the corresponding phenotype according to the laws of Mendelian genetics. Two possible uses can be made for such transgenic animals: as models for research and as a source for useful materials such as large quantities of therapeutic proteins where gene expression takes place randomly throughout the body and the proteins may be secreted in milk. This technique can be useful in producing human serum albumin and alpha-trypsin in larger animal species. Another use of transgenic animals is in supplying organs for transplantation. For example, if a pig is transformed with a human gene so that the cells in its organs express a human surface protein, it is expected that the hyperacute rejection upon transplant of pig organs into humans would be blocked or reduced.

The Oncomouse was developed in the 1980s at Harvard Medical School, through DuPont funding. It was patented by Harvard and licensed exclusively to DuPont. "Onco" is derived from oncogene, a name geneticists give to a damaged or mutated gene, which can cause cancer if these genes are responsible for regulation of cell growth. When oncogene meets mouse, the result is the Oncomouse, and when two such mice breed, the cancer-causing genes are passed to the offspring, which are thus predisposed to developing cancer at an accelerated rate. Scientists study the interplay between oncogenes in the mice as a model for studying cancer in humans.

Currently the Oncomouse is patented in U.S., Europe, and Japan but denied in Canada where the litigation went all the way to Supreme Court.

TRANSGENIC PLANTS

Unlike animal cells, plant cells have external cell wall that is difficult to penetrate when introducing genetic material. It is also difficult for the vector to move around in the cell because of the cellular environment. Novel techniques like placing DNA molecules on the surface of micronized glass beads physically shot into cells are thus used. Once transformed, the plants can be bred in the normal process. The purpose of transgenic plants is to produce higher yields, improve nutritional quality, and lower the cost of production. For example, one early product was a transgenic tomato Flavr Savr (Calgene, Davis, CA) that did not do well in the market. Insect and virus-resistant crops are one of the targets of plant transgenic research. Maize contains a gene from *Bacillus thuringensis*, which produces a toxin harmful to insects but not to mammals, as a result, the larva of the corn borer is killed by eating the plant and insecticide treatment may be avoided.

PATENTING STRATEGIES

Pharmaceutical and biotechnology scientists face several major challenges in designing their research:

- Does the research create a product that is prohibited by statute to be patented; a thorough process, a law of physics, an object of little utility, or another prohibited area of patentability? Obviously, the end goal is not always to secure a patent for a product; a proprietary process need not be patented if it is possible to keep it protected, something that is becoming very difficult to ensure as the information flow becomes easier between individuals and around the world.
- Is the research likely to lead to a novel product or process meaning something that has never existed before? Novel is not necessary patentable as we go through the legality of patenting process; this is, however, one of the fundamental requirement.
- Is the novel research unobvious to those with ordinary skill in the art? This aspect of patenting is most confusing and often leads to most rejections of patent applications. Researchers need to study existing art (what is called prior art) before designing experiments to ensure that they can create sufficient features in the invention to take it out of

the obviousness arena. What is needed here is a demonstration that there was an inventive step, or in ordinary words, something was actually discovered and that it was not something that could have been easily discovered. A lot of experimentation goes into demonstrating unusual results to obviate the assertion of obviousness by the patent examiners.

- Can the claim made withstand court challenge? Even though these areas of interpretations are beyond what a scientist would be expected to have any expertise, a keen understanding of the scope of claims is essential; a patent with too broad a claim is not necessarily a good patent just as much as vice versa. The patent disclosure must support the claim adequately.
- Does the disclosure in the patent meet the legal requirements of patent allowance? In the U.S., the patentee must disclose a best mode, the best formula, and the best approach to use the research outcome. There is no need to disclose an industrial model but a workable model. Keeping the information out of a patent can be a double-edge sword.
- Is it possible to create a sequel to a successful research product? It is not unusual for the companies to keep some portions of the research aside and out of a patent to be able to claim it later. This can be a dangerous practice. If prior art appears in the interim then all research is lost and even one's own patent can be taken as a prior art.
- Is it possible to continue the patent coverage by designing products around an issued patent? This is most critical to the pharmaceutical and biotechnology industry. Good examples of this practice include changes in the formulation to improve the product such as Abbott did when its patent on calcitriol came to expiry; the company changed the specification on the level of oxygen in the solution. What it meant was that there would be no generic equivalent to Abbott's calcitriol, though the generic forms may not be any less active. SmithKline Beecham's remarkable patenting of amoxicillin and clavulanic combination is a good example of intelligent patenting; you will find not only patents for specific combination of the two antibiotics but of a score of different dosage forms; one patent is based only on the hardness of the tablet. This type of research requires a keen understanding of the patenting process.
- Is it possible to invent around a patent or a publication? Once sildenafil citrate became a success or once statins became the choice treatment for lowering cholesterol, the drug companies rushed to make similar products; obviously, there were problems in prior art. What is already disclosed cannot be obviated. The researchers are then faced with a challenge to find solutions novel enough to be patented; some degree of reverse engineering is required. However, as we see the results, they did succeed. However, with each patent issuing the field gets narrower as to what can be patented. Scientists often get bogged down with the science and do not realize that to receive a patent on an invention there is no need to explain how it works. In fact, there need not even be an explanation how it came into existence or how it worked. Just the fact that there is a working example is sufficient. In many instances even a working example is not required. A new drug may be subject to Food and Drug Administration comments before the U.S. Patent Office allows the claims, however, it is not required of the patent office. On the other hand, the patent office need not accept the approval by the regulatory authorities as a proof of the utility, a key requirement for patentability.

Obviously, good research in an industrial environment is research that yields good profits, and to achieve marketability and profitability from the research, the product must be either patentable or of a type that could not be reverse-engineered if proprietary techniques are relied upon. The challenges to scientists are great with expanding technology and stiffer competition to produce new products. One way to take these challenges head on is to understand the art of patenting as well as the science. Keeping abreast with the knowledge is critical, and scientists are strongly urged to hone their skills in the use of computers to search the literature.

Appendix I

Recombinant DNA and
Monoclonal Antibody
Products Approved by FDA

Product	Company	Application	FDA Approval Date	Description
Actimmune® (interferon gamma-1b)	InterMune Pharmaceuticals, Inc.	Treatment of chronic granulomatous disease; Treatment of severe, malignant osteopetrosis	Dec 1990 Feb 2000	Actimmune® (Interferon gamma-1b), a biologic response modifier, is a single-chain polypeptide containing 140 amino acids. Production of Actimmune is achieved by fermentation of a genetically engineered *Escherichia coli* bacterium containing the DNA that encodes for the human protein. Purification of the product is achieved by conventional column chromatography. Actimmune is a highly purified sterile solution consisting of noncovalent dimers of two identical 16,465 dalton monomers; with a specific activity of 20 million International Units (IU)/mg (2×10^6 IU per 0.5 mL), which is equivalent to 30 million units/mg. Actimmune is a sterile, clear, colorless solution filled in a single-dose vial for subcutaneous injection. Each 0.5 mL of Actimmune contains: 100 mcg (2 million IU) of Interferon gamma-1b formulated in 20 mg mannitol, 0.36 mg sodium succinate, 0.05 mg polysorbate 20 and sterile water for injection. *Note that the above activity is expressed in International Units (1 million IU/50mcg). This is equivalent to what was previously expressed as units (1.5 million U/50mcg).*
Activase®/Cathflo® Activase® (alteplase; tissue plasminogen activator)	Genentech, Inc.	Treatment of acute myocardial infarction; Acute massive pulmonary embolism; Acute ischemic stroke within first three hours of symptom onset; Dissolution of clots in central venous access devices	Nov 1987 Jun 1990 Jun 1996 Sep 2001	Activase, Alteplase, is a tissue plasminogen activator produced by recombinant DNA technology. It is a sterile, purified glycoprotein of 527 amino acids. It is synthesized using the complementary DNA (cDNA) for natural human tissue-type plasminogen activator obtained from a human melanoma cell line. The manufacturing process involves the secretion of the enzyme alteplase into the culture medium by an established mammalian cell line (Chinese hamster ovary cells) into which the cDNA for alteplase has been genetically inserted. Fermentation is carried out in a nutrient medium containing the antibiotic gentamicin, 100 mg/L. However, the presence of the antibiotic is not detectable in the final product. Phosphoric acid or sodium hydroxide may be used prior to lyophilization for pH adjustment. Activase is a sterile, white to off-white, lyophilized powder for intravenous administration after reconstitution with sterile water for injection, USP.

Quantitative Composition of the Lyophilized Product

	100 mg Vial	50 mg Vial
Alteplase	100 mg (58 million IU)	50 mg (29 million IU)
L-Arginine	3.5 g	1.7 g
Phosphoric Acid	1 g	0.5 g
Polysorbate 80	≤ 11 mg	≤ 4 mg
Vacuum	No	Yes

Biological potency is determined by an *in vitro* clot lysis assay and is expressed in International Units as tested against the WHO standard. The specific activity of Activase is 580,000 IU/mg. Powder for reconstitution for use in central venous access devices Cathflo™ Activase® [Alteplase] is a tissue plasminogen activator (t-PA) produced by recombinant DNA technology. It is a sterile, purified glycoprotein of 527 amino acids. It is synthesized using the complementary DNA (cDNA) for natural human tissue-type plasminogen activator (t-PA) obtained from an established human cell line. The

Product	Company	Indication	Date	Description
Advate® (Recombinant antihemophilic factor produced without any added human or animal plasma proteins and albumin)	Baxter Healthcare Corp.	Hemophilia A	Jul 2003	

manufacturing process involves secretion of the enzyme Alteplase into the culture medium by an established mammalian cell line (Chinese hamster ovary cells) into which the cDNA for Alteplase has been genetically inserted. Fermentation is carried out in a nutrient medium containing the antibiotic gentamicin sulfate, 100 mg/L. The presence of the antibiotic is not detectable in the final product. Cathflo Activase is a sterile, white to pale yellow, lyophilized powder for intracatheter instillation for restoration of function to central venous access devices following reconstitution with sterile water for injection, USP. Each vial of Cathflo Activase contains 2.2 mg of Alteplase (which includes a 10% overfill), 77 mg of L-arginine, 0.2 mg of polysorbate 80, and phosphoric acid for pH adjustment. Each reconstituted vial will deliver 2 mg of Cathflo Activase, at a pH of approximately 7.3.

Advate® Antihemophilic Factor (Recombinant), Plasma/Albumin-Free Method (rAHF-PFM) is a purified glycoprotein consisting of 2332 amino acids that is synthesized by a genetically engineered Chinese hamster ovary (CHO) cell line. In culture, the CHO cell line expresses recombinant antihemophilic factor (rAHF) into the cell culture medium. The rAHF is purified from the culture medium using a series of chromatography columns. The cornerstone of the purification process is an immunoaffinity chromatography step in which a monoclonal antibody directed against Factor VIII is employed to selectively isolate the rAHF from the medium. The cell culture and purification processes used in the manufacture of ADVATE rAHF-PFM employ no additives of human or animal origin. The production process includes a dedicated, viral inactivation solvent-detergent treatment step. The rAHF synthesized by the CHO cells has the same biological effects as Antihemophilic Factor (Human) [AHF (Human)]. Structurally the recombinant protein has a similar combination of heterogeneous heavy and light chains as found in AHF (Human). Advate rAHF-PFM is formulated as a sterile, nonpyrogenic, white to off-white powder for intravenous injection. Advate rAHF-PFM is available in single-dose vials that contain nominally 250, 500, 1000, or 1500 International Units (IU) per vial. When reconstituted with the appropriate volume of diluent, the product contains the following stabilizers in maximal amounts: 38 mg/mL mannitol, 10 mg/mL trehalose, 108 mEq/L sodium, 12 mM histidine, 12 mM Tris, 1.9 mM calcium, 0.17 mg/mL polysorbate-80, and 0.10 mg/mL glutathione. Von Willebrand Factor (vWF) is co-expressed with FVIII and helps to stabilize it in culture. The final product contains no more than 2 ng vWF/IU rAHF, which will not have any clinically relevant effect in patients with von Willebrand's disease. The product contains no preservative. Each vial of Advate rAHF-PFM is labeled with the AHF activity expressed in IU per vial. Biological potency is determined by an in vitro assay, which employs a Factor VIII concentrate standard that is referenced to a World Health Organization (WHO) International Standard for Factor VIII: C concentrates. The specific activity of Advate rAHF-PFM is 4000 to 10,000 IU mg of protein.

Product	Company	Application	FDA Approval Date	Description
Aldurazyme® (laronidase; recombinant enzyme replacement)	BioMarin Pharmaceuticals Inc. and Genzyme	Mucopolysaccharidosis-1	Apr 2003	Aldurazyme® (laronidase) is a polymorphic variant of the human enzyme, _-L-iduronidase that is produced by recombinant DNA technology in a Chinese hamster ovary cell line. _-L-iduronidase (glycosaminoglycan _-L-iduronohydrolase, EC 3.2.1.76) is a lysosomal hydrolase that catalyses the hydrolysis of terminal _-L-iduronic acid residues of dermatan sulfate and heparan sulfate. Laronidase is a glycoprotein with a molecular weight of approximately 83 kD. The predicted amino acid sequence of the recombinant form, as well as the nucleotide sequence that encodes it, are identical to a polymorphic form of human _-L-iduronidase. The recombinant protein is comprised of 628 amino acids after cleavage of the N-terminus and contains 6 N-linked oligosaccharide modification sites. Two oligosaccharide chains terminate in mannose-6-phosphate sugars. Aldurazyme has a specific activity of approximately 172 U/mg. Aldurazyme, for intravenous infusion, is supplied as a sterile, nonpyrogenic, colorless to pale yellow, clear to slightly opalescent solution that must be diluted prior to administration in 0.9% sodium chloride injection, USP containing 0.1% albumin (human). The solution in each vial contains a nominal laronidase concentration of 0.58 mg/mL and a pH of approximately 5.5. The extractable volume of 5.0 mL from each vial provides 2.9 mg laronidase, 43.9 mg sodium chloride, 63.5 mg sodium phosphate monobasic monohydrate, 10.7 mg sodium phosphate dibasic heptahydrate, and 0.05 mg polysorbate 80. Aldurazyme does not contain preservatives; vials are for single use only.
Amevive® (alefacept; recombinant, dimeric fusion protein; targets CD45RO+ T-cells)	Biogen Idec	Moderate to severe chronic plaque psoriasis	Jan 2003	Amevive® (alefacept) is an immunosuppressive dimeric fusion protein that consists of the extracellular CD2-binding portion of the human leukocyte function antigen-3 (LFA-3) linked to the Fc (hinge, CH2 and CH3 domains) portion of human IgG1. Alefacept is produced by recombinant DNA technology in a Chinese hamster ovary (CHO) mammalian cell expression system. The molecular weight of alefacept is 91.4 kilodaltons. Amevive is supplied as a sterile, white to off-white, preservative-free, lyophilized powder for parenteral administration. After reconstitution with 0.6 mL of the supplied sterile water for injection, USP, the solution of Amevive is clear, with a pH of approximately 6.9. Amevive is available in two formulations. Amevive for intramuscular injection contains 15 mg alefacept per 0.5 mL of reconstituted solution. Amevive for intravenous injection contains 7.5 mg alefacept per 0.5 mL of reconstituted solution. Both formulations also contain 12.5 mg sucrose, 5.0 mg glycine, 3.6 mg sodium citrate dihydrate, and 0. 06 mg citric acid monohydrate per 0.5 mL.
Apidra® (insulin glulisine rDNA origin)	Aventis	Apidra is indicated for the treatment of adult patients with diabetes mellitus for the control of hyperglycemia. Apidra has a more rapid onset of action and a shorter duration of	April 2004	Apidra™ (insulin glulisine [rDNA origin]) is a human insulin analog that is a rapid-acting, parenteral blood glucose lowering agent. Insulin glulisine is produced by recombinant DNA technology utilizing a nonpathogenic laboratory strain of *Escherichia coli* (K12). Insulin glulisine differs from human insulin in that the amino acid asparagine at position B3 is replaced by lysine and the lysine in position B29 is replaced by glutamic acid. Chemically, it is 3^B-lysine-29^B-glutamic acid — human insulin, has the empirical formula $C_{258}H_{384}N_{64}O_{78}S_6$, and a molecular weight of 5823. Apidra is a sterile, aqueous, clear, and

Product	Manufacturer	Date	Indication	Description
			action than regular human insulin. Apidra should normally be used in regimens that include a longer-acting insulin or basal insulin analog.	colorless solution. Each milliliter of Apidra (insulin glulisine injection) contains 100 IU (3.49 mg) insulin glulisine, 3.15 mg m-cresol, 6 mg tromethamine, 5 mg sodium chloride, 0.01 mg polysorbate 20, and water for injection. Apidra has a pH of approximately 7.3. The pH is adjusted by addition of aqueous solutions of hydrochloric acid or sodium hydroxide.
Aranesp™ (darbepoetin alfa)	Amgen	Sep 2001 Jul 2002	Anemia associated with chronic renal failure; Chemotherapy-induced anemia in patients with nonmyeloid malignancies	Aranesp™ is an erythropoiesis stimulating protein closely related to erythropoietin that is produced in Chinese hamster ovary (CHO) cells by recombinant DNA technology. Aranesp is a 165-amino acid protein that differs from recombinant human erythropoietin in containing 5 N-linked oligosaccharide chains, whereas recombinant human erythropoietin contains 3. The 2 additional N-glycosylation sites result from amino acid substitutions in the erythropoietin peptide backbone. The additional carbohydrate chains increase the approximate molecular weight of the glycoprotein from 30,000 to 37,000 Da. Aranesp is formulated as a sterile, colorless, preservative-free protein solution for intravenous (IV) or subcutaneous (SC) administration. Single-dose vials are available containing either 25, 40, 60, 100, or 200 mcg of Aranesp. Two formulations contain excipients as follows: *Polysorbate solution* contains 0.05 mg polysorbate 80, 2.12 mg sodium phosphate monobasic monohydrate, 0.66 mg sodium phosphate dibasic anhydrous, and 8.18 mg sodium chloride in water for injection, USP (per 1 mL) at pH 6.2 ± 0.2. *Albumin solution* contains 2.5 mg albumin (human), 2.23 mg sodium phosphate monobasic monohydrate, 0.53 mg sodium phosphate dibasic anhydrous, and 8.18 mg sodium chloride in sterile water for injection, USP (per 1 mL) at pH 6.0 ± 0.3.
Avonex® (Interferon beta-1a; recombinant)	Biogen Idec	May 1996 Feb 2003	Treatment of relapsing-remitting forms of multiple sclerosis; Treatment after initial MS attack if a brain MRI scan shows abnormalities characteristic of the disease	Avonex® (Interferon beta-1a) is produced by recombinant DNA technology. Interferon beta-1a is a 166 amino acid glycoprotein with a predicted molecular weight of approximately 22,500 daltons. It is produced by mammalian cells (Chinese hamster ovary cells) into which the human interferon beta gene has been introduced. The amino acid sequence of Avonex is identical to that of natural human interferon beta. Using the World Health Organization (WHO) natural interferon beta standard, Second International Standard for Interferon, Human Fibroblast (Gb-23-902-531), Avonex has a specific activity of approximately 200 million international units (IU) of antiviral activity per mg; 30 mcg of Avonex contains 6 million IU of antiviral activity. The activity against other standards is not known. Avonex is formulated as a sterile, white to off-white lyophilized powder for intramuscular injection after reconstitution with supplied diluent or sterile water for injection, USP, preservative-free. Each 1.0 mL (1.0 cc) of reconstituted Avonex contains 30 mcg of Interferon beta-1a, 15 mg albumin human, USP, 5.8 mg sodium chloride, USP, 5.7 mg dibasic sodium phosphate, USP, and 1.2 mg monobasic sodium phosphate, USP, at a pH of approximately 7.3.
BeneFix™ (coagulation factor IX)	Wyeth	Feb 1997	Treatment of hemophilia B	BeneFix®, coagulation factor IX recombinant is a purified protein produced by recombinant DNA technology for use in therapy of factor IX deficiency, known as hemophilia B or Christmas disease. Coagulation factor IX (recombinant) is a glycoprotein with an approximate molecular mass of 55,000 Da consisting of 415 amino acids in a single chain. It has a primary amino acid sequence that is identical to the Ala[148] allelic form of plasma

Continued.

Product	Company	Application	FDA Approval Date	Description
				derived factor IX, and has structural and functional characteristics similar to those of endogenous factor IX. BeneFix is produced by a genetically engineered Chinese hamster ovary (CHO) cell line that is extensively characterized and shown to be free of infectious agents. The stored cell banks are free of blood or plasma products. The CHO cell line secretes recombinant factor IX into a defined cell culture medium that does not contain any proteins derived from animal or human sources, and the recombinant factor IX is purified by a chromatography purification process that does not require a monoclonal antibody step and yields a high-purity, active product. A membrane filtration step that has the ability to retain molecules with apparent molecular weights > 70,000 (such as large proteins and viral particles) is included for additional viral safety. BeneFix is predominantly a single component by SDS-polyacrylamide gel electrophoresis evaluation. The potency (in international units, IU) is determined using an in vitro one-stage clotting assay against the World Health Organization (WHO) International Standard for factor IX concentrate. One international unit is the amount of factor IX activity present in 1 mL of pooled, normal human plasma. The specific activity of BeneFix is greater than or equal to 200 IU per mg of protein. BeneFix is not derived from human blood and contains no preservatives or added animal or human components. BeneFix is inherently free from the risk of transmission of human blood-borne pathogens such as HIV, hepatitis viruses, and parvovirus. BeneFix is formulated as a sterile, nonpyrogenic, lyophilized powder preparation. BeneFix is intended for intravenous (IV) injection. It is available in single-use vials containing the labeled amount of factor IX activity, expressed in international units (IU). Each vial contains nominally 250, 500, or 1000 IU of coagulation factor IX (recombinant). After reconstitution of the lyophilized drug product, the concentrations of excipients in the 500 and 1000 IU dosage strengths are 10 mM L-histidine, 1% sucrose, 260 mM glycine, 0.005% polysorbate 80. The concentrations after reconstitution in the 250 IU dosage strength are half those of the other two dosage strengths. The 500 and 1000 IU dosage strengths are isotonic after reconstitution, and the 250 IU dosage strength has half the tonicity of the other two dosage strengths after reconstitution. All dosage strengths yield a clear, colorless solution upon reconstitution.
Betaseron® (Interferon beta-1b)	Berlex Laboratories and Chiron Corp.	Treatment of relapsing-remitting multiple sclerosis; New labeling includes data from studies in patients with secondary progressive multiple sclerosis; and the indications section reflects Betaseron is indicated for treatment of relapsing	Aug 1993 Mar 2003	Betaseron® (Interferon beta-1b) is a purified, sterile, lyophilized protein product produced by recombinant DNA techniques and formulated for use by injection. Interferon beta-1b is manufactured by bacterial fermentation of a strain of *Escherichia coli* that bears a genetically engineered plasmid containing the gene for human interferon beta$_{ser17}$. The native gene was obtained from human fibroblasts and altered in a way that substitutes serine for the cysteine residue found at position 17. Interferon beta-1b is a highly purified protein that has 165 amino acids and an approximate molecular weight of 18,500 Da. It does not include the carbohydrate side chains found in the natural material. The specific activity of Betaseron is approximately 32 million international units (IU)/mg Interferon beta-1b. Each vial

Product	Company	Date	Indication	Description
			forms of MS to reduce the frequency of clinical exacerbations	contains 0.3 mg of Interferon beta-1b. The unit measurement is derived by comparing the antiviral activity of the product to the World Health Organization (WHO) reference standard of recombinant human interferon beta. Dextrose and albumin human, USP (15 mg each/vial) are added as stabilizers. Prior to 1993, a different analytical standard was used to determine potency. It assigned 54 million IU to 0.3 mg Interferon beta-1b. Lyophilized Betaseron is a sterile, white to off-white powder intended for subcutaneous injection after reconstitution with the diluent supplied (sodium chloride, 0.54% solution).
Bexxar® (tositumomab and I-131 tositumomab; monoclonal antibody targeting the CD20 antigen and radiolabeled version of the antibody)	Corixa Corp. and GlaxoSmithKline	Jun 2003	CD20-positive, follicular non-Hodgkin's lymphoma whose cancer is refractory to Rituxan® and has relapsed following chemotherapy	The Bexxar® therapeutic regimen (tositumomab and iodine I 131 tositumomab) is an antineoplastic radioimmunotherapeutic monoclonal antibody-based regimen composed of the monoclonal antibody, Tositumomab, and the radiolabeled monoclonal antibody, Iodine I 131 tositumomab. Tositumomab is a murine IgG_{2a} lambda monoclonal antibody directed against the CD20 antigen, which is found on the surface of normal and malignant B lymphocytes. Tositumomab is produced in an antibiotic-free culture of mammalian cells and is composed of two murine gamma 2a heavy chains of 451 amino acids each and two lambda light chains of 220 amino acids each. The approximate molecular weight of tositumomab is 150 kD. Tositumomab is supplied as a sterile, pyrogen-free, clear to opalescent, colorless to slightly yellow, preservative-free liquid concentrate. It is supplied at a nominal concentration of 14 mg/mL tositumomab in 35 mg and 225 mg single-use vials. The formulation contains 10% (w/v) maltose, 145 mM sodium chloride, 10 mM phosphate, and water for injection, USP. The pH is approximately 7.2. Iodine I 131 tositumomab is a radio-iodinated derivative of Tositumomab that has been covalently linked to iodine-131. Unbound radio-iodine and other reactants have been removed by chromatographic purification steps. Iodine I 131 tositumomab is supplied as a sterile, clear, preservative-free liquid for IV administration. The dosimetric dosage form is supplied at nominal protein and activity concentrations of 0.1 mg/mL and 0.61 mCi/mL (at date of calibration), respectively. The therapeutic dosage form is supplied at nominal protein and activity concentrations of 1.1 mg/mL and 5.6 mCi/mL (at date of calibration), respectively. The formulation for the dosimetric and the therapeutic dosage forms contains 5.0% to 6.0% (w/v) povidone, 1–2 mg/mL maltose (dosimetric dose) or 9–15 mg/mL maltose (therapeutic dose), 0.85–0. 95 mg/mL sodium chloride, and 0.9–1.3 mg/mL ascorbic acid. The pH is approximately 7.
Bioclate™ (antihemophilic factor)	Aventis Behring	Dec 1993	Treatment of hemophilia A for the prevention and control of hemorrhagic episodes; perioperative management of patients with hemophilia A	Antihemophilic factor (recombinant). Bioclate™ is a glyco-protein synthesized by a genetically engineered Chinese hamster ovary (CHO) cell line. In culture the CHO cell line secretes recombinant antihemophilic factor (rAHF) into the cell culture medium. The rAHF is purified from the culture medium utilizing a series of chromatography columns. A key step in the purification process is an immunoaffinity chromatography methodology in which a purification matrix prepared by immobilization of a monoclonal antibody directed to factor VIII is utilized to selectively isolate the rAHF in the medium. The rAHF

Continued.

Product	Company	Application	FDA Approval Date	Description
BioTropin™ (human growth hormone)	Biotech General	Treatment of human growth hormone deficiency in children	May 1995	BioTropin™ (Somatropin) consists of a sequence of 191 amino acids and a molecular weight of about 22,125 Da. It is identical to that of endogenous, pituitary-derived human growth hormone, also known as somatropin manufactured by recombinant process in *E. coli*. Human growth hormone controls many physiological functions that are essential for normal growth and development. When the hormone is deficient in children, the result is hypopituitarianism. hGH release is controlled by the pituitary gland, and it is responsible for stimulating tissue repair, cell replacement, cell and growth. BioTropin was developed by Biotechnology General as a recombinant human growth hormone indicated for the long-term treatment of children who have growth failure due to an inadequate secretion of normal endogenous growth hormone. Studies have shown that a weekly dose of Biotropin divided into daily injections increases growth rate. For pediatric patients the recommended starting dosage is .025 to .035 mg/kg/day.
Campath® (alemtuzumab)	Ilex Oncology, Inc., Millennium Pharmaceuticals, Inc., and Berlex Laboratories, Inc.	B-cell chronic lymphocytic leukemia in patients who have been treated with alkylating agents and who have failed fludarabine therapy	May 2001	Campath® (alemtuzumab) is a recombinant DNA–derived humanized monoclonal antibody (Campath-1H) that is directed against the 21–28 kD cell surface glycoprotein, CD52. CD52 is expressed on the surface of normal and malignant B and T lymphocytes, NK cells, monocytes, macrophages, and tissues of the male reproductive system. The Campath-1H antibody is an IgG1 kappa with human variable framework and constant regions, and complementarity-determining regions from a murine (rat) monoclonal antibody (Campath-1G). The Campath-1H antibody has an approximate molecular weight of 150 kD. Campath is produced in mammalian cell (Chinese hamster ovary) suspension culture in a medium containing neomycin. Neomycin is not detectable in the final product. Campath is a sterile, clear, colorless, isotonic pH 6.8 to 7.4 solution for injection. Each single use ampoule of Campath contains 30 mg alemtuzumab, 24.0 mg sodium chloride, 3.5 mg dibasic sodium phosphate, 0.6 mg potassium chloride, 0.6 mg monobasic potassium phosphate, 0.3 mg polysorbate 80, and 0.056 mg disodium edetate. No preservatives are added.

produced has the same biological effects as antihemophilic factor (human) [AHF(Human)] and structurally has a similar combination of heterogeneous heavy and light chains as found in AHF (human). Bioclate is formulated as a sterile, nonpyrogenic, off-white to faint yellow lyophilized powder preparation of concentrated recombinant AHF for intravenous injection and is available in single-dose bottles, which contain nominally 250, 500, 1000 IU per bottle. When reconstituted with the appropriate volume of diluent, it contains the following stabilizers in maximum amounts: 12.5 mg/mL albumin (Human), 1.5 mg/mL polyethylene glycol (3350), 180 mEq/L sodium, 55 mM histidine, 1.5 pg/AHF IU polysorbate-80, and 0.20 mg/mL calcium. Von Willebrand Factor (vWF) is coexpressed with the Antihemophilic Factor (Recombinant) and helps to stabilize it. The final product contains not more than 2 ng vWF/IU rAHF, which will not have any clinically relevant effect in patients with von Willebrand's disease. The product contains no preservative.

CEA-Scan® (arcitumomab; technetium-99 labeled)	Immunomedics, Inc.	Imaging agent for metastatic colorectal cancer	Jun 1996

CEA-Scan® is a radiodiagnostic agent consisting of a murine monoclonal antibody Fab' fragment, arcitumomab, formulated to be labeled with Technetium Tc 99m. The active component, arcitumomab, is a Fab' fragment generated from IMMU-4, a murine IgG$_1$ monoclonal antibody produced in murine ascitic fluid supplied to Immunomedics, Inc., by Charles River Laboratories. IMMU-4 is purified from the ascitic fluid and is digested with pepsin to produce F(ab')$_2$ fragments and subsequently reduced to produce the 50,000-dalton arcitumomab. Each vial contains the nonradioactive materials necessary to prepare one patient dose. CEA-Scan is a sterile, lyophilized formulation, containing 1.25 mg of arcitumomab and 0.29 mg stannous chloride per vial, with potassium sodium tartrate tetrahydrate, sodium acetate trihydrate, sodium chloride, acetic acid, glacial, hydrochloric acid, and sucrose. The imaging agent, Technetium Tc 99m CEA-Scan, Technetium Tc 99m Arcitumomab, is formed by reconstitution of the contents of the CEA-Scan vial with 30 mCi of Tc 99m sodium per technetate in 1 ml of sodium chloride for injection, USP. The resulting solution is pH 5 to 7 and for intravenous use only.

Cerezyme® (imiglucerase; recombinant form of beta-glucocerebrosidase)	Genzyme	Treatment of type 1 Gaucher's disease	May 1994

Cerezyme® (imiglucerase for injection) is an analogue of the human enzyme, (beta)-glucocerebrosidase produced by recombinant DNA technology. (beta)-Glucocerebrosidase ((beta)-D-glucosyl-N-acylsphingosine glucohydrolase, E.C.3.2.1.45) is a lysosomal glycoprotein enzyme that catalyzes the hydrolysis of the glycolipid glucocerebroside to glucose and ceramide. Cerezyme is produced by recombinant DNA technology using mammalian cell culture (Chinese hamster ovary). Purified imiglucerase is a monomeric glycoprotein of 497 amino acids, containing 4 N-linked glycosylation sites (Mr = 60,430). Imiglucerase differs from placental glucocerebrosidase by one amino acid at position 495 where histidine is substituted for arginine. The oligosaccharide chains at the glycosylation sites have been modified to terminate in mannose sugars. The modified carbohydrate structures on imiglucerase are somewhat different from those on placental glucocerebrosidase. These mannose-terminated oligosaccharide chains of imiglucerase are specifically recognized by endocytic carbohydrate receptors on macrophages, the cells that accumulate lipid in Gaucher disease. Cerezyme is supplied as a sterile, nonpyrogenic, white to off-white lyophilized product. The quantitative composition of the lyophilized drug is provided in the following table:

Ingredient	200 Unit Vial	400 Unit Vial
Imiglucerase (total amount)	212 units	424 units
Mannitol	170 mg	340 mg
Sodium citrates	70 mg	140 mg
(trisodium citrate)	52 mg	104 mg
(disodium hydrogen citrate)	18 mg	36 mg
Polysorbate 80, NF	0.53 mg	1.06 mg

Citric acid or sodium hydroxide may have been added at the time of manufacture to adjust pH. This provides a respective withdrawal dose of 200 and 400 units of imiglucerase. An enzyme unit (U) is defined as the amount of enzyme that catalyzes the hydrolysis of one

Continued.

Product	Company	Application	FDA Approval Date	Description
Comvax™ (*Haemophilus* B conjugate [meningococcal conjugate] and hepatitis B [recombinant] vaccine)	Merck & Co., Inc.	Vaccination against *Haemophilus influenzae* type B and against all known subtypes of hepatitis B in infants born to HbsAg-negative mothers	Oct 1996	Comvax™ [Haemophilus b Conjugate (Meningococcal Protein Conjugate) and Hepatitis B (Recombinant) Vaccine] is a sterile bivalent vaccine made of the antigenic components used in producing PedvaxHIB [Haemophilus B Conjugate Vaccine (Meningococcal Protein Conjugate)] and RECOMBIVAX HB [Hepatitis B Vaccine (Recombinant)]. These components are the *Haemophilus influenzae* type B capsular polysaccharide [polyribosylribitol phosphate (PRP)] that is covalently bound to an outer membrane protein complex (OMPC) of *Neisseria meningitidis* and hepatitis B surface antigen (HBsAg) from recombinant yeast cultures. *Haemophilus influenzae* type B and *Neisseria meningitidis* serogroup B are grown in complex fermentation media. The primary ingredients of the phenol-inactivated fermentation medium for *Haemophilus influenzae* include an extract of yeast, nicotinamide adenine dinucleotide, hemin chloride, soy peptone, dextrose, and mineral salts and for *Neisseria meningitidis* include an extract of yeast, amino acids, and mineral salts. The PRP is purified from the culture broth by purification procedures, which include ethanol fractionation, enzyme digestion, phenol extraction, and diafiltration. The OMPC from *Neisseria meningitidis* is purified by detergent extraction, ultracentrifugation, diafiltration, and sterile filtration. The PRP-OMPC conjugate is prepared by the chemical coupling of the highly purified PRP (polyribosylribitol phosphate) of *Haemophilus influenzae* type B (*Haemophilus* B. Ross strain) to an OMPC of the B11 strain of *Neisseria meningitidis* serogroup B. The coupling of the PRP to the OMPC is necessary for enhanced immunogenicity of the PRP. This coupling is confirmed by analysis of the components of the conjugate following chemical treatment that yields a unique amino acid. After conjugation, the aqueous bulk is then adsorbed onto an amorphous aluminum hydroxyphosphate sulfate adjuvant (previously referred to as aluminum hydroxide). HBsAg is produced in recombinant yeast cells. A portion of the hepatitis B virus gene, coding for HBsAg, is cloned into yeast, and the vaccine for hepatitis B is produced from cultures of this recombinant yeast strain according to methods developed in the Merck Research Laboratories. The antigen is harvested and purified from fermentation cultures of a recombinant strain of the yeast *Saccharomyces cerevisiae* containing the gene for the *adw* subtype of HBsAg. The fermentation process involves growth of *Saccharomyces cerevisiae* on a complex fermentation medium that consists of an extract of yeast, soy peptone, dextrose, amino acids, and mineral salts. The HBsAg protein is released from the yeast cells by mechanical cell disruption and detergent

micromole of the synthetic substrate para-nitrophenyl-(beta)-D-glucopyranoside (pNP-Glc) per minute at 37°C. The product is stored at 2 to 8°C (36 to 46°F). After reconstitution with sterile water for injection, USP, the imiglucerase concentration is 40 U/mL for final concentrations and volumes). Reconstituted solutions have a pH of approximately 6.1. In addition, Haemaccel® (cross-linked gelatin polypeptides), which is used as a stabilizing agent during the manufacturing process, may also be present in very small amounts in the final product.

extraction, and purified by a series of physical and chemical methods, which includes ion and hydrophobic chromatography and diafiltration. The purified protein is treated in phosphate buffer with formaldehyde and then coprecipitated with alum (potassium aluminum sulfate) to form bulk vaccine adjuvanted with amorphous aluminum hydroxyphosphate sulfate. The vaccine contains no detectable yeast DNA, and 1% or less of the protein is of yeast origin. The individual PRP-OMPC and HBsAg adjuvanted bulks are combined to produce Comvax. Each 0.5 mL dose of Comvax is formulated to contain 7.5 mcg PRP conjugated to approximately 125 mcg OMPC, 5 mcg HBsAg, approximately 225 mcg aluminum as amorphous aluminum hydroxyphosphate sulfate, and 35 mcg sodium borate (decahydrate) as a pH stabilizer, in 0.9% sodium chloride. The vaccine contains not more than 0.0004% (w/v) residual formaldehyde. The potency of the PRP-OMPC component is measured by quantitating the polysaccharide concentration by an HPLC method. The potency of the HBsAg component is measured relative to a standard by an *in vitro* immunoassay The product contains no preservative. Comvax is a sterile suspension for intramuscular injection.

Product	Company	Approval date	Indication	Description
Elitek® (rasburicase)	Sanofi-Synthelabo	Jul 2002	Management of plasma uric acid levels in pediatric chemotherapy patients	Elitek® (rasburicase) is a recombinant urate-oxidase enzyme produced by a genetically modified *Saccharomyces cerevisiae* strain. The cDNA coding for rasburicase was cloned from a strain of *Aspergillus flavus*. Rasburicase is a tetrameric protein with identical subunits of a molecular mass of about 34 kDa. The molecular formula of the monomer is $C_{1521}H_{2383}N_{417}O_{462}S_7$. The monomer, made up of a single 301 amino acid polypeptide chain, has no intra- or interdisulfide bridges and is N-terminal acetylated. The drug product is a sterile, white to off-white, lyophilized powder intended for intravenous administration following reconstitution. Elitek is supplied in 3 mL colorless, glass vials containing 1.5 mg rasburicase, 10.6 mg mannitol, 15.9 mg L-alanine, and between 12.6 and 14.3 mg of dibasic sodium phosphate. The diluent solution for reconstitution, supplied in a 2 mL clear, glass ampule, is composed of 1.0 mL sterile water for injection, USP, and 1.0 mg poloxamer 188. The product reconstituted with diluent is a clear, colorless solution.
Enbrel® (Etanercept; recombinant product; dimeric fusion protein consisting of tumor necrosis factor receptor linked to the Fc portion of human IgG1)	Amgen and Wyeth	Nov 1998 May 1999 Jun 2000 Jan 2002 Jul 2003 Aug 2003	Treatment of moderate to severely active rheumatoid arthritis in patients who have had an inadequate response to one or more disease-modifying antirheumatic drugs; Treatment of polyarticular course juvenile rheumatoid arthritis; Treatment as a first-line therapy for moderate to severe active rheumatoid arthritis; Reduction of signs and	Enbrel® (etanercept) is a dimeric fusion protein consisting of the extracellular ligand-binding portion of the human 75 kDa (p75) tumor necrosis factor receptor (TNFR) linked to the Fc portion of human IgG1. The Fc component of etanercept contains the C_H2 domain, the C_H3 domain and hinge region, but not the C_H1 domain of IgG1. Etanercept is produced by recombinant DNA technology in a Chinese hamster ovary (CHO) mammalian cell expression system. It consists of 934 amino acids and has an apparent molecular weight of approximately 150 kDa. Enbrel is supplied as a sterile, white, preservative-free, lyophilized powder for parenteral administration after reconstitution with 1 mL of the supplied sterile bacteriostatic water for injection, USP (containing 0.9% benzyl alcohol). Following reconstitution, the solution of Enbrel is clear and colorless, with a pH of 7.4 ± 0.3. Each single-use vial of Enbrel contains 25 mg etanercept, 40 mg mannitol, 10 mg sucrose, and 1.2 mg tromethamine.

Continued.

Product	Company	Application	FDA Approval Date	Description
		symptoms of active arthritis in patients with psoriatic arthritis; Improvement of physical function in patients with moderately to severely active rheumatoid arthritis; Ankylosing spondylitis; Expanded psoriatic arthritis label claiming blockage of progression of structural damage		
Engerix-B® (hepatitis B vaccine)	GlaxoSmithKline	Hepatitis B vaccine; Adults with chronic hepatitis C infection	Sep 1989 Aug 1998	Engerix-B® [Hepatitis B Vaccine (Recombinant)] is a noninfectious recombinant DNA hepatitis B vaccine developed and manufactured by GlaxoSmithKline Biologicals. It contains purified surface antigen of the virus obtained by culturing genetically engineered *Saccharomyces cerevisiae* cells, which carry the surface antigen gene of the hepatitis B virus. The surface antigen expressed in *Saccharomyces cerevisiae* cells is purified by several physicochemical steps and formulated as a suspension of the antigen adsorbed on aluminum hydroxide. The procedures used to manufacture *Engerix-B* result in a product that contains no more than 5% yeast protein. No substances of human origin are used in its manufacture. *Engerix-B* is supplied as a sterile suspension for intramuscular administration. The vaccine is ready for use without reconstitution; it must be shaken before administration since a fine white deposit with a clear colorless supernatant may form on storage. *Pediatric/Adolescent*. Each 0.5 mL of vaccine consists of 10 mcg of hepatitis B surface antigen adsorbed on 0.25 mg aluminum as aluminum hydroxide. The pediatric/adolescent vaccine is formulated without preservatives. The pediatric formulation contains a trace amount of thimerosal (< 0.5 mcg mercury) from the manufacturing process, sodium chloride (9 mg/mL), and phosphate buffers (disodium phosphate dihydrate, 0.98 mg/mL; sodium dihydrogen phosphate dihydrate, 0.71 mg/mL). *Adult* Each 1 mL adult dose consists of 20 mcg of hepatitis B surface antigen adsorbed on 0.5 mg aluminum as aluminum hydroxide. The adult vaccine is formulated without preservatives. The adult formulation contains a trace amount of thimerosal (< 1.0 mcg mercury) from the manufacturing process, sodium chloride (9 mg/mL), and phosphate buffers (disodium phosphate dihydrate, 0.98 mg/mL; sodium dihydrogen phosphate dihydrate, 0.71 mg/mL).

Epogen® (epoietin alfa)

Amgen

Treatment of anemia associated with chronic renal failure and anemia in Retrovir-treated HIV-infected patients; Pediatric use

Jun 1989
Jul 1999

Erythropoietin is a glycoprotein that stimulates red blood cell production. It is produced in the kidney and stimulates the division and differentiation of committed erythroid progenitors in the bone marrow. Epogen® (Epoetin alfa), a 165 amino acid glycoprotein manufactured by recombinant DNA technology, has the same biological effects as endogenous erythropoietin. It has a molecular weight of 30,400 Da and is produced by mammalian cells into which the human erythropoietin gene has been introduced. The product contains the identical amino acid sequence of isolated natural erythropoietin. Epogen is formulated as a sterile, colorless liquid in an isotonic sodium chloride/sodium citrate buffered solution or a sodium chloride/sodium phosphate buffered solution for intravenous (IV) or subcutaneous (SC) administration. *Single-dose, Preservative-free Vial:* Each 1 mL of solution contains 2000, 3000, 4000, or 10,000 Units of Epoetin alfa, 2.5 mg albumin (human), 5.8 mg sodium citrate, 5.8 mg sodium chloride, and 0.06 mg citric acid in sterile water for injection, USP (pH 6.9 ± 0.3). This formulation contains no preservative. *Single-dose, Preservative-free Vial:* 1 mL (40,000 Units/mL). Each 1 mL of solution contains 40,000 Units of Epoetin alfa, 2.5 mg albumin (human), 1.2 mg sodium phosphate monobasic monohydrate, 1.8 mg sodium phosphate dibasic anhydrate, 0.7 mg sodium citrate, 5.8 mg sodium chloride, and 6.8 mg citric acid in sterile water for injection, USP (pH 6.9 ± 0.3). This formulation contains no preservative. *Multidose, Preserved Vial:* 2 mL (20,000 Units, 10,000 Units/mL). Each 1 mL of solution contains 10,000 Units of Epoetin alfa, 2.5 mg albumin (human), 1.3 mg sodium citrate, 8.2 mg sodium chloride, 0.11 mg citric acid, and 1% benzyl alcohol as preservative in sterile water for injection, USP (pH 6.1 ± 0.3). *Multidose, Preserved Vial:* 1 mL (20,000 Units/mL). Each 1 mL of solution contains 20,000 Units of Epoetin alfa, 2. 5 mg albumin (human), 1.3 mg sodium citrate, 8.2 mg sodium chloride, 0.11 mg citric acid, and 1% benzyl alcohol as preservative in sterile water for injection, USP (pH 6.1 ± 0.3).

Fabrazyme® (Algasidase beta; recombinant enzyme replacement)

Genzyme

Fabry's disease

Apr 2003

Fabrazyme® is a recombinant human α-galactosidase A enzyme with the same amino acid sequence as the native enzyme. Purified agalsidase beta is a homodimeric glycoprotein with a molecular weight of approximately 100 KD. The mature protein is comprised of two subunits of 398 amino acids (approximately 51 KD), each of which contains three N-linked glycosylation sites. α-galactosidase A catalyzes the hydrolysis of globotriaosylceramide (GL-3) and other α-galactylterminated neutral glycosphingolipids, such as galabiosylceramide and blood group B substances to ceramide dihexoside and galactose. The specific activity of Fabrazyme is approximately 70 U/mg (one unit is defined as the amount of activity that results in the hydrolysis of 1 µmole of a synthetic substrate, p-nitrophenyl-α-D-galactopyranoside, per minute under the assay conditions). Fabrazyme is produced by recombinant DNA technology in a Chinese hamster ovary mammalian cell expression system. Fabrazyme is intended for intravenous infusion. It is supplied as a sterile, nonpyrogenic, white to off-white lyophilized cake or powder for reconstitution with sterile water for injection, USP. Each vial contains 37 mg of agalsidase beta as well as 222 mg mannitol, 20.4 mg sodium phosphate monobasic monohydrate, and 59.2 mg sodium phosphate dibasic heptahydrate. Following reconstitution as directed, 35 mg of agalsidase beta (7 mL) may be extracted from each vial.

Product	Company	FDA Approval Date	Application	Description
Follistim™ (follitropin beta)	Organon (unit of Akzo Nobel)	Sep 1997 Feb 2002	Recombinant follicle-stimulating hormone for treatment of infertility; Induction of spermatogenesis in men with primary and secondary hypogonadotropic hypogonadism in whom the cause of infertility is not due to primary testicular failure	Follistim® (follitropin beta for injection) contains human follicle-stimulating hormone (hFSH), a glycoprotein hormone, which is manufactured by recombinant DNA (rDNA) technology. Follitropin beta has a dimeric structure containing two glycoprotein subunits (alpha and beta). Both the 92 amino acid alpha chain and the 111 amino acid beta chain have complex heterogeneous structures arising from two N-linked oligosaccharide chains. Follitropin beta is synthesized in a Chinese hamster ovary (CHO) cell line that has been transfected with a plasmid containing the two subunit DNA sequences encoding for hFSH. The purification process results in a highly purified preparation with a consistent hFSH isoform profile and high specific activity. The biological activity is determined by measuring the increase in ovary weight in female rats. The intrinsic luteinizing hormone (LH) activity in follitropin beta is less than 1 IU per 40,000 IU FSH. The compound is considered to contain no LH activity. The amino acid sequence and tertiary structure of the product are indistinguishable from that of human follicle-stimulating hormone (hFSH) of urinary source. Also, based on available data derived from physiochemical tests and bioassay, follitropin beta and follitropin alfa, another recombinant follicle-stimulating hormone product, are indistinguishable. Follistim is presented as a sterile, freeze-dried cake, intended for subcutaneous or intramuscular administration after reconstitution with sterile water for injection. USP. Each vial of Follistim contains 75 IU of FSH activity plus 25.0 mg sucrose, NF; 7.35 mg sodium citrate dihydrate, USP; 0.10 mg polysorbate 20, NF, and hydrochloric acid, NF or sodium hydroxide, NF to adjust the pH in a sterile, lyophilized form. The pH of the reconstituted preparation is approximately 7.0. The recombinant protein in Follistim has been standardized for FSH *in vivo* bioactivity in terms of the First International Reference Preparation for human menopausal gonadotropins (code 70/45). issued by the World Health Organization Expert Committee on Biological Standardization (1982). Under current storage conditions, Follistim may contain up to 20% of oxidized follitropin beta. In clinical trials with Follistim, serum antibodies to FSH or anti-CHO cell derived proteins were not detected in any of the treated patients after exposure to Follistim for up to three cycles. Therapeutic Class: Infertility. As determined by the Ph. Eur. Test for FSH *in vivo* bioactivity and on the basis of the molar extinction coefficient at 277 nm ([egr]$_s$: mg^{-1} cm^{-1}) = 1. 066.
FORTEO® (teriparatide)	Eli Lilly and Company	Nov 2002	Treatment of osteoporosis in postmenopausal women at high risk of fracture, and to increase bone mass in men with primary or hypogonadal osteoporosis who are at high risk of fracture	Forteo® [teriparatide (rDNA origin) injection] contains recombinant human parathyroid hormone (1-34), [rhPTH(1-34)], which has an identical sequence to the 34 N-terminal amino acids (the biologically active region) of the 84-amino acid human parathyroid hormone. Teriparatide has a molecular weight of 4117.8 Da. Teriparatide (rDNA origin) is manufactured by Eli Lilly and Company using a strain of *Escherichia coli* modified by recombinant DNA technology. Forteo is supplied as a sterile, colorless, clear, isotonic solution in a glass cartridge that is preassembled into a disposable pen device for subcutaneous injection. Each prefilled delivery device is filled with 3.3 mL to deliver 3 mL. Each mL contains 250 mcg teriparatide (corrected for acetate, chloride, and water

Product	Company	Indication	Date	Description
GenoTropin® (human somatropin)	Pharmacia	Treatment of growth hormone deficiency in children; Growth hormone deficiency in adults; Long-term treatment of growth failure in children born small for gestational age who fail to catch up by age 2	Aug 1995 Nov 1997 Jul 2001	content), 0.41 mg glacial acetic acid, 0.10 mg sodium acetate (anhydrous), 45.4 mg mannitol, 3.0 mg Metacresol, and sterile water for injection, USP. In addition, hydrochloric acid solution 10% or sodium hydroxide solution 10% may have been added to adjust the product to pH 4. Each cartridge preassembled into a pen device delivers 20 mcg of teriparatide per dose each day for up to 28 days. GenoTropin® Lyophilized Powder contains somatropin [rDNA origin], which is a polypeptide hormone of recombinant DNA origin. It has 191 amino acid residues and a molecular weight of 22,124 Da. The amino acid sequence of the product is identical to that of human growth hormone of pituitary origin (somatropin). GenoTropin is synthesized in a strain of $Escherichia\ coli$ that has been modified by the addition of the gene for human growth hormone. GenoTropin is a sterile white lyophilized powder intended for subcutaneous injection. GenoTropin 1.5 mg is dispensed in a two-chamber cartridge. The front chamber contains recombinant somatropin 1.5 mg (approximately 4.5 IU), glycine 27.6 mg, sodium dihydrogen phosphate anhydrous 0.3 mg, and disodium phosphate anhydrous 0.3 mg; the rear chamber contains 1.13 mL sterile water for injection, USP. GenoTropin 5.8 mg is dispensed in a two-chamber cartridge. The front chamber contains recombinant somatropin 5.8 mg (approximately 17.4 IU), glycine 2.2 mg, mannitol 1.8 mg, sodium dihydrogen phosphate anhydrous 0.32 mg, and disodium phosphate anhydrous 0.31 mg; the rear chamber contains 0.3% m-Cresol (as a preservative) and mannitol 45 mg in 1.14 mL sterile water for injection, USP. GenoTropin 13.8 mg is dispensed in a two-chamber cartridge. The front chamber contains recombinant somatropin 13.8 mg (approximately 41.4 IU), glycine 2.3 mg, mannitol 14.0 mg, sodium dihydrogen phosphate anhydrous 0.47 mg, and disodium phosphate anhydrous 0.46 mg; the rear chamber contains 0.3% m-Cresol (as a preservative) and mannitol 32 mg in 1.13 mL water for injection. GenoTropin Miniquick® is dispensed as a single-use syringe device containing a two-chamber cartridge. GenoTropin Miniquick is available as individual doses of 0.2 mg to 2.0 mg in 0.2-mg increments. The front chamber contains recombinant somatropin 0.22 to 2.2 mg (approximately 0.66 to 6.6 IU), glycine 0.23 mg, mannitol 1.14 mg, sodium dihydrogen phosphate 0.05 mg, and disodium phosphate anhydrous 0.027 mg; the rear chamber contains mannitol 12.6 mg in sterile water for injection, USP. 0.275 mL. GenoTropin is a highly purified preparation. The reconstituted recombinant somatropin solution has an osmolality of approximately 300 mOsm/kg, and a pH of approximately 6.7. The concentration of the reconstituted solution varies by strength and presentation.
Geref®	Serono S. A.	Treatment of growth hormone deficiency in children with growth failure	Oct 1997	Sermorelin acetate is the acetate salt of an amidated synthetic 29-amino acid peptide (GRF 1-29 NH$_2$) that corresponds to the amino-terminal segment of the naturally occurring human growth hormone-releasing hormone (GHRH or GRF) consisting of 44 amino acid residues. The free base of sermorelin has the empirical formula $C_{149}H_{246}N_{44}O_{42}S$ and a molecular weight of 3358 Da. Geref® is a sterile, nonpyrogenic, lyophilized powder intended for subcutaneous injection after reconstitution with sodium chloride injection, USP. The reconstituted solution has a pH of 5.0 to 5.5. Geref is available in vials. The *Continued.*

Product	Company	Application	FDA Approval Date	Description
				quantitative composition per vial is: 0.5 mg vial. Each vial contains 0.5 mg sermorelin (as the acetate) and 5 mg mannitol. The pH is adjusted with dibasic sodium phosphate and monobasic sodium phosphate buffer. 1.0 mg vial: Each vial contains 1.0 mg sermorelin (as the acetate) and 5 mg mannitol. The pH is adjusted with dibasic sodium phosphate and monobasic sodium phosphate buffer.
GlucaGen® (glucagon)	Novo Nordisk	Treatment of severe hypoglycemic reactions in insulin-treated diabetics and for diagnostic use	Jun 1998	GlucaGen® [glucagon (rDNA origin) for injection], manufactured by Novo Nordisk A/S, is produced by expression of recombinant DNA in a saccharomyces cerevisiae vector with subsequent purification. The chemical structure of the glucagon in GlucaGen is identical to naturally occurring human glucagon and to glucagon extracted from beef and pork pancreas. Glucagon with the empirical formula of $C_{153}H_{225}N_{41}O_{49}S$, and a molecular weight of 3483, is a single-chain polypeptide containing 29 amino acid residues. GlucaGen 1 mg (1 IU) is supplied as a sterile, lyophilized white powder in a 2 ml vial, accompanied by sterile water for reconstitution (1 ml) also in a 2 ml vial. Glucagon, as supplied at pH 2.5 to 3.5, is soluble in water. Active ingredient in each vial: glucagon is hydrochloride 1 mg (corresponding to 1 IU). Other ingredients: lactose monohydrate (107 mg). When the glucagon powder is reconstituted with sterile water for reconstitution, it forms a solution of 1 mg (1 IU)/ml glucagon for subcutaneous (sc), intramuscular (im), or intravenous (iv) injection. GlucaGen is an antihypoglycemic agent and a gastrointestinal motility inhibitor. Glucagon for injection (rDNA origin) is a polypeptide hormone identical to human glucagon that increases blood glucose and relaxes smooth muscle of the gastrointestinal tract. Glucagon is synthesized in a special nonpathogenic laboratory strain of *Escherichia coli* bacteria that has been genetically altered by the addition of the gene for glucagon. Glucagon is a single-chain polypeptide that contains 29 amino acid residues and has a molecular weight of 3483. The empirical formula is $C_{153}H_{225}N_{43}O_{49}S$. Crystalline glucagon is a white to off-white powder. It is relatively insoluble in water but is soluble at a pH of less than 3 or more than 9. 5. Glucagon is available for use intravenously, intramuscularly, or subcutaneously in a kit that contains a vial of sterile glucagon and a syringe of sterile diluent. The vial contains 1 mg (1 unit) of glucagon and 49 mg of lactose. Hydrochloric acid may have been added during manufacture to adjust the pH of the glucagon. One International Unit of glucagon is equivalent to 1 mg of glucagon. The diluent syringe contains 12 mg/mL of glycerin, water for injection, and hydrochloric acid.
Gonal-F® (follitropin alfa)	Serono S. A.	Treatment of infertility in women not due to primary ovarian failure; Treatment of infertility in men and women	Sep 1998 Jun 2000	Gonal-F® (follitropin alfa for injection) is a human follicle stimulating hormone (FSH) preparation of recombinant DNA origin, which consists of two noncovalently linked, nonidentical glycoproteins designated as the (alpha)- and (beta)-subunits. The (alpha)- and (beta)-subunits have 92 and 111 amino acids, respectively, and their primary and tertiary structure are indistinguishable from those of human follicle stimulating hormone. Recombinant FSH production occurs in genetically modified Chinese hamster ovary (CHO) cells cultured in bioreactors. Purification by immunochromatography using an

Helixate® FS
(antihemophilic factor)

Aventis Behring

Feb 1994
Jun 2000

Factor VIII for treatment of hemophilia A; Second-generation factor VIII formulated with sucrose for treatment of hemophilia A

antibody specifically binding FSH results in a highly purified preparation with a consistent FSH isoform profile and a high specific activity. The biological activity of follitropin alfa is determined by measuring the increase in ovary weight in female rats. The *in vivo* biological activity of follitropin alfa has been calibrated against the second International Reference Preparation for Human Menopausal Gonadotrophins established in September 1964 by the Expert Committee on Biological Standards of the World Health Organization. Gonal-F contains no luteinizing hormone (LH) activity. Based on available data derived from physicochemical tests and bioassays, follitropin alfa and follitropin beta, another recombinant follicle stimulating hormone product, are indistinguishable. Gonal-F is a sterile, lyophilized powder intended for subcutaneous injection after reconstitution with either sterile water for injection, USP for single-dose ampules or bacteriostatic water for injection (0.9% benzyl alcohol), USP for multiple dose vials. Each container of Gonal-F contains either 37.5 IU, 75 IU, 150 IU (single dose), or 1200 IU (multidose). Each ampule of Gonal-F contains either 37.5 IU, 75 IU, or 150 IU recombinant FSH, 30 mg sucrose, 1.11 mg dibasic sodium phosphate, and 0.45 mg monobasic sodium phosphate monohydrate. O-phosphoric acid or sodium hydroxide may be used prior to lyophilization for pH adjustment. Under current storage conditions, Gonal-F may contain up to 15% of oxidized follitropin alfa.

Helixate® FS antihemophilic factor (recombinant) is a sterile, stable, purified, nonpyrogenic, dried concentrate that has been manufactured using recombinant DNA technology. Helixate FS is intended for use in the treatment of classical hemophilia (hemophilia A), and is produced by baby hamster kidney (BHK) cells into which the human factor VIII (FVIII) gene has been introduced. The cell culture medium contains human plasma protein solution (HPPS) and recombinant insulin, but does not contain any proteins derived from animal sources. Helixate FS is a highly purified glycoprotein consisting of multiple peptides including an 80 kD and various extensions of the 90 kD subunit. It has the same biological activity as FVIII derived from human plasma. Compared to its predecessor product Helixate® antihemophilic factor (recombinant), Helixate FS incorporates a revised purification and formulation process that eliminates the addition of albumin (human). The purification process includes an effective solvent/detergent virus inactivation step in addition to the use of the classical purification methods of ion exchange chromatography, monoclonal antibody immunoaffinity chromatography, along with other chromatographic steps designed to purify recombinant FVIII and remove contaminating substances. Helixate FS is formulated with sucrose (0.9 to 1.3%), glycine (21 to 25 mg/mL), and histidine (18 to 23 mM) as stabilizers in the final container in place of albumin (human), as used in Helixate, and is then lyophilized. The final product also contains calcium chloride (2 to 3 mM), sodium (27 to 36 mEq/L), chloride (32 to 40 mEq/L), polysorbate 80 (not more than [NMT] 35 µg/mL), imidazole (NMT 20 µg/1000 IU), tri-n-butyl phosphate (NMT 5 µg/1000 IU), and copper (NMT 0.6 µg/1000 IU). The product contains no preservatives. The amount of sucrose in each

Continued.

Product	Company	Application	FDA Approval Date	Description
				vial is 28 mg. Intravenous administration of sucrose contained in Helixate FS will not affect blood glucose levels. Each vial of Helixate FS contains the labeled amount of recombinant FVIII in international units (IU). One IU, as defined by the World Health Organization standard for blood coagulation FVIII, human, is approximately equal to the level of FVIII activity found in 1 mL of fresh pooled human plasma. Helixate FS must be administered by the intravenous route.
Herceptin® (trastuzumab)	Genentech, Inc.	Treatment of patients with metastatic breast cancer whose tumors overexpress the HER2 protein	Sep 1998	Herceptin® (Trastuzumab) is a recombinant DNA–derived humanized monoclonal antibody that selectively binds with high affinity in a cell-based assay (Kd = 5 nM) to the extracellular domain of the human epidermal growth factor receptor 2 protein, HER2. The antibody is an IgG_1 kappa that contains human framework regions with the complementarity-determining regions of a murine antibody (4D5) that binds to HER2. The humanized antibody against HER2 is produced by a mammalian cell (Chinese hamster ovary) [CHO] suspension culture in a nutrient medium containing the antibiotic gentamicin. Gentamicin is not detectable in the final product. Herceptin is a sterile, white to pale yellow, preservative-free lyophilized powder for intravenous (IV) administration. The nominal content of each Herceptin vial is 440 mg Trastuzumab, 9.9 mg L-histidine HCl, 6.4 mg L-histidine, 400 mg (alpha), (alpha)-trehalose dihydrate, and 1.8 mg polysorbate 20, USP. Reconstitution with only 20 mL of the supplied bacteriostatic water for injection (BWFI), USP, containing 1.1% benzyl alcohol as a preservative, yields a multi-dose solution containing 21 mg/mL Trastuzumab, at a pH of approximately 6.
Humalog® (insulin)	Eli Lilly and Company	Treatment of diabetes	Jun 1996	Humalog® (insulin lispro, rDNA origin) is a human insulin analog that is a rapid-acting, parenteral blood glucose-lowering agent. Chemically, it is Lys(B28), Pro(B29) human insulin analog, created when the amino acids at positions 28 and 29 on the insulin B-chain are reversed. Humalog is synthesized in a special nonpathogenic laboratory strain of *Escherichia coli* bacteria that has been genetically altered by the addition of the gene for insulin lispro. Insulin lispro has the empirical formula $C_{257}H_{383}N_{65}O_{77}S_6$ and a molecular weight of 5808, both identical to that of human insulin. The vials and cartridges contain a sterile solution of Humalog for use as an injection. Humalog injection consists of zinc-insulin lispro crystals dissolved in a clear aqueous fluid. Each milliliter of Humalog injection contains insulin lispro 100 Units, 16 mg glycerin, 1.88 mg dibasic sodium phosphate, 3.15 mg *m*-cresol, zinc oxide content adjusted to provide 0.0197 mg zinc ion, trace amounts of phenol, and water for injection. Insulin lispro has a pH of 7.0 to 7.8. Hydrochloric acid 10% or sodium hydroxide 10% may be added to adjust pH.

Product	Company	Date	Indication	Description
Humatrope® (Somatotropin)	Eli Lilly and Company	Aug 1996 Mar 1997 Jul 2003	Treatment of growth hormone deficiency in children; Somatotropin deficiency syndrome in adults; Long-term treatment of children of short stature (unknown cause)	Humatrope® (Somatotropin, rDNA Origin, for Injection) is a polypeptide hormone of recombinant DNA origin. Humatrope has 191 amino acid residues and a molecular weight of about 22,125 Da. The amino acid sequence of the product is identical to that of human growth hormone of pituitary origin. Humatrope is synthesized in a strain of *Escherichia coli* that has been modified by the addition of the gene for human growth hormone. Humatrope is a sterile, white lyophilized powder intended for subcutaneous or intramuscular administration after reconstitution. Humatrope is a highly purified preparation. Phosphoric acid or sodium hydroxide may have been added to adjust the pH. Reconstituted solutions have a pH of approximately 7.5. This product is oxygen sensitive. Each vial of Humatrope contains 5 mg somatotropin (15 IU or 225 nanomoles); 25 mg mannitol; 5 mg glycine; and 1.13 mg dibasic sodium phosphate. Each vial is supplied in a combination package with an accompanying 5-mL vial of diluting solution. The diluent contains sterile water for injection with 0.3% metacresol as a preservative and 1.7% glycerin. The cartridges of somatotropin contain either 6 mg (18 IU), 12 mg (36 IU), or 24 mg (72 IU) of somatotropin. The 6 mg, 12 mg, and 24 mg cartridges contain respectively: mannitol 18 mg, 36 mg, and 72 mg; glycine 6 mg, 12 mg, and 24 mg; dibasic sodium phosphate 1.36 mg, 2.72 mg, and 5.43 mg. Each cartridge is supplied in a combination package with an accompanying syringe containing approximately 3 mL of diluting solution. The diluent contains sterile water for injection; 0.3% metacresol as a preservative; and 1.7%, 0.29%, and 0.29% glycerin in the 6 mg, 12 mg, and 24 mg cartridges respectively.
Humira™ (adalimumab)	Cambridge Antibody Technologies and Abbott Laboratories	Dec 2002	Patients with moderately to severely active rheumatoid arthritis who have had insufficient response to one or more traditional disease modifying antirheumatic drugs	Humira™ (adalimumab) is a recombinant human IgG1 monoclonal antibody specific for human tumor necrosis factor (TNF). Humira was created using phage display technology resulting in an antibody with human derived heavy and light chain variable regions and human IgG1 constant regions. Humira is produced by recombinant DNA technology in a mammalian cell expression system and is purified by a process that includes specific viral inactivation and removal steps. It consists of 1330 amino acids and has a molecular weight of approximately 148 kilodaltons. Humira is supplied in single-use, 1 mL prefilled glass syringes, and also 2 mL glass vials as a sterile, preservative-free solution for subcutaneous administration. The solution of Humira is clear and colorless, with a pH of about 5.2. Each syringe delivers 0.8 mL (40 mg) of drug product. Each vial contains approximately 0.9 mL of solution to deliver 0.8 mL (40 mg) of drug product. Each 0.8 mL Humira contains 40 mg adalimumab, 4.93 mg sodium chloride, 0.69 mg monobasic sodium phosphate dihydrate, 1.22 mg dibasic sodium phosphate dihydrate, 0.24 mg sodium citrate, 1.04 mg citric acid monohydrate, 9.6 mg mannitol, 0.8 mg polysorbate 80, and sterile water for injection, USP. Sodium hydroxide added as necessary to adjust pH.

Product	Company	Application	FDA Approval Date	Description
Humulin® (human insulin)	Eli Lilly And Company	Treatment of diabetes	Oct 1982	Humulin® is synthesized in a special nondisease-producing laboratory strain of *Escherichia coli* bacteria that has been genetically altered by the addition of the gene for human insulin production. Humulin consists of zinc-insulin crystals dissolved in a clear fluid. Humulin has had nothing added to change the speed or length of its action. It takes effect rapidly and has a relatively short duration of activity (4 to 12 hours) as compared with other insulins. The time course of action of any insulin may vary considerably in different individuals or at different times in the same individual. As with all insulin preparations, the duration of action of Humulin is dependent on dose, site of injection, blood supply, temperature, and physical activity. Humulin is a sterile solution and is for subcutaneous injection. It should not be used intramuscularly. The concentration of Humulin is 100 Units/mL (U-100).
Infergen® (interferon alfacon-1)	InterMune Pharmaceuticals, Inc., and Amgen	Treatment of hepatitis C (HCV) in patients 18 years or older with compensated liver disease who have anti-HCV serum antibodies or the presence of HCV RNA; Subsequent treatment of HCV-infected patients who have tolerated an initial course of interferon therapy	Oct 1997 Dec 1999	Interferon alfacon-1 is a recombinant nonnaturally occurring type-I interferon. The 166-amino acid sequence of interferon alfacon-1 was derived by scanning the sequences of several natural interferon alpha subtypes and assigning the most frequently observed amino acid in each corresponding position. Four additional amino acid changes were made to facilitate the molecular construction, and a corresponding synthetic DNA sequence was constructed using chemical synthesis methodology. Interferon alfacon-1 differs from interferon alfa-2b at 20/166 amino acids (88% homology), and comparison with interferon-beta shows identity at over 30% of the amino acid positions. Interferon alfacon-1 is produced in *Escherichia coli* cells that have been genetically altered by insertion of a synthetically constructed sequence that codes for interferon alfacon-1. Prior to final purification, interferon alfacon-1 is allowed to oxidize to its native state, and its final purity is achieved by sequential passage over a series of chromatography columns. This protein has a molecular weight of 19,434 Da. Infergen® is the Amgen Inc. trademark for interferon alfacon-1. Infergen is a sterile clear colorless preservative-free liquid formulated with 100 mM sodium chloride and 25 mM sodium phosphate at pH 7.0 ± 0.2. The product is available in single-use vials and prefilled syringes containing 9 mcg and 15 mcg interferon alfacon-1 at a fill volume of 0.3 mL and 0.5 mL, respectively. Infergen vials and prefilled syringes contain 0.03 mg/mL interferon alfacon-1, 5.9 mg/mL sodium chloride, and 3.8 mg/mL sodium phosphate in water for injection, USP. The Infergen SingleJect® prefilled syringe has a glass barrel and a 26 gauge, 5/8 inch needle. Infergen is to be administered undiluted by subcutaneous (SC) injection. Formulation, filling, and packaging operations for Infergen are performed by Amgen Puerto Rico, a wholly owned subsidiary of Amgen Inc.

Infuse™ Bone Graft/LT-CAGE™ (device utilizing recombinant human bone morphogenetic protein [rhBMP-2])

Wyeth and Medtronic Sofamor Danek

For use in spinal fusion surgery to treat certain types of spinal degenerative disease

Jul 2002

Infuse™ Bone Graft and the LT-CAGE™ Lumbar Tapered Fusion Device, used in combination to treat degenerative disc disease, represent a revolutionary new approach to spinal fusion surgery. Infuse Bone Graft contains a genetically engineered version of a protein that occurs naturally. This protein has been isolated in the laboratory and then purified and reproduced using recombinant DNA technology. The resulting recombinant human protein is known as rhBMP-2, and when combined with an absorbable collagen sponge, is marketed by Medtronic Sofamor Danek under the trade name Infuse Bone Graft. Infuse Bone Graft is packaged with a collagen sponge and sterile water for reconstitution. Prior to surgery, the powdered rhBMP-2 is mixed with the sterile water to create a liquid solution. The collagen sponge, which is used to carry the rhBMP-2 solution, is cut and sized to fit inside two LT-CAGE devices. The sponges are soaked with the rhBMP-2 protein for at least 15 minutes, rolled up, and placed inside the cages. Surgeons remove the damaged disc from the patient's spine and prepare the adjacent vertebrae for the insertion of the cages. Surgeons implant the cages with the sponge soaked in Infuse Bone Graft, in the space between the vertebrae, and the rhBMP-2 promotes the growth of bone to fuse the spine at that location.

Intron A® (alpha-interferon)

Schering-Plough Corp.

Treatment of hairy cell leukemia; Genital warts; AIDS-related Kaposi's sarcoma; Non-A, non-B hepatitis; Hepatitis B; Chronic malignant melanoma; Extended therapy for chronic viral hepatitis C; Treatment for follicular lymphoma in conjunction with chemotherapy; Treatment of hepatitis B in pediatric patients

Jun 1986
Jun 1988
Nov 1988
Feb 1991
Jul 1992
Dec 1995
Mar 1997
Nov 1997
Aug 1998

Intron A® Interferon alfa-2b, recombinant for intramuscular, subcutaneous, intralesional, or intravenous injection is a purified sterile recombinant interferon product. Interferon alfa-2b, recombinant for injection has been classified as an alfa interferon and is a water-soluble protein with a molecular weight of 19,271 Da produced by recombinant DNA techniques. It is obtained from the bacterial fermentation of a strain of *Escherichia coli* bearing a genetically engineered plasmid containing an interferon alfa-2b gene from human leukocytes. The fermentation is carried out in a defined nutrient medium containing the antibiotic tetracycline hydrochloride at a concentration of 5 to 10 mg/L; the presence of this antibiotic is not detectable in the final product. The specific activity of interferon alfa-2b, recombinant is approximately 2.6×10^8 IU/mg protein as measured by the HPLC assay.

Powder for Injection

Vial Strength	mL Diluent	Final Concentration after Reconstitution million IU/mL.*	mg Intron A† Interferon alfa-2b, recombinant	Route of Administration
3 MIU	1	3	0.012	IM, SC, IV
5 MIU	1	5	0.019	IM, SC, IV
10 MIU	2	5	0.038	IM, SC, IV, IL++
18 MIU	1	18	0.069	IM, SC, IV
25 MIU	5	5	0.096	IM, SC, IV
50 MIU	1	50	0.192	IM, SC, IV

* Each mL. also contains 20 mg glycine, 2.3 mg sodium phosphate dibasic, 0.55 mg sodium phosphate monobasic, and 1.0 mg human albumin.

Continued.

Product	Company	Application	FDA Approval Date	Description

Description

† Based on the specific activity of approximately 2.6×10^8 IU/mg protein, as measured by HPLC assay.

†† The 10 MIU vial for intralesional use should be reconstituted with 1 mL of the provided diluent.

Prior to administration, the Intron A powder for injection is to be reconstituted with the provided diluent for Intron A Interferon alfa-2b, recombinant for injection (bacteriostatic water for injection) containing 0.9% benzyl alcohol as a preservative. Intron A powder for injection is a white to cream-colored powder.

Solution Vials for Injection

Vial Strength	Final Concentration*	mg Intron A† Interferon alfa-2b, recombinant	Route of Administration
3 MIU	3 million IU/0.5 mL	0.012	IM, SC
5 MIU	5 million IU/0.5 mL	0.019	IM, SC, IL
10 MIU	10 million IU/1.0 mL	0.038	IM, SC, IL
18‡ MIU multidose	3 million IU/0.5 mL	0.088	IM, SC
25¶ MIU multidose	5 million IU/0.5 mL	0.123	IM, SC, IL

* Each mL contains 7.5 mg sodium chloride, 1.8 mg sodium phosphate dibasic, 1.3 mg sodium phosphate monobasic, 0.1 mg edetate disodium, 0.1 mg polysorbate 80, and 1.5 mg m-cresol as a preservative.

† Based on the specific activity of approximately 2.6×10^8 IU/mg protein as measured by HPLC assay.

‡ This is a multidose vial which contains a total of 22.8 million IU of interferon alfa-2b, recombinant per 3.8 mL in order to provide the delivery of six 0.5-mL doses, each containing 3 million IU of Intron A interferon alfa-2b, recombinant for injection (for a label strength of 18 million IU).

¶ This is a multidose vial which contains a total of 32.0 million IU of interferon alfa-2b, recombinant per 3.2 mL in order to provide the delivery of five 0.5-mL doses, each containing 5 million IU of Intron A interferon alfa-2b, recombinant for injection (for a label strength of 25 million IU).

Solution in Multidose Pens for Injection

Pen Strength	Final Concentration*	Intron A Dose Delivered million IU/mL*	mg Intron A† (6 doses, 0.2 mL each)	Route of Administration
18 MIU	22.5 MIU/1.5 mL	3 MIU/dose	0.087	SC
30 MIU	37.5 MIU/1.5 mL	5 MIU/dose	0.144	SC
60 MIU	75 MIU/1.5 mL	10 MIU/dose	0.288	SC

* Each mL also contains 7.5 mg sodium chloride, 1.8 mg sodium phosphate dibasic, 1.3 mg sodium phosphate monobasic, 0.1 mg edetate disodium, 0.1 mg polysorbate 80, and 1.5 mg m-cresol as a preservative.

† Based on the specific activity of approximately 2.6×10^8 IU/mg protein as measured by HPLC assay.

These packages do not require reconstitution prior to administration. Intron A solution for injection is a clear, colorless solution.

Kineret™ (anakinra)   Amgen   Nov 2001   Moderately to severely active rheumatoid arthritis in adult patients who have failed disease-modifying antirheumatic drugs

Kineret™ (anakinra) is a recombinant, nonglycosylated form of the human interleukin-1 receptor antagonist (IL-1Ra). Kineret differs from native human IL-1Ra in that it has the addition of a single methionine residue at its amino terminus. Kineret consists of 153 amino acids and has a molecular weight of 17.3 kilodaltons. It is produced by recombinant DNA technology using an *E. coli* bacterial expression system. Kineret is supplied in single use 1 mL, prefilled glass syringes with 27 gauge needles as a sterile, clear, colorless-to-white, preservative-free solution for daily subcutaneous (SC) administration. Each 1 mL prefilled glass syringe contains: 0.67 mL (100 mg) of anakinra in a solution (pH 6.5) containing sodium citrate (1.29 mg), sodium chloride (5.48 mg), disodium EDTA (0.12 mg), and polysorbate 80 (0.70 mg) in sterile water for injection, USP

Kogenate® FS (antihemophilic factor)   Bayer Corp.   Sep 1989   Jun 2000   Factor VIII for treatment of hemophilia A; Second-generation factor VIII formulated with sucrose for treatment of hemophilia A

Kogenate® FS antihemophilic factor (recombinant) is a sterile, stable, purified, nonpyrogenic, dried concentrate that has been manufactured using recombinant DNA technology. Kogenate FS is intended for use in the treatment of classical hemophilia (hemophilia A), and is produced by baby hamster kidney (BHK) cells into which the human factor VIII (FVIII) gene has been introduced. The cell culture medium contains human plasma protein solution (HPPS) and recombinant insulin, but does not contain any proteins derived from animal sources. Kogenate FS is a highly purified glycoprotein consisting of multiple peptides including an 80 kD and various extensions of the 90 kD subunit. It has the same biological activity as FVIII derived from human plasma. Compared to its predecessor product Kogenate Antihemophilic Factor (Recombinant), Kogenate FS incorporates a revised purification and formulation process that eliminates the addition of albumin (human). The purification process includes an effective solvent/detergent virus inactivation step in addition to the use of the classical purification

Continued.

Product	Company	Application	FDA Approval Date	Description
				methods of ion exchange chromatography, monoclonal antibody immunoaffinity chromatography, along with other chromatographic steps designed to purify recombinant FVIII and remove contaminating substances. Kogenate FS is formulated with sucrose (0.9 to 1.3%), glycine (21 to 25 mg/mL), and histidine (18 to 23 mM) as stabilizers in the final container in place of albumin (human) as used in Kogenate and is then lyophilized. The final product also contains calcium chloride (2 to 3 mM), sodium (27 to 36 mEq/L), chloride (32 to 40 mEq/L), polysorbate 80 (not more than [NMT] 35 µg/mL), imidazole (NMT 20 µg/1000 IU), tri-n-butyl phosphate (NMT 5 µg/1000 IU), and copper (NMT 0.6 µg/1000 IU). The product contains no preservatives. The amount of sucrose in each vial is 28 mg. Intravenous administration of sucrose contained in Kogenate FS will not affect blood glucose levels. Each vial of Kogenate FS contains the labeled amount of recombinant FVIII in international units (IU). One IU, as defined by the World Health Organization standard for blood coagulation FVIII, human, is approximately equal to the level of FVIII activity found in 1 mL of fresh pooled human plasma. Kogenate FS must be administered by the intravenous route. Antihemophilic Factor (Recombinant) Kogenate® (Bayer Biological) Antihemophilic Factor (Recombinant), Kogenate is a sterile, stable, purified, nonpyrogenic, dried concentrate which has been manufactured by recombinant DNA technology. Kogenate is intended for use in therapy of classical hemophilia (hemophilia A). Kogenate is produced by baby hamster kidney (BHK) cells into which the human factor VIII (FVIII) gene has been introduced. Kogenate is a highly purified glycoprotein consisting of multiple peptides including an 80 kD and various extensions of the 90 kD subunit. It has the same biological activity as FVIII derived from human plasma. In addition to the use of the classical purification methods of ion exchange chromatography and size exclusion chromatography, monoclonal antibody immunoaffinity chromatography is utilized along with other steps designed to purify recombinant factor VIII (rAHF) and remove contaminating substances. The final preparation is stabilized with albumin (human) and lyophilized. The concentration of Kogenate is approximately 100 IU/mL. The product contains no preservatives. Each vial of Kogenate contains the labeled amount of rAHF in International Units (IU). One IU, as defined by the World Health Organization standard for blood coagulation factor VIII, human, is approximately equal to the level of factor VIII activity found in 1.0 mL of fresh pooled human plasma. The final product when reconstituted as directed contains the following excipients: 10 to 30 mg glycine/mL, not more than (NMT) 500 µg imidazole/1000 IU, NMT 600 µg polysorbate 80/1000 IU, 2 to 5 mM calcium chloride, 100 to 130 mEq/L sodium, 100 to 130 mEq/L chloride, and 4 to 10 mg albumin (human)/mL. Kogenate must be administered by the intravenous route.

Product	Company	Indication	Date	Description
Lantus® (insulin glargine)	Aventis	Biosynthetic basal insulin for adult and pediatric patients with type 2 diabetes	Apr 2000	Lantus® (insulin glargine [rDNA origin] injection) is a sterile solution of insulin glargine for use as an injection. Insulin glargine is a recombinant human insulin analog that is a long-acting (up to 24-hour duration of action), parenteral blood-glucose-lowering agent. Lantus is produced by recombinant DNA technology utilizing a nonpathogenic laboratory strain of *Escherichia coli* (K12) as the production organism. Insulin glargine differs from human insulin in that the amino acid asparagine at position A21 is replaced by glycine and two arginines are added to the C-terminus of the B-chain. Chemically, it is 21^A-Gly-30^{B}a-L-Arg-30^{B}b-L-Arg-human insulin and has the empirical formula $C_{267}H_{404}N_{72}O_{78}S_6$ and a molecular weight of 6063. Lantus consists of insulin glargine dissolved in a clear aqueous fluid. Each milliliter of Lantus (insulin glargine injection) contains 100 IU (3.6378 mg) insulin glargine, 30 mcg zinc, 2.7 mg m-cresol, 20 mg glycerol 85%, and water for injection. The pH is adjusted by addition of aqueous solutions of hydrochloric acid and sodium hydroxide. It has a pH of approximately 4.
Leukine®/Leukine® Liquid (granulocyte macrophage colony-stimulating factor)	Berlex Laboratories	Treatment of autologous bone marrow transplantation; Treatment of white blood cell toxicities following induction chemotherapy in older patients with acute myelogenous leukemia; For use following allogenic bone marrow transplantation from HLA-matched related donors; For use mobilizing peripheral blood progenitor cells and for use after PBPC transplantation; Treatment of autologous bone marrow transplantation; treatment of white blood cell toxicities following induction chemotherapy in older patients with acute myelogenous leukemia; for use following allogenic bone marrow transplantation from HLA-matched related donors; for	Mar 1991 Sep 1995 Nov 1995 Dec 1995 Nov 1996	Leukine® (sargramostim) is a recombinant human granulocyte-macrophage colony stimulating factor (rhu GM-CSF) produced by recombinant DNA technology in a yeast (*S. cerevisiae*) expression system. GM-CSF is a hematopoietic growth factor that stimulates proliferation and differentiation of hematopoietic progenitor cells. Leukine is a glycoprotein of 127 amino acids characterized by 3 primary molecular species having molecular masses of 19,500, 16,800, and 15,500 Da. The amino acid sequence of Leukine differs from the natural human GM-CSF by a substitution of leucine at position 23, and the carbohydrate moiety may be different from the native protein. Sargramostim has been selected as the proper name for yeast-derived rhu GM-CSF. The Leukine Liquid presentation is formulated as a sterile, preserved (1.1% benzyl alcohol), injectable solution (500 mcg/mL) in a vial. Lyophilized Leukine is a sterile, white, preservative-free powder (250 mcg) that requires reconstitution with 1 mL sterile water for injection, USP or 1 mL bacteriostatic water for injection, USP. Leukine Liquid and reconstituted lyophilized Leukine are clear, colorless liquids suitable for subcutaneous injection or intravenous infusion. Leukine Liquid contains 500 mcg (2.8 × 10^6 IU/mL) sargramostim and 1.1% benzyl alcohol in a 1 mL solution. The vial of lyophilized Leukine contains 250 mcg (1.4 × 10^6 IU/vial) sargramostim. The Leukine Liquid vial and reconstituted lyophilized Leukine vial also contain 40 mg/mL mannitol, USP; 10 mg/mL sucrose, NF; and 1.2 mg/mL tromethamine, USP, as excipients. Biological potency is expressed in International Units (IU) as tested against the WHO First International Reference Standard. The specific activity of Leukine is approximately 5.6 × 10^6 IU/mg.

Continued.

Product	Company	Application	FDA Approval Date	Description
		use mobilizing peripheral blood progenitor cell (Leukine® Liquid) ready-to-use formulation in a multidose vial		
LYMErix™ (OspA lipoprotein)	SmithKline Beecham Biologicals (subsidiary of GlaxoSmithKline)	Prevention of Lyme disease	Dec 1998	LYMErix™ [Lyme Disease Vaccine (Recombinant OspA)] is a noninfectious recombinant vaccine developed and manufactured by GlaxoSmithKline Biologicals. The causative agent of Lyme disease is *Borrelia burgdorferi*; in North America, all Lyme disease is due to *Borrelia burgdorferi sensu stricto*. The vaccine contains lipoprotein OspA, an outer surface protein of *Borrelia burgdorferi sensu stricto ZS7*, as expressed by *Escherichia coli*. Lipoprotein OspA is a single polypeptide chain of 257 amino acids with lipids covalently bonded to the N terminus. No substance of animal origin is used in the commercial manufacturing process. Fermentation media consist primarily of inorganic salts and vitamins, with small quantities of antifoam (contains silicon), kanamycin sulfate (an aminoglycoside antibiotic), and yeast extract. Silicon and kanamycin are removed to levels below detection (< 7 ppm and < 10 ppb, respectively). The vaccine is adsorbed onto aluminum hydroxide. LYMErix is supplied as a sterile suspension in single-dose vials and prefilled syringes for intramuscular administration. The vaccine is ready for use without reconstitution; it must be shaken before administration to ensure a uniform turbid white suspension. Each 0.5 mL dose of vaccine consists of 30 mcg of lipoprotein OspA adsorbed onto 0.5 mg aluminum as aluminum hydroxide adjuvant. Each dose of the vaccine preparation contains 10 mM phosphate buffered saline and 2.5 mg of 2-phenoxyethanol, a bacteriostatic agent. The potency of the vaccine is evaluated by immunizing mice with LYMErix [Lyme Disease Vaccine (Recombinant OspA)] and measuring their serum antibody response to OspA by ELISA.
Mylotarg™ (gemtuzumab ozogamicin)	Celltech Pharmaceuticals and Wyeth	Human antibody linked to calicheamicin (chemotherapeutic) for treatment of CD33 positive acute myeloid leukemia in patients 60 and older in first relapse who are not considered candidates for cytotoxic chemotherapy	May 2000	Mylotarg™ (gemtuzumab ozogamicin for injection) is a chemotherapy agent composed of a recombinant humanized IgG4, kappa antibody conjugated with a cytotoxic antitumor or antibiotic, calicheamicin, isolated from fermentation of a bacterium, *Micromonospora echinospora* ssp. *calichensis*. The antibody portion of Mylotarg binds specifically to the CD33 antigen, a sialic acid-dependent adhesion protein found on the surface of leukemic blasts and immature normal cells of myelomonocytic lineage, but not on normal hematopoietic stem cells. The anti-CD33 hP67.6 antibody is produced by mammalian cell suspension culture using a myeloma NS0 cell line and is purified under conditions that remove or inactivate viruses. Three separate and independent steps in the hP67.6 antibody purification process achieves retrovirus inactivation and removal. These include low pH treatment, DEAE-Sepharose chromatography, and viral filtration. Mylotarg contains amino acid sequences of which approximately 98.3% are of human origin. The constant region and framework regions contain human sequences, while the complementarity-determining regions are derived from a murine antibody (p67.6) that

Product	Company	Date	Indication	Description
				binds CD33. This antibody is linked to N-acetyl-gamma calicheamicin via a bifunctional linker. Gemtuzumab ozogamicin has approximately 50% of the antibody loaded with 4 to 6 moles calicheamicin per mole of antibody. The remaining 50% of the antibody is not linked to the calicheamicin derivative. Gemtuzumab ozogamicin has a molecular weight of 151 to 153 kDa. Mylotarg (gemtuzumab ozogamicin for injection) is a sterile, white, preservative-free lyophilized powder containing 5 mg of drug conjugate (protein equivalent) in a 20-mL amber vial. The drug product is light sensitive and must be protected from direct and indirect sunlight and unshielded fluorescent light during the preparation and administration of the infusion. The inactive ingredients are: dextran 40; sucrose; sodium chloride; monobasic and dibasic sodium phosphate.
Natrecor® (nesiritide)	Scios, Inc.	Aug 2001	Acutely decompensated congestive heart failure with shortness of breath at rest or with minimal activity	Natrecor® (nesiritide) is a sterile, purified preparation of a new drug class, human B-type natriuretic peptide (hBNP), and is manufactured from *E. coli* using recombinant DNA technology. Nesiritide has a molecular weight of 3464 g/mol and an empirical formula of $C_{143}H_{244}N_{50}O_{42}S_4$. Nesiritide has the same 32 amino acid sequence as the endogenous peptide, which is produced by the ventricular myocardium. Natrecor is formulated as the citrate salt of rhBNP and is provided in a sterile, single-use vial. Each 1.5-mg vial contains a white- to off-white lyophilized powder for intravenous (IV) administration after reconstitution. The quantitative composition of the lyophilized drug per vial is: nesiritide 1.58 mg, mannitol 20.0 mg, citric acid monohydrate 2.1 mg, and sodium citrate dihydrate 2.94 mg.
Neulasta™ (pegfilgrastim)	Amgen	Jan 2002	Reduction of incidence of infection as manifested by febrile neutropenia in nonmyeloid cancer patients receiving certain chemotherapies	Neulasta™ (pegfilgrastim) is a covalent conjugate of recombinant methionyl human G-CSF (Filgrastim) and monomethoxypoly-ethylene glycol. Filgrastim is a water-soluble 175 amino acid protein with a molecular weight of approximately 19 kDa. Filgrastim is obtained from the bacterial fermentation of a strain of *Escherichia coli* transformed with a genetically engineered plasmid containing the human G-CSF gene. To produce pegfilgrastim, a 20 kDa monomethoxypolyethylene glycol molecule is covalently bound to the N-terminal methionyl residue of Filgrastim. The average molecular weight of pegfilgrastim is approximately 39 kDa. Neulasta is supplied in 0.6 mL, prefilled syringes for subcutaneous (SC) injection. Each syringe contains 6 mg pegfilgrastim (based on protein weight), in a sterile, clear, colorless, preservative-free solution (pH 4.0) containing acetate (0.35 mg), sorbitol (30.0 mg), polysorbate 20 (0.02 mg), and sodium (0.02 mg) in water for injection, USP.
Neumega® (oprelvekin)	Wyeth	Nov 1997	Prevention of severe chemotherapy-induced thrombocytopenia in cancer patients	Interleukin eleven (IL-11) is a thrombopoietic growth factor that directly stimulates the proliferation of hematopoietic stem cells and megakaryocyte progenitor cells and induces megakaryocyte maturation resulting in increased platelet production. IL-11 is a member of a family of human growth factors, which includes human growth hormone, granulocyte colony-stimulating factor (G-CSF), and other growth factors. Oprelvekin, the active ingredient in Neumega, is produced in *Escherichia coli* by recombinant DNA methods. The protein has a molecular mass of approximately 19,000 Da and is nonglycosylated. *Continued.*

Product	Company	Application	FDA Approval Date	Description
				The polypeptide is 177 amino acids in length and differs from the 178 amino acid length of native IL-11 only in lacking the amino-terminal proline residue. This alteration has not resulted in measurable differences in bioactivity either *in vitro* or *in vivo*. Neumega is available for subcutaneous administration in single-use vials containing 5 mg of Oprelvekin (specific activity approximately 8×10^6 Units/mg) as a sterile, lyophilized powder with 23 mg Glycine, USP, 1.6 mg dibasic sodium phosphate heptahydrate, USP, and 0.55 mg monobasic sodium phosphate monohydrate, USP. When reconstituted with 1 mL of sterile water for injection, USP, the resulting solution has a pH of 7. 0 and a concentration of 5 mg/mL.
Neupogen® (filgrastim)	Amgen	Treatment of chemotherapy-induced neutropenia; Bone marrow transplant accompanied by neutropenia; Severe chronic neutropenia; Autologous bone marrow transplant engraftment or failure; Mobilization of autologous PBPCs after chemotherapy	Feb 1991 Jun 1994 Dec 1994 Dec 1995 Apr 1998	Filgrastim is a human granulocyte colony-stimulating factor (G-CSF), produced by recombinant DNA technology. Neupogen® is the Amgen Inc. trademark for filgrastim, which has been selected as the name for recombinant methionyl human granulocyte colony-stimulating factor (r-metHuG-CSF). Neupogen is a 175 amino acid protein manufactured by recombinant DNA technology. Neupogen is produced by *Escherichia coli* bacteria into which has been inserted the human granulocyte colony-stimulating factor gene. Neupogen has a molecular weight of 18,800 Da. The protein has an amino acid sequence that is identical to the natural sequence predicted from human DNA sequence analysis, except for the addition of an N-terminal methionine necessary for expression in *E. coli*. Because Neupogen is produced in *E. coli*, the product is nonglycosylated and thus differs from G-CSF isolated from a human cell. Neupogen is a sterile, clear, colorless, preservative-free liquid for parenteral administration containing filgrastim at a specific activity of $1.0 \pm 0. 6 \times 10^8$ U/mg (as measured by a cell mitogenesis assay). The product is available in single-use vials and prefilled syringes. The single-use vials contain either 300 mcg or 480 mcg filgrastim at a fill volume of 1.0 mL or 1.6 mL, respectively. The single-use prefilled syringes contain either 300 mcg or 480 mcg filgrastim at a fill volume of 0.5 mL or 0.8 mL, respectively. See table below for product composition of each single-use vial or prefilled syringe.

	300 mcg/ 1.0 mL Vial	480 mcg/ 1.6 mL Vial	300 mcg/ 0.5 mL Syringe	480 mcg/ 0.8 mL Syringe
Filgrastim	300 mcg	480 mcg	300 mcg	480 mcg
Acetate	0.59 mg	0.94 mg	0.295 mg	0.472 mg
Sorbitol	50.0 mg	80.0 mg	25.0 mg	40.0 mg
Tween® 80	0.004%	0.004%	0.004%	0. 004%
Sodium	0.035 mg	0.056 mg	0.0175 mg	0.028 mg
Water for Injection USP q. s. ad	1.0 mL	1.6 mL	0.5 mL	0.8 mL

Norditropin® (somatropin) — Novo Nordisk — Treatment of growth hormone deficiency in children — May 1995

Norditropin® is the Novo Nordisk Pharmaceuticals, Inc. registered trademark for somatropin, a polypeptide hormone of recombinant DNA origin. The hormone is synthesized by a special strain of *E. coli* bacteria that has been modified by the addition of a plasmid that carries the gene for human growth hormone. Norditropin contains the identical sequence of 191 amino acids constituting the naturally occurring pituitary human growth hormone with a molecular weight of about 22,000 Da. Norditropin cartridges are supplied as solutions in ready-to-administer cartridges with a volume of 1.5 mL. Each Norditropin cartridge contains the following:

Component	5 mg/1.5 mL	10 mg/1.5 mL	15 mg/1.5 mL
Somatropin	5 mg	10 mg	15 mg
Histidine	1 mg	1 mg	1.7 mg
Poloxamer 188	4.5 mg	4.5 mg	4.5 mg
Phenol	4.5 mg	4.5 mg	4.5 mg
Mannitol	60 mg	60 mg	58 mg
HCl/NaOH	q.s.	q.s.	q.s.
Water for Injection	ad 1.5 mL	ad 1.5 mL	ad 1.5 mL

Novolin L® (insulin; zinc suspension) — Novo Nordisk — Treatment of diabetes — Jun 1991

This vial contains Novolin L®, commonly known as Lente® Human Insulin Zinc Suspension (recombinant DNA origin). The concentration of this product is 100 U/mL insulin. It is a cloudy or milky suspension of 70% crystalline and 30% amorphous human insulin. The insulin substance (the cloudy material) settles at the bottom of the vial, therefore, the vial must be gently agitated or rotated so that the contents are uniformly mixed before a dose is withdrawn. Novolin L has an intermediate duration of action. The effect of Novolin L begins approximately 2.5 hours after injection. The effect is maximal between 7 and 15 hours and ends approximately 22 hours after injection. The time course of action of any insulin may vary considerably in different individuals or at different times in the same individual. Because of this variation, the time periods listed here should be considered as general guidelines only. This human insulin (recombinant DNA origin) is structurally identical to the insulin produced by the human pancreas. This human insulin is produced by recombinant DNA technology utilizing *Saccharomyces cerevisiae* (bakers yeast) as the production organism.

Novolin N® (insulin; isophane suspension) — Novo Nordisk — Treatment of diabetes — Jul 1991

This vial contains Novolin® N, commonly known as NPH, Human Insulin Isophane Suspension (recombinant DNA origin). The concentration of this product is 100 U/mL insulin. It is a cloudy or milky suspension of human insulin with protamine and zinc. The insulin substance (the cloudy material) settles at the bottom of the vial, therefore, the vial must be gently agitated or rotated so that the contents are uniformly mixed before a dose is withdrawn. Novolin N has an intermediate duration of action. The effect of Novolin N begins approximately 1.5 hours after injection. The effect is maximal between 4 and 12 hours. The full duration of action may last up to 24 hours after injection. The time course of action of any insulin may last up to 24 hours after injection. The time course of action of any insulin may vary considerably in different individuals, or at different times in the same individual. Because of this variation, the time periods listed here should

Continued.

Product	Company	Application	FDA Approval Date	Description
				be considered as general guidelines only. This human insulin (recombinant DNA origin) is structurally identical to the insulin produced by the human pancreas. This human insulin is produced by recombinant DNA technology utilizing *Saccharomyces cerevisiae* (bakers yeast) as the production organism. Novolin N Prefilled® contains NPH, Human Insulin Isophane Suspension (recombinant DNA origin). The concentration of this product is 100 U/mL insulin. It is a cloudy or milky suspension of human insulin with protamine and zinc. The insulin substance (the cloudy material) settles to the bottom of the insulin reservoir, therefore, the syringe must be rotated up and down so that the contents are uniformly mixed before a dose is given. Novolin N has an intermediate duration of action. The effect of Novolin N begins approximately 1.5 hours after injection. The effect is maximal between 4 and approximately 12 hours. The full duration of action may last up to 24 hours after injection.
Novolin R® (insulin, regular)	Novo Nordisk	Treatment of diabetes	Jun 1991	This vial contains Novolin® R commonly known as Regular, Human Insulin Injection (recombinant DNA origin). The concentration of this product is 100 U/mL insulin. It is a clear, colorless solution which has a short duration of action. The effect of Novolin R begins approximately .5 hour after injection. The effect is maximal between 2.5 and 5 hours and ends approximately 8 hours after injection. The time course of action of any insulin may vary considerably in different individuals or at different times in the same individual. Because of this variation, the time periods listed here should be considered as general guidelines only. This human insulin (recombinant DNA origin) is structurally identical to the insulin produced by the human pancreas. This human insulin is produced by recombinant DNA technology utilizing *Saccharomyces cerevisiae* (bakers yeast) as the production organism.
Novolin® (insulin)	Novo Nordisk	Treatment of diabetes	Oct 1982	This vial contains Novolin® commonly known as Regular, Human Insulin Injection (recombinant DNA origin). The concentration of this product is 100 U/mL insulin. It is a clear, colorless solution that has a short duration of action. The effect of Novolin R begins approximately .5 hour after injection. The effect is maximal between 2.5 and 5 hours and ends approximately 8 hours after injection. The time course of action of any insulin may vary considerably in different individuals or at different times in the same individual. Because of this variation, the time periods listed here should be considered as general guidelines only. This human insulin (recombinant DNA origin) is structurally identical to the insulin produced by the human pancreas. This human insulin is produced by recombinant DNA technology utilizing *Saccharomyces cerevisiae* (bakers yeast) as the production organism. Insulin should be stored in a cold place, preferably in a refrigerator, but not in the freezing compartment. *Do not let it freeze.* Keep the insulin vial in its carton so that it will stay clean and protected from light. If refrigeration is not possible, the bottle of insulin you are currently using can be kept unrefrigerated as long as it is kept as cool as possible and away from heat and sunlight. Never use Novolin if it becomes viscous (thickened) or cloudy; use it only if it is clear and colorless. Novolin R Prefilled® contains

Novolin® 70/30 (70% insulin isophane suspension and 30% regular insulin)	Novo Nordisk	Jun 1991	Regular, Human Insulin Injection (recombinant DNA origin). The concentration of this product is 100 U/mL insulin. It is a clear, colorless solution which has a short duration of action. The effect of Novolin begins approximately .5 hour after injection. The effect is maximal between 2.5 and 5 hours and ends approximately 8 hours after injection. This human insulin (recombinant DNA origin) is structurally identical to the insulin produced by the human pancreas. This human insulin is produced by recombinant DNA technology utilizing *Saccharomyces cerevisiae* (bakers yeast) as the production organism. Novolin 70/30 Prefilled® contains Novolin® 70/30, a mixture of 70% NPH, Human Insulin Isophane Suspension (recombinant DNA origin) and 30% Regular, Human Insulin Injection (recombinant DNA origin) USP. The concentration of this product is 100 U/mL insulin. It is a cloudy or milky suspension of human insulin with protamine and zinc. The insulin substance (the cloudy material) settles to the bottom of the insulin reservoir, therefore, the syringe must be rotated up and down so that the contents are uniformly mixed before a dose is given. Novolin 70/30 has an intermediate duration of action. The effect of Novolin 70/30 begins approximately .5 hour after injection. The effect is maximal between 2 and approximately 12 hours. The full duration of action may last up to 24 hours after injection. The time course of action of any insulin may vary considerably in different individuals or at different times in the same individual. Because of the variation, the time periods listed here should be considered as general guidelines only. Storage: Novolin Prefilled insulin syringes should be stored in a cold place, preferably in a refrigerator, but not in the freezing compartment. *Do not let it freeze.* Keep Novolin Prefilled in the carton so that they will stay clean and protected from light. Novolin 70/30 Prefilled and Novolin N Prefilled can be kept unrefrigerated for 1 week. Novolin R Prefilled can be kept unrefrigerated for 1 month. Unrefrigerated syringes must be used within this time period or discarded. Be sure to protect syringes from sunlight and extreme heat or cold. Never use any Novolin R Prefilled if the insulin becomes viscous (thickened or cloudy); use it only if it is clear and colorless. Never use any Novolin 70/30 Prefilled or Novolin N Prefilled if the precipitate (the white deposit) has become lumpy or granular in appearance or has formed a deposit of solid particles on the wall of the insulin reservoir. This insulin should not be used if the liquid in the insulin reservoir remains clear after it has been mixed. Never use insulin after the expiration date printed on the label and carton.
NovoLog® (insulin aspart)	Novo Nordisk	May 2000 Dec 2001	NovoLog® (insulin aspart [rDNA origin] injection) is a human insulin analog that is a rapid-acting, parenteral blood glucose-lowering agent. NovoLog is homologous with regular human insulin with the exception of a single substitution of the amino acid proline by aspartic acid in position B28 and is produced by recombinant DNA technology utilizing *Saccharomyces cerevisiae* (bakers yeast) as the production organism. Insulin aspart has the empirical formula $C_{256}H_{381}N_{65}O_{79}S_6$ and a molecular weight of 5825.8. NovoLog is a sterile, aqueous, clear, and colorless solution that contains insulin aspart (B28 asp regular human insulin analog) 100 U/mL, glycerin 16 mg/mL, phenol 1.50 mg/mL, metacresol 1.72 mg/mL, zinc 19.6 μg/mL, disodium hydrogen phosphate dihydrate 1.25 mg/mL, and sodium chloride 0.58 mg/mL. NovoLog has a pH of 7.2 to 7.6. Hydrochloric acid 10% or sodium hydroxide 10% may be added to adjust pH.

	Insulin analog for adults with diabetes mellitus; For pump therapy in diabetes		

Continued.

Product	Company	Application	FDA Approval Date	Description
NovoSeven® (coagulation factor VIIa)	Novo Nordisk	Treatment of bleeding episodes in hemophilia A or B patients with inhibitors to factor VIII or factor IX	Mar 1999	NovoSeven® is recombinant human coagulation factor VIIa (rFVIIa), intended for promoting hemostasis by activating the extrinsic pathway of the coagulation cascade. NovoSeven is a vitamin K-dependent glycoprotein consisting of 406 amino acid residues (MW 50 K Dalton). NovoSeven is structurally similar to human plasma-derived factor VIIa. The gene for human factor VII is cloned and expressed in baby hamster kidney (BHK) cells. Recombinant FVII is secreted into the culture media (containing newborn calf serum) in its single-chain form and then proteolytically converted by autocatalysis to the active two-chain form, rFVIIa, during a chromatographic purification process. The purification process has been demonstrated to remove exogenous viruses (MuLV, SV40, Pox virus, Reovirus, BEV, IBR virus). No human serum or other proteins are used in the production or formulation of NovoSeven. NovoSeven is supplied as a sterile, white lyophilized powder of rFVIIa in single-use vials. Each vial of lyophilized drug contains the following:

Contents	1.2 mg (60 KIU) Vial	4.8 mg (240 KIU) Vial
rFVIIa	1200 µg	4800 µg
Sodium chloride*	5.84 mg	23.36 mg
Calcium chloride dihydrate*	2.94 mg	11.76 mg
Glycylglycine	2.64 mg	10.56 mg
Polysorbate 80	0.14 mg	0.56 mg
Mannitol	60.0 mg	240.0 mg

* Per mg of rFVIIa: 0.44 mEq sodium, 0.06 mEq calcium.

After reconstitution with the appropriate volume of sterile water for injection, USP (not supplied), each vial contains approximately 0.6 mg/mL. NovoSeven (corresponding to 600 µg/mL). The reconstituted vials have a pH of approximately 5.5 in sodium chloride (3 mg/mL), calcium chloride dihydrate (1.5 mg/mL), glycylglycine (1.3 mg/mL), polysorbate 80 (0.1 mg/mL), and mannitol (30 mg/mL). The reconstituted product is a clear colorless solution that contains no preservatives. NovoSeven contains trace amounts of proteins derived from the manufacturing and purification processes such as mouse IgG (maximum of 1.2 ng/mg), bovine IgG (maximum of 30 ng/mg), and protein from BHK-cells and media (maximum of 19 ng/mg).

Product	Company	Application	FDA Approval Date	Description
Nutropin Depot™ (sustained-release formulation of somatropin)	Alkermes, Inc., and Genentech, Inc.	Growth hormone deficiency	Dec 1999	Nutropin Depot™ [somatropin (rDNA origin) for injectable suspension] is a long-acting dosage form of recombinant human growth hormone (rhGH). Somatropin has 191 amino acid residues and a molecular weight of 22,125 Da. The amino acid sequence of the product is identical to that of pituitary-derived human growth hormone. The protein is synthesized by a specific laboratory strain of *E. coli* as a precursor consisting of the rhGH molecule preceded by the secretion signal from an *E. coli* protein. This precursor is

directed to the plasma membrane of the cell. The signal sequence is removed and the native protein is secreted into the periplasm so that the protein is folded appropriately as it is synthesized. Somatropin is a highly purified preparation. Biological potency is determined using a cell proliferation bioassay. The Nutropin Depot formulation consists of micronized particles of rhGH embedded in biocompatible, biodegradable polylactide-coglycolide (PLG) microspheres. Nutropin Depot is packaged in vials as a sterile, white to off-white, preservative-free, free-flowing powder. Before administration, the powder is suspended in Diluent for Nutropin Depot (a sterile aqueous solution). Each 13.5 mg 3 cc single-use vial of Nutropin Depot contains 13.5 mg somatropin, 1.2 mg zinc acetate, 0.8 mg zinc carbonate, and 68.9 mg PLG. Each 18 mg 3 cc single-use vial of Nutropin Depot contains 18 mg somatropin, 1.6 mg zinc acetate, 1.1 mg zinc carbonate, and 91.8 mg PLG. Each 22.5 mg 3 cc single-use vial of Nutropin Depot contains 22.5 mg somatropin, 2.0 mg zinc acetate, 1.4 mg zinc carbonate, and 114.8 mg PLG. Each dosage size contains an overage of rhGH microspheres to ensure delivery of labeled contents. Each 1.5 mL single-use vial of Diluent for Nutropin Depot contains 30 mg/mL carboxymethylcellulose sodium salt, 1 mg/mL polysorbate 20, 9 mg/mL sodium chloride, and sterile water for injection; pH 5.8 to 7.2.

NUTROPIN® (Genentech)[somatropin (rDNA origin) for injection] Nutropin® [somatropin (rDNA origin) for injection] is a human growth hormone (hGH) produced by recombinant DNA technology. Nutropin has 191 amino acid residues and a molecular weight of 22,125 Da. The amino acid sequence of the product is identical to that of pituitary-derived human growth hormone. The protein is synthesized by a specific laboratory strain of *E. coli* as a precursor consisting of the rhGH molecule preceded by the secretion signal from an *E. coli* protein. This precursor is directed to the plasma membrane of the cell. The signal sequence is removed and the native protein is secreted into the periplasm so that the protein is folded appropriately as it is synthesized. Nutropin is a highly purified preparation. Biological potency is determined using a cell proliferation bioassay. Nutropin is a sterile, white, lyophilized powder intended for subcutaneous administration after reconstitution with bacteriostatic water for injection, USP (benzoyl alcohol preserved). The reconstituted product is nearly isotonic at a concentration of 5 mg/mL growth hormone (GH) and has a pH of approximately 7.4. Each 5 mg Nutropin vial contains 5 mg (approximately 15 IU) somatropin, lyophilized with 45 mg mannitol, 1.7 mg sodium phosphates (0.4 mg sodium phosphate monobasic, 1.3 mg sodium phosphate dibasic), and 1.7 mg glycine. Each 10 mg Nutropin vial contains 10 mg (approximately 30 IU) somatropin, lyophilized with 90 mg mannitol, 3.4 mg sodium phosphates (0.8 mg sodium phosphate monobasic and 2.6 mg sodium phosphate dibasic), and 3.4 mg glycine. Bacteriostatic water for injection, USP, is sterile water containing 0.9 percent benzoyl alcohol per mL as an antimicrobial preservative packaged in a multidose vial. The diluent pH is 4.5 to 7.0.

Product	Company	Application	FDA Approval Date	Description
Nutropin®/Nutropin AQ® (somatropin)	Genentech, Inc.	Treatment of growth hormone deficiency in children; Treatment of growth hormone deficiency in adults; Growth failure associated with chronic renal insufficiency prior to kidney transplantation; Short stature associated with Turner Syndrome; To improve spine bone mineral density observed in childhood-onset adult growth hormone-deficient patients and to increase serum alkaline phosphatase	Nov 1993 Jan 1994 Jan 1996 Dec 1996 Dec 1999	Nutropin AQ® [somatropin (rDNA origin) injection] is a human growth hormone (hGH) produced by recombinant DNA technology. Nutropin AQ has 191 amino acid residues and a molecular weight of 22,125 Da. The amino acid sequence of the product is identical to that of pituitary-derived human growth hormone. The protein is synthesized by a specific laboratory strain of *E. coli* as a precursor consisting of the rhGH molecule preceded by the secretion signal from an *E. coli* protein. This precursor is directed to the plasma membrane of the cell. The signal sequence is removed and the native protein is secreted into the periplasm so that the protein is folded appropriately as it is synthesized. Nutropin AQ is a highly purified preparation. Biological potency is determined using a cell proliferation bioassay. Nutropin AQ may contain not more than 15% deamidated growth hormone (GH) at expiration. The deamidated form of GH has been extensively characterized and has been shown to be safe and fully active. Nutropin AQ is a sterile liquid intended for subcutaneous administration. The product is nearly isotonic at a concentration of 5 mg of GH per mL and has a pH of approximately 6.0. Each 2 mL vial contains 10 mg (approximately 30 IU) somatropin, formulated in 17.4 mg sodium chloride, 5 mg phenol, 4 mg polysorbate 20, and 10 mM sodium citrate.
Ontak® (denileukin diftitox)	Ligand Pharmaceuticals, Inc.	Treatment of patients with persistent or recurrent cutaneous T-cell lymphoma whose malignant cells express the CD25 component of the interleukin-2 receptor	Feb 1999	Ontak® (denileukin diftitox), a recombinant DNA-derived cytotoxic protein composed of the amino acid sequences for diphtheria toxin fragments A and B (Met$_1$-Thr$_{387}$)-His followed by the sequences for interleukin-2 (IL-2; Ala$_1$-Thr$_{133}$), is produced in an *E. coli* expression system. Ontak has a molecular weight of 58 kDa. Neomycin is used in the fermentation process but is undetectable in the final product. The product is purified using reverse phase chromatography followed by a multistep diafiltration process. Ontak is supplied in single use vials as a sterile, frozen solution intended for intravenous (IV) administration. Each 2 mL vial of Ontak contains 300 mcg of recombinant denileukin diftitox in a sterile solution of citric acid (20 mM), EDTA (0.05 mM) and polysorbate 20 (<1%) in water for injection, USP. The solution has a pH of 6.9 to 7.2.
Orthoclone OKT3® (muromomab-CD3)	Ortho Biotech, Inc. (subsidiary of Johnson & Johnson)	Reversal of acute kidney transplant rejection	Jun 1986	Orthoclone OKT3® (muromonab-CD3) sterile solution is a murine monoclonal antibody to the CD3 antigen of human T-cells, which functions as an immunosuppressant. It is for intravenous use only. The antibody is a biochemically purified IgG2a immunoglobulin with a heavy chain of approximately 50,000 Da and a light chain of approximately 25,000 Da. It is directed to a glycoprotein with a molecular weight of 20,000 in the human T-cell surface, which is essential for T-cell functions. Because it is a monoclonal antibody preparation, Orthoclone OKT3 sterile solution is a homogeneous, reproducible antibody product with consistent, measurable reactivity to human T-cells. Each 5 mL ampule of Orthoclone OKT3 sterile solution contains 5 mg (1 mg/mL) of muromonab-CD3 in a clear colorless solution, which may contain a few fine translucent protein particles. Each ampule contains a buffered solution (pH 7.0 + 0.5) of monobasic sodium phosphate (2.25 mg), dibasic sodium phosphate (9.0 mg), sodium chloride (43 mg), and polysorbate 80 (1.0 mg) in water for injection. The proper name, muromonab-CD3, is derived from the

Ovidrel®

descriptive term murine monoclonal antibody. The CD3 designation identifies the specificity of the antibody as the cell differentiation (CD) cluster 3 defined by the First International Workshop on Human Leukocyte Differentiation Antigens.

Ovidrel® (choriogonadotropin alfa for injection) is a sterile lyophilized powder composed of choriogonadotropin alfa (recombinant human Chorionic Gonadotropin, r-hCG), sucrose, and phosphoric acid. The drug substance is produced by recombinant DNA techniques. Choriogonadotropin alfa is a water soluble glycoprotein consisting of two noncovalently linked subunits — designated (alpha) and (beta) — consisting of 92 and 145 amino acid residues, respectively, with carbohydrate moieties linked to ASN-52 and ASN-78 (on alpha subunit) and ASN-13, ASN-30, SER-121, SER-127, SER-132, and SER-138 (on beta subunit). The primary structure of the (alpha)-chain of r-hCG is identical to that of the (alpha)-chain of hCG, FSH, and LH. The glycoform pattern of the (alpha)-subunit of r-hCG is closely comparable to urinary derived hCG (u-hCG), the differences mainly being due to the branching and sialicylation extent of the oligosaccharides. The (beta)-chain has both O- and N-glycosylation sites and its structure and glycosylation pattern are also very similar to that of u-hCG. The production process involves expansion of genetically modified Chinese hamster ovary (CHO) cells from an extensively characterized cell bank into large-scale cell culture processing. Choriogonadotropin alfa is secreted by the CHO cells directly into the cell culture medium that is then purified using a series of chromatographic steps. This process yields a product with a high level of purity and consistent product characteristics including glycoforms and biological activity. The biological activity of choriogonadotropin alfa is determined using the seminal vesicle weight gain test in male rats described in the Chorionic Gonadotrophins monograph of the European Pharmacopoeia. The *in vivo* biological activity of choriogonadotropin alfa has been calibrated against the third international reference preparation IS75/587 for chorionic gonadotropin. Ovidrel is a sterile, lyophilized powder intended for subcutaneous (SC) injection after reconstitution with sterile water for injection, USP. Each vial of Ovidrel contains 285 mcg of choriogonadotropin alfa, 30 mg sucrose, 0.98 mg phosphoric acid, and sodium hydroxide (for pH adjustment) which, when reconstituted with the diluent, will deliver 250 mcg of recombinant human Chorionic Gonadotropin. The pH of the reconstituted solution is 6.5 to 7.5.

Pediarix™ (diphtheria and tetanus toxoids and acellular pertussis adsorbed, hepatitis B [recombinant] and inactivated polio-virus vaccine combined)

GlaxoSmithKline

Dec 2002

Prevention of diphtheria, tetanus, pertussis, hepatitis B, and polio

Pediarix™ [Diphtheria and Tetanus Toxoids and Acellular Pertussis Adsorbed, Hepatitis B (Recombinant) and Inactivated Poliovirus Vaccine Combined] is a noninfectious, sterile, multivalent vaccine for intramuscular administration manufactured by GlaxoSmithKline Biologicals. It contains diphtheria and tetanus toxoids, 3 pertussis antigens (inactivated pertussis toxin [PT], filamentous hemagglutinin [FHA], and pertactin [69 kDa outer membrane protein]), hepatitis B surface antigen, plus poliovirus Type 1 (Mahoney), Type 2 (MEF-1), and Type 3 (Saukett). The diphtheria toxoid, tetanus toxoid, and pertussis antigens are the same as those in Infanrix® (Diphtheria and Tetanus Toxoids and Acellular Pertussis Vaccine Adsorbed). The hepatitis B surface antigen is the same as that in Engerix-B® [Hepatitis B Vaccine (Recombinant)]. The diphtheria toxin is produced by growing *Corynebacterium diphtheriae* in Fenton medium containing a bovine extract. Tetanus

Continued.

Product	Company	Application	FDA Approval Date	Description
				toxin is produced by growing *Clostridium tetani* in a modified Latham medium derived from bovine casein. The bovine materials used in these extracts are sourced from countries the U.S. Department of Agriculture (USDA) has determined neither have nor are are at risk of bovine spongiform encephalopathy (BSE). Both toxins are detoxified with formaldehyde, concentrated by ultrafiltration, and purified by precipitation, dialysis, and sterile filtration. The 3 acellular pertussis antigens (PT, FHA, and pertactin) are isolated from *Bordetella pertussis* culture grown in modified Stainer-Scholte liquid medium. PT and FHA are isolated from the fermentation broth; pertactin is extracted from the cells by heat treatment and flocculation. The antigens are purified in successive chromatographic and precipitation steps. PT is detoxified using glutaraldehyde and formaldehyde. FHA and pertactin are treated with formaldehyde. The hepatitis B surface antigen (HBsAg) is obtained by culturing genetically engineered *Saccharomyces cerevisiae* cells, which carry the surface antigen gene of the hepatitis B virus, in synthetic medium. The surface antigen expressed in the *S. cerevisiae* cells is purified by several physiochemical steps, which include precipitation, ion exchange chromatography, and ultrafiltration. The purified HBsAg undergoes dialysis with cysteine to remove residual thimerosal. The inactivated poliovirus component of Pediarix is an enhanced potency component. Each of the three strains of poliovirus is individually grown in VERO cells, a continuous line of monkey kidney cells, cultivated on microcarriers. Calf serum and lactalbumin hydrolysate are used during VERO cell culture or virus culture. Calf serum is sourced from countries the USDA has determined neither have nor are at risk of BSE. After clarification, each viral suspension is purified by ultrafiltration, diafiltration, and successive chromatographic steps, and inactivated with formaldehyde. The three purified viral strains are then pooled to form a trivalent concentrate. The diphtheria, tetanus, and pertussis antigens are individually adsorbed onto aluminum hydroxide; hepatitis B component is adsorbed onto aluminum phosphate. All antigens are then diluted and combined to produce the final formulated vaccine. Each 0.5-mL dose is formulated to contain 25 Lf of diphtheria toxoid, 10 Lf of tetanus toxoid, 25 mcg of inactivated PT, 25 mcg of FHA, 8 mcg of pertactin, 10 mcg of HBsAg, 40 D-antigen Units (DU) of Type 1 poliovirus, 8 DU of Type 2 poliovirus, and 32 DU of Type 3 poliovirus. Diphtheria and tetanus toxoid potency is determined by measuring the amount of neutralizing antitoxin in previously immunized guinea pigs. The potency of the acellular pertussis components (PT, FHA, and pertactin) is determined by enzyme-linked immunosorbent assay (ELISA) on sera from previously immunized mice. Potency of the hepatitis B component is established by HBsAg ELISA. The potency of the inactivated poliovirus component is determined by using the D-antigen ELISA and by a poliovirus neutralizing cell culture assay on sera from previously immunized rats. Each 0.5-mL dose also contains 2.5 mg of 2-phenoxyethanol as a preservative, 4.5 mg of NaCl, and aluminum adjuvant (not more than 0.85 mg aluminum by assay). Each dose also contains ~100 mcg of residual formaldehyde and ~100 mcg of polysorbate 80 (Tween 80). Thimerosal is used at the

early stages of manufacture and is removed by subsequent purification steps to below the analytical limit of detection (< 25 ng of mercury/20 mcg HBsAg), which upon calculation is < 12. 5 ng mercury per dose. Neomycin sulfate and polymyxin B are used in the polio vaccine manufacturing process and may be present in the final vaccine at ~0.05 ng neomycin and ~0.01 ng polymyxin B per dose. The procedures used to manufacture the HBsAg antigen result in a product that contains ~5% yeast protein. The vaccine must be well shaken before administration and is a turbid white suspension after shaking. Diphtheria and Tetanus Toxoids Adsorbed Bulk Concentrate (For Further Manufacturing) is manufactured by Chiron Behring GmbH & Co., Marburg, Germany. The acellular pertussis antigens, the hepatitis B surface antigen, and the inactivated poliovirus antigens are manufactured by GlaxoSmithKline Biologicals, Rixensart, Belgium. Formulation, filling, testing, packaging, and release of the vaccine are performed by GlaxoSmithKline Biologicals Manufacturing (wholly owned subsidiary of GlaxoSmithKline Biologicals).

Product	Company	Indication	Dates	Description
Pegasys® (peginterferon alfa-2a)	Roche and Nektar Therapeutics, Inc.	Chronic hepatitis C patients with compensated liver disease who have not been previously treated with alpha interferon; Combination therapy with Ribavirin in patients with chronic hepatitis C who have compensated liver disease and have not been previously treated with alpha interferon	Oct 2002 Dec 2002	Pegasys®, peginterferon alfa-2a, is a covalent conjugate of recombinant alfa-2a interferon (approximate molecular weight [MW] 20,000 Da) with a single branched bismonomethoxy polyethylene glycol (PEG) chain (approximate MW 40,000 Da). The PEG moiety is linked at a single site to the interferon alfa moiety via a stable amide bond to lysine. Peginterferon alfa-2a has an approximate molecular weight of 60,000 Da. Interferon alfa-2a is produced using recombinant DNA technology in which a cloned human leukocyte interferon gene is inserted into and expressed in *Escherichia coli*. Each vial contains approximately 1.2 mL of solution to deliver 1.0 mL of drug product. Subcutaneous (SC) administration of 1.0 mL delivers 180 μg of drug product (expressed as the amount of interferon alfa-2a), 8.0 mg sodium chloride, 0.05 mg polysorbate 80, 10.0 mg benzoyl alcohol, 2.62 mg sodium acetate trihydrate, and 0.05 mg acetic acid. The solution is colorless to light yellow and the pH is 6.0 ± 0.01.
PEG-Intron™ (pegylated version of interferon alfa-2b)	Enzon, Inc., and Schering-Plough Corp.	Monotherapy for chronic hepatitis C; Combination therapy with Rebetol for treatment of hepatitis C in patients with compensated liver disease	Jan 2001 Aug 2001	PEG-Intron™, peginterferon alfa-2b Powder for Injection, is a covalent conjugate of recombinant alfa interferon with monomethoxy polyethylene glycol (PEG). The molecular weight of the PEG portion of the molecule is 12,000 Da. The average molecular weight of the PEG-Intron molecule is approximately 31,000 Da. The specific activity of pegylated interferon alfa-2b is approximately 0.7×10^8 IU/mg protein. Interferon alfa-2b, the starting material used to manufacture PEG-Intron, is a water-soluble protein with a molecular weight of 19,271 Da produced by recombinant DNA techniques. It is obtained from the bacterial fermentation of a strain of *Escherichia coli* bearing a genetically engineered plasmid containing an interferon gene from human leukocytes. PEG-Intron is a white to off-white lyophilized powder supplied in 2-mL vials for subcutaneous use. Each vial contains either 74 μg, 118.4 μg, 177.6 μg, or 222 μg of PEG-Intron, and 1.11 mg dibasic sodium phosphate anhydrous, 1.11 mg monobasic sodium phosphate dihydrate, 59.2 mg sucrose, and 0.074 mg polysorbate 80. Following reconstitution with 0.7 mL of the supplied diluent (sterile water for injection, USP), each vial contains PEG-Intron at strengths of either 100 μg/mL, 160 μg/mL, 240 μg/mL, or 300 μg/mL.

Product	Company	Application	FDA Approval Date	Description
Procrit® (epoietin alfa)	Ortho Biotech, Inc.	Treatment of anemia in AZT-treated HIV-infected patients; Anemia in cancer patients on chemotherapy; For use in anemic patients scheduled to undergo elective noncardiac, nonvascular surgery	Dec 1990 Apr 1993 Dec 1996	Erythropoietin is a glycoprotein which stimulates red blood cell production. It is produced in the kidney and stimulates the division and differentiation of committed erythroid progenitors in the bone marrow. Procrit® (Epoetin alfa), a 165 amino acid glycoprotein manufactured by recombinant DNA technology, has the same biological effects as endogenous erythropoietin. It has a molecular weight of 30,400 Da and is produced by mammalian cells into which the human erythropoietin gene has been introduced. The product contains the identical amino acid sequence of isolated natural erythropoietin. Procrit is formulated as a sterile, colorless, liquid in an isotonic sodium chloride/sodium citrate or a sodium chloride/sodium phosphate buffered solution for intravenous (IV) or subcutaneous (SC) administration. *Single-Dose, Preservative-Free Vial:* 1 mL (2000, 3000, 4000, or 10,000 Units/mL). Each 1 mL of solution contains 2000, 3000, 4000, or 10,000 Units of Epoetin alfa, 2.5 mg albumin (human), 5.8 mg sodium citrate, 5.8 mg sodium chloride, and 0.06 mg citric acid in water for injection, USP (pH 6.9 ± 0.3). This formulation contains no preservative. *Single-Dose, Preservative-Free Vial:* 1 mL (40,000 Units/mL). Each 1 mL of solution contains 40,000 Units of Epoetin alfa, 2.5 mg albumin (human), 1.164 mg sodium phosphate monobasic monohydrate, 1.766 mg sodium phosphate dibasic anhydrate, 0.696 mg sodium citrate, 5.78 mg sodium chloride, and 6.8 mcg citric acid in water for injection, USP (pH 6.9 ± 0.3). This formulation contains no preservative. *Multidose, Preserved Vial:* 2 mL (20,000 Units, 10,000 Units/mL). Each 1 mL of solution contains 10,000 Units of Epoetin alfa, 2.5 mg albumin (human), 1.3 mg sodium citrate, 8.2 mg sodium chloride, 0.11 mg citric acid, and 1% benzoyl alcohol as preservative in water for injection, USP (pH 6.1 ± 0.3). *Multidose, Preserved Vial:* 1 mL (20,000 Units/mL). Each 1 mL of solution contains 20,000 Units of Epoetin alfa, 2.5 mg albumin (human), 1.3 mg sodium citrate, 8.2 mg sodium chloride, 0.11 mg citric acid, and 1% benzoyl alcohol as preservative in water for injection, USP (pH 6.1 ± 0.3).
Proleukin, IL-2® (aldesleukin)	Chiron Corp.	Treatment of kidney carcinoma; Treatment of metastatic melanoma	May 1992 Jan 1998	Proleukin® (aldesleukin) for injection, a human recombinant interleukin-2 product, is a highly purified protein with a molecular weight of approximately 15,300 Da. The chemical name is des-alanyl-1, serine-125 human interleukin-2. Proleukin, a lymphokine, is produced by recombinant DNA technology using a genetically engineered *E. coli* strain containing an analog of the human interleukin-2 gene. Genetic engineering techniques were used to modify the human IL–2 gene, and the resulting expression clone encodes a modified human interleukin-2. This recombinant form differs from native interleukin-2 in the following ways: (a) Proleukin is not glycosylated because it is derived from *E. coli;* (b) the molecule has no N-terminal alanine; the codon for this amino acid was deleted during the genetic engineering procedure; (c) the molecule has serine substituted for cysteine at amino acid position 125; this was accomplished by site-specific manipulation during the genetic engineering procedure; and (d) the aggregation state of Proleukin is likely to be different from that of native interleukin-2. The *in vitro* biological activities

of the native nonrecombinant molecule have been reproduced with Proleukin. Proleukin is supplied as a sterile, white to off-white, lyophilized cake in single-use vials intended for intravenous (IV) administration. When reconstituted with 1.2 mL sterile water for injection, USP, each mL contains 18 million IU (1.1 mg) Proleukin, 50 mg mannitol, and 0.18 mg sodium dodecyl sulfate, buffered with approximately 0.17 mg monobasic and 0.89 mg dibasic sodium phosphate to a pH of 7.5 (range 7.2 to 7.8). The manufacturing process for Proleukin involves fermentation in a defined medium containing tetracycline hydrochloride. The presence of the antibiotic is not detectable in the final product. Proleukin contains no preservatives in the final product. Proleukin biological potency is determined by a lymphocyte proliferation bioassay and is expressed in International Units (IU) as established by the World Health Organization 1st International Standard for Interleukin-2 (human). The relationship between potency and protein mass is as follows: 18 million (18×10^6) IU Proleukin = 1.1 mg protein.

ProstaScint® (Capromab Pendetide) is the murine monoclonal antibody, 7E11-C5. 3, conjugated to the linker-chelator, glycyl-tyrosyl-(N,-diethylenetriaminepentaacetic acid)-lysine hydrochloride (GYK-DTPA-HCl). The 7E11-C5.3 antibody is of the IgG1, kappa subclass (IgG1K). This antibody is directed against a glycoprotein expressed by prostate epithelium known as prostate specific membrane antigen (PSMA). The PSMA epitope recognized by monoclonal antibody (MAb) 7E11-C5.3 is located in the cytoplasmic domain. Expression of this glycoprotein has not been demonstrated on any other adenocarcinomas or transitional cell cancers tested. The antibody is produced by serum-free *in vitro* cultivation of cells and purified by sequential protein isolation and chromatographic separation procedures. Each ProstaScint kit consists of two vials that contain all of the nonradioactive ingredients necessary to produce a single unit dose of Indium In 111 ProstaScint, an immunoscintigraphic agent for administration by intravenous injection only. The ProstaScint vial contains 0.5 mg of capromab pendetide in 1 mL of sodium phosphate buffered saline solution adjusted to pH 6; a sterile, pyrogen-free, clear, colorless solution that may contain some translucent particles. The vial of sodium acetate buffer contains 82 mg of sodium acetate in 2 mL of water for injection adjusted to pH 5 to 7 with glacial acetic acid; it is a sterile, pyrogen-free, clear, and colorless solution. Neither solution contains a preservative. Each kit also includes one sterile 0.22 μm Millex® GV filter, prescribing information, and two identification labels. The sodium acetate solution must be added to the sterile, nonpyrogenic high-purity Indium In 111 Chloride solution to buffer it prior to radiolabeling ProstaScint. The immunoscintigraphic agent Indium In 111 Capromab Pendetide (Indium In 111 ProstaScint) is formed after radiolabeling with Indium In 111. Physical characteristics of Indium In 111 Indium In 111 decay by electron capture with a physical half-life of 67.2 hours (2.8 days).

Product	Company	Date	Indication
ProstaScint® (indium In 111 capromab pendetide)	Cytogen Corp.	Oct 1996	Imaging agent for newly diagnosed patients with biopsy-proven prostate cancer

Product	Company	Application	FDA Approval Date	Description
Protropin® (somatrem)	Genentech, Inc.	Treatment of growth hormone deficiency in children	Oct 1985	Protropin® (somatrem for injection), is a polypeptide hormone produced by recombinant DNA technology. Protropin has 192 amino acid residues and a molecular weight of about 22,000 Da. The product contains the identical sequence of 191 amino acids constituting pituitary-derived human growth hormone plus an additional amino acid, methionine, on the N-terminus of the molecule. Protropin is synthesized in a special laboratory strain of *E. coli* bacteria that has been modified by the addition of the gene for human growth hormone production. Protropin is a highly purified preparation. Biological potency is determined using a cell proliferation bioassay. Protropin is a sterile, white, lyophilized powder intended for intramuscular or subcutaneous administration after reconstitution with bacteriostatic water for injection, USP (benzoyl alcohol preserved). Each 5 mg Protropin vial contains 5 mg (approximately 15 IU) somatrem, lyophilized with 40 mg mannitol, and 1.7 mg sodium phosphates (0.1 mg sodium phosphate monobasic and 1.6 mg sodium phosphate dibasic). Each 10 mg Protropin vial contains 10 mg (approximately 30 IU) somatrem, lyophilized with 80 mg mannitol, and 3.4 mg sodium phosphates (0.2 mg sodium phosphate monobasic, and 3.2 mg sodium phosphate dibasic). Phosphoric acid may be used for pH adjustment. Bacteriostatic water for injection, USP, is a sterile water containing 0.9% benzoyl alcohol per mL as an antimicrobial preservative packaged in a multidose vial. The diluent pH is 4.5 to 7.0. In 1985, the Food and Drug Administration approved Protropin as a replacement therapy for the long-term treatment of children with growth failure due to inadequate growth hormone (hGH or GH) secretion (GH deficiency). Protropin is a synthetic hormone produced by Genentech that is nearly identical to natural GH. Protropin will be phased out by the end of 2004 and replaced by Nutropin family of products (see above).
Pulmozyme® (dornase alfa)	Genentech, Inc.	Treatment of mild to moderate cystic fibrosis; Treatment of advanced cystic fibrosis; Pediatric use in infants 3 months to 2 years and children 2 to 4 years old	Dec 1993 Dec 1996 Mar 1998	Pulmozyme® (dornase alfa) inhalation solution is a sterile, clear, colorless, highly purified solution of recombinant human deoxyribonuclease I (rhDNase), an enzyme that selectively cleaves DNA. The protein is produced by genetically engineered Chinese hamster ovary (CHO) cells containing DNA encoding for the native human protein, deoxyribonuclease I (DNase). Fermentation is carried out in a nutrient medium containing the antibiotic gentamicin, 100 to 200 mg/L. However, the presence of the antibiotic is not detectable in the final product. The product is purified by tangential flow filtration and column chromatography. The purified glycoprotein contains 260 amino acids with an approximate molecular weight of 37,000 Da. The primary amino acid sequence is identical to that of the native human enzyme. Pulmozyme is administered by inhalation of an aerosol mist produced by a compressed air driven nebulizer system (see Clinical Experience; Dosage and Administration). Each Pulmozyme single-use ampule will deliver 2.5 mL of the solution to the nebulizer bowl. The aqueous solution contains 1.0 mg/mL dornase alfa, 0.15 mg/mL calcium chloride dihydrate and 8.77 mg/mL sodium chloride. The solution contains no preservative. The nominal pH of the solution is 6.3.

| Raptiva™ (Efalizumab; selective, reversible T-cell blocker [subcutaneous injection; self-administered]) | Xoma, Ltd. and Genentech, Inc. | Chronic moderate to severe plaque psoriasis in adults | Oct 2003 | Raptiva™ (efalizumab) is an immunosuppressive recombinant humanized IgG1 kappa isotype monoclonal antibody that binds to human CD11a. Efalizumab has a molecular weight of approximately 150 kDa and is produced in a Chinese hamster ovary mammalian cell expression system in a nutrient medium containing the antibiotic gentamicin. Gentamicin is not detectable in the final product. Raptiva is supplied as a sterile, white to off-white, lyophilized powder in single-use glass vials for subcutaneous (SC) injection. Reconstitution of the single-use vial with 1.3 mL of the supplied sterile water for injection (non-USP) yields approximately 1.5 mL of solution to deliver 125 mg per 1.25 mL (100 mg/mL) of Raptiva. The sterile water for injection supplied does not comply with USP requirement for pH. After reconstitution, Raptiva is a clear to pale yellow solution with a pH of approximately 6.2. Each single-use vial of Raptiva contains 150 mg of efalizumab, 123.2 mg of sucrose, 6.8 mg of L-histidine hydrochloride monohydrate, 4.3 mg of L-histidine, and 3 mg of polysorbate 20 and is designed to deliver 125 mg of efalizumab in 1.25 mL. |
| Rebetron™ (combination of ribavirin and alpha interferon) | Schering-Plough Corp. | Combination therapy for treatment of chronic hepatitis C in patients with compensated liver disease who have relapsed following alpha-interferon treatment; Treatment of chronic hepatitis C in patients with compensated liver disease previously untreated with alpha interferon therapy | Jun 1998 Dec 1998 | Rebetol® is Schering Corporation's brand name for ribavirin, a nucleoside analog with antiviral activity. The chemical name of ribavirin is 1-(beta)-D-ribofuranosyl-1H-1,2,4-triazole-3-carboxamide and has the following structural formula: $C_8H_{12}N_4O_5$; Ribavirin is a white, crystalline powder. It is freely soluble in water and slightly soluble in anhydrous alcohol. The molecular weight is 244. 21. Rebetol capsules consist of a white powder in a white, opaque, gelatin capsule. Each capsule contains 200 mg ribavirin and the inactive ingredients microcrystalline cellulose, lactose monohydrate, croscarmellose sodium, and magnesium stearate. The capsule shell consists of gelatin and titanium dioxide. The capsule is printed with edible blue pharmaceutical ink, which is made of shellac, anhydrous ethyl alcohol, isopropyl alcohol, n-butyl alcohol, propylene glycol, ammonium hydroxide, and FD&C; blue #2 aluminum lake. Intron A® is Schering Corporation's brand name for interferon alfa-2b, recombinant, a purified, sterile, recombinant interferon product. Interferon alfa-2b recombinant has been classified as an alpha interferon and is a water-soluble protein composed of 165 amino acids with a molecular weight of 19,271 Da produced by recombinant DNA techniques. It is obtained from the bacterial fermentation of a strain of *Escherichia coli* bearing a genetically engineered plasmid containing an interferon alfa-2b gene from human leukocytes. The fermentation is carried out in a defined nutrient medium containing the antibiotic tetracycline hydrochloride at a concentration of 5 to 10 mg/L; the presence of this antibiotic is not detectable in the final product. Intron A Injection is a clear, colorless solution. The 3 million IU vial of Intron A Injection contains 3 million IU of interferon alfa-2b, recombinant per 0.5 mL. The 18 million IU multidose vial of Intron A Injection contains a total of 22.8 million IU of interferon alfa-2b, recombinant per 3.8 mL (3 million IU/0.5 mL) in order to provide the delivery of six 0.5-mL doses, each containing 3 million IU of Intron A (for a label strength of 18 million IU). The 18 million IU Intron A Injection multidose pen contains a total of 22.5 million IU of interferon alfa-2b, recombinant per 1.5 mL (3 million IU/0.2 mL) in order to provide the delivery of six 0.2-mL doses, each containing 3 million IU of Intron A (for a label strength of 18 million IU). Each mL also contains 7.5 mg sodium |

Continued.

Product	Company	Application	FDA Approval Date	Description
				chloride, 1.8 mg sodium phosphate dibasic, 1.3 mg sodium phosphate monobasic, 0.1 mg edetate disodium, 0.1 mg polysorbate 80, and 1.5 mg m-cresol as a preservative. Based on the specific activity of approximately 2.6×10^8 IU/mg protein as measured by HPLC assay, the corresponding quantities of interferon alfa-2b, recombinant in the vials and pen described above are approximately 0.012 mg, 0.088 mg, and 0.087 mg protein, respectively. Mechanism of Action Ribavirin/Interferon alfa-2b, recombinant: The mechanism of inhibition of hepatitis C virus (HCV) RNA by combination therapy with Rebetol and Intron A has not been established.
Rebif® (interferon beta 1-a)	Serono S. A., and Pfizer, Inc.	Relapsing forms of multiple sclerosis	Mar 2002	Rebif® (interferon beta-1a) is a purified 166 amino acid glycoprotein with a molecular weight of approximately 22,500 Da. It is produced by recombinant DNA technology using genetically engineered Chinese hamster ovary cells into which the human interferon beta gene has been introduced. The amino acid sequence of Rebif is identical to that of natural fibroblast derived human interferon beta. Natural interferon beta and interferon beta-1a (Rebif) are glycosylated with each containing a single N-linked complex carbohydrate moiety. Using a reference standard calibrated against the World Health Organization natural interferon beta standard (Second International Standard for Interferon, Human Fibroblast GB 23 902 531), Rebif has a specific activity of approximately 270 million International Units (MIU) of antiviral activity per mg of interferon beta-1a determined specifically by an *in vitro* cytopathic effect bioassay using WISH cells and Vesicular Stomatitis virus. Rebif 44 mcg contains approximately 12 MIU of antiviral activity using this method. Rebif (interferon beta-1a) is formulated as a sterile solution in a prefilled syringe intended for subcutaneous (SC) injection. Each 0.5 ml (0.5 cc) of Rebif contains either 44 mcg or 22 mcg of interferon beta-1a, 4 or 2 mg albumin (human) USP, 27.3 mg mannitol USP, 0.4 mg sodium acetate, water for injection, USP.
Recombinate® rAHF (antihemophilic factor)	Baxter Healthcare Corp.	Blood-clotting factor VIII for the treatment of hemophilia A	Feb 1992	Recombinate®, Antihemophilic Factor (Recombinant) (rAHF) is a glycoprotein synthesized by a genetically engineered Chinese hamster ovary (CHO) cell line. In culture, the CHO cell line secretes recombinant antihemophilic factor (rAHF) into the cell culture medium. The rAHF is purified from the culture medium utilizing a series of chromatography columns. A key step in the purification process is an immunoaffinity chromatography methodology in which a purification matrix, prepared by immobilization of a monoclonal antibody directed to factor VIII, is utilized to selectively isolate the rAHF in the medium. The synthesized rAHF produced by the CHO cells has the same biological effects as antihemophilic factor (human) [AHF (Human)]. Structurally the protein has a similar combination of heterogenous heavy and light chains as found in AHF (Human). Recombinate rAHF is formulated as a sterile, nonpyrogenic, off-white to faint yellow, lyophilized powder preparation of concentrated recombinant AHF for intravenous injection. Recombinate rAHF is available in single-dose bottles, which contain nominally 250, 500, and 1000 International Units (IU) per bottle. When reconstituted with the appropriate volume of diluent, the product contains the following stabilizers in maximum

amounts: 12.5 mg/mL albumin (human), 0.20 mg/mL calcium, 1.5 mg/mL polyethylene glycol (3350), 180 mEq/L sodium, 55 mM histidine, 1.5 μg/AHF IU polysorbate-80. Von Willebrand Factor (vWF) is coexpressed with the antihemophilic factor (recombinant) and helps to stabilize it. The final product contains not more than 2 ng vWF/IU rAHF, which will not have any clinically relevant effect in patients with von Willebrand disease. The product contains no preservative. Manufacturing of recombinate rAHF is shared by Baxter Healthcare Corporation, Hyland Immuno and Genetics Institute, Inc. The recombinant Antihemophilic Factor Concentrate (For Further Manufacturing Use). is produced by Baxter Healthcare Corporation. Hyland Immuno and Genetics Institute (For Further Manufacturing Use) and subsequently formulated and packaged at Baxter Healthcare Corporation. Hyland Immuno. Each bottle of recombinate rAHF is labeled with the AHF activity expressed in IU per bottle. Biological potency is determined by an *in vitro* assay, which is referenced to the World Health Organization (WHO) International Standard for Factor VIII:C Concentrate.

Recombivax HB® hepatitis B vaccine (recombinant) is a noninfectious subunit viral vaccine derived from hepatitis B surface antigen (HBsAg) produced in yeast cells. A portion of the hepatitis B virus gene, coding for HBsAg, is cloned into yeast, and the vaccine for hepatitis B is produced from cultures of this recombinant yeast strain according to methods developed in the Merck Research Laboratories. The antigen is harvested and purified from fermentation cultures of a recombinant strain of the yeast *Saccharomyces cerevisiae* containing the gene for the *adw* subtype of HBsAg. The HBsAg protein is released from the yeast cells by cell disruption and purified by a series of physical and chemical methods. The vaccine contains no detectable yeast DNA but may contain not more than 1% yeast protein. The vaccine produced by the Merck method has been shown to be comparable to the plasma-derived vaccine in terms of animal potency (mouse, monkey, and chimpanzee) and protective efficacy (chimpanzee and human). The vaccine against hepatitis B, prepared from recombinant yeast cultures, is free of association with human blood or blood products. Each lot of hepatitis B vaccine is tested for safety, in mice and guinea pigs, and for sterility. Recombivax HB is a sterile suspension for intramuscular injection. However, for persons at risk of hemorrhage following intramuscular injection, the vaccine may be administered subcutaneously. Recombivax HB hepatitis B vaccine (recombinant) is supplied in three formulations. Pediatric/Adolescent Formulation (With and Without Preservative), 10 mcg/mL: each 0.5 mL dose contains 5 mcg of hepatitis B surface antigen. Adult Formulation, 10 mcg/mL: each 1 mL dose contains 10 mcg of hepatitis B surface antigen. Dialysis Formulation, 40 mcg/mL: each 1 mL dose contains 40 mcg of hepatitis B surface antigen. Formulations that contain a preservative include thimerosal, a mercury derivative, at 1:20,000 or 50 mcg/mL. All formulations have been treated with formaldehyde prior to adsorption onto aluminum hydroxide. In each formulation, hepatitis B surface antigen is adsorbed onto approximately 0.5 mg of aluminum (provided as aluminum hydroxide) per mL of vaccine. The vaccine is of the *adw* subtype. Recombivax HB is indicated for vaccination of persons at risk of infection

Continued.

Recombivax-
HB®Recombivax HB
Dialysis Formulation
(hepatitis B vaccine)

Merck & Company, Inc.

Vaccination against hepatitis
B; hepatitis B vaccine for
adolescents and high-risk
infants; adults; dialysis;
pediatrics

Jul 1986
Jan 1987
Jan 1989
Jun 1993

Product	Company	Application	FDA Approval Date	Description
				from hepatitis B virus including all known subtypes. Recombivax HB dialysis formulation is indicated for vaccination of adult predialysis and dialysis patients against infection caused by all known subtypes of hepatitis B virus.
ReFacto® (antihemophilic factor)	Wyeth	Control and prevention of hemophilia A and short-term prophylaxis to reduce bleeding episodes	Mar 2000	ReFacto® antihemophilic factor (recombinant) is a purified protein produced by recombinant DNA technology for use in therapy of factor VIII deficiency. ReFacto is a glycoprotein with an approximate molecular mass of 170 kDa consisting of 1438 amino acids. It has an amino acid sequence that is comparable to the 90 + 80 kDa form of factor VIII, and posttranslational modifications that are similar to those of the plasma-derived molecule. ReFacto has *in vitro* functional characteristics comparable to those of endogenous factor VIII. ReFacto is produced by a genetically engineered Chinese hamster ovary (CHO) cell line. The CHO cell line secretes B-domain deleted recombinant factor VIII into a defined cell culture medium that contains human serum albumin and recombinant insulin, but does not contain any proteins derived from animal sources. The protein is purified by a chromatography purification process that yields a high-purity, active product. The potency expressed in International Units (IU) is determined using the European Pharmacopoeial chromogenic assay against the WHO standard. The specific activity of ReFacto is 11,200 to 15,500 IU per milligram of protein. ReFacto is not purified from human blood and contains no preservatives or added human components in the final formulation. ReFacto is formulated as a sterile, nonpyrogenic, lyophilized powder preparation for intravenous (IV) injection. It is available in single-use vials containing the labeled amount of factor VIII activity (IU). Each vial contains nominally 250, 500, or 1000 IU of ReFacto per vial. The formulated product is a clear colorless solution upon reconstitution and contains sodium chloride, sucrose, L-histidine, calcium chloride, and polysorbate 80.
Refludan® (lepirudin)	Berlex Laboratories	For anticoagulation in patients with heparin-induced thrombocytopenia and associated thromboembolic disease in order to prevent further thromboembolic complications	Mar 1998	Refludan® [lepirudin (rDNA) for injection] is a highly specific direct inhibitor of thrombin. Lepirudin (chemical designation: [Leu¹, Thr²]-63-desulfohirudin) is a recombinant hirudin derived from yeast cells. The polypeptide composed of 65 amino acids has a molecular weight of 6979.5 Da. Natural hirudin is produced in trace amounts as a family of highly homologous isopolypeptides by the leech *Hirudo medicinalis*. The biosynthetic molecule (lepirudin) is identical to natural hirudin except for substitution of leucine for isoleucine at the N-terminal end of the molecule and the absence of a sulfate group on the tyrosine at position 63. The activity of lepirudin is measured in a chromogenic assay. One antithrombin unit (ATU) is the amount of lepirudin that neutralizes one unit of World Health Organization preparation 89/588 of thrombin. The specific activity of lepirudin is approximately 16,000 ATU/mg. Its mode of action is independent of antithrombin III. Platelet factor 4 does not inhibit lepirudin. One molecule of lepirudin binds to one molecule of thrombin and thereby blocks the thrombogenic activity of thrombin. As a result, all thrombin-dependent coagulation assays are affected, e.g., activated partial thromboplastin time (aPTT) values increase in a dose-dependent fashion. Refludan is

		supplied as a sterile, white, freeze-dried powder for injection or infusion and is freely soluble in sterile water for injection USP or 0.9% sodium chloride injection USP. Each vial of Refludan contains 50 mg lepirudin. Other ingredients are 40 mg mannitol and sodium hydroxide for adjustment of pH to approximately 7.	
Regranex® Gel (gel becaplermin)	Ortho-McNeil and Chiron Corp.	Platelet-derived growth factor for treatment of diabetic foot ulcers	Dec 1997
		Regranex® Gel contains becaplermin, a recombinant human platelet-derived growth factor (rhPDGF-BB) for topical administration. Becaplermin is produced by recombinant DNA technology by insertion of the gene for the B chain of platelet-derived growth factor (PDGF) into the yeast, *Saccharomyces cerevisiae*. Becaplermin has a molecular weight of approximately 25 kDa and is a homodimer composed of two identical polypeptide chains that are bound together by disulfide bonds. Becaplermin Concentrate is produced by Chiron Corp. and supplied to OMJ Pharmaceuticals under a shared manufacturing arrangement. Regranex Gel is a nonsterile, low bioburden, preserved, sodium carboxymethylcellulose-based (CMC) topical gel, containing the active ingredient becaplermin and the following inactive ingredients: sodium chloride, sodium acetate trihydrate, glacial acetic acid, water for injection, and methylparaben, propylparaben, and m-cresol as preservatives and l-lysine hydrochloride as a stabilizer. Each gram of Regranex Gel contains 100 µg of becaplermin.	
Remicade® (infliximab; recombinantly produced, chimeric monoclonal antibody)	Centocor, Inc. (subsidiary of Johnson & Johnson)	Short-term management of moderately to severely active Crohn's disease including those patients with fistulae; Treatment of patients with rheumatoid arthritis who have had inadequate response to methotrexate alone; Improving physical function in patients with moderately to severely active rheumatoid arthritis who have had an inadequate response to methotrexate; Reducing signs and symptoms, and inducing and maintaining clinical remission in patients with moderately to severely active Crohn's disease who have had an inadequate response to conventional therapy;	Aug 1998 Nov 1999 Feb 2002 Jun 2002 Apr 2003
		Remicade® (infliximab) is a chimeric IgG1k monoclonal antibody with an approximate molecular weight of 149,100 Da. It is composed of human constant and murine variable regions. Infliximab binds specifically to human tumor necrosis factor alpha (TNF(alpha)) with an association constant of $10^{10}\ M^{-1}$. Infliximab is produced by a recombinant cell line cultured by continuous perfusion and is purified by a series of steps that includes measures to inactivate and remove viruses. Remicade is supplied as a sterile, white, lyophilized powder for intravenous infusion. Following reconstitution with 10 mL of sterile water for injection, USP, the resulting pH is approximately 7.2. Each single-use vial contains 100 mg infliximab, 500 mg sucrose, 0.5 mg polysorbate 80, 2.2 mg monobasic sodium phosphate, monohydrate, and 6.1 mg dibasic sodium phosphate, dihydrate. No preservatives are present.	

Continued.

Product	Company	Application	FDA Approval Date	Description
ReoPro™ (abciximab)	Centocor, Inc. (subsidiary of Johnson & Johnson) and Eli Lilly and Company	Reduction of draining enterocutaneous and rectovaginal fistulas and for maintaining fistula closure in patients with fistulizing Crohn's disease Reduction of acute blood clot-related complications for high-risk angioplasty patients; Reduction of acute blood clot complications for all patients undergoing any coronary intervention; treatment of unstable angina not responding to conventional medical therapy when percutaneous coronary intervention is planned within 24 hours	Dec 1994 Dec 1997	Abciximab, ReoPro®, is the Fab fragment of the chimeric human-murine monoclonal antibody 7E3. Abciximab binds to the glycoprotein (GP) IIb/IIIa receptor of human platelets and inhibits platelet aggregation. Abciximab also binds to the vitronectin ((alpha)$_v$beta$_3$) receptor found on platelets and vessel wall endothelial and smooth muscle cells. The chimeric 7E3 antibody is produced by continuous perfusion in mammalian cell culture. The 47,615 Da Fab fragment is purified from cell culture supernatant by a series of steps involving specific viral inactivation and removal procedures, digestion with papain and column chromatography. ReoPro is a clear, colorless, sterile, nonpyrogenic solution for intravenous (IV) use. Each single use vial contains 2 mg/mL of abciximab in a buffered solution (pH 7.2) of 0.01 M sodium phosphate, 0.15 M sodium chloride, and 0.001% polysorbate 80 in water for injection. No preservatives are added.
Retavase™ (reteplase)	Centocor, Inc. (subsidiary of Johnson & Johnson)	Management of acute myocardial infarction in adults	Oct 1996	Retavase® (Reteplase) is a nonglycosylated deletion mutein of tissue plasminogen activator (tPA), containing the kringle 2 and the protease domains of human tPA. Retavase contains 355 of the 527 amino acids of native tPA (amino acids 1-3 and 176-527). Retavase is produced by recombinant DNA technology in *E. coli*. The protein is isolated as inactive inclusion bodies from *E. coli*, converted into its active form by an *in vitro* folding process, and purified by chromatographic separation. The molecular weight of Reteplase is 39,571 Da. Potency is expressed in units (U) using a reference standard specific for Retavase and is not comparable with units used for other thrombolytic agents. Retavase is a sterile, white, lyophilized powder for intravenous bolus injection after reconstitution with sterile water for injection, USP (without preservatives). Following reconstitution, the pH is 6.0 ± 0.3. Retavase is supplied as a 10.4 unit vial to ensure sufficient drug for administration of each 10 unit injection. Each single-use vial contains: Reteplase 18.1 mg Tranexamic Acid 8.32 mg Dipotassium Hydrogen Phosphate 136.24 mg Phosphoric Acid 51.27 mg Sucrose 364.0 mg Polysorbate 80 5.20 mg

Product	Manufacturer	Indication	Date	Description
Rituxan™ (rituximab)	IDEC Pharmaceuticals Corp. and Genentech, Inc.	Treatment of relapsed or refractory low-grade or follicular, CD20-positive B-cell non-Hodgkin's lymphoma	Nov 1997	The Rituxan™ (Rituximab) antibody is a genetically engineered chimeric murine/human monoclonal antibody directed against the CD20 antigen found on the surface of normal and malignant B lymphocytes. The antibody is an IgG_1 kappa immunoglobulin containing murine light- and heavy-chain variable region sequences and human constant region sequences. Rituximab is composed of two heavy chains of 451 amino acids and two light chains of 213 amino acids (based on cDNA analysis) and has an approximate molecular weight of 145 kDa. Rituximab has a binding affinity for the CD20 antigen of approximately 8.0 nM. The chimeric anti-CD20 antibody is produced by mammalian cell (Chinese hamster ovary) suspension culture in a nutrient medium containing the antibiotic gentamicin. Gentamicin is not detectable in the final product. The anti-CD20 antibody is purified by affinity and ion exchange chromatography. The purification process includes specific viral inactivation and removal procedures. Rituximab drug product is manufactured from either bulk drug substance manufactured by Genentech, Inc. (U.S. License No. 1048), or utilizing formulated bulk Rituximab supplied by IDEC Pharmaceuticals Corporation (U.S. License No. 1235) under a shared manufacturing arrangement. Rituxan is a sterile, clear, colorless, preservative-free liquid concentrate for IV administration. Rituxan is supplied at a concentration of 10 mg/mL in either 100 mg (10 mL) or 500 mg (50 mL) single-use vials. The product is formulated for IV administration in 9.0 mg/mL sodium chloride, 7.35 mg/mL sodium citrate dihydrate, 0.7 mg/mL polysorbate 80, and sterile water for injection. The pH is adjusted to 6.5.
Roferon-A® (interferon alfa-2a)	Hoffmann-La Roche, Inc.	Treatment of hairy cell leukemia; AIDS-related Kaposi's sarcoma; Chronic phase Philadelphia chromosome positive chronic myelogenous leukemia; Hepatitis C	Jun 1986 Nov 1988 Oct 1995 Nov 1995	Roferon-A® (Interferon alfa-2a, recombinant) is a sterile protein product for use by injection. Roferon-A is manufactured by recombinant DNA technology that employs a genetically engineered *Escherichia coli* bacterium containing DNA that codes for the human protein. Interferon alfa-2a, recombinant is a highly purified protein containing 165 amino acids, and it has an approximate molecular weight of 19,000 Da. Fermentation is carried out in a defined nutrient medium containing the antibiotic tetracycline hydrochloride, 5 mg/L. However, the presence of the antibiotic is not detectable in the final product. Roferon-A is supplied as an injectable solution in a vial or a prefilled syringe. Each glass syringe barrel contains 0.5 mL of product. In addition, there is a needle which is .5 inch in length. Single Use Injectable Solution: 3 million IU (11.1 mcg/mL) Roferon-A per vial — The solution is colorless and each mL contains 3 MIU of interferon alfa-2a, recombinant, 7.21 mg sodium chloride, 0.2 mg polysorbate 80, 10 mg benzoyl alcohol as a preservative, and 0.77 mg ammonium acetate. 6 million IU (22.2 mcg/mL) Roferon-A per vial — The solution is colorless and each mL contains 6 MIU of interferon alfa-2a, recombinant, 7.21 mg sodium chloride, 0.2 mg polysorbate 80, 10 mg benzoyl alcohol as a preservative, and 0.77 mg ammonium acetate. 9 million IU (33.3 mcg/0.9 mL) Roferon-A per vial — The solution is colorless and each 0.9 mL contains 9 MIU of interferon alfa-2a, recombinant, 6.49 mg sodium chloride, 0.18 mg polysorbate 80, 9 mg benzoyl alcohol as a preservative, and 0.69 mg ammonium acetate. For single dose administration, withdraw 0.9 mL using a 1 mL syringe. Also can be used as a multidose vial. 36 million IU (133.3 mcg/mL) Roferon-A per vial — The solution is colorless and each mL contains 36 MIU of interferon alfa-2a, recombinant, 7.21 mg

Continued.

Product	Company	Application	FDA Approval Date	Description
				sodium chloride, 0.2 mg polysorbate 80, 10 mg benzoyl alcohol as a preservative, and 0.77 mg ammonium acetate. Single Use Prefilled Syringes: 3 million IU (11.1 mcg/0.5 mL) Roferon-A per syringe — The solution is colorless and each 0.5 mL contains 3 MIU of interferon alfa-2a, recombinant, 3.605 mg sodium chloride, 0.1 mg polysorbate 80, 5 mg benzoyl alcohol as a preservative, and 0.385 mg ammonium acetate. 6 million IU (22.2 mcg/0.5 mL) Roferon-A per syringe — The solution is colorless and each 0.5 mL contains 6 MIU of interferon alfa-2a, recombinant, 3.605 mg sodium chloride, 0.1 mg polysorbate 80, 5 mg benzoyl alcohol as a preservative, and 0.385 mg ammonium acetate. 9 million IU (33.3 mcg/0.5 mL) Roferon-A per syringe — The solution is colorless and each 0.5 mL contains 9 MIU of interferon alfa-2a, recombinant, 3.605 mg sodium chloride, 0.1 mg polysorbate 80, 5 mg benzoyl alcohol as a preservative, and 0.385 mg ammonium acetate. Multidose Injectable Solution: 9 million IU (33.3 mcg/0.9 mL) Roferon-A per vial — The solution is colorless and each 0.9 mL contains 9 MIU of interferon alfa-2a, recombinant, 6.49 mg sodium chloride, 0.18 mg polysorbate 80, 9 mg benzoyl alcohol as a preservative, and 0.69 mg ammonium acetate. Also can be used as a single use vial. 18 million IU (66.7 mcg/3 mL) Roferon-A per vial — The solution is colorless and each mL contains 6 MIU of interferon alfa-2a, recombinant, 7.21 mg sodium chloride, 0.2 mg polysorbate 80, 10 mg benzoyl alcohol as a preservative, and 0.77 mg ammonium acetate. Each 0.5 mL contains 3 MIU of interferon alfa-2a, recombinant. Based on the specific activity of 2.7×10^8 IU/mg protein, the corresponding quantities of interferon alfa-2a, recombinant in the vials described above are approximately 3 MIU (11.1 mcg/mL), 6 MIU (22.2 mcg/mL), 9 MIU (33.3 mcg/0.9 mL), 18 MIU (66.7 mcg/3 mL), and 36 MIU (133.3 mcg/mL). The route of administration for the vial is subcutaneous or intramuscular; the route of administration for the prefilled syringe is subcutaneous only.
Saizen® (human growth hormone)	Serono S. A.	Treatment of growth hormone deficiency in children	Oct 1996	Saizen® [somatropin (rDNA origin) for injection] is a human growth hormone produced by recombinant DNA technology. Saizen has 191 amino acid residues and a molecular weight of 22,125 Da. Its amino acid sequence and structure are identical to the dominant form of human pituitary growth hormone. Saizen is produced by a mammalian cell line (mouse C127) that has been modified by the addition of the human growth hormone gene. Saizen, with the correct three-dimensional configuration, is secreted directly through the cell membrane into the cell-culture medium for collection and purification. Saizen is a highly purified preparation. Biological potency is determined by measuring the increase in body weight induced in hypophysectomized rats. Saizen is a sterile, nonpyrogenic, white, lyophilized powder intended for subcutaneous or intramuscular injection after reconstitution with bacteriostatic water for injection, USP (0. 9% benzoyl alcohol). The reconstituted solution has a pH of 6.5 to 8.5. Saizen is available in 5 mg and 8.8 mg vials. The quantitative composition per vial is 5 mg (approximately 15 IU) vial. Each vial

Product	Description	Manufacturer	Indication	Date
Serostim®	contains 5.0 mg somatropin (approximately 15 IU), 34.2 mg sucrose, and 1.165 mg O-phosphoric acid. The pH is adjusted with sodium hydroxide or O-phosphoric acid. Each vial contains 8.8 mg somatropin (approximately 26.4 IU), 60.2 mg sucrose and 2.05 mg O-phosphoric acid. The pH is adjusted with sodium hydroxide or O-phosphoric acid. The diluent is bacteriostatic water for injection, USP containing 0.9% benzoyl alcohol added as an antimicrobial preservative. Serostim® [somatropin (rDNA origin) for injection] is a human growth hormone produced by recombinant DNA technology. Serostim has 191 amino acid residues and a molecular weight of 22,125 Da. Its amino acid sequence and structure are identical to the dominant form of human pituitary growth hormone. Serostim is produced by a mammalian cell line (mouse C127) that has been modified by the addition of the human growth hormone gene. Serostim is secreted directly through the cell membrane into the cell-culture medium for collection and purification. Serostim is a highly purified preparation. Biological potency is determined by measuring the increase in the body weight induced in hypophysectomized rats. Serostim is available in 4 mg, 5 mg, and 6 mg vials for single dose administration. Serostim is also available in 8.8 mg vials for multidose administration. Each 4 mg vial contains 4.0 mg (approximately 12 IU) somatropin, 27.3 mg sucrose, 0.9 mg phosphoric acid. Each 5 mg vial contains 5.0 mg (approximately 15 IU) somatropin, 34.2 mg sucrose, 1.2 mg phosphoric acid. Each 6 mg vial contains 6.0 mg (approximately 18 IU) somatropin, 41.0 mg sucrose, 1.4 mg phosphoric acid. Each 8.8 mg vial contains 8.8 mg (approximately 26. 4 IU) somatropin, 60.19 mg sucrose, 2.05 mg phosphoric acid. The pH is adjusted with sodium hydroxide or phosphoric acid to give a pH of 7.4 to 8.5 after reconstitution.			
Simulect® (basiliximab)	Simulect® (basiliximab) is a chimeric (murine/human) monoclonal antibody (IgG 1) produced by recombinant DNA technology, that functions as an immunosuppressive agent, specifically binding to and blocking the interleukin-2 receptor (alpha)-chain (IL-2R(alpha), also known as CD25 antigen) on the surface of activated T-lymphocytes. Based on the amino acid sequence, the calculated molecular weight of the protein is 144 kDa. It is a glycoprotein obtained from fermentation of an established mouse myeloma cell line genetically engineered to express plasmids containing the human heavy and light chain constant region genes and mouse heavy and light chain variable region genes encoding the RFT5 antibody that binds selectively to the IL-2R(alpha). The active ingredient, basiliximab, is water soluble. The drug product, Simulect, is a sterile lyophilisate, which is available in 6 mL colorless glass vials. Each vial contains 20 mg basiliximab, 7.21 mg monobasic potassium phosphate, 0.99 mg disodium hydrogen phosphate (anhydrous), 1.61 mg sodium chloride, 20 mg sucrose, 80 mg mannitol, and 40 mg glycine, to be reconstituted in 5 mL. of sterile water for injection, USP. No preservatives are added.	Novartis Pharmaceutical Corp.	Prevention of acute rejection episodes in kidney transplant recipients; Prevention of rejection in combination with triple immunosuppressive therapy in renal transplant; use in pediatric renal transplant; and use of IV bolus injection	May 1998 Mar 2001

Product	Company	Application	FDA Approval Date	Description
Somavert® (Pegvisomant; pegylated version of a recombinant human growth hormone analog structurally altered to act as a GH receptor antagonist)	Nektar Therapeutics and Pfizer, Inc.	Acromegaly	Mar 2003	Somavert® contains pegvisomant for injection, an analog of human growth hormone (GH) that has been structurally altered to act as a GH receptor antagonist. Pegvisomant is a protein of recombinant DNA origin containing 191 amino acid residues to which several polyethylene glycol (PEG) polymers are covalently bound (predominantly 4 to 6 PEG/protein molecule). The molecular weight of the protein of pegvisomant is 21,998 Da. The molecular weight of the PEG portion of pegvisomant is approximately 5000 Da. The predominant molecular weights of pegvisomant are thus approximately 42,000, 47,000, and 52,000 Da. The schematic shows the amino acid sequence of the pegvisomant protein (PEG polymers are shown attached to the 5 most probable attachment sites). Pegvisomant is synthesized by a specific strain of *Escherichia coli* bacteria that has been genetically modified by the addition of a plasmid that carries a gene for GH receptor antagonist. Biological potency is determined using a cell proliferation bioassay. Somavert is supplied as a sterile, white lyophilized powder intended for subcutaneous injection after reconstitution with 1 mL of sterile water for injection, USP. Somavert is available in single-dose sterile vials containing 10, 15, or 20 mg of pegvisomant protein (approximately 10, 15, and 20 U activity, respectively). Vials containing 10, 15, and 20 mg of pegvisomant protein correspond to approximately 21, 32, and 43 mg pegvisomant, respectively. Each vial also contains 1.36 mg of glycine, 36.0 mg of mannitol, 1.04 mg of sodium phosphate dibasic anhydrous, and 0.36 mg of sodium phosphate monobasic monohydrate. Somavert is supplied in packages that include a plastic vial containing diluent. Sterile water for injection, USP, is a nonpyrogenic preparation of water for injection that contains no bacteriostat, antimicrobial agent, or added buffer, and is supplied in single-dose containers to be used as a diluent.
Synagis™ (Palivizumab; recombinantly produced, humanized monoclonal antibody)	MedImmune, Inc.	Prevention of serious lower respiratory tract disease caused by respiratory syncytial virus (RSV) in pediatric patients at high risk of RSV disease; FDA cleared addition of new safety and efficacy data supporting the drug's use in young children with hemodynamically significant congenital heart disease	Jun 1998 Sep 2003	Synagis® (palivizumab) is a humanized monoclonal antibody (IgG1) produced by recombinant DNA technology, directed to an epitope in the A antigenic site of the F protein of respiratory syncytial virus (RSV). Palivizumab is a composite of human (95%) and murine (5%) antibody sequences. The human heavy chain sequence was derived from the constant domains of human IgG1 and the variable framework regions of the V H genes Cor and Cess. The human light chain sequence was derived from the constant domain of C and the variable framework regions of the V L gene K104 with J-4. The murine sequences were derived from a murine monoclonal antibody, Mab 1129, in a process which involved the grafting of the murine complementarity determining regions into the human antibody frameworks. Synagis is composed of two heavy chains and two light chains and has a molecular weight of approximately 148,000 Da. Synagis is supplied as a sterile lyophilized product for reconstitution with sterile water for injection. Reconstituted Synagis is to be administered by intramuscular injection only. Upon reconstitution, Synagis contains the following excipients: 47 mM histidine, 3.0 mM glycine, and 5.6% mannitol and the active ingredient, palivizumab, at a concentration of 100 mg/mL solution. The reconstituted solution should appear clear or slightly opalescent.

Product	Manufacturer	Indication	Date	Description
Thyrogen® (thyrotropin alfa)	Genzyme	Adjunctive diagnostic tool for serum thyroglobulin (Tg) testing with or without radioiodine imaging in the follow-up of patients with thyroid cancer	Dec 1998	Thyrogen® (thyrotropin alfa for injection) contains a highly purified recombinant form of human thyroid stimulating hormone (TSH), a glycoprotein that is produced by recombinant DNA technology. Thyrotropin alfa is synthesized in a genetically modified Chinese hamster ovary cell line. Thyrotropin alfa is a heterodimeric glycoprotein comprised of two noncovalently linked subunits, an alpha subunit of 92 amino acid residues containing two N-linked glycosylation sites and a beta subunit of 118 residues containing one N-linked glycosylation site. The amino acid sequence of thyrotropin alfa is identical to that of human pituitary thyroid stimulating hormone. Both thyrotropin alfa and naturally occurring human pituitary thyroid stimulating hormone are synthesized as a mixture of glycosylation variants. Unlike pituitary TSH, which is secreted as a mixture of sialylated and sulfated forms, thyrotropin alfa is sialylated but not sulfated. The biological activity of thyrotropin alfa is determined using both an *in vivo* bioassay and an *in vitro* bioassay. The *in vivo* bioassay measures an increase in thyroxine (T_4) level in response to the intraperitoneal injection of thyrotropin alfa after suppression of endogenous TSH levels in mice. The *in vitro* assay measures the amount of cAMP produced by a bovine thyroid-derived microsome preparation in response to thyrotropin alfa. The specific activity of thyrotropin alfa is calibrated against the World Health Organization (WHO) human pituitary derived TSH reference standard, NIBSC 84/703. The biological activity of thyrotropin alfa has been determined to be no less than 4 IU/mg by the *in vitro* bioassay. Thyrogen is supplied as a sterile, nonpyrogenic, white to off-white lyophilized product, intended for intramuscular (IM) administration after reconstitution with sterile water for injection, USP. Each vial of Thyrogen contains 1.1 mg thyrotropin alfa ($\geq$ 4 IU), 36 mg mannitol, 5.1 mg sodium phosphate, and 2.4 mg sodium chloride. After reconstitution with 1.2 mL of sterile water for injection, USP, the thyrotropin alfa concentration is 0.9 mg/mL. The pH of the reconstituted solution is approximately 7.0.
TNKase™ (tenecteplase)	Genentech, Inc.	Treatment of acute myocardial infarction	Jun 2000	Tenecteplase is a tissue plasminogen activator (tPA) produced by recombinant DNA technology using an established mammalian cell line (Chinese hamster ovary cells). Tenecteplase is a 527 amino acid glycoprotein developed by introducing the following modifications to the complementary DNA (cDNA) for natural human tPA: a substitution of threonine 103 with asparagine, and a substitution of asparagine 117 with glutamine, both within the kringle 1 domain, and a tetra-alanine substitution at amino acids 296 to 299 in the protease domain. Cell culture is carried out in nutrient medium containing the antibiotic gentamicin (65 mg/L). However, the presence of the antibiotic is not detectable in the final product (limit of detection is 0.67 μg/vial). TNKase™ is a sterile, white to off-white, lyophilized powder for single intravenous (IV) bolus administration after reconstitution with sterile water for injection, USP. Each vial of TNKase nominally contains 52.5 mg tenecteplase, 0.55 g L-arginine, 0.17 g phosphoric acid, and 4.3 mg polysorbate 20, which includes a 5% overfill. Each vial will deliver 50 mg of tenecteplase.

Product	Company	Application	FDA Approval Date	Description
Twinrix® (hepatitis A inactivated and hepatitis B [recombinant] vaccine)	SmithKline Beecham Biologicals (unit of GlaxoSmithKline)	Immunization against hepatitis A and B viruses	May 2001	Twinrix® [Hepatitis A Inactivated and Hepatitis B (Recombinant) Vaccine] is a sterile bivalent vaccine containing the antigenic components used in producing Havrix® (Hepatitis A Vaccine, Inactivated) and Engerix-B® [Hepatitis B Vaccine (Recombinant)]. Twinrix is a sterile suspension of inactivated hepatitis A virus (strain HM175) propagated in MRC-5 cells and combined with purified surface antigen of the hepatitis B virus. The purified hepatitis B surface antigen (HBsAg) is obtained by culturing genetically engineered *Saccharomyces cerevisiae* cells, which carry the surface antigen gene of the hepatitis B virus, in synthetic media containing inorganic salts, amino acids, dextrose, and vitamins. Bulk preparations of each antigen are adsorbed separately onto aluminum salts and then pooled during formulation. A 1.0 mL dose of vaccine contains not less than 720 ELISA Units of inactivated hepatitis A virus and 20 mcg of recombinant HBsAg protein. One dose of vaccine also contains 0.45 mg of aluminum in the form of aluminum phosphate and aluminum hydroxide as adjuvants, amino acids, 5.0 mg 2-phenoxyethanol as a preservative, sodium chloride, phosphate buffer, polysorbate 20, water for injection, traces of formalin (not more than 0.1 mg), a trace amount of thimerosal (< 1 mcg mercury) from the manufacturing process, and residual MRC-5 cellular proteins (not more than 2.5 mcg). Neomycin sulfate, an aminoglycoside antibiotic, is included in the cell growth media; only trace amounts (not more than 20 ng/dose) remain following purification. The manufacturing procedures used to manufacture Twinrix result in a product that contains no more than 5% yeast protein. Twinrix [Hepatitis A Inactivated and Hepatitis B (Recombinant) Vaccine] is supplied as a sterile suspension for intramuscular administration. The vaccine must be shaken before administration to ensure a uniform suspension. After shaking, the vaccine is a homogenous white turbid suspension.
Velosulin® BR (insulin; buffered formulation)	Novo Nordisk	Diabetes	Jul 1999	Velosulin® BR is a clear solution of insulin in a phosphate buffer. The concentration of this product is 100 U/mL insulin. This human insulin is structurally identical to the insulin produced by the pancreas in the human body. This structural identity is obtained by recombinant-DNA technology utilizing *Saccharomyces cerevisiae* (bakers yeast) as the production organism. When a U-100 insulin syringe is used to deliver the insulin, the effect of Velosulin BR begins approximately .5 hour after the injection. The effect lasts up to approximately 8 hours with a maximal effect between the 1st and 3rd hour. The time course of action of any insulin may vary considerably in different individuals, or at different times in the same individual, or when using an external insulin infusion pump to deliver the insulin. Because of this variation, the time periods listed here should be considered as general guidelines only when using U-100 insulin syringes to deliver the insulin.

Product	Company	Indication	Date	Description
Xigris™ (drotrecogin alfa)	Eli Lilly and Company	Severe, life-threatening sepsis	Nov 2001	Xigris™ (drotrecogin alfa (activated)) is a recombinant form of human activated protein C. An established human cell line possessing the complementary DNA for the inactive human protein C zymogen secretes the protein into the fermentation medium. Fermentation is carried out in a nutrient medium containing the antibiotic geneticin sulfate. Geneticin sulfate is not detectable in the final product. Human protein C is enzymatically activated by cleavage with thrombin and subsequently purified. Drotrecogin alfa (activated) is a serine protease with the same amino acid sequence as human plasma-derived activated protein C. Drotrecogin alfa (activated) is a glycoprotein of approximately 55 kDa molecular weight, consisting of a heavy chain and a light chain linked by a disulfide bond. Drotrecogin alfa (activated) and human plasma-derived activated protein C have the same sites of glycosylation, although some differences in the glycosylation structures exist. Xigris is supplied as a sterile, lyophilized, white to off-white powder for intravenous infusion. The 5 and 20 mg vials of Xigris contain 5.3 mg and 20.8 mg of drotrecogin alfa (activated), respectively. The 5 and 20 mg vials of Xigris also contain 40.3 and 158.1 mg of sodium chloride, 10.9 and 42.9 mg of sodium citrate, and 31.8 and 124.9 mg of sucrose, respectively.
Xolair® (Omalizumab; recombinant DNA-derived humanized monoclonal antibody targeting immunoglobulin-E [subcutaneous])	Genentech, Tanox, Inc. and Novartis Pharmaceuticals	Moderate to severe persistent asthma in adults and adolescents	Jun 2003	Xolair® (Omalizumab) is a recombinant DNA-derived humanized IgG1_ monoclonal antibody that selectively binds to human immunoglobulin E (IgE). The antibody has a molecular weight of approximately 149 kDa. Xolair is produced by a Chinese hamster ovary cell suspension culture in a nutrient medium containing the antibiotic gentamicin. Gentamicin is not detectable in the final product. Xolair is a sterile, white, preservative-free, lyophilized powder contained in a single-use vial that is reconstituted with sterile water for injection (SWFI), USP, and administered as a subcutaneous (SC) injection. A Xolair vial contains 202.5 mg of omalizumab, 145.5 mg sucrose, 2.8 mg L-histidine hydrochloride monohydrate, 1.8 mg L-histidine, and 0.5 mg polysorbate 20, and is designed to deliver 150 mg of omalizumab in 1.2 mL after reconstitution with 1.4 mL SWFI, USP.
Zenapax® (daclizumab)	Hoffmann-La Roche, Inc., and Protein Design Labs	Humanized monoclonal antibody for prevention of kidney transplant rejection	Dec 1997	Zenapax® (Daclizumab) is an immunosuppressive, humanized IgG1 monoclonal antibody produced by recombinant DNA technology that binds specifically to the alpha subunit (p55 alpha, CD25, or Tac subunit) of the human high-affinity interleukin-2 (IL-2) receptor that is expressed on the surface of activated lymphocytes. Daclizumab is a composite of human (90%) and murine (10%) antibody sequences. The human sequences were derived from the constant domains of human IgG1 and the variable framework regions of the Eu myeloma antibody. The murine sequences were derived from the complementarity-determining regions of a murine anti-Tac antibody. The molecular weight predicted from DNA sequencing is 144 kDa. Zenapax 25 mg/5 mL is supplied as a clear, sterile, colorless concentrate for further dilution and intravenous administration. Each milliliter of Zenapax contains 5 mg of daclizumab and 3.6 mg sodium phosphate monobasic monohydrate, 11 mg sodium phosphate dibasic heptahydrate, 4.6 mg sodium chloride, 0.2 mg polysorbate 80, and may contain hydrochloric acid or sodium hydroxide to adjust the pH to 6.9. No preservatives are added.

Product	Company	Application	FDA Approval Date	Description
Zevalin™ (ibritumomab tiuxetan)	IDEC Pharmaceuticals Corp.	Relapsed or refractory low-grade, follicular, or transformed B-cell non-Hodgkin's lymphoma	Feb 2002	Kits for the Preparation of Indium-111 (In–111) Ibritumomab Tiuxetan (In–111 ZEVALIN) and Yttrium-90 (Y–90) Ibritumomab Tiuxetan (Y-90 ZEVALIN) In–111 Ibritumomab Tiuxetan and Y–90 Ibritumomab Tiuxetan are components of the Zevalin™ therapeutic regimen. Zevalin (ibritumomab tiuxetan) is the immunoconjugate resulting from a stable thiourea covalent bond between the monoclonal antibody ibritumomab and the linker-chelator tiuxetan [N-[2-bis(carboxymethy)amino]-3-(p-isothiocyanatophenyl)-propyl]-[N-[2-bis(carboxymethyl)amino]-2-(methyl)-ethyl]glycine. This linker-chelator provides a high affinity, conformationally restricted chelation site for Indium-111 or Yttrium-90. The approximate molecular weight of ibritumomab tiuxetan is 148 kDa. The antibody moiety of Zevalin is ibritumomab, a murine IgG$_1$ kappa monoclonal antibody directed against the CD20 antigen, which is found on the surface of normal and malignant B lymphocytes. Ibritumomab is produced in Chinese hamster ovary cells and is composed of two murine gamma 1 heavy chains of 445 amino acids each and two kappa light chains of 213 amino acids each.
Zorbitive™ (**Serostim**®) (Somatotropin)	Serono S. A.	Treatment of cachexia (AIDS-wasting); Short bowel syndrome	Aug 1996 Dec 2003	Serostim® [somatropin (rDNA origin) for injection] is a human growth hormone produced by recombinant DNA technology. Serostim has 191 amino acid residues and a molecular weight of 22,125 Da. Its amino acid sequence and structure are identical to the dominant form of human pituitary growth hormone. Serostim is produced by a mammalian cell line (mouse C127) that has been modified by the addition of the human growth hormone gene. Serostim is secreted directly through the cell membrane into the cell-culture medium for collection and purification. Serostim is a highly purified preparation. Biological potency is determined by measuring the increase in the body weight induced in hypophysectomized rats. Serostim is available in 4 mg, 5 mg, and 6 mg vials for single-dose administration. Serostim is also available in 8.8 mg vials for multidose administration. Each 4 mg vial contains 4.0 mg (approximately 12 IU) somatropin, 27.3 mg sucrose, 0.9 mg phosphoric acid. Each 5 mg vial contains 5.0 mg (approximately 15 IU) somatropin, 34.2 mg sucrose, and 1.2 mg phosphoric acid. Each 6 mg vial contains 6.0 mg (approximately 18 IU) somatropin, 41.0 mg sucrose, and 1.4 mg phosphoric acid. Each 8.8 mg vial contains 8.8 mg (approximately 26.4 IU) somatropin, 60.2 mg sucrose, and 2.05 mg phosphoric acid. The pH is adjusted with sodium hydroxide or phosphoric acid to give a pH of 7.4 to 8.5 after reconstitution.

Appendix II
Glossary of Terms

ABBREVIATIONS (USP)

7-AAD	7-amino-actinomycin D
AABB	American Association of Blood Banks
AATB	American Association of Tissue Banks
AAV	adeno-associated virus
ADA	amino deaminase
BSE	bovine spongiform encephalopathy (mad cow disease)
CBER	FDA Center for Biologics Evaluation and Research
CDER	FDA Center for Drug Evaluation and Research
cDNA	complementary DNA
CDRH	Center for Devices and Radiological Health
cfu	colony-forming unit
cGMP	current Good Manufacturing Practice
CSF	colony-stimulating factor
DNA	deoxyribonucleic acid
ELISA	enzyme-linked immunosorbent assay
FACS	fluorescence-activated cell sorter
FBS	fetal bovine serum
GM-CSF	granulocyte–macrophage colony-stimulating factor
GVHD	graft versus host disease
HLA	human leukocyte antigen
HRSA	Health Research Services Administration
HSV	herpes simplex virus
kb	kilobase
NIH	National Institutes of Health
NMDR	National Marrow Donor Registry
PBPC	peripheral blood progenitor cell
PCR	polymerase chain reaction
QC–QA	quality control–quality assurance
RCA	replication-competent adenovirus
RCR	replication-competent retrovirus
RCV	replication-competent virus
rDNA	recombinant DNA
RNA	ribonucleic acid
SDS-PAGE	sodium dodecyl sulfate polyacrylamide gel electrophoresis
TCID50	tissue culture infectious dose, 50%

Absorption Removing a particular antibody or antigen from a sample (from serum, for example) by adding the corresponding antigen or antibody to that sample.

Acceptance criteria Numerical limits, ranges, or other suitable measures for acceptance of the results of analytical procedures that the drug substance or drug product or materials at other stages of manufacture should meet.

Action limit An internal (in-house) value used to assess the consistency of the process at less critical steps. Generally the action limits are tighter than the specification limits; however, to comply with cGMP and GLP requirements, action limits must be listed in the testing SOP and an action plan listed for values going beyond action limits (the corrective action), though they remain within.

Additive A substance added to another in relatively small amounts to effect a desired change in properties.

Adsorption The binding of molecules to a surface as a result of a chemical or physioelectric interaction between the membrane surface or the chromatographic resin and the molecule. A nonspecific adherence of substances in solution or suspension to cells or other particulate matter.

Adventitious agents Acquired, sporadic, or accidental contaminants. Examples include: bacteria, yeast, mold, mycoplasma, or viruses that can potentially contaminate prokaryote or eukaryote cells used in production. Potential sources of adventitious organisms include the serum used in cell culture media, persistently or latently infected cells, or the environment.

Adventitious virus Unintentionally introduced contaminant virus. See also Virus.

Aerobe An aerobic organism is one that grows in the presence of oxygen. A strict aerobe grows only under such a condition.

Affinity The thermodynamic quantity defining the energy interaction or binding of two molecules, usually that of antibody with its corresponding antigenic determinant. See also Affinity chromatography.

Affinity chromatography (AC) A chromatography separation method based on a chemical interaction specific to the target species. In AC, a biospecific adsorbent is prepared by coupling a specific ligand (such as a protein, peptide, or nickel) for the molecule of interest to a solid support. The inherent high specificity of ligand/target interactions makes AC particularly suitable for the capture stage of downstream processing. As a result, the types of affinity methods are: biosorption — site recognition (e.g., monoclonal antibody, Protein A); hydrophobic interaction — contacts between nonpolar regions in aqueous solutions; dye-ligand specific binding of macromolecules to triazine and triphenylmethane dyes; metal chelate — matrix-bound chelate complexes with target molecule by exchanging low molecular weight metal bound ligands; and covalent — disulfide bonding reversible under mild conditions.

Agarose High-molecular-weight polysaccharide used as a separation medium in bead form for biochromatography.

Aggregate A clustered mass of individual cells — solid, fluffy, or pelletized — that can clog the pores of filters or other fermentation apparatus.

Agrobacterium tumefaciens A bacterial plant pathogen, commonly found in soil, that contains a plasmid used to introduce desired sections of DNA into plants.

Air diffusion rate The rate at which air diffuses through the wetted pores of a membrane at a given differential pressure. Measuring the air diffusion rate is a method used to check the integrity of a membrane filter.

Alpha helix and beta strand In a protein, certain domains may form specific structures such as alpha helix and beta strand, which constitute the secondary structure of the protein. An alpha helix has the following features: every 3.6 residues make one turn, the distance between two turns is 0.54 nm, the C = O (or N–H) of one turn is hydrogen bonded to

N-H (or C = O) of the neighboring turn. In a beta strand, the torsion angle of N – Ca–C – N in the backbone is about 120 degrees.

Amino acid composition analysis Used to determine the amino acid composition or the protein quantity. A two-step process involving a complete hydrolysis (chemical or enzymatic) of the protein into its component amino acids followed by chromatographic separation and quantitation via HPLC. The complete amino acid composition of the peptide or protein should include accurate values for methionine, cysteine, and tryptophan. The amino acid composition presented should be the average of at least three separate hydrolysates of each lot number. Integral values for those amino acid residues generally found in low quantities, such as tryptophan or methionine, could be obtained and used to support arguments of purity.

Amino acid sequencing A partial sequencing (8 to15 residues) of amino acids within a protein or polypeptide by either amino-terminal or carboxy-terminal sequencing. This method is used to obtain information about the primary structure of the protein, its homogeneity, and the presence or absence of polypeptide cleavages. The sequence data determined by HPLC analysis is presented in tabular form and should include the total yield for every amino acid at each sequential cleavage cycle. Full sequence is often done by sequencing the peptide fragments isolated from HPLC fractionation. Amino acid sequencing is a required test in BP/EP for listed monographs of therapeutic proteins.

Amino acids An amino acid is defined as the molecule containing an amino group (NH_2), a carboxyl group (COOH), and an R group. It has the following general formula, R–CH(NH2)–COOH. The R group differs among various amino acids. In a protein, the R group is also called a side chain. There are over 300 naturally occurring amino acids on earth, but the number of different amino acids in proteins is only 20.

Anaerobe An anaerobic organism grows in the absence of air or oxygen. Some anaerobic organisms are killed by brief exposure to oxygen, whereas oxygen may just retard or stop the growth of others.

Anion exchange The ion exchange procedure used for the separation of anions. The tetra-alkylammonium group is a typical strong anion exchange functional group.

Antibiotic resistance The gene coding for antibiotic resistance is needed for identifying transformants and to ensure antibiotic selective pressure, that is, only cells that harbor an expression vector will divide, thus preventing plasmid loss. Genes conferring ampicillin, tetracycline, or kanamycin resistance are commonly used in expression vectors. Ampicillin resistance is mostly used only on a laboratory scale because the lactamase, which confers the resistance, degrades ampicillin and thus the selective pressure is lost after a few generations of cell growth. Furthermore, ampicillin has been thought to be potentially allergenic and is therefore usually not the antibiotic of choice in the production of biotherapeutics intended for human use. The U.S. FDA and other regulatory authorities discourage use of β-lactam antibiotics

Antibody A protein molecule having a characteristic structure consisting of two types of peptide chains: heavy (H) and light (L). Antibodies contain areas (binding sites) that specifically fit into and can bind to its corresponding determinant site on an antigen, which has induced the production of that antibody by the B-lymphocytes and plasma cells in a living species.

Antifoam agent A chemical added to the fermentation broth to reduce surface tension and counteract the foaming that can be caused by mixing, sparging, or stirring.

Antigen A foreign protein or carbohydrate, which when introduced into an organism, activates specific receptors on the surface immunocompetent T- and B-lymphocytes. After interaction between antigen and receptors, there usually will be induction of an immune response, i.e., production of antibodies capable of reacting specifically with determinant sites on the antigen.

Antigen determinant   The specific part of a structure of an antigen that will induce an immune response, i.e., it will fit to the receptors on T- and B-lymphocytes and will also be able to react with the antibodies produced.

Antigenicity   The capacity of a substance to function as an antigen — to trigger an immune response. Any agent, often a large molecule that stimulates production, of an antibody that will react specifically with it. Each antigen may contain more than one site capable of binding to a particular antibody. An immunogen can cause the production of a number of antibodies with different specificities. Antigenicity of therapeutic proteins is one of the major issues in the comparability of generic therapeutic proteins.

Antiserum   Blood serum that contains antibodies against a particular antigen or immunogen. This frequently means serum from an animal that has been inoculated with the antigen.

Apoptosis   Apoptosis describes the molecular and morphological changes that characterize controlled cellular self-destruction, often called "programmed cell death."

Artificial chromosome   Synthesized DNA in chromosomal form for use as an expression vector.

Ascites   Liquid accumulations in the peritoneal cavity. Monoclonal antibodies can be purified from the ascites of mice that carry a transplanted hybridoma.

Aseptic   Sterile, free from bacteria, viruses, and contaminants such as foreign DNA.

Association constant   A reaction between antibody and its determinant that comprises a measure of affinity. The constant is quantitated by mass action law rate constants for association and for dissociation.

Asymmetric membrane   A membrane that is made such that the pore size increases through the membrane matrix.

Asymmetry   See Asymmetry factor.

Asymmetry factor   Factor describing the shape of a chromatographic peak. Theory assumes a Gaussian shape and that peaks are symmetrical. The peak asymmetry factor is the ratio (at 10% of the peak height) of the distance between the peak apex and the backside of the chromatographic curve to the distance between the peak apex and the front side of the chromatographic curve. A value > 1 is a tailing peak, while a value < 1 is a fronting peak.

Attenuated   Weakened (attenuated) viruses often used as vaccines; they can no longer produce disease but still stimulate a strong immune response similar to the natural virus. Examples include oral polio, measles, mumps, and rubella vaccines.

Autoclave, Autoclavability   An autoclave is a device that uses saturated steam at a specified pressure over time to kill microorganisms and thus achieve sanitization or sterilization. Because many materials change properties when exposed to moisture, heat, and pressure, products destined for this process must be specially engineered for autoclavability.

Autoradiography   Detection of radioactively labeled molecules on X- ray film.

Avidity   The total binding strength between all available binding sites of an antibody molecule and the corresponding determinants present on antigen.

Bacillus subtilis   A microbe commonly found in soil and vegetation, normally considered non-pathogenic, sometimes used in recombinant microbial fermentation.

Back flushing, backwash   Backflushing is used to elute strongly held compounds at the head of the column by reversing the flow direction of the mobile phase through a chromatographic column. In case of membranes reversing the permeate flow can mechanically clean the column.

Bacterial expression   The most common microbial source for recombinant protein production is *E. coli* because of its well-understood genetics. *B. subtilis* and its relatives have been used, mainly because of their greater tendency to secrete proteins into their environment. Various *Streptomyces* species are under study in recombinant fermentation, but so far they have demonstrated low expression levels. *Pseudomonas fluorescens* may have greater potential. But *E. coli* remains one of the most attractive because of its ability to grow rapidly and at high density on inexpensive substrates, its well-characterized genetics, and the availability of an increasingly large number of cloning vectors and mutant host strains. Bacterial genes are contained in a circular genome and on small circular pieces of extragenomic double-stranded DNA elements called *plasmids* in their nucleus-free cells. Self-replicating plasmids contain regulatory regions (promoter regions and origins of replication) that make them ideal candidates for use in genetic engineering. They can be manipulated using restriction enzymes, cloning vectors (such as bacteriophage viruses), and relatively simple procedures. Certain gene segments with the ability to promote (promoters), direct, or terminate transcription of the foreign DNA are often involved as well.

Bacteriophage   A virus that infects bacteria, sometimes used as a vector. The lambda bacteriophage is frequently used as a vector in recombinant gene experiments. Examples include: dsDNA phages with contractile tails, such as T4; dsDNA phages with long flexible tails are most commonly used in DNA cloning; dsDNA phages with stubby tails, such as p22; ssDNA phages, such as phi X 174; and ssRNA phages, such as MS2.

Baculovirus   A class of insect virus used as vectors for recombinant protein expression in insects; baculovirus is noninfective to humans.

Baseline   The more or less constant signal observed when only the mobile phase passes through the detector. This steady baseline portion of the chromatogram is the reference from which quantitative measurements can be made.

Base pair   Two bases on different strands of nucleic acid that join together. In DNA, cytosine (C) always pairs with guanine (G) and adenine (A) always links to thymine (T). In RNA molecules, adenine joins to uracil (U).

Batch culture   Large-scale cell culture in which cell inoculum is cultured to a maximum density in a tank or airlift fermenter, harvested, and processed as a batch.

Batch fermentation mode   The most commonly used type of fermentation, in which microbes are added to a sterile nutrient broth and allowed to ferment without the addition of further nutrients (except oxygen). A batch fermentation is a closed system where microbes are added to a sterilized nutrient solution in the fermenter, then allowed to incubate. Nothing more is added except oxygen (most microorganisms used in biotechnology are aerobic species), an antifoam agent (to prevent bubble formation), and acid or base to control the solution pH. Consequently, the mixture changes constantly as a result of cellular metabolism, with waste products accumulating and biomass increasing over time. Four growth phases follow inoculation: a lag phase (microorganisms physicochemically equilibrating with their environment), a log phase (cells have adapted to their new surroundings and begin doubling their number logarithmically), a stationary phase (available food has been used up and growth slows or stops; this is when metabolites or recombinant proteins are best harvested), and a death phase (their energy depleted, the cells die off). Doubling times during the log phase vary according to the size and complexity of the microbe: bacteria double in less than an hour, yeasts in 1 or 2 hours, filamentous fungi in 2 to 6 hours. In fed-batch fermentation nutrients are added in increments as growth progresses. Certain ingredients are present at inoculation, and they continue to be added in small doses throughout production.

Bed volume $V = (\times r2) \times h$ where, r = inner radius of the column tube; h = the height of the column tube.

Beta ratio   A standard method of rating a filter's ability to remove particles. Beta (x) = # particles > size (x) upstream / # particles > size (x) downstream where, x = particle size in microns.

Binding   The process by which some components in a feed solution adhere to the membrane. Binding can be desirable in some instances, but often, as in the case of protein binding during sterile filtration, can result in a loss of valuable product.

Binding capacity   The binding capacity describes the actual amount of a sample that will bind to the medium packed in a column under defined conditions. It is determined by saturating a gel with sample and then measuring the amount of sample that binds. Parameters like pH, ionic strength, the counter-ion, and the sample all influence the available capacity. Available capacity will change depending on the experimental conditions. It is essential to take these conditions into consideration when comparing the available capacities of different chromatography media.

Binding site   The part of the antibody molecule that will specifically bind antigen.

Bioactivity   (1) A protein's ability to function correctly after it has been delivered to the active site of the body (*in vivo*). (2) The level of specific activity or potency as determined by animal model, cell culture, or *in vitro* biochemical assay.

Bioavailability   Measure of the true rate and the total amount of drug that reaches the target tissue after administration.

Biologic   A therapeutic agent derived from living things.

Biological activity   The specific ability or capacity of the product to achieve a defined biological effect. Potency is the quantitative measure of the biological activity.

Biological containment   Characteristics of an organism that limit its survival or multiplication in the environment.

Biological response modifier   Generic term for hormones, neuroactive compounds, and immunoreactive compounds that act at the cellular level; many are possible candidates for biotechnological production.

Biopharmaceutical   A therapeutic product created through the genetic manipulation of living things, including (but not limited to) proteins and monoclonal antibodies, peptides, and other molecules that are not chemically synthesized, along with gene therapies, cell therapies, and engineered tissues.

Bioprocessing   Using organisms or biologically derived macromolecules to carry out enzymatic reactions or to manufacture products.

Bioreactor   A vessel capable of supporting a cell culture in which a biological transformation takes place (also called a fermenter or reactor). Typically the vessel contains microbes or other cells grown under controlled conditions of temperature, aeration, mixing, acidity, and sterility. Classically, it represented fermentation when bacteria were used; still differentiated forms from other cells are used.

Biosafety test   A class of tests that determine whether a chromatographic media or filter's material of construction can induce systemic toxicity, skin irritation, sensitization reaction, or other biological responses. These test are often completed by labs in vivo or in vitro.

Biosensors   The powerful recognition systems of biological chemicals (enzymes, antibodies, DNA) are coupled to microelectronics to enable rapid, accurate low-level detection of such substances as sugars and proteins (such as hormones) in body fluids, pollutants in water, and gases in air.

Blinded   When a filter is blinded, it means that particles have filled the pores and the flow through the filter from the feed side to the permeate side is reduced or stopped.

Blotting methods and applications Following gel electrophoresis, probes are often used to detect specific molecules from the mixture. However, probes cannot be applied directly to the gel. The problem can be solved by three types of blotting methods: see Southern blotting, Northern blotting, and Western blotting.

Broth   The contents of a microbial bioreactor: cells, nutrients, waste, and so on.

Bubble point   The minimum pressure required to overcome the capillary forces and surface tension of a liquid in a fully wetted membrane filter. The bubble point value is determined by observing when bubbles first begin to emerge on the permeate side or downstream side of a fully wetted membrane filter when pressurized with a gas on the feed (upstream) side of the membrane filter.

Buffer A mixture of an acid and its conjugate base; its pH changes slowly upon the addition of small amounts of acid or base.

Buffer exchange Filtration process used for the removal of smaller ionic solutes, whereby the feed solution is washed, usually repeatedly, and one buffer is removed and replaced with an alternative buffer.

Calibrator A term in clinical chemistry commonly referring to the standard used to "calibrate" an instrument or used in construction of a standard (calibrator) curve.

Capillary electrophoresis Used as a complement to high-performance liquid chromatography (HPLC), particularly for peptide mapping. This technique is faster and will often separate peptides that coelute using HPLC. Separation is accomplished by relative mobility of the peptides in a buffer in response to an electrical current.

Capture step The initial purification of the target molecule from crude or clarified source material. The objectives are the rapid isolation, stabilization, and concentration of the desired molecule. The initial chromatographic purification step following harvest with the purpose of removing cells.

Carbohydrate analysis Used to determine the consistency of the composition of the covalently bound monosaccharides in glycoproteins. Unlike the polypeptide chain of the glycoprotein where production is controlled by the genetic code, the oligosaccharides are synthesized by posttranslational enzymes. Microheterogeneity of the carbohydrate chains is common. Determination can be accomplished on underivatized sugars after hydrolysis by high-performance liquid chromatography separation with pulsed amperometric detection or by gas chromatography after derivatization.

Cartridge or cartridge filter A filtration or separation device having a membrane encapsulated within a housing. The housing normally has feed and permeate ports and in the case of cross-flow filters, a retentate port. All of these ports may be used to control the flow parameters of fluid into and out of the housing and through the membrane.

Cartridge pressure drop The differential pressure between cartridge inlet and outlet.

Cascade effects A series of events that result from one initial cause.

Cassette A device used for cross-flow filtration, typically in a rectangular form comprised of stacked flat sheets of membrane integrally bonded together. Most cassettes are typically designed to fit into a standard cassette holder where the feed, permeate and any retentate ports mate with appropriate fittings on the cassette holders.

Catabolites Waste products of catabolism, by which organisms convert substances into excreted compounds.

Cation exchange chromatography The form of ion exchange chromatography that uses resins or packings with functional groups that can separate cations. A sulphonic acid would be an example of a strong cation exchange group; a carboxylic acid would be a weak cation exchange group.

Cell culture Cells taken from a living organism and grown under controlled conditions ("in culture"). Methods used to maintain cell lines or strains. The in vitro growth of cells isolated from multicellular organisms. These cells are usually of one type.

Cell differentiation The process whereby descendants of a common parental cell achieve and maintain specialization of structure and function.

Cell fusion The formation of a hybrid cell with nuclei and cytoplasm from different cells, produced by fusing two cells of the same or different species.

Cell harvesting The process of concentrating (dewatering) the cell mass after fermentation. Cell slurries in excess of 70% wet cell weight are achievable. The cells may also be washed to prepare them for further processing, such as freezing or lysing. Unlike clarification processing, with cell harvesting, the cells are the target material.

Cell lines   Cells that acquire the ability to multiply indefinitely *in vitro*. When cells from the first culture (taken from the organism) are used to make subsequent cultures, a cell line is established. Thanks to genetic or other manipulations, immortal cell lines can replicate indefinitely.

Cell substrate   Cells used to manufacture product.

Cells, type of   All cells are divided into two types: prokaryotic cells and eukaryotic cells. The basic component of living organisms is composed of cells with the ability to multiply. All cells contain cytoplasm, a plasma membrane, and DNA.

Central dogma   The flow of genetic information is generally in the direction: DNA RNA Protein. This rule was dubbed the "central dogma," because it was thought that the same principle would apply to all organisms. However, we now know that for RNA viruses, the flow of genetic information starts from RNA.

cGMP   The current Good Manufacturing Practice. The minimum requirements by law for the manufacture, processing, packaging, holding, or distribution of a material as established in Title 21 of the Code of Federal Regulations. Examples are Part 211 for Finished Pharmaceuticals, Part 606 for Blood and Blood Components, Part 820 for Medical Devices and Quality System Regulations (QCR).

Channel length   The total length that the feed solution must travel along a flat cassette to reach the retentate outlet.

Chaperones   Proteins that help other proteins fold correctly, either by preventing them from folding incorrectly or by catalyzing their correct formation, used to maximize the usable protein produced by a variety of expression systems.

Chemical compatibility or resistance   The ability of the components of a packed column or a filter to resist chemicals that can influence its performance. For example, some chemicals could cause the filter to shed particles, swell, or dissolve filter components. Repeatable performance requires that filters are resistant to all the chemicals that they are exposed to at a given concentration, temperature, and total exposure time.

Chemokines   Chemokines are the cytokines that may activate or chemoattract leukocytes. Each chemokine contains 65 ~ 120 amino acids, with molecular weight of 8 ~ 10 kD. Their receptors belong to G-protein-coupled receptors. Since the entry of HIV into host cells requires chemokine receptors, their antagonists are being developed to treat AIDS.

Chemostat   A growth chamber that keeps a bacterial culture at a specific volume and rate of growth by limiting nutrient medium and removing spent culture.

Chemotaxis   Net-oriented movement in a concentration gradient of certain compounds. Various sugars and amino acids can serve as attractants, while some substances such as acid or alkali serve as repellents in microbial chemotaxis. White blood cells and macrophages demonstrate chemotactic movement in the presence of bacterial products, complement proteins and antigen activated T-cells to contribute to the local inflammatory reaction and resistance to pathogens.

Chimeric transgene   A transgene that contains sequences derived from two different genes from two different species.

Chromatogram   A plot of detector signal output versus time, elution volume, or column volume during the chromatographic process.

Chromatographic column   Vessel, typically in cylindrical shape including attached accessory parts like valves, for harboring the chromatography medium.

Chromosome   A long and complex DNA chain containing the genetic information (genes) of a cell. Prokaryotes contain only a single chromosome; eukaryotes have more than one, made up of a complex of DNA, RNA, and protein. The exact number of chromosomes is species-specific. Humans have 23 pairs.

CIP   Clean in place. A way to clean large vessels (tanks, piping, and associated equipment) without moving them or taking them apart, using a high-pressure rinsing treatment, sometimes followed by steam-in-place (SIP) sanitization.

Circular dichroism   With optical rotary dispersion, one of the optical spectrophotometric methods used to determine secondary structure and to quantitate the specific structure forms (a-helix, B-pleated sheet, and random coil) within a protein. The resultant spectra are compared to that of the natural protein form or to the reference standard for the recombinant.

Cistron   The smallest unit of genetic material that is responsible for the synthesis of a specific polypeptide.

Cleaning frequency   The number of chromatographic runs, after a cleaning cycle has to occur.

Clean room   A room in which the concentration of airborne particulate matter is controlled at specific limits to facilitate the manufacture of sterile and high-purity products. Clean rooms are classified according to the number of particles per volume of air.

Clearance   Demonstrated removal according to specified parameters.

Clogging   The process in which solids block the filter or the chromatographic column.

Clone   To duplicate exactly, whether a gene or a whole organism; or an organism that is a genetically identical copy of another organism. A cell line stemming from a single ancestral cell and normally expressing all the same genes.

Cloning vectors   Methods of transferring desired genes to organisms that will be used to express them. Cloning vectors are used to make recombinant organisms. Vector is an agent that can carry a DNA fragment into a host cell. If it is used for reproducing the DNA fragment, it is called a cloning vector. If it is used for expressing certain genes in the DNA fragment, it is called an "expression vector." Commonly used vectors include plasmid, Lambda phage, cosmid, and yeast artificial chromosome (YAC). Plasmids are circular, double-stranded DNA molecules that exist in bacteria and in the nuclei of some eukaryotic cells. They can replicate independently of the host cell. The size of plasmids ranges from a few kb to near 100 kb. A typical plasmid vector contains a polylinker which can recognize several different restriction enzymes, an ampicillin-resistance gene (ampr) for selective amplification, and a replication origin (ORI) for proliferation in the host cell. A plasmid vector is made from natural plasmids by removing unnecessary segments and adding essential sequences. To clone a DNA sample, the same restriction enzyme must be used to cut both the vector and the DNA sample. Therefore, a vector usually contains a sequence (polylinker) that can recognize several restriction enzymes so that the vector can be used for cloning a variety of DNA samples. A plasmid vector must also contain a drug-resistance gene for selective amplification. After the vector enters into a host cell, it may proliferate with the host cell. However, since the transformation efficiency of plasmids in E. coli is very low, most E. coli cells that proliferate in the medium would not contain the plasmids. Therefore, we must find a way to allow only the transformed E. coli to proliferate. Typically, antibiotics are used to kill E. coli cells that do not contain the vectors. The transformed E. coli cells are protected by the ampicillin-resistance gene (ampr), which can express the enzyme, β-lactamase, to inactivate the antibiotic ampicillin.

Codon   Group of three nucleotide bases in DNA or RNA that determines the composition of one amino acid in "building" a protein and also can code for chain termination.

Cohesion termini   DNA molecule with single-stranded ends with exposed (cohesive) complementary bases.

Column back pressure   The pressure of a chromatography system is measured right after the system pump. This pressure is called system back pressure. The additional pressure if a column is attached to the system is called column back pressure.

Column dead volume (Vd) The volume outside of the column packing itself. The interstitial volume (intraparticle volume + interparticle volume) plus extra column volume (contributed by injector, detector, connecting tubing, and end-fittings) all combine to create the dead volume. This volume can be determined by injecting an inert compound (i.e., a compound that does not interact with the column packing). Also abbreviated V0 or Vm.

Column equilibration To achieve a stable and equal distribution of a desired buffer, a column packed with a chromatography medium has to be run in the respective buffer to a point where pH, conductivity, and UV, measured at the column outlet, are identical to the respective values of the applied buffer.

Column performance The performance of a column can be determined by checking the HETP and the asymmetry factor.

Complementary DNA (cDNA) DNA that is complementary to messenger RNA; used for cloning or as a probe in DNA hybridization studies.

Complementary DNA (cDNA) Library The advantage of cDNA library is that it contains only the coding region of a genome. To prepare a cDNA library, the first step is to isolate the total mRNA from the cell type of interest. Because eukaryotic mRNAs consist of a poly-A tail, they can easily be separated. Then the enzyme reverse-transcriptase is used to synthesize a DNA strand complementary to each mRNA molecule. After the single-stranded DNA molecules are converted into double-stranded DNA molecules by DNA polymerase, they are inserted into vectors and cloned.

Composite membrane A membrane that is made up of two or more layers those are usually chemically or structurally different.

Concentrate Also called retentate. The part of the process solution that does not pass through a cross flow membrane filter.

Concentration Cross-flow filtration process in which the components that do not pass through the membrane remain in the feed loop and increase in concentration.

Concentration factor The concentration factor equals the ratio of the initial feed volume to retentate volume after separation. For example, if the initial flow volume is 1000 mL and the final retentate volume is 10 mL, the concentration factor is 10 times.

Concentration polarization The build up of molecules of dissolved substances (solutes) on the surface of the membrane filter during filtration. The concentration polarization layer increases resistance to filtrate flow and reduces the permeate flux, thus decreasing filtration efficiency.

Concurrent process validation Establishing documented evidence that a process does what it purports to do based on information generated during actual implementation of the process.

Conductivity Measurement of a substances ability to conduct an electric current. Measured in Siemens/cm. See also Ionic strength.

Conjugated proteins Covalently bonded to prosthetic groups such as glycoprotein and metalloprotein.

Constitutive promoter A DNA sequence that controls gene expression and is always available.

Contaminants Any adventitiously introduced materials (e.g., chemical, biochemical, or microbial species) not intended to be part of the manufacturing process of the drug substance or drug product.

Continuous fermentation mode Continuous fermentation is an open system. Sterile nutrient solution is continuously introduced while an equal amount of waste products are removed. Cell growth may or may not be adjusted: In the chemostat in the steady state, cell growth is controlled by adjusting the concentration of one substrate. In the turbidistat, cell growth is kept constant by using turbidity to monitor the biomass concentration and that the rate of feed of nutrient solution is appropriately adjusted. The nutrients involved can include carbohydrates, fatty acids, amino acids, and sources of nitrogen and sulfur. Sugars such as glucose, lactose, sucrose, and starch provide carbohydrates and nitrogen. Vitamins, minerals, or growth factors may be necessary for some microbe species. Stirring and mixing adds an air supply, removes carbon dioxide, and distributes nutrients, but an antifoam chemical agent is necessary to keep excess bubbles from forming. Fermentation is a multiphasic reaction in which gaseous components (N_2, O_2, and CO_2) must be mixed continuously with the liquid medium and solid cells. For optimal yields, the whole process must be carried out at a constant temperature.

Continuous mode An open system of fermentation in which nutrient solution is continuously added and removed from the fermenter.

Cosmid (cosmid vector) An artificially constructed plasmid vector that contains a specific bacteriophage gene, which allows it to carry up to 45,000 base pairs of desired DNA. A vector that is similar to a plasmid but it also contains the cohesive sites (cos site) of bacteriophage lambda to permit insertion of large fragments of DNA and in vitro packaging into a phage. The cosmid vector is a combination of the plasmid vector and the COS site, which allows the target DNA to be inserted into the head.

Counterion In an ion-exchange process, the ion in solution used to displace the ion of interest from the ionic site. In ion pairing, it is the ion of opposite charge added to the mobile phase to form a neutral ion pair in solution.

Creutzfeldt-Jakob disease A disease affecting the human nervous system, believed to be caused by a prion that also causes bovine spongiform encephalopathy (BSE) or mad cow disease in cattle.

Cross-flow filtration Also called tangential flow filtration. In cross-flow filtration (CFF), the feed solution flows parallel to the surface of the membrane. Driven by pressure, some of the feed solution passes through the membrane filter. Most of the solution is circulated back to the feed tank. The movement of the feed solution across the membrane surface helps to remove the buildup of foulants on the surface.

Cross-flow rate Also called retentate flow rate. The flow rate of solution that remains in the feed loop as measured in the retentate line.

Cross-linking During the process of copolymerization of resins to form a three-dimensional matrix, a difunctional monomer is added to form cross-linkages between adjacent polymer chains. The degree of cross-linking is determined by the amount of this monomer added to the reaction. For example, divinylbenzene is a typical cross-linking agent for polystyrene ion-exchange resins. The swelling and diffusion characteristics of a resin are governed by its degree of cross-linking.

Cross reaction Antibodies against an antigen A can react with other antigens if the latter has one or more determinants in common with the determinants present on the antigen A or carry one or more determinants that are structurally very similar to the determinants present on antigen A.

Cryopreservation Maintenance of frozen cells, usually in liquid nitrogen.

Cutoff Nominally, the smallest entity that will pass through a separations device to become permeate (filtrate) larger particles (where retention is > 90%) are thus "cut off" from the permeate. Actual cutoff values of any given device or lot of devices usually must be determined empirically. See also Molecular weight cut off (MWCO) and Nominal molecular weight cutoff (NMWC).

Cytokines A protein that acts as a chemical messenger to stimulate cell migration, usually toward where the protein was released. Interleukins, lymphokines, and interferons are the most common. Small, nonimmunoglobulin proteins produced by monocytes and lymphocytes that serve as intercellular communicators after binding to specific receptors on the responding cells. Cytokines regulate a variety of biological activities. Cytokines regulate immunity, inflammation, apoptosis, and hematopoiesis.

Cytopathic Damaging to cells, causing them to exhibit signs of disease.

Cytopathic effect Morphological alterations of cell lines produced when cells are infected with a virus. Examples of cytopathic effects include cell rounding and clumping, fusion of cell membranes, enlargement or elongation of cells, or lysis of cells.

Cytoplasm The protoplasm of a cell outside the nucleus (inside the nucleus is it called nucleoplasm). Protoplasm is a semifluid, viscous, translucent mixture of water, proteins, lipids, carbohydrates, and inorganic salts found in all plant and animal cells.

Cytostat Something that retards cellular activity and production. This can refer to cytostatic agents or to machinery, such as those that would freeze cells.

Cytotoxic Damaging to cells.

Dalton The unit of molecular weight, equal to the weight of a hydrogen atom.

Darcy's law In 1856, a French hydraulic engineer named Henry Darcy published an equation for flow through a porous medium that today bears his name. $Q = KA (h1–h2)/L$ where, Q = volumetric flow rate (m3/s or ft3/s); A = flow area perpendicular to L (m2 or ft2); K = hydraulic conductivity (m/s or ft/s); L = flow path length (m or ft); h = hydraulic head (m or ft); $h1–h2$ = denotes the change in h over the path L.

Dead-ended filtration Also called normal flow filtration. In dead-ended filtration, liquid flows perpendicular to the filtration media, and all of the feed passes through.

Degassing The process of removing dissolved gas from the mobile phase before or during use. Dissolved gas may come out of a solution in the detector cell and cause baseline spikes and noise. Dissolved air can affect electrochemical detectors (by reaction) or fluorescence detectors (by quenching). Degassing is carried out by heating the solvent or by vacuum (in a vacuum flask), or on-line using evacuation of a tube made from a gas-permeable substance such as PTFE, or by helium sparging.

Degradation products Molecular variants resulting from changes in the desired product or product-related substances brought about over time or by the action of, e.g., light, temperature, pH, water, or by reaction with an excipient or the immediate container/closure system. Such changes may occur as a result of manufacture or storage (e.g., deamidation, oxidation, aggregation, proteolysis). Degradation products may be either product-related substances or product-related impurities.

Denaturation Unfolding of a protein molecule into a generally bioinactive form. Also the disruption of DNA duplex into two separate strands.

Depth filter A thick filter that captures contaminants within its structure. A membrane filter primarily captures contaminates on its surface.

Depyrogenate The removal of pyrogens (lipopolysaccharides) from a process solution.

Desalting Technique in which low-molecular-weight salts and other compounds are removed from nonionic and high-molecular-weight compounds. An example is the use of a reversed-phase packing to retain sample compounds by hydrophobic effects but to allow salts to pass through nonretained. Use of a size-exclusion chromatography column to exclude large molecules and retain lower-molecular-weight salts is another example. See also Diafiltration.

Desired product The protein that has the expected structure, or the protein that is expected from the DNA sequence and anticipated posttranslational modification (including glycoforms), and from the intended downstream modification to produce an active biological molecule.

Desorption The opposite of adsorption, i.e., from the ion exchanger essentially two possibilities exist to desorb sample molecules: reducing the net charge by changing pH or adding a competing ion to "block" the charges on the ion exchanger.

Developmentally regulated promoters A DNA sequence that controls gene expression and is available only at certain times or stages.

Diafiltration Diafiltration is a unit operation that incorporates ultrafiltration membranes to remove salts or other microsolutes from a solution. Small molecules are separated from a solution while retaining larger molecules in the retentate. Microsolutes are generally so easily washed through the membrane that for a fully permeated species about 3 volumes of diafiltration water will eliminate 95% of the microsolute.

Dialysis Removal of small molecules from a solution of macromolecules by allowing them to diffuse through a semipermeable membrane into water or a buffer solution. This osmotic pressure separations method is controlled by the concentration gradient of salts across the membrane.

Differential pressure In cross-flow filtration; the pressure drop along the cartridge between the feed (inlet) port and the retentate (outlet) port.

Diffusion Movement of gas molecules caused by a concentration gradient.

Direct flow filtration Filtration process where the entire feed stream flows through the filter's media. Also referred to as normal flow filtration and dead-end filtration.

DNA (deoxyribonucleic acid) The nucleic acid based on deoxyribose (a sugar) and the nucleotides G, A, T, and C. Occurring in a corkscrew-ladder shape, it is the primary component of chromosomes, which thus carry inheritable characteristics of life. The basic biochemical component of the chromosomes and the support of heredity. DNA contains the sugar deoxyribose and is the nucleic acid in which genetic information is stored (apart from some viruses). A DNA molecule has two strands, held together by the hydrogen bonding between their bases. Due to the specific base pairing, DNA's two strands are complementary. If we know the sequence of one strand, we can deduce the sequence of another strand. For this reason, a DNA database needs to store only the sequence of one strand. By convention, the sequence in a DNA database refers to the sequence of the 5′ to 3′ strand (left to right). In a DNA molecule, the two strands are not parallel, but intertwined with each other. Each strand looks like a helix. The two strands form a "double helix" structure, which was first discovered by James D. Watson and Francis Crick in 1953. In this structure, also known as the B form, the helix makes a turn every 3.4 nm, and the distance between two neighboring base pairs is 0.34 nm. Hence, there are about 10 pairs per turn. The intertwined strands make two grooves of different widths, referred to as the major groove and the minor groove, which may facilitate binding with specific proteins. In a solution with higher salt concentrations or with alcohol added, the DNA structure may change to an A form, which is still right-handed, but every 2.3 nm makes a turn and there are 11 base pairs per turn. Another DNA structure is called the Z form, because its bases seem to zigzag. Z DNA is left-handed. One turn spans 4.6 nm, comprising 12 base pairs. The DNA molecule with alternating G-C sequences in alcohol or high salt solution tends to have such structure.

DNA cloning Production of many identical copies of a defined DNA fragment. DNA cloning is a technique for reproducing DNA fragments. It can be achieved by either cell based or polymerase chain reaction (PCR)-based technique. In the cell-based approach, a vector is required to carry the DNA fragment of interest into the host cell.

DNA fingerprinting Sequences of nucleic acids in specific areas (loci) on a DNA molecule are polymorphic, meaning that the genes in those locations may differ from person to person. DNA fragments can be cut from those sequences using restriction enzymes. Fragments from various samples can be analyzed to determine whether they are from the same person. The technique of analyzing restriction fragment length polymorphism (RFLP) is called DNA typing or DNA fingerprinting.

DNA hybridization (dot blot) analysis Detection of DNA to the nanogram level using hybridization of cellular DNA with specific DNA probes. Manifestation can be by 32P labeling, chemiluminescence, or chromogenic- or avidin-biotin assays.

DNA library Set of cloned DNA fragments that together represent the entire genome or the transcription of a particular tissue.

DNA polymerase An enzyme that catalyses the synthesis of double-stranded DNA from single-stranded DNA.

DNA replication DNA molecules are synthesized by DNA polymerases from deoxyribonucleoside triphosphate (dNTP). The chemical reaction is similar to the synthesis of RNA strands. Both DNA and RNA polymerases can extend nucleic acid strands only in the 5′ to 3′ direction. However, the two strands in a DNA molecule are antiparallel. Therefore, only one strand (leading strand) can be synthesized continuously by the DNA polymerase. The other strand (lagging strand) is synthesized segment by segment. DNA replication is triggered by the expression of all required proteins, such as DNA polymerase, DNA primase, and cyclin. In yeast, the transcription factor regulating the expression of these proteins is called MCB binding factor. In mammals, the corresponding transcription factor is E2F.

DNA screening Once a particular DNA fragment is identified, it can be isolated and amplified to determine its sequence. If we know the partial sequence of a gene and want to determine its entire sequence, the probe should contain the known sequence so that the detected DNA fragment may contain the gene of interest.

DNase An enzyme which produces single- stranded nicks in DNA. DNase is used in nick translation.

DNA sequencing The Sanger method being used today was pioneered by Fred Sanger in the 1970s. It is also known as the Dideoxy method, because a small amount of dideoxynucleotides is mixed with normal deoxynucleotides during sequencing. The dideoxynucleotides lack both 2′ and 3′ hydroxyl groups, while the deoxynucleotides lack only the 2′ hydroxyl group. The 3′ hydroxyl group is essential for forming the phosphodiester bond that connects two nucleotides. Therefore, the dideoxynucleotide will be the terminator of a polynucleotide chain since it lacks the essential 3′ hydroxyl group. The Sanger method may sequence a DNA fragment containing up to 500 nucleotides. For large-scale sequencing (such as the entire human genome), a strategy known as the shotgun sequencing is commonly used. In this approach, the DNA molecule of interest is randomly chopped into numerous small pieces. After these small pieces are sequenced, the whole sequence is assembled by their common overlaps.

DNA synthesis The formation of DNA by the sequential addition of nucleotide bases.

DNA vaccine A nucleic acid vaccine where genes coding for specific antigenic proteins are injected to produce those antigens and trigger an immune response.

Downstream processing Starting with a feed stream free of cells and cell debris, the purification sequences involving chromatography and membrane separations to achieve final product purity. Capture, intermediary purification, or polishing comprise the purification part of the process.

Drain valve Valve for draining off material in a filter housing usually at the lowest point.

Drug master file (DMF) A submission to FDA that can be used to provide detailed information about facilities, or articles used in the manufacturing, processing, packaging, and storing of one or more human drugs.

Drug product (DP) A pharmaceutical product type that contains a drug substance, generally in association with excipients.

Drug substance (DS) The material that is subsequently formulated with excipients to produce the drug product. It can be composed of the desired product, product-related substances, and product- and process-related impurities. It may also contain excipients including other components, such as buffers.

Dynamic binding capacity Dynamic capacity describes the amount of sample that will bind to a gel packed in a column run under defined conditions. The dynamic capacity for any media is highly dependent on running conditions, sample preparation, and even origin of the sample. In general the lower the flow rates, the higher the dynamic capacity. As the flow rate approaches zero, the dynamic capacity approaches the available capacity. Dynamic binding capacities are determined by loading a sample containing a known concentration of the target molecule, and monitoring for the molecule in the column flow-through while applying sample.

Edman degradation A type of protein sequencing from the amino terminus.

Effective area In a membrane separations device, the active area of the membrane exposed to flow.

Efficacy The ability of a substance (such as a protein therapeutic) to produce a desired clinical effect; its strength, and effectiveness.

Efficiency Description of the peak width and shape. The efficiency of a column is usually expressed as a plate number and an asymmetry factor.

Effluent The stream of fluid leaving the filter.

Electrophoresis Methods in which molecules or molecular complexes are separated on the basis of their relative ability to migrate when placed in an electric field. An analyte is placed on an electrophoretic support, then separated by charge (isoelectric focusing) or by molecular weight (SDS-PAGE). Visualization is accomplished by staining of the protein with nonselective (Coomassie blue) or selective (silver) staining techniques. The dye-binding method using Coomassie blue is a quantifiable technique when a laser densitometer is used to read the gels. The silver stain method is much more sensitive and therefore used for detection of low levels of protein impurities, but due to variability of staining from protein to protein, it cannot be used for quantitation.

ELISA See Enzyme linked immunosorbent assay.

Eluate Combination of mobile phase and solute exiting column, also called effluent.

Elution The removal of adsorbed material from an adsorbent such as the removal of a product from an enzyme bound on a column.

Endogenous Growing or developing from a cell or organism, or arising from causes within the organism.

Endogenous pyrogen assay An in vitro assay based on the release of endogenous pyrogen produced by endotoxin from human monocytes. This assay appears to be more sensitive than the USP rabbit pyrogen test, but is much less sensitive than the limulus amoebocyte lysate assay. It does have the advantage that it can detect all substances that cause a pyrogenic response from human monocytes.

Endogenous virus Viral entity whose genome is part of the germ line of the species of origin of the cell line and is covalently integrated into the genome of the animal from which the parental cell line was derived. For the purposes of this document, intentionally introduced, nonintegrated viruses such as EBV are used to immortalize cell substrates or bovine papilloma virus that fit in this category.

Endonuclease (1) A restriction enzyme that breaks up nucleic acid molecules at specific sites along their length. Such enzymes are naturally produced by microorganisms as a defense against foreign nucleic acids. (2) Enzymes that cleave bonds within nucleic acid molecules.

Endoplasmic reticulum A highly specialized and complex network of branching, interconnecting tubules (surrounded by membranes) found in the cytoplasm of most animal and plant cells. The rough endoplasmic reticulum is where ribosomes make proteins. It appears "rough" because it is covered with ribosomes. The smooth endoplasmic reticulum is the site for synthesis and metabolism of lipids, and it is involved in detoxifying chemicals such as drugs and pesticides.

Endotoxin The outer cell wall of gram-negative bacteria. A poison in the form of a fat/sugar complex (lipopolysaccharide) that forms a part of the cell wall of some types of bacteria.

It is released only when the cell is ruptured and can cause septic shock and tissue damage. Pharmaceuticals are tested routinely for endotoxins. A heat stable lipopolysaccharide associated with the outer membrane of certain gram negative bacteria. It is not secreted and is released only when the cells are disrupted.

Enhancers Enhancers are the positive regulatory elements located either upstream or downstream of the transcriptional initiation site. However, most of them are located upstream. In prokaryotes, enhancers are quite close to the promoter, but eukaryotic enhancers could be far from the promoter. An enhancer region may contain one or more elements recognized by transcriptional activators.

Enzyme linked immunosorbent assay (ELISA) A multiantigen test for unknown residual (host) cellular protein and confirmation of desired protein. It may be used to determine the potency of a product. It is extremely specific and sensitive, basically simple, and inexpensive. It requires a reference standard preparation of host cell protein impurities to serve as an immunogen for preparation of polyclonal antibodies used for the assay.

Enzymes Proteins that catalyze biochemical reactions by causing or speeding up reactions without being changed in the process themselves. Enzymes are the catalysts of biochemical reactions in the cell and include such examples as oxidoreductases, transferases, hydrolases, proteases, nucleases, phosphatases, lysases, isomerases, and ligases.

Epithelium (epithelial) The layer(s) of cells between an organism or its tissues or organs and their environment (skin cells, inner linings of lungs or digestive organs, outer linings of kidneys, and so on).

Ethylene oxide (EtO) sterilization A sterilization process still common for biomedical products, in which a product is subjected to steam and highly toxic ethylene oxide gas. Because many materials change properties when exposed to moisture and EtO by-products, products destined for this process must be specially engineered for EtO sterilization.

Eukaryote A complex organism whose cells contain a membrane-bound nucleus. Sometimes spelled *eucaryote*. The eukaryotic cell contains a nucleus. Eukaryotes include protista, fungi, animals, and plants. The eukaryotic cell contains organelles, which are defined as membrane-bound structures such as nucleus, mitochondria, chloroplasts, endoplasmic reticulum (ER), Golgi apparatus, lysosomes, vacuoles, peroxisomes, etc. For animal cells, the cell surface consists of the plasma membrane only, but plant cells have an additional layer called cell wall, which is made up of cellulose and other polymers. All biological membranes, including plasma membranes and all organelle membranes, contain lipids and proteins. The lipids found in biomembranes are mainly phospholipids and cholesterol. In the plasma membrane and some of organelle membranes, proteins and phospholipids are attached to carbohydrates, forming glycoproteins and glycolipids, respectively.

Excipient An ingredient added intentionally to the drug substance which should not have pharmacological properties in the quantity used.

Exclusion limit In size-exclusion chromatography (SED), the upper limit of molecular weight (or size), beyond which molecules will elute at the same retention volume, called the exclusion volume. Many SEC packings are referred to by their exclusion limit.

Exclusion volume (Ve) The retention volume of a molecule on a size-exclusion chromatography (SED) packing; all molecules larger than the size of the largest pore are totally excluded and elute at the interstitial volume of the column.

Exogenous Developing from outside, originating externally. Exogenous factors can be external factors such as food and light that affect an organism.

Exonucleases Enzymes that catalyze the removal of nucleotides from the ends of a DNA molecule.

Expanded bed adsorption (EBA) mode Expanded bed mode is a single pass operation in which desired proteins are purified from crude, containing feed-stock with particles without the need for separate clarification, concentration, and initial purification. The expansion of the adsorbent bed creates a distance between the adsorbent particles, i.e., increased voidage (void volume fraction) in the bed, which allows for unhindered passage of cells, cell debris, and other particles during application of crude feed to the column. Expanded bed adsorption is a unit operation that uses adsorbents and columns for recovering proteins directly from crude feedstock. The system of expanded bed adsorption comprises several distinct steps. First, the settled bed is expanded by the upward liquid flow of equilibration buffer; the crude feed, a mixture of soluble proteins, contaminants, cells and cell debris, is passed upward through the expanded bed. Target proteins are captured on the adsorbent media while particles and contaminants pass through the expanded bed. Loosely bound material is washed out with the upward flow of buffer; a change to elution buffer while maintaining the upward flow desorbs the target protein in expanded bed mode. Alternatively, if flow is reversed, the adsorbent particles will quickly settle and the proteins can be desorbed by an elution buffer as in conventional packed bed chromatography. The mode used for elution, expanded bed or settled bed, depends on the characteristics of the feed. After elution the adsorbent is cleaned by a predefined clean-in-place (CIP) solution, followed by either regeneration with application buffer for further use or equilibrated in storage solution.

Express To translate a cell's genetic information, stored in its DNA (gene), into a specific protein.

Expression construct The expression vector that contains the coding sequence of the recombinant protein and the elements necessary for its expression.

Expression system Organisms chosen to manufacture (by expression) a protein of interest through recombinant DNA technology.

Expression vector A way of delivering foreign genes to a host, creating a recombinant organism that will express the desired protein.

Extractables Substances that may dissolve or leach from a membrane during filtration and contaminate the process solution. For example, the leachates might include wetting agents in the membrane, membrane-cleaning solutions, or substances from the materials used to encase the membrane.

Fed-batch mode Fermentation in which substrate is added incrementally throughout the process.

Feed Material or solution that you apply on chromatography column or introduce into a membrane separation system device.

Feed pressure The pressure measured at the feed port of a separation device such as a chromatographic column, a cartridge, or cassette.

Feed stream flow rate Volumetric flow rate of the feed. Measured in volume per unit time.

Fermentation An anaerobic bioprocess, fermentation is used in various industrial processes for the manufacture of products such as alcohols, acids, and cheese by the action of yeasts, molds, and bacteria. The fermentation process is also used in the production of monoclonal antibodies. Whereas the use of fermentation goes back several millennia, its use as an expression system began in 1973 with the first genetic engineering experiment: A gene from the African clawed toad was inserted into laboratory *Escherichia coli* bacteria. Besides the familiar alcoholic beverages, products made by microbial fermentation (some recombinant, others not) are far-ranging: from ethanol, dyes, and other chemicals to enzymes, foods and food additives, vitamins, soy products, vaccines for animals and people, antibiotics and antifungal agents, steroids, diagnostic agents, and enzyme inhibitors. Bacteria and yeast grow fast in low-cost media; offer high expression levels of the proteins they can make, which they sometimes secrete into their circulating medium; and both can withstand rough treatment compared with animal cells. Fermentation of recombinant cell lines begins with genetic engineering of microbes classified "generally recognized as safe" (GRAS), such as *E. coli, Bacillus subtilis, Streptomyces* species, and *Saccharomyces cerevisiae* and *Schizosaccharomyces pombe* yeasts.

Fermenter A bioreactor used to grow bacteria or yeasts in liquid culture. See also Fermentation.

Fiber More correctly called hollow fiber membrane.

Filter area The surface area of filter media inside a separation device.

Filter efficiency Filter efficiency represents the percentage of particles that are removed from the fluid by the filter.

Filtrate Also called permeate. The portion of the process fluid that passes through the membrane.

Filtrate flow rate The instantaneous volume per unit time of filtrate produced by a system, typically measured on a filtrate flow meter.

Filtration Removal of particles, normally solids, from a fluid. These can be contaminants or valuable products.

Filtration efficiency A filter's ability to remove particles of the specified size, expressed as a percentage or as a beta ratio.

Flanking control regions Noncoding nucleotide sequences that are adjacent to the 5' and 3' end of the coding sequence of the product that contain important elements that affect the transcription, translation, or stability of the coding sequence. These regions include, e.g., promoter, enhancer, and splicing sequences, and do not include origins of replication and antibiotic resistance genes.

Floc A fluffy aggregate that resembles a woolly cloud.

Flowpath length, nominal flowpath length The total length that a feed solution travels from inlet to outlet. Flowpath length is an important parameter to consider when doing any process development, system design, or scale-up or scale-down experiments. The flow path length and other fluid channel geometries such as lumen diameter or channel height can impact the fluid dynamics of the system and will directly impact pump requirements and differential pressure of the filtration step.

Flow rate The volumetric or linear rate of flow of mobile phase through a chromatography column.

Flux The volume of solution flowing through a given membrane area during a given time. Expressed as LMH (liters per square meter per hour).

Flux rate in LMH Flux rate in LMH = [permeate flow (ml/min) ÷ cassette surface area (m2)] × 0.06.

Formulation Conversion of drug substance (the API) to drug product.

Fouling Accumulation of material on the surface of the chromatography media or on the membrane that can slow and alter the process.

Fractionation Separation of molecules in a solution based on differences in the properties of the molecules.

Frit The porous element at either end of a column that serves to contain the column packing. It is placed at the very ends of the column tube or, more commonly, in the end-fitting. Frits are made from stainless steel or other inert metal or plastic, such as porous PTFE or polypropylene.

Fungal fermentation Fungal fermentation can manufacture many recombinant therapeutic proteins. Yeasts offer certain advantages over bacteria as a recombinant expression system such as their ability as eukaryotic organisms to perform certain posttranslational modifications on the proteins they make. *Streptomyces cerevisiae* (baker's or brewer's yeast) is the fungal species most commonly found in fermentation processes, recombinant or not. It is the one with which people have the most experience (thousands of years' worth) and thus the best understanding (the full genome was sequenced in 1996). *S. cerevisiae* has been genetically engineered to produce a wide range of proteins: antigens to hepatitis B, influenza, and polio; human growth hormone and insulin; antibodies and antibody fragments; human growth factors; interferon and interleukin; blood components such as human serum albumin; and tissue plasminogen activator. Other species that have been studied include *S. pombe* and *Pichia pastoris.* In yeast, the expression of recombinant proteins to at least 150 mg/L in shake flasks. Coexpression of a necessary enzyme has helped some yeasts produce correctly folded collagen molecules. Some heterologous proteins can be lethal to the yeast cells that make them — but a methanol-induced promoter has been developed to meet that challenge. Once the yeast culture has reached a certain cell density, changing its growth medium to methanol induces expression of the therapeutic protein in large amounts (effectively ending the batch). Similar inducible promoter genes have been used with bacteria and *S. cerevisiae,* but *P. pastoris* only works with methanol, and it is the only one that does.

Fusion of protoplast   Fusion of two cells whose walls have been eliminated, making it possible to redistribute the genetic heritage of microorganisms.

Fusion partner   The gene for a protein that can be joined to the gene for a medically useful protein to optimize production in bacterial fermentation expression systems. When making a small protein or peptide in E. coli, it is often necessary to produce the protein fused to a larger protein to get high levels of stable expression. The resulting fusion protein must be cleaved (chemically or enzymatically broken) to yield the desired protein or peptide. The nonproduct fusion partner is left over and usually thrown away.

Gamma sterilization   A type of sterilization process accomplished by bombarding the object to be sterilized with electron beam, X-ray, or 60 Co or 137 Cs irradiators. All generate forms of gamma rays, radiant energy at short wavelength (0.1 nm or less). The governing standard is ISO 11137-Sterilization of Healthcare Products — Requirements for Validation and Routine Control — Radiation Sterilization. Because some product materials can be adversely affected by gamma radiation, objects destined for gamma sterilization must be engineered specifically for this process.

Gel electrophoresis   Gel electrophoresis is a technique for separating charged molecules with different sizes. Two kinds of gels are commonly used: agarose and polyacrylamide. Agarose gels can be applied to a wider range of sizes than polyacrylamide gels. By using standard agarose electrophoresis, nuclei acids up to 50 kb may be separated. If pulsed field gel electrophoresis is used, the upper limit can be extended to 10 Mb. Polyacrylamide gels may separate nucleic acids that differ in length by only 1 nucleotide if their length is less than 500 bp. In a gel (either agarose or polyacrylamide), the negatively charged DNA fragments move toward the positive electrode at a rate inversely proportional to their length. After the electric field is applied for a certain period, DNA fragments with different lengths will be separated, which can be visualized by autoradiography or by treatment with a fluorescent dye (e.g., ethidium bromide). The relationship between the size of a DNA fragment and the distance it migrates in the gel is logarithmic. Therefore, from the band positions, the lengths of DNA fragments can be determined. Also used is a two-dimensional (or 2-D) gel electrophoresis.

Gel filtration   A separation method based on the molecular size or the hydrodynamic volume of the components being separated. This can be accomplished with the proteins in their natural state or denatured with detergents. Also called size exclusion chromatography (SEC).

Gel layer   During the filtration process, the thin layer of particles or molecules that may build up at the membrane surface. It is also referred to as the concentration polarization layer. High transmembrane pressure can lead to an increase in the thickness of the gel layer and negatively impact the filtration process by reducing flux and inhibiting passage though the membrane.

Gene   The basic unit of heredity, which plays a part in the expression of a specific characteristic. The expression of a gene is the mechanism by which the genetic information that it contains is transcribed and translated to obtain a protein. A gene is a part of the DNA molecule that directs the synthesis of a specific polypeptide chain. It is composed of many codons. When the gene is considered as a unit of function in this way, the term cistron is often used. By definition, a gene includes the entire nucleic acid sequence necessary for the expression of its product (peptide or RNA). Such sequence may be divided into regulatory region and transcriptional region. The regulatory region could be near or far from the transcriptional region. The transcriptional region consists of exons and introns. Exons encode a peptide or functional RNA. Introns will be removed after transcription. "Gene family" refers to a set of genes with homologous sequences.

Gene regulatory elements Transcriptional regulation is mediated by the interaction between transcription factors and their DNA binding sites, which are the *cis*-acting elements, whereas the sequences encoding transcription factors are transacting elements. The *cis*-acting elements may be divided into the following four types: promoters, enhancers, silencers, and response elements. The transcription region consists of exons and introns. The regulatory elements include promoter, response element, enhancer, and silencer. Downstream refers to the direction of transcription and upstream is opposite to the transcription direction. The numbering of base pairs in the promoter region is as follows. The number increases along the direction of transcription, with "+1" assigned for the initiation site. There is no "0" position. The base pair just upstream of +1 is numbered "−1," not "0."

Genetic code Protein synthesis is based on the sequence of mRNA, which is made up of nucleotides, while proteins are made up of amino acids. There must be a specific relationship between the nucleotide sequence and amino acid sequence. This relationship is the so-called genetic code, which was deciphered by Marshall Nirenberg and his colleagues in early 1960s. One of their approaches is shown below. Three nucleotides (a codon) code for one amino acid. Synthesis of a peptide always starts from methionine (Met), coded by AUG. The stop codon (UAA, UAG, or UGA) signals the end of a peptide. This applies to mRNA sequences. For DNA, U (uracil) is replaced by T (thymine). In a DNA molecule, the sequence from an initiating codon (ATG) to a stop codon (TAA, TAG or TGA) is called an open reading frame (ORF), which is likely (but not always) to encode a protein or polypeptide. The genetic code is not randomly assigned. If an amino acid is coded by several codons, they often share the same sequence in the first two positions and differ in the third position. Such assignment is accomplished by the design of wobble position, but "*the evolutionary dynamic that shaped the code remains a mystery.*" The standard genetic code applies to most, but not all, cases. Exceptions have been found in the mitochondrial DNA of many organisms and in the nuclear DNA of a few lower organisms.

Genetic engineering A technique used to modify the genetic information in a living cell, reprogramming it for a desired purpose (such as the production of a substance it would not naturally produce). Altering the genetic structure of an organism (adding foreign genes, removing native genes, or both) through technological means rather than traditional breeding.

Gene expression An organism may contain many types of somatic cells, each with a distinct shape and function. However, they all have the same genome. The genes in a genome do not have any effect on cellular functions until they are "expressed." Different types of cells express different sets of genes, thereby exhibiting various shapes and functions. The essential steps involved in expression of protein genes are transcription where a DNA strand is used as the template to synthesize an RNA strand, which is called the primary transcript; RNA processing that modifies the primary transcript to generate a mature mRNA (for protein genes) or a functional tRNA or rRNA; for RNA genes (tRNA and rRNA), the expression is complete after a functional tRNA or rRNA is generated.

However, protein genes require additional steps of nuclear transport where mRNA is transported from the nucleus to the cytoplasm for protein synthesis and finally protein synthesis in the cytoplasm where mRNA binds to ribosomes and synthesizes a polypeptide based on the sequence of mRNA.

Gene transfer The use of genetic or physical manipulation to introduce foreign genes into host cells to achieve desired characteristics in progeny.

Genome All the genes carried by a cell. "Genome" is the total genetic information of an organism. For most organisms, it is the complete DNA sequence. For RNA viruses, the genome is the complete RNA sequence, since their genetic information is encoded in RNA. The genomes of prominent organisms are given below:

Organism	Genome Size (Mb)	Gene Number
Hepatitis D virus	0.0017	1
Hepatitis B virus	0.0032	4
HIV-1	0.0092	9
Bacteriophage 1	0.0485	80
Escherichia coli	4.6392	4400
S. cerevisiae (yeast)	12.155	6300
C. elegans (nematode)	97	19000
D. melanogaster (fruit fly)	137	13600
Mus musculus (mouse)	3000	30000–70000
Homo sapiens (human)	3000	30000–70000

Note: 1 Mb = 1 million base pairs (for double-stranded DNA or RNA) or 1 million bases (for single-stranded DNA or RNA).

Genomic library The genomic library is normally made by lambda phage vectors, instead of plasmid vectors because the entire human genome is about 3×10^9 bp long, while a plasmid or lambda phage vector may carry up to 20 kb fragments. This would require 1.5×10^5 recombinant plasmids or lambda phages. When plating *E. coli* colonies on a 3-inch petri dish, the maximum number to allow isolation of individual colonies is about 200 colonies per dish. Thus, at least 700 petri dishes are required to construct a human genomic library. By contrast, as many as 5×10^4 lambda phage plagues can be screened on a typical petri dish. This requires only 30 petri dishes to construct a human genomic library. Another advantage of lambda phage vector is that its transformation efficiency is about 1000 times higher than the plasmid vector. Preparation of the genomic library using lambda phage vectors is basically the cloning of all DNA fragments representing the entire genome.

Genotype The genetic composition of an organism (including expressed and nonexpressed genes), which may not be readily apparent.

Germ cell The "sex cells" in higher animals and plants that carry only half of the organism's genetic material and can combine to develop into new living things.

GLP (Good Laboratory Practice) Regulations issued by the FDA describing practices for conducting nonclinical laboratory studies.

Glycoprotein Protein to which groups of sugars become attached. Human blood group proteins, cell wall proteins, and some hormones are examples of glycoproteins.

Glycosylation (1) Adding one or more carbohydrate molecules onto a protein (a glycoprotein) after it has been built by the ribosome; a posttranslational modification. (2) The addition of one or more oligosaccharide groups to a protein. The covalent attachment of sugars to an amino acid in the protein portion of a glycoprotein.

GMPs Good Manufacturing Practices required by FDA regulations. cGMP stands for current Good Manufacturing Practices.

Golgi body A cell organelle consisting of stacked membranes where posttranslational modifications of proteins are performed; also called Golgi apparatus.

Gradient elution Technique for the separation of molecules by increasing mobile phase strength (i.e., conductivity, etc.) over time during the chromatographic separation. Gradients can be continuous or stepwise.

Growth hormone A protein produced in the pituitary gland to control cell growth.

Hapten A low molecular weight substance that alone can react with its corresponding antibody. In order to be immunogenic, haptens are bonded to molecules having molecular weights greater than 5000. An example would be the hapten digoxin covalently bonded to bovine serum albumin, forming the digoxin-BSA immunogen.

Hemocytometer A device for counting blood cells.

HETP Height equivalent to a theoretical plate. A carryover from distillation theory: a measure of a column's efficiency. For a typical HPLC column well-packed with 5 μm particles, HETP (or H) values are usually between 0.01 and 0.03 mm. HETP = L/N, where, L = column length; N = the number of theoretical plates.

High-affinity antibody Antibodies with a high affinity for antigen. These antibodies are predominantly IgG and produced during a secondary response to antigen. Cells producing a high-affinity antibody can be triggered by low concentration of antigen.

High performance liquid chromatography (HPLC) A separation technique that uses small particle size, narrow bore columns, and high inlet pressures to achieve separation in short periods of time with high resolution. Any form of column chromatography that uses a liquid mobile phase can be extended to HPLC. An instrumental separation technique used to characterize or determine the purity of a therapeutic protein by passing the product (or its component peptides or amino acids) in liquid form over a chromatographic column containing a solid support matrix. The mode of separation, i.e., reversed phase, ion exchange, gel filtration, or hydrophobic interaction, is determined by the column matrix and the mobile phase. Detection is usually by UV absorbance or by electrochemical means.

Hold-up volume Quantity of fluid remaining within the filtration media after draining the system.

Hollow fiber The tube-like structure made from a membrane and sealed inside a cross-flow cartridge where the feed stream flows into the inner diameter of one end of the hollow fiber and the retentate (the material that does not permeate through the walls of the hollow fiber) flows out the other end. The material that passes through the membrane (walls of the hollow fiber) is called permeate. In hollow-fiber bioreactor cell culture system cells are separated from the medium using semipermeable membranes arranged into hollow fibers.

Hormone A protein released by an endocrine gland to travel in the blood and act on tissues at another location in the body.

Host A cell whose metabolism is used for the growth and reproduction of a virus, plasmid, or other form of foreign DNA.

Host-related impurities Impurities related to the culturing of cells (e.g., cell debris, nucleic acids, host cell proteins, cell culture media components, endotoxins) or transgenic milk components.

Housing The mechanical structure that surrounds and supports the membrane or filter element. The housing normally has feed, retentate, and permeate ports that direct the flow of process fluids into and out of the filter assembly.

HPLC High-performance liquid chromatography or high-pressure liquid chromatography, a commonly used method for separating liquid mixtures.

Hybridoma An immortalized cell line (usually derived by fusing B-lymphocyte cells with myeloma tumor cells) that secretes desirable antibodies.

Hybridoma technology Fusion between an antibody forming cell (lymphocyte) and a malignant myeloma cell ("immortal"), which will result in a continuously growing cell clone (hybridoma), that can produce antibodies of a single specificity. Hybrid cells made by combining tumor cells and plasma cells; the combination of normal B-lymphocytes and myeloma cells is commonly used in cell-culture expression systems to produce monoclonal antibodies.

Hydrophilic "Water-loving": refers both to stationary phases that are compatible with water and to water soluble molecules in general. Most chromatography media used to separate proteins are hydrophilic in nature and should not attract or denature protein in the aqueous environment.

Hydrophobic "Water-hating": refers both to stationary phases that are not compatible with water and to molecules in general that have little affinity for water. Hydrophobic molecules have few polar functional groups: most are hydrocarbons or have high hydrocarbon content.

Hydrophobic interaction chromatography (HIC) A technique in which reversed-phase packings are used to separate molecules by virtue of the interactions between their hydrophobic moieties and the hydrophobic sites on the surface. High salt concentrations are used in the mobile phase; separations are effected by changing the salt concentration. The technique is analogous to salting out molecules from solution. Gradients are run by decreasing the salt concentration over time. HIC is accomplished in high salt medium by binding the hydrophobic portions of a protein to a slightly hydrophobic surface containing such entities as phenyl, or short-chain hydrocarbons. The protein can be eluted in a decreasing salt gradient, with the most hydrophobic proteins eluting from the column last.

Immortalize To alter cells (either chemically or genetically) so that they can reproduce indefinitely.

Immunoassay A qualitative or quantitative assay technique based on the measure of interaction of high-affinity antibody with antigen used to identify and quantify proteins.

Immunoblotting A technique for transferring antibody/antigen from a gel to a nitrocellulose filter on which they can be complexed with their complementary antigen/antibody.

Immunodiffusion (double, Ouchterlony technique) A technique in which an antigen and antibody are placed in two adjacent wells cut into a medium such as agar. As they diffuse through the medium, they form visible precipitation lines of antigen/antibody complexes at the point where the respective concentrations are at the optimum ratio for lattice formation.

Immunodiffusion (single) An identity diffusion technique whereby the product (antigen) is placed in a well cut into a medium such as agar containing its complementary antibody. The product diffuses into the medium forming a ring shaped precipitate whose density is a function of antigen concentration.

Immunospecificity A performance characteristic determined by conducting cross-reactivity studies with structurally similar substances that may be present in the analyte matrix. Specificity studies are determined with each new lot of polyclonal antibodies used in the immunoassay. For monoclonal antibody, each subsequent new lot is usually characterized by biochemical and biophysical techniques in lieu of comprehensive specificity studies.

Immunotoxin Monoclonal antibodies coupled with toxins that are capable of delivering the toxin moiety to a target cell.

Impurity (1) Impurities are intrinsic unwanted compounds of a respective sample. (2) Any component present in the drug substance or drug product that is not the desired product, a product-related substance, or an excipient including buffer components. It may be either process- or product-related.

Inactivation   Reduction of virus infectivity caused by chemical or physical modification.

Inclusion bodies   Very high levels of heterologous proteins expressed in bacteria may lead to the formation of inclusion bodies. In such cases, the protein molecules clump together (aggregate) in the cytoplasm to create irregular organelle-like structures (about 1 μm in diameter). This presents a good-news–bad-news scenario: Dense inclusion bodies are easily separated from broken cells by centrifugation, thus facilitating product purification after the cells are homogenized. But the aggregated, misfolded proteins are also insoluble, which can make further processing difficult. Organic solvents, detergents, or chaotropic substances can be used to denature those clumps and solubilize the proteins. But the next problem encountered is that their three-dimensional structure is almost always wrong by that point. To get correct, biologically active proteins, a renaturation step must follow: Inclusion bodies are dissolved using chaotropes, then diluted so the proteins can properly refold. A few bacterial expression options are available that avoid the inclusion body issue entirely. For example, some species secrete products rather than retaining them within cellular walls. Cultivation of E. coli at lower temperatures (30°C rather than 37°C) sometimes prevents aggregation of heterologous proteins. Coexpression of chaperone proteins (or increased production of innate cofactors) that encourage proper folding of the biotherapeutic molecule may also help. And combining the gene for the protein of interest with one expressing a highly soluble native cytoplasmic protein (a fusion partner) may offer an answer. But the resulting fusion proteins must be chemically or enzymatically cleaved in downstream processing so the fusion partner can be purified away.

Inducer   A chemical or conditional change that activates the expression leading to the production of a desired product. A small molecule that interacts with a regulator protein and triggers gene transcription.

In-house working reference material   A material prepared similarly to the primary reference material that is established solely to assess and control subsequent lots for the individual attribute in question. It is always calibrated against the in-house primary reference material.

Inlet   The initial part of the column or a filtration device, where the solvent and sample enter. In case of a chromatographic column there is usually an inlet frit that holds the packing in place and, in some cases, protects the packed bed.

Inlet pressure   The pressure driving a fluid into the feed port of a separation device.

Inoculate   To introduce cells into a culture medium.

Inoculum   Material (usually cells) introduced into a culture medium.

In situ **hybridization**   Hybridization with an appropriate probe carried out directly on a chromosome preparation or histological section.

Installation qualification (IQ)   The installation qualification provides a systematic method to check the system/equipment static attributes prior to normal operation. A detailed description of the system should be included as a part of IQ. This description includes all important major/minor components of the system. The availability of the applicable SOPs must be verified. These include system/equipment operation, maintenance, cleaning, and sanitization.

Integration site   The site where one or more copies of the expression construct is integrated into the host cell genome.

Interferons   A cytokine that inhibits virus reproduction. Interferons also affect growth and development (differentiation) in certain normal and tumor cells. Interferons are the cytokines that can "interfere" with viral growth. They also have the ability to inhibit proliferation and modulate immune responses. Four types of interferons have been identified: IFN-α, IFN-β, IFN-ω, and IFN-γ.

Interleukins   Interleukins are the cytokines that act specifically as mediators between leukocytes. The following table shows the major source and effects of various types of interleukins.

	Major source	**Major effects**
IL-1	Macrophages	Stimulation of T-cells and antigen-presenting cells. B-cell growth and antibody production. Promotes hematopoiesis (blood cell formation).
IL-2	Activated T-cells	Proliferation of activated T cells.
IL-3	T-lymphocytes	Growth of blood cell precursors.
IL-4	T-cells and mast cells	B-cell proliferation. IgE production.
IL-5	T-cells and mast cells	Eosinophil growth.
IL-6	Activated T-cells	Synergistic effects with IL-1 or TNF-α.
IL-7	Thymus and bone marrow stromal cells	Development of T-cell and B cell precursors.
IL-8	Macrophages	Chemoattracts neutrophils.
IL-9	Activated T-cells	Promotes growth of T-cells and mast cells.
IL-10	Activated T-cells, B-cells, and monocytes	Inhibits inflammatory and immune responses.
IL-11	Stromal cells	Synergistic effects on hematopoiesis.
IL-12	Macrophages, B-cells	Promotes T_H1 cells while suppressing T_H2 functions.
IL-13	T_H2 cells	Similar to IL-4 effects.
IL-15	Epithelial cells and monocytes	Similar to IL-2 effects.
IL-16	CD8 T-cells	Chemoattracts CD4 T cells.
IL-17	Activated memory T-cells	Promotes T-cell proliferation.
IL-18	Macrophages	Induces IFN-γ production.

Intermediary purification Chromatographic purification step(s) following capture with the purpose of removing cell culture and process-related impurities.

Intermediate purification step Further removal of bulk impurities with the main objectives of concentration and purification.

Interspersed repeats Interspersed repeats are repeated DNA sequences located at dispersed regions in a genome. They are also known as mobile elements or transposable elements. A stretch of DNA sequence may be copied to a different location through DNA recombination. After many generations, such sequences (the repeat unit) could spread over various regions. In mammals, the most common mobile elements are LINEs and SINEs. LINEs stands for long interspersed nuclear elements. Its basic organization is shown below. All mobile elements contain direct repeats. The most common LINEs in humans are the L1 family. A human genome contains about 60,000 to 100,000 L1 elements. SINEs stands for short interspersed nuclear elements. Its length is about 300 bp. In humans, the most abundant SINEs are the Alu family. A human genome contains about 700,000 to 1,000,000 Alu sites. Although most LINEs and SINEs are located in extragenic regions, some of them are located in introns. For example, the human retinoblastoma gene (RB gene) is as long as 180 kb, consisting of 27 exons. Its introns contain many Alu and a few L1 elements.

In vitro (1) An experiment performed in a test tube, petri dish, or other lab apparatus with parts of a living organism, such as testing a drug with tissue samples. From Latin, meaning "in glass." (2) Performed in the laboratory rather than in a living organism (*in vivo*). Biological reactions taking place outside the body in an artificial system.

In vitro **cell age** A measure of the period between thawing of the MCB vial(s) and harvest of the production vessel measured by elapsed chronological time in culture, population doubling level of the cells, or passage level of the cells when subcultivated by a defined procedure for dilution of the culture.

In vivo An experiment performed using a living organism. From Latin, meaning "in live [subjects]." Biological reaction taking place inside a living cell or organism.

Ion exchange chromatography (IEC) A mode of chromatography in which ionic substances are separated on cationic or anionic sites of the packing. The sample ion (and usually a counterion) will exchange with ions already on the ionogenic group of the packing. Retention is based on the affinity of different ions for the site and on a number of other solution parameters (pH, ionic strength, counterion type, etc.). A gradient-driven separation based on the charge of the protein and its relative affinity for the chemical backbone of the column. Anion/cation exchange is commonly used for proteins. A mode of chromatography in which ionic substances are separated on cationic or anionic sites of the packing. Separation in IEC is based upon the selective, reversible adsorption of charged molecules to an immobilized ion exchange group of the opposite charge. An ion exchanger consists of an insoluble porous matrix to which charged groups have been covalently bound.

Ionic strength The weight concentration of ions in solution, computed by multiplying the concentration of each ion in solution (C) by the corresponding square of the charge on the ion (Z) summing this product for all ions in solution and dividing by 2.

Isocratic elution Use of a constant-composition mobile phase in liquid chromatography.

Isoelectric focusing (IEF) An electrophoretic method that separates proteins by their pI. They move through a pH gradient medium in an electric field until they are located at their isoelectric point where they carry no net charge. Prior to reaching their pI, protein mobility also depends upon size, conformation, steepness of pH gradient, and the voltage gradient. This method is used to detect incorrect or altered forms of a protein as well as protein impurities.

Isoelectric point The isoelectric point is the pH of a solution or dispersion at which the net charge on the macromolecules or colloidal particles is zero.

lac **operon** The *lac* operon governs the production of enzymes for metabolizing lactose. In the absence of lactose, the repressor substance binds to the operator, inhibiting the production of three enzymes. Lactose, however, represses the repressor, allowing the enzymes to be produced. The *lac* operon of *E. coli* consists of three genes: *lacZ*, *lacY*, and *lacA*, encoding β-galactosidase, lactose permease, and thiogalactoside transacetylase, respectively. Lactose permease is located on the cell membrane, capable of pumping lactose into the cell. β-galactosidase can convert lactose into glucose and galactose. Thiogalactoside transacetylase is responsible for degrading small molecules.

lac **repressor** In the absence of lactose, transcription of the *lac* operon is inhibited by the *lac* repressor. The lactose can bind to the *lac* repressor, preventing it from interacting with its DNA binding site. Hence, in a medium containing lactose, the *lac* operon is quickly transcribed, producing the enzymes to generate glucose, which is the major energy source for *E. coli*.

Lambda λ phages The λ phages are viruses that can infect bacteria. The major advantage of the λ phage vector is its high transformation efficiency, about 1000 times more efficient than the plasmid vector. The λ phages are commonly used in DNA cloning. They have two life cycles: lytic and lysogenic. In the lytic cycle, λ phages replicate rapidly and eventually cause lysis of the host cell. In the lysogenic cycle, the viral DNA circularizes and integrates into the host DNA. Then, λ phages may replicate with the host cell. Under certain conditions (e.g., ultraviolet irradiation of cells), the λ phages may transform from the lysogenic cycle to the lytic cycle. This transformation is mainly controlled by two proteins: cI (also known as λ repressor) and Cro. Increase in cI proteins promotes the lysogenic cycle, whereas increase in Cro proteins promotes the lytic cycle.

Leakage Leakage occurs when resin-derived substances (ligands or other compounds) disintegrate from the matrix.

Library, genome or cDNA DNA library is a collection of cloned DNA fragments. There are two types of DNA libraries. The genomic library contains DNA fragments representing the entire genome of an organism. The cDNA library contains only complementary DNA molecules synthesized from mRNA molecules in a cell.

Ligase   Enzyme used to join DNA molecules. An enzyme that causes fragments of DNA or RNA to link together; used with restriction enzymes to create recombinant DNA.

Limulus amoebocyte lysate (LAL) test   A sensitive test for the presence of endotoxins using the ability of the endotoxin to cause a coagulation reaction in the blood of a horseshoe crab. The LAL test is easier, quicker, less costly, and much more sensitive than the rabbit test, but it can detect only endotoxins and not all types of pyrogens and must therefore be thoroughly validated before being used to replace the USP rabbit pyrogen test. Various forms of the LAL test include a gel clot test, a colorimetric test, a chromogenic test, and a turbidimetric test.

Linear velocity   The velocity of the mobile phase moving through the column, expressed in cm/h. Related to flow rate by the cross-sectional area of the column.

Locus   The site of a gene on a chromosome.

Lumen   The inner open space or cavity of a single hollow fiber element that is used in the construction of hollow fiber cartridges.

Lymphocytes   White blood cells that produce antibodies.

Lymphokines   Substances released predominantly from T-lymphocytes after reaction with the specific antigen. Lymphokines are biologically highly active and will cause chemotaxis and activation of macrophages and other cell mediated immune reactions. Gamma-interferon is a lymphokine.

Lyophilization   Freeze-drying, used for the long-term preservation of microorganisms and some finished therapeutics.

Lysis   The process whereby a cell wall breakdown occurs releasing cellular content into the surrounding environment. Destruction of bacteria by infective phage.

Lysosomes   Cell organelles containing enzymes, responsible for degrading proteins and other materials ingested by the cell.

MAb   Monoclonal antibody: A highly specific, purified antibody that recognizes only a single antigen.

Macrokinetics   Movement of whole cells and their media within a bioreactor.

Macrovoid   A generally undesirable open space in a membrane filter that is appreciably larger than the average of the pore openings in a given filter. Macrovoids can lead to pinhole defects resulting in unwanted passage that directly impacts final product yield. Macrovoids can also impact the overall membrane strength and thus the device's ability to maintain integrity under pressure.

Mass spectrometry   A technique useful in primary structure analysis by determining the molecular mass of peptides and small proteins. Often used with peptide mapping to identify variants in the peptide composition. Useful to locate disulfide bonds and to identify posttranslational modifications.

Master cell bank (MCB)   An aliquot of a single pool of cells that generally has been prepared from the selected cell clone under defined conditions, dispensed into multiple containers, and stored under defined conditions. The MCB is used to derive all working cell banks (WCB). The testing performed on a new MCB (from a previous initial cell clone, MCB, or WCB) should be the same as for the MCB unless justified.

Media   A (usually sterile) preparation made for the growth, storage, maintenance, or transport of microorganisms or other cells.

Media exchange   A filtration step used to exchange one type of media for an alternative type of media during an aseptic cell culture separation.

Media migration Media migration occurs when solid components of a filter (particles, adhesives, etc.) break free of the filter and enter the process solution.

Medium (media) The component of a separation device. For example, the chromatographic matrix in a chromatography column or the membrane in a membrane cassette.

Meiosis Cell division in which the daughter cells have half the number of chromosomes as the parent cell.

Membrane A thin layer of a highly engineered material with pores used to separate particles, biological matter, and molecules from a solution.

Membrane recovery The degree to which the original performance of a membrane can be restored by cleaning.

Membrane test A process, based on membrane bubble point characteristics, for testing the integrity of the membranes.

Messenger RNA (mRNA) RNA that serves as the template for protein synthesis; it carries the transcribed genetic code from the DNA to the protein synthesizing complex to direct protein synthesis.

Metabolites Chemical by-products of metabolism, the chemical process of life.

Microbiology The study of microscopic life such as bacteria, viruses, and yeast.

Microcarrier A microscopic particle (often, a 200-μm polymer bead) that supports cell attachment and growth in suspension culture.

Microencapsulated Surrounded by a thin, protective layer of biodegradable substance referred to as a microsphere.

Microfiltration The process of removing particles from a liquid by passing it through a porous membrane under pressure. Microfiltration is a pressure-driven membrane-based separation process in which particles and dissolved macromolecules larger than 0.1 μm are rejected (collected). The process removes particles, primarily from liquids, by passing the liquid sample through a microporous membrane. MF usually refers to the removal of particles between 0.1 microns to 5 or 10 microns in size.

Microheterogeneity Slight differences in large, complex macromolecules that result in a population of closely related but not identical structures. Protein microheterogeneity can arise from many sources: genetic variants, proteolytic activity in cells, during translation into protein, during attachment of sugars, and during commercial production.

Microinjection Manually using tiny needles to inject microscopic material (such as DNA) directly into cells or cell nuclei; computer screens provide a magnified view; a technique by which part of one cell is injected into another cell, as DNA into ova or other cells to create transgenic animals.

Microkinetics Movement of chemicals into, out of, and within the cell.

Micron (micrometer, μm) One one-millionth of one meter.

Microporous membrane A thin, porous film or hollow fiber having pores ranging from 0.01 to 10 μm. Science and industry use microporous membranes to separate suspended matter from liquids.

Microtubules Cellular organelles common in microorganisms: thin tubes that make structures involved in cellular movement.

Minimum exposure time The shortest period for which a treatment step will be maintained.

Mitochondria (Mitochondrion singular) Animal-cell organelles that reproduce using their own DNA. They metabolize nutrients to provide the cell with energy and are believed to have once been symbiotic bacteria. Chloroplasts are their plant-cell equivalents; cellular organelle responsible for oxidative metabolism and phosphorylation in eukaryotic cells, widely believed to have originated as a symbiotic bacterium.

Mobile phase The solvent that moves the solute through the column.

Molecular weight cut off (MWCO) The size designation in Daltons for ultrafiltration membranes. The molecular weight of the globular protein that is 90% retained by the membrane. No industry standard exists, hence the MWCO ratings of different manufacturers are not always comparable.

Monoclonal antibodies (MAb) Antibodies that are produced by a cellular clone and are all identical.

Motif The motif is a characteristic domain structure consisting of two or more helices or strands. Common examples include coiled coil, helix-loop-helix, zinc finger, leucine zipper, etc. Many proteins also contain specific domains such as the SH2 (Src homology 2) domain.

Multicellular organisms Referring to organisms composed of more than one cell — often billions of them, arranged in various organs, tissues, and systems.

Multimerization of genes Low yields often result due to the susceptibility of the peptides to proteolysis. Fusion peptide improves stability but often this is only a small portion of the fusion protein, still resulting in low yields of the target peptide. One way of increasing the molar ratio, and hence increasing the amount of peptide produced, is to produce a fusion protein with multiple copies of the target peptide. An additional beneficial effect is often obtained by this strategy, since the gene multimerization has also been shown to increase the proteolytic stability of the produced peptides. When the gene multimerization strategy is employed to increase the production yield, subsequent processing of the gene product to obtain the native peptide is needed. By flanking a peptide gene with codons encoding methionine, CNBr cleavage of the fusion protein, containing multiple repeats of the peptide, has successfully been used for obtaining native peptide at high yield. A pentapeptide multimerized to 3, 14, and 28 copies, fused to dihydrofolate reductase, is engineered to be separated by trypsin cleavage.

Mutagen An agent (chemicals, radiation) that causes mutations in DNA.

Mutagenesis The induction of genetic mutation by physical or chemical means to obtain a characteristic desired by researchers.

Mutation A change in the genetic material, either of a single base pair (point mutation) or in the number or structure of the chromosomes. A permanent change in DNA sequence or chromosomal structure.

Mycoplasma Parasitic microorganisms that infect mammals, possessing some characteristics of both bacteria and viruses.

Myeloma Lymphocytic cancer; a malignancy normally found in bone marrow. Tumor cell line derived from a lymphocyte.

Nanofiltration Separation processes targeted for solutes having molecular weights from 500 Da to 1000 Da.

Necrosis Localized nonapoptotic death of cells and tissues.

NF-κB This regulator of transcription consists of two subunits: p50 (green) and p65 (red). They belong to the Rel family.

Nick A break in the sugar–phosphate backbone of a DNA or RNA strand.

Nick translation In vitro method used to introduce radioactively labeled nucleotides into DNA.

Nominal filter rating A rating that indicates the percentage of particles of a specific size or molecules of a specific molecular weight that will be removed by a filter. No industry standard exists; hence the ratings from manufacturer to manufacturer are not always comparable.

Nominal molecular weight cutoff In ultrafiltration, the molecular weight size of a protein or other solute (in thousands of Daltons) that will be retained to 90% by the membrane.

Nonendogenous virus Virus from external sources present in the MCB. See also Virus.

Nonspecific model virus A virus used for characterization of viral clearance of the process when the purpose is to characterize the capacity of the manufacturing process to remove or inactivate viruses in general, i.e., to characterize the robustness of the purification process.

Normal flow filtration Also called dead-ended filtration. In normal flow filtration, liquid flows perpendicular to the filter media, and all of the feed passes through.

Normalized water permeability (NWP) The water flux rate at 20°C. Flux (normalized to 20°C) = Cassette flux measured temp. (°C) × 20°C ÷ measured temperature (°C).

Northern blot (blotting) Technique for transferring RNA fragments from an agarose gel to a nitrocellulose filter on which they can be hybridized to a complementary DNA. Northern blotting is used for detecting RNA fragments, instead of DNA fragments. The technique is called "Northern" simply because it is similar to "Southern," not because it was invented by a person named "Northern." In the Southern blotting, DNA fragments are denatured with alkaline solution. In the Northern blotting, RNA fragments are treated with formaldehyde to ensure linear conformation.

Nuclear transfer Moving a part or all of an organism's genetic information into an unfertilized egg (whose nucleus had previously been removed); can be used for cloning or to produce transgenic animals (if the genes put into the egg have been recombined with genes from others species).

Nuclear transport After RNA molecules (mRNA, tRNA and rRNA) are produced in the nucleus, they must be exported to the cytoplasm for protein synthesis. On the other hand, many proteins operating in the nucleus must be imported from the cytoplasm. The traffic through the nuclear envelope is mediated by a protein family that can be divided into exportins and importins. Binding of a molecule (a "cargo") to exportins facilitates its export to the cytoplasm. Importins facilitate import into the nucleus.

Nucleic acids DNA or RNA: long, chainlike molecules composed of nucleotides.

Nucleic acid chain In a nucleic acid chain, two nucleotides are linked by a phosphodiester bond, which may be formed by the condensation reaction similar to the formation of the peptide bond.

Nucleotides Molecules composed of a nitrogen-rich base, phosphoric acid, and a sugar. The bases can be adenine (A), cytosine (C), guanine (G), thymine (T), or uracil (U). A nucleotide is composed of three parts: pentose, base, and phosphate group. In DNA or RNA, a pentose is associated with only one phosphate group, but a cellular-free nucleotide (such as ATP) may contain more than one phosphate group. If all phosphate groups are removed, a nucleotide becomes a nucleoside. In cells, a free nucleotide may contain one, two, or three phosphate groups. The energy carrier ATP (adenosine triphosphate) has three phosphate groups; ADP (adenosine diphosphate) has two; AMP (adenosine monophosphate) has one. If all phosphate groups are removed, a nucleotide becomes a nucleoside such as adenosine.

Nucleus The largest organelle, a sphere that contains all the cell's genetic material and a nucleolus that builds ribosomes.

Oleophobic Membranes that repel nonpolar fluids such as oil and lubricants.

Oligonucleotides Short segments of DNA or RNA, i.e., a chain of a few nucleotides.

Oncogene A gene that, when expressed as a protein, can lead cells to become cancerous, usually by removing the normal constraints on its growth.

Operation qualification (OQ) The documented evidence that the system or equipment performs as intended throughout all anticipated operating ranges. The OQ protocol contains the procedures to verify specific dynamic attributes of a system or equipment throughout its operating range, which may include worst case conditions. Applicable standard operating procedures and training procedures are documented in the appropriate protocol section. The executed operational qualification protocol verifies that the system or equipment performs as intended.

Operator gene A gene that switches on adjacent structural gene(s).

Operon A segment of DNA containing adjacent genes including structural genes and an operator gene and a regulatory gene. Complete unit of bacterial gene expression consisting of a regulator gene(s), control elements (promoter and operator) and adjacent structural gene(s).

Organelle A structurally discrete component that performs a certain function inside a eukaryotic cell.

Organism A single, autonomous living thing. Bacteria and yeasts are organisms; mammalian and insect cells used in culture are not.

Overload In preparative chromatography, the overload condition is defined as the mass of sample injected onto the column at which efficiency and resolution begin to be affected if the sample size is further increased.

p53 (LocusLink) Involved in control of transcription, this is a tumor suppressor protein, also known as "Guardian of the Genome." It plays an important role in cell cycle control and apoptosis. Defective p53 could allow abnormal cells to proliferate, resulting in cancer. As many as 50% of all human tumors contain p53 mutants.

Packed bed mode A traditional chromatography mode, where the resin is confined between the bottom of the column and the flow adapter.

Particle size distribution The distribution of particle sizes (number or weight fraction) in a fluid.

PCR See Polymerase chain reaction.

Peak shape Describes the profile of a chromatographic peak. Theory assumes a Gaussian peak shape (perfectly symmetrical); peak asymmetry factor describes shape as a ratio.

Peptide bond Chemical bond between the carboxyl (–COOH) group of one amino acid and the amino (–NH2) group of another.

Peptide mapping A powerful technique that involves the breakdown of proteins into peptides using highly specific enzymes. The enzymes cleave the proteins at predictable and reproducible amino acid sites and the resultant peptides are separated via high-performance liquid chromatography or electrophoresis. A sample peptide map is compared to a map done on a reference sample as a confirmational step in the identity profiling of a product. It is also used for confirmation of disulfide bonds, location of carbohydrate attachment, sequence analysis, and for identification of impurities and protein degradation.

Peptides The peptide is a chain of amino acids linked together by peptide bonds. Polypeptides usually refer to long peptides, whereas oligopeptides are short peptides (< 10 amino acids). Proteins are made up of one or more polypeptides with more than 50 amino acids. The primary structure of a protein refers to its amino acid sequence. The amino acid in a peptide is also called a residue. Proteins consisting of fewer than 40 amino acids.

Performance qualification (PQ) The documented evidence that the system, equipment, or process is capable of consistently producing a safe product of high quality. The PQ protocol describes the procedures that verify the specific capabilities of a process equipment/system through the use of simulation material or actual product.

Permeate Also called filtrate. The portion of a process fluid that passes through a membrane.

Phenotype The part of an organism's genotype that is expressed and thus is generally apparent by observation.

Pilot plant A medium-scale bioprocessing facility used as an intermediate in scaling up processes from the laboratory to commercial production.

Pilot plant scale The production of a recombinant protein by a procedure fully representative of and simulating that to be applied on a full commercial manufacturing scale. The methods of cell expansion, harvest, and product purification should be identical except for the scale of production.

Plaque Clear area in a plated bacterial culture due to lysis by a phage.

Plasmid A circular molecule of DNA that can replicate autonomously of other replicons and is commonly dispensable to the cell; used in genetic engineering. Hereditary material that is not part of a chromosome. Plasmids are extrachromosomal, circular, and self-replicating and found in the cytoplasm of cells (naturally in bacteria and some yeasts). They can be used as vectors (along with viruses) for introducing up to 10,000 base-pairs of foreign DNA into recipient cells.

Plasmid cloning Process by which a plasmid is used to import recombinant DNA into a host cell for cloning. In DNA cloning, a DNA fragment that contains a gene of interest is inserted into a cloning vector or plasmid.

Plasmid insertion Plasmids are similar to viruses, but lack a protein coat and cannot move from cell to cell in the same fashion as a virus. Plasmid vectors are small circular molecules of double stranded DNA derived from natural plasmids that occur in bacterial cells. A piece of DNA can be inserted into a plasmid if both the circular plasmid and the source of DNA have recognition sites for the same restriction endonuclease. The plasmid and the foreign DNA are cut by this restriction endonuclease (EcoRI in this example; see also Restriction enzymes), producing intermediates with sticky and complementary ends. Those two intermediates recombine by base-pairing and are linked by the action of DNA ligase. A new plasmid containing the foreign DNA as an insert is obtained. A few mismatches may occur, producing an undesirable recombinant.

Plasmid plastid Any of several types of cellular organelle found in plants and algae but not in animals or prokaryotes.

Plate number Refers to theoretical plates in a packed column.

PLC Programmable logic controller, a purpose-made device for industrial control. Microprocessors, now common in desktop computers, were originally devised in the 1970s for PLCs or for the types of operations common to PLCs (polling or checking sensors and activating/deactivating valves and switches compared against programmed presets or default levels).

Pleating Folding filter media to increase the surface area that can be fitted into a given separation device.

Point of breakthrough The breakthrough volume is useful in determining the total sample capacity of the column for a particular solute.

Polishing step Final removal of trace impurities to gain high-level purity of end product. The final chromatographic purification step(s) with the purpose of removing product-related impurities.

Polyclonal Derived from different types of cells.

Polyhedrin Protein some viruses use to protect themselves from ultraviolet light.

Polymerase An enzyme that catalyzes the production of nucleic acid molecules.

Polymerase chain reaction (PCR) *In vitro* technique for amplifying nucleic acid. The technique involves a series of repeated cycles of high temperature denaturation, low temperature oligonucleotide primer annealing, and intermediate temperature chain extension. Nucleic acid can be amplified a million-fold after 25 to 30 cycles. PCR is a cell-free method of DNA cloning. It is much faster and more sensitive than cell-based cloning.

Pore Small interconnecting passage through the membrane. The size and irregular path of a pore determines the removal rating of a membrane.

Pore size distribution The range of pore sizes in a membrane. The tighter the pore size distribution, the better control one has over the filtration process.

Porosity A measurement of the open space in a membrane. Also called open area or voids volume.

Posttranslational processing Protein processing done by the Golgi bodies after proteins have been constructed by ribosomes. Enzymatic processing of a protein such as the addition of carbohydrate moieties or the removal of a signal sequence to direct a protein through a cell or organelle membrane. Endoplasmic reticuli (ER) are either smooth or rough. These membrane-bound networks of branching, interconnected tubules are like little manufacturing plants inside the cells of most eukaryotes. The smooth ER synthesizes and metabolizes lipid molecules and helps detoxify cells. The rough ER is covered with ribosomes, which are the site of protein synthesis, where RNA from the cell nucleus is translated into amino acid sequences based on the genetic code. Bacteria have ribosomes, but they do not have ER. Yeasts have most of the same organelles as other eukaryotes (plants and animals), but they do not function quite the same way. In a eukaryotic cell, protein synthesis does not stop at the amino acid chain. Complex posttranslational modifications are performed by the Golgi apparati in a way that has barely begun to be understood by cellular biologists. These stacked-membrane structures put the finishing touch on glycoproteins and other complex polypeptides. It is not well understood how they differentiate one from the other or how they recognize molecules.

Potency The measure of the biological activity using a suitably quantitative biological assay (also called potency assay or bioassay), based on the attribute of the product that is linked to the relevant biological properties.

Prefiltration Removal of coarse particles/contaminants prior to final normally finer filtration.

Pressure An increase in the force exerted on something above standard atmospheric conditions, measured as gauge pressure (psig, barg).

Pressure, absolute Gauge pressure plus 14.7 psi (1 bar).

Pressure drop The difference in pressure between two points.

Pressure-flow rate curve To determine the optimal packing flow rate and pressure, a pressure versus flow rate curve for each lot of chromatography media is performed.

Pretreatment The chemical or physical cleaning of a fluid prior to filtration or chromatography.

Prions Resembling viruses, these pathogens are composed only of protein, with no detectable nucleic acid.

Probes A probe is a piece of DNA or RNA used to detect specific nucleic acid sequences by hybridization (binding of two nucleic acid chains by base pairing). They are radioactively labeled so that the hybridized nucleic acid can be identified by autoradiography. The size of probes ranges from a few nucleotides to hundreds of kilobases. Long probes are usually made by cloning. Originally they may be double-stranded, but the working probes must be single-stranded. Short probes (oligonucleotide probes) can be made by chemical synthesis.

Process characterization of viral clearance Viral clearance studies in which nonspecific "model" viruses are used to assess the robustness of the manufacturing process to remove or inactivate viruses.

Process-related impurities Target protein derivatives (e.g., des-amido forms, oxidized forms, scrambled forms, di- and polymeric forms). Impurities that are derived from the manufacturing process. They may be derived from cell substrates (e.g., host cell proteins, host cell DNA), cell culture (e.g., inducers, antibiotics, or media components), or downstream processing (e.g., processing reagents or column leachables).

Process-scale chromatography The chromatographic procedure and equipment used in industrial production are referred to process scale.

Process validation Establishing documented evidence that provides a high degree of assurance that a specific process will consistently produce a product meeting its predetermined specifications and quality attributes.

Production cells Cell substrate used to manufacture product.

Product-related impurities Molecular variants of the desired product (e.g., precursors, certain degradation products arising during manufacture, or storage) that do not have properties comparable to those of the desired product with respect to activity, efficacy, and safety.

Prokaryote An organism (e.g., bacterium, virus, blue-green algae) whose DNA is not enclosed within a nuclear membrane or whose cell contains neither a membrane-bound nucleus nor other membrane-bound organelles such as mitochondria and plastids. Includes the "true bacteria" and the archaens. Sometimes spelled *procaryote.*

Promoters DNA sequence that initiates transcription of a gene to produce mRNA, used in genetic engineering to direct cells to manufacture a protein of interest. Promoter is the DNA region where the transcription initiation takes place. In prokaryotes, the sequence of a promoter is recognized by the sigma (σ) factor of the RNA polymerase. In eukaryotes, it is recognized by specific transcription factors. *E. coli* has five sigma factors:
- Sigma 70: Regulate expression of most genes.
- Sigma 32: Regulate expression of heat shock proteins.
- Sigma 28: Regulate expression of flagellar operon (involved in cell motion).
- Sigma 38: Regulate gene expression against external stresses.
- Sigma 54: Regulate gene expression for nitrogen metabolism.

Prospective validation Validation conducted prior to the distribution of either a new product or a product made under a revised manufacturing process, where the revisions may have affected the product's characteristics. It is also to ensure that the finished product meets all release requirements for functionality and safety.

Protease Enzyme that speeds the breakdown of proteins into amino acids.

Protein Macromolecules whose structures are coded in an organism's DNA. Each is a chain of more than 40 amino acids folded back upon itself in a particular way. A polypeptide consisting of amino acids. In their biologically active states, proteins function as catalysts in metabolism and, to some extent, as structural elements of cells and tissues. See also Enzymes, Interleukin, Interferon.

Protein passage The passage of protein into the permeate stream.

Protein quantification Quantitation of the total amount of protein can be done by a number of assays. There is no one method that is better than the rest; each has its own disadvantages ranging from the amount of protein required to do the test to a problem with variability between proteins. Some of the types include Lowry, Bicinchonic Acid (BCA), Bradford, Biuret, Kjeldahl, and ultraviolet spectroscopy.

Protein sorting Proteins are synthesized on ribosomes that are located mainly in the cytosol. Only a small number of ribosomes are located in mitochondria and chloroplasts. Proteins synthesized on these ribosomes can be directly incorporated into the compartments within these organelles. However, most mitochondrial and chloroplast proteins are encoded by nuclear DNA and synthesized on cytosolic ribosomes. These and all other proteins synthesized in the cytosol must be transported to appropriate locations in the cell. This is made possible by the specific signal sequence in the newly synthesized peptide.

Protein synthesis The process of protein synthesis goes through following steps:

Initiation: Peptide synthesis always starts from methionine (Met). Therefore, the initial aminoacyl-tRNA is Met-tRNA$_i^{Met}$, where the subscript "i" specifies "initiation." In bacteria, the methionine of the initial aminoacyl-tRNA has been modified by the addition of a formyl group (HCO) to its amino group. The modified methionine is called formylmethionine (fMet), which is unique for bacteria. Thus, fMet is an obvious foreign substance in eukaryotes. It can elicit a strong immune response. In humans, the immune response elicited by the peptide "fMet-Leu-Phe" is about a thousand times greater than "Met-Leu-Phe."

Elongation: A ribosome contains two major tRNA-binding sites: A site and P site. After the large subunit joins the initiation complex, the initial Met-tRNA$_i^{Met}$ enters the P site and the newly arrived aminoacyl-tRNA is always placed at the A site ("A" for "aminoacyl"). Then, methionine is transferred to the new aminoacyl-tRNA, forming a "peptidyl-tRNA" where a peptide is attached to the tRNA. Subsequently, the empty tRNA at the P site is ejected from the ribosome and the peptidyl-tRNA jumps to the P site ("P" for "peptidyl"). During this translocation step, the ribosome also moves one codon down the mRNA chain. Similar steps are repeated in the next cycles of elongation.

Termination: Protein synthesis will terminate when the ribosome arrives at one of three stop codons. The termination process is assisted by special proteins called termination factors, which recognize the stop codons. Their association stimulates the release of the peptidyl-tRNA from the ribosome. Subsequently, the released peptidyl-tRNA divides into tRNA and a newly synthesized peptide chain. The ribosome also divides into the large and small subunits, ready for synthesizing another peptide.

Protein transport A protein destined for the nucleus or cytoplasm contains a specific sequence that can be recognized directly by importin/exportin or through an adaptor protein.

Proteolytic Capable of lysing (denaturing, or breaking down) proteins.

Proteomics Study of proteome, which contains all proteins in a cell at a particular time. Although all cells in an organism have the same genome, they usually have different proteomes.

PSI Pounds per square inch. A unit of pressure. 1 PSI = 6.78 kPa.

Pyrogen A substance (e.g., endotoxin) that produces a fever within a warm-blooded animal when injected into the bloodstream. Filtration materials of construction that come in contact with injectable liquids must meet pyrogenicity standards.

Pyrogenicity The tendency for some bacterial cells or parts of cells to cause inflammatory reactions in the body, which may detract from their usefulness as pharmaceutical products.

Quality assurance The activity of providing evidence that all the information necessary to determine that the product is fit for the intended use meets cGMP requirements. The quality assurance department executes this function.

Rabbit pyrogen test (USP) An assay for the presence of pyrogens (not restricted to endotoxins as is the limulus amoebocyte lysate test) involving the injection of the test material into rabbits that are well controlled and of known history. The rabbits are then monitored for a rise in temperature over a period of 3 hours.

Radioimmunoassay (RIA) A generic term for immunoassays having a radioactive label (tag) on either the antigen or antibody. Common labels include I125 and H3, which are used for assay detection and quantitation. Classical RIAs are competitive binding assays, where the antigen and tagged antigen compete for a limited fixed number of binding sites on the antibody. The antibody bound tagged complex is inversely proportional to the concentration of the antigen.

Recirculation rate Same as retentate flow rate.

Recombinant Containing genetic material from another organism. Genetically altered microorganisms are usually referred to as recombinant, whereas plants and animals so modified are called transgenic. See also Transgenics.

Recombinant DNA DNA that contains genes from different sources that have been combined by methods of genetic engineering as opposed to traditional breeding experiments.

Recombinant proteins production Many proteins that may be used for medical treatment or for research are normally expressed at very low concentrations. Through recombinant DNA technology, a large quantity of proteins can be produced. This involves the cloning of the gene encoding the desired protein into an "expression vector," which must contain a promoter so that the protein can be expressed.

Recovery The amount of solute (sample) that elutes from a chromatography column or can be collected in the retentate or permeate solution of a filtration device relative to the amount applied.

rDNA Technology The rDNA technology relates generally to the manipulation of genetic materials and, more particularly, to recombinant procedures, making possible the production of polypeptides possessing part or all of the primary structural conformation or one or more of the biological properties of naturally-occurring proteins such as erythropoietin.

Reequilibration The equilibration phase after a chromatographic run.

Reference standards International or national standards.

Regeneration Returning the packing in the column to its initial state after gradient elution. Mobile phase is passed through the column stepwise or in a gradient. The stationary phase is solvated to its original condition. In ion-exchange chromatography, regeneration involves replacing ions taken up in the exchange process with the original ions that occupied the exchange sites. Regeneration can also refer to bringing back any column to its original state (e.g., the removal of impurities with a strong solvent).

Relevant genotypic and phenotypic markers Those markers permitting the identification of the strain of the cell line that should include the expression of the recombinant protein or presence of the expression construct.

Relevant virus Virus used in process evaluation studies that is either the identified virus or of the same species as the virus that is known, or likely to contaminate the cell substrate or any other reagents or materials used in the production process.

Residence time The time required for an incremental unit of feed solution to pass through a separations device.

Resin See Medium.

Resolution (Rs) The resolution is defined as the distance between chromatographic peak maxima compared with the average base width of the two peaks. The resolution is a measure of the relative separation between two peaks. Ability of a chromatography media to separate chromatographic peaks. It is usually expressed in terms of the separation of two peaks. Resolution can be calculated as follows: $Rs = 1.18 \times (tR2 - tR1) / (wh1 + wh2)$ where, wh1 = peak width at half height (in units of time) of the first peak; wh2 = peak width at half height (in units of time) of the second peak; tR1 and tR2 refer to the retention times of the first respectively the second peak A value of 1 is considered to be the minimum for a measurable separation to occur and to allow good quantification. Values of 1.7 or larger are generally desirable for rugged methods. Resolution is more important in analytical techniques than in preparatory techniques.

Response elements Response elements are the recognition sites of certain transcription factors. Most of them are located within 1 kb from the transcriptional start site.

Restriction enzyme Bacterial enzyme that cuts DNA molecules at the location of particular sequences of base pairs. The role of these enzymes in bacteria is to "restrict" the invasion of foreign DNA by cutting it into pieces. Hence, these enzymes are known as restriction enzymes. Restriction enzymes, also called restriction nucleases (e.g., EcoRI from *E. coli*), surround the DNA molecule at the point it seeks (sequence GAATTC). It cuts one strand of the DNA double helix at one point and the second strand at a different, complementary point (between the G and the A base). The separated pieces have single stranded "sticky-ends," which allow the complementary pieces to combine.

Restriction map Linear arrangement of various restriction enzyme sites.

Restriction site Base sequence recognized by an enzyme.

Retentate The portion of the feed solution that does not pass through a cross flow membrane filter.

Retention The ability of a separation device to retain particles of a given size.

Retention time The time between injection and the appearance of the peak maximum.

Retention volume The volume of mobile phase required to elute a substance from the column. $VR = Vm - KD\ Vs$ where, Vm = void volume; KD = distribution coefficient; Vs = stationary phase volume.

Retrospective validation Validation of a process for a product already in distribution based upon establishing documented evidence. The review and analysis of historical manufacturing and product testing data that verifies a specific process can be consistently produced meeting its predetermined specifications and quality attributes.

Retrovirus RNA virus that replicates via conversion into a DNA duplex.

Reverse osmosis Type of cross-flow filtration used for removal of very small solutes (< 1000 Daltons) and salts. It uses a semipermeable membrane under high pressure to separate water from ionic materials. High pressure is necessary to overcome the natural osmotic pressure created by the concentration gradient across the membrane.

Reverse phase chromatography A chromatographical separation method based on a column stationary phase coated to give a nonpolar hydrophobic surface. Analyte retention is proportional to hydrophobic reactions between solute and surface. Retention is roughly proportional to the length of the bonded carbon chain. Reversed phase chromatography (RPC) is in theory closely related to hydrophobic interaction chromatography. This is the most common HPLC mode. Mobile phase utilizes water and a water-miscible organic solvent such as methanol or acetonitrile. There are many variations of RPC in which various mobile phase additives are used to gain a different selectivity.

Reverse transcriptase An enzyme that catalyzes the synthesis of DNA from RNA.

Ribosome Cell organelles that translate RNA to build proteins.

RNA polymerase An enzyme that catalyzes the synthesis of RNA in transcription.

RNA processing RNA processing is to generate a mature mRNA (for protein genes) or a functional tRNA or rRNA from the primary transcript.

Robustness The robustness of a procedure is a measure of its capacity to remain unaffected by small, but deliberate variations in method parameters and provides an indication of its reliability during normal usage.

Roller bottle A container with large growth surfaces in which cells can be grown in a confluent monolayer. The bottles are rotated or agitated to keep cells in suspension, but they require extensive handling, labor, and media. In large-scale vaccine production, roller bottles have been replaced by microcarrier culture systems that offer the advantage of scale up.

Running buffer The solution used to perform a chromatographic run.

Sanitization A cleaning process that destroys most living (pathogenic) microorganisms.

Sanitizing agent An agent introduced into a system to kill organisms and prevent the growth of organisms.

Scale up To take a biopharmaceutical manufacturing process from the laboratory scale to a scale at which it is commercially feasible.

SDS PAGE (sodium dodecyl sulfate polyacrylamide gel electrophoresis) An electrophoretic separation of proteins based on their molecular weights. A uniform net negative charge is imposed on the molecules by the addition of SDS. Under these conditions, migration toward the anode through a gel matrix allows separation via size, not charge, with the smaller molecules migrating the longest distance. This technique is not reliable for sizes below a MW of ca. 8000. Proteins are observed via Coomassie blue or silver staining or can be further transferred to membranes for antigen/antibody specificity testing.

Seed stock The initial inoculum, or the cells placed in growth medium from which other cells will grow.

Selectivity Same as separation factor or relative retention ratio. The separation factor is a measure of the time or distance between the maxima of two peaks. If a = 1, then the peaks have the same retention and coelute. a = k2 / k1 where, k1 = retention factor of the first peak; k2 = retention factor of the second peak.

Separation During operation, the separation device divides a liquid or gas feed stream into separate components.

Sequence The precise order of bases in a nucleic acid or amino acids in a protein.

Serum The watery portion of an animal or plant fluid (such as blood) remaining after coagulation. When cheese is made, whey is the milk serum that is left.

Shear rate A ratio of velocity and distance expressed in units of s^1. The shear rate for a hollow fiber cartridge is based on the flow rate through the fiber lumen and can be calculated as follows: $g = 4q/r^3$ where g = shear rate, s^1; q = flow rate through the fiber lumen cm^3s^1; r = fiber radius, cm.

Sieving Removal of particles from a feed stream as a result of entrapment within the depth of the membrane pore structure.

Silencers Silencers are the DNA elements that interact with repressors (proteins) to inhibit transcription. In prokaryotes, silencers are known as operators, found in many genes such as *lac* operon and *trp* operon. In a few cases, a DNA element may act either as enhancer or silencer, depending on the binding protein. For example, certain genes contain an element called E box (consensus CACGTG), which can bind either Max/Myc dimer or Max/Mad dimer. The Max/Myc dimer activates transcription, whereas the Max/Mad dimer suppresses transcription of these genes.

SIP Steam in place or sterilize in place.

Size-exclusion chromatography (SEC) A chromatographic technique in which analytes are excluded from the stationary phase, and thus separated, based on their size.

Size-exclusion membrane separation Mechanism for removing particles from a feed stream. Based strictly on the size of the particles versus the pore size that the feed stream is being filtered through. Retained particles are held back because they are larger than the pore opening.

Slurry A thick mixture of adsorbent and solvent used to pour columns. Excess solvent is drained out as the adsorbent settles and more slurry is added until the column is filled.

Solute An ionic or organic compound dissolved in a solvent, for example, the sugar in a cup of coffee is a solute.

Somatic cell In higher organisms, a cell that (unlike germ cells) carries the full genetic makeup of an organism.

Southern blot (blotting) Technique for transferring DNA fragments from an agarose gel to a nitrocellulose filter on which they can be hybridized to a complementary DNA. Southern blotting is a technique for detecting specific DNA fragments in a complex mixture. The technique was invented in mid-1970s by Edward Southern. It has been applied to detect restriction fragment length polymorphism (RFLP) and variable number of tandem repeat polymorphism (VNTR). The latter is the basis of DNA fingerprinting.

Sparge To spray. A sparger is the component of a fermenter that sprays air into the broth.

Specification A list of tests, references to analytical procedures, and appropriate acceptance criteria that are numerical limits, ranges, or other criteria for the tests described. It establishes the set of criteria to which a drug substance, drug product, or materials at other stages of its manufacture should conform to be considered acceptable for its intended use. Conformance to specification means that the drug substance and drug product, when tested according to the listed analytical procedures, will meet the acceptance criteria. Specifications are critical quality standards that are proposed and justified by the manufacturer and approved by regulatory authorities as conditions of approval.

Specific model virus Virus that is closely related to the known or suspected virus (same genus or family), having similar physical and chemical properties to those of the observed or suspected virus.

Spiking Adding a known amount of substance being measured to a sample in order to determine the original sample concentration by the known addition technique or to determine the accuracy of a direct measurement technique.

Starling flow A portion of filtrate (permeate) that is driven back through the membrane in the reverse direction near the outlet of the cartridge, due to the high permeability of these membranes in the presence of permeate pressure. This phenomenon is most often associated with the operation of microfiltration membranes using permeate flow control.

Steam-in-place (SIP) The process of sterilizing a tank or process device, such as a hollow fiber cartridge, with steam, without removing the device from the separation system.

Stepwise elution Use of eluents of different compositions during the chromatographic run. These eluents are added in a stepwise manner.

Sterilization A process that removes/destroys all (pathogenic) microorganisms from a solution or a solution processing system.

Strain A population of cells all descended from a single cell. A group of organisms of the same species having distinctive characteristics, but not usually considered a separate breed or variety.

Substrate Reactive material, the substance on which an enzyme acts.

Substratum The solid surface on which a cell moves or on which cells grow.

Supernatant Material floating on the surface of a liquid mixture (often the liquid component that has the lowest density).

Surface area In an adsorbent, refers to the total area of the solid surface as determined by an accepted measurement technique such as the BET method using nitrogen adsorption.

Surface filter A filter in which particles larger than the pores are retained on the surface of the filter.

Surfactant Any substance that changes the nature of a surface, such as lowering the surface tension of water.

Suspension Particles floating in (not necessarily on) a liquid medium, or the mix of particles and liquid itself.

Swelling, shrinking Process in which chromatographic resins increase or decrease their volume because of their solvent environment. Swelling is dependent upon the degree of crosslinking; low-cross-linking resins will swell and shrink more than highly cross-linked resins. If swelling occurs in a packed column blockage, increased back pressure can occur, and column efficiency can be affected.

Symbiotic Living together for mutual benefit.

Synthesis Creating products through chemical and enzymatic reactions.

Tailing The phenomenon in which the normal Gaussian peak has an asymmetry factor > 1. The peak will have skew in trailing edge. Tailing is caused by sites on the packing that have a stronger-than-normal retention for the solute.

Tandem repeats Tandem repeats are an array of consecutive repeats of DNA sequence. They include three subclasses: satellites, minisatellites, and microsatellites. The name "satellites" comes from their optical spectra. The size of a satellite DNA ranges from 100 kb to over 1 Mb. In humans, a well-known example is the alphoid DNA located at the centromere of all chromosomes. Its repeat unit is 171 bp and the repetitive region accounts for 3 to 5% of the DNA in each chromosome. Other satellites have a shorter repeat unit. Most satellites in humans or in other organisms are located at the centromere.

Tangential flow filtration Also called cross flow filtration. In tangential flow filtration, the feed solution flows parallel to the surface of the membrane. Driven by pressure, some of the feed solution passes through the membrane filter. Most of the solution is circulated back to the feed tank. The movement of the feed solution across the face of the membrane surface helps to remove the buildup of foulants on the surface.

Telomerase In eukaryotes, the chromosome ends are called telomeres, which have at least two functions: to protect chromosomes from fusing with each other and to solve the end-replication problem. In the absence of telomerase, the telomere will become shorter after each cell division. When it reaches a certain length, the cell may cease to divide and die. Therefore, telomerase plays a critical role in the aging process.

T-helper cells T-lymphocytes with the specific capacity to help other cells, such as B-lymphocytes, to make antibodies. T-helper cells are also required for the induction of other T-lymphocyte activities. Synonym is T inducer cell, T4 cell, or CD4 lymphocyte.

Theoretical plate (N) Column efficiency is expressed by the number of theoretical plates (N). The number of theoretical plates can be calculated using the equation below. Theoretical plates is a concept, and a column does not contain anything resembling physical distillation plates or any other similar feature. Theoretical plate numbers are an indirect measure of peak width for a peak at a specific retention time. Columns with high plate numbers are considered to be more efficient (i.e., higher column efficiency) than columns with lower plate numbers. A column with a high number of plates will have a narrower peak at a given retention time than a column with a lower number of plates. Length of column relating to this concept is called height equivalent to a theoretical plate (HETP). $N = 5.55 \times (tR / w1/2)2$ or $N = 16 \times (tR / wb)2$, Where, tR = retention time, and w1/2 and wb = width of the peak at half the peak height (hp/2).

Thermal stability The ability of a membrane and filtering device to maintain its performance during and after exposure to elevated temperatures; for example, elevated temperature experienced during high-temperature processing or steam sterilization.

Three-dimensional structure The three-dimensional (3D) structure is also called the tertiary structure. If a protein molecule consists of more than one polypeptide, it also has the quaternary structure, which specifies the relative positions among the polypeptides (subunits) in a protein.

Throughput The volume of solution that will pass through a separations device before the filtrate output drops to an unacceptable level. It is also the rate at which a separations system will generate filtrate.

Tissue culture Growing plant or animal tissues outside of the body, as in a nutrient medium in a laboratory; similar to cell culture, but cells are maintained in their structured, tissue form.

Titer A measured sample or to draw a measured, representative sample from a larger amount is to titrate.

Titer reduction The measurement of a filter's ability to remove microbes or virus from a fluid.

Topoisomers During replication, the unwinding of DNA may cause the formation of tangling structures, such as supercoils or catenanes. The major role of topoisomerases is to prevent DNA tangling.

Transcription The first stage in the expression of a gene by means of genetic information being transmitted from the DNA in the chromosomes to messenger RNA. Transcription is a process in which one DNA strand is used as a template to synthesize a complementary RNA. In eukaryotes, there are three classes of RNA polymerases: I, II, and III. In prokaryotes, binding of the polymerase's σ factor to promoter can catalyze unwinding of the DNA double helix. The most important σ factor is Sigma 70, whose structure has been determined by X-ray crystallography, but its complex with DNA has not been solved. After the DNA strands have been separated at the promoter region, the core polymerase (ααββ′) can then start to synthesize RNA based on the sequence of the DNA template strand.

Transduction Transfer of genes from one bacterium to another using a phage (virus).

Transfection Permanently changing a cell using viral DNA.

Transformation Permanent genetic change following incorporation of new DNA.

Transgene A foreign gene incorporated by transformation into the germline.

Transgenics The alteration of plant or animal DNA so that it contains a gene from another organism. There are two types of cells in animals and plants: germ line cells (the sperm and egg in animals, pollen and ovule in plants) and somatic cells (all of the other cells). It is the germline DNA that is altered in transgenic animals and plants, so those alterations are passed on to offspring. Transgenic animals are used to produce therapeutics, to study disease, or to improve livestock strains. Transgenic plants have been created for increased resistance to disease and insects as well as to make biopharmaceuticals.

Translation The process by which information transferred from DNA by RNA specifies the sequence of amino acids in a polypeptide (protein) chain.

Transmembrane Pressure (TMP) The force that drives liquid flow through a cross flow membrane. During filtration, the feed side of the membrane is under higher pressure than the permeate side. The pressure difference forces liquid through the membrane. TMP = {(feed pressure + retentate pressure) / 2} − permeate pressure.

Transplastomic Transformation of plastids.

tRNA translation Translation is a process by which the nucleotide sequence of mRNA is converted into the amino acid sequence of a peptide. It starts from the initiation codon and then follows the mRNA sequence in a strictly "three nucleotides for one amino acid" manner.

Trypsin Trypsin allows the growth of cells as independent microorganisms distinct from tissue culture by causing cell disaggregation. Excised tissue is softened and treated with a proteolytic enzyme, normally trypsin, then washed and suspended in a growth medium to produce a primary culture. Subculturing from the primary culture usually involves treatment with an antitrypsin (such as serum) to produce a secondary culture. Cell lines are established by repeated culture through cycles of growth, trypsinization, and subculture.

Trypsin T-suppressor cells T-lymphocytes with specific capacity to inhibit T- helper cell function.

Tryptic fragment analysis Quantitating the resultant fragments caused by tryptic digestion.

Tubule Tube-like structure (larger ID fibers than hollow fibers) made from ultrafiltration or microfiltration membrane and sealed inside a crossflow cartridge. When in use, the feed stream flows into one end of the tubule and the retentate (the material that does not permeate through the walls of the tubule) flows out the other end. The material that does flow through the membrane (walls of the tubule) is called the permeate.

Tumor necrosis factors Tumor necrosis factors are the cytokines produced mainly by macrophages and T-lymphocytes that help regulate the immune response and hematopoiesis (blood cell formation). There are two types of TNF: TNF-α— also called cachectin, produced by macrophages and TNF-β — also called lymphotoxin, produced by activated CD4+ T-cells.

Turbidity The measure of relative sample clarity of a liquid. Measurements are based on the amount of light transmitted in straight lines through a sample. The more light that is scattered by fine solids or colloids, the less clear (and more turbid) the solution. Often reported in NTU (nephelometric turbidity unit).

Turbidostat A variation on a chemostat. Whereas a chemostat is designed for constant input of medium, a turbidostat is designed to keep the organisms at a constant concentration. A turbidity sensor measures the concentration of organisms in the culture and adds additional medium when a preset value is exceeded. A continuous-mode fermenter in which fresh medium is introduced to keep turbidity constant whey acidic proteins non-casein milk proteins containing eight characteristically spaced cysteine residues.

Turbulent flow field The state that results from mixing the contents of a fermenter or bioreactor to provide oxygen to the cells. That must be balanced against the shear that causes cell damage and death.

Two-dimensional gel electrophoresis A type of electrophoresis in which proteins are separated, first in one direction by charge followed by a size separation in the perpendicular direction.

Ultrafiltration The separation of macrosolutes based on their molecular weight or size. Ultrafiltration is a pressure-driven, convective process using semipermeable membranes to separate macrosolutes based on their molecular weight or size. By removing solvent from solution, solute is concentrated or enriched. UF membranes may also be used for diafiltration to remove salts or other microspecies from solution via repeated or continuous dilution and reconcentration.

Unicellular Composed of only a single cell.

Unprocessed bulk One or multiple pooled harvests of cells and culture media. When cells are not readily accessible, the unprocessed bulk would constitute fluid harvested from the fermenter.

Upstream The feed side of a separation process. Microbial fermentation, insect cell culture mammalian cell culture, animal care, or plant cultivation.

Upstream processing Cellular separations including cell lysates, cell harvesting, clarification, and cell culture perfusion.

UV spectroscopy A quantitation technique for proteins using their distinctive absorption spectra due to the presence of side-chain chromophores (phenylalanine, tryptophan, and tyrosine). Since this absorbance is linear, highly purified proteins can be quantitated by calculations using their molar extinction coefficient.

Vaccines Preparations of antigens from killed or modified organisms that elicit immune response (production of antibodies) to protect a person or animal from the disease-causing agent.

Vacuolation In cell and tissue culture, excess fluid, debris (aggregates), or gas (from sparging) can form inside a cell vacuole. A vacuole is a cavity within the cell that can be relatively clear and fluid filled, gas filled (as in a number of blue-green algae), or food filled (as in protozoa).

Validation Validation is establishing documented evidence that provides a high degree of assurance that a specific system (an interacting or interdependent group of items that function together to achieve a specific function), process, or facility will consistently produce a product meeting its predetermined specifications and quality attributes. Validation can be subdivided into three activities: installation, operational, and performance qualifications.

Validation change control A formal monitoring system by which qualified representatives review proposed or actual changes that might affect validated status and take preventive or corrective action to ensure that the system retains its validated state of control.

Validation protocol A validation protocol is a documented set of instructions designed to confirm specific static or dynamic attributes of the installation, operation, or performance of a utility/system, equipment, or process.

Vector The plasmid, virus, or other vehicle used to carry a DNA sequence into the cell of another species.

Vessel jacket A temperature control method consisting of a double wall outside the main vessel wall. Liquid or steam flows through the jacket to heat (or cool) the fluid in the vessel. Because biopharmaceutical products are so sensitive and vessel jackets can cause uneven heating (hot or cold spots), shell-and-tube or plate-and-frame heat exchangers are more common in biopharmaceutical production systems.

Viability Life and health, ability to grow and reproduce; a measure of the proportion of live cells in a population.

Viral clearance The removal of viral contamination using specialized membranes or chromatography. In order to ensure that therapeutic drugs derived from certain sources are fully rid of any viral contamination, these protein solutions undergo viral clearance to inactivate or remove viral materials.

Virus The simplest form of life: RNA or DNA wrapped in a shell of protein, sometimes with a means of injecting that genetic material into a host organism (infection). Viruses cannot reproduce on their own, but require the aid of a host.

Virus-like particles   Structures visible by electron microscopy that morphologically appear to be related to known viruses.

Virus removal   Physical separation of virus particles from the intended product.

Viscosity   A measurement of a fluid's resistance to shear. A slow-flowing liquid such as gear oil has a higher viscosity than a free-flowing liquid such as mineral spirits. In a given separation process, higher-viscosity, Newtonian fluids, have a lower flow rate through a cartridge than do lower-viscosity fluids.

Void time   The time for elution of an unretained peak (tm or t0).

Void volume (Vi)   The total volume of mobile phase in the column (the remainder of the column is taken up by packing material). It can be determined by injecting an unretained substance that measures void volume plus extra column volume. Also referred to as interstitial volume. Instead of Vi, V0 or Vm are sometimes used as symbols. For example, for nonrigid gels like Superose™, Sephacryl™, and other gel filtration gels, one can estimate the void volume of a column to be approximately 30% of the total bed volume. Also, it is the amount of open space within membrane filter media.

Volumetric flow rate   Units for measuring quantities of a substance by the volume they take up — usually at standard atmospheric (cubic feet, cubic meters).

Wall effect   The consequence of the looser packing density near the walls of the rigid column. Mobile phase has a tendency to flow slightly faster near the wall because of the decreased permeability. The solute molecules that happen to be near the wall are carried along faster than the average of the solute band, and consequently, band spreading results.

Water flux   Measurement of the amount of water that flows through a cartridge. Clean water flux refers to the flux measurement made under standardized conditions on a new (and cleaned) membrane cartridge.

Water-for-injection   Very pure water suitable for medical uses.

Western blot (blotting)   This test is used to detect contaminating cell substrates and to evaluate recombinant polypeptides. After electrophoretic separation, the negatively charged proteins (the antigens) are electrophoretically transferred from the polyacrylamide gel onto a nitrocellulose membrane positioned on the anode side of the gel. Following incubation of the membrane with a specific antibody, they are labeled with another antibody for detection. Western blotting is used to detect a particular protein in a mixture. The probe used is therefore not DNA or RNA, but antibodies. The technique is also called "immunoblotting."

Wetting   The process of filling pores of a hydrophobic membrane with water. Typical methods include use of alcohol as a wetting solution or high pressure to drive air out.

Wobble pairing   See tRNA translation

Working cell bank (WCB)   The WCB is prepared from aliquots of a homogeneous suspension of cells obtained from culturing the master cell bank (MCB) under defined culture conditions. A WCB is created from the MCB by reviving the live cells: thawing and then culturing them on agar medium. From a frozen bank, it may take 2 days to grow enough new cells to begin fermentation. From a lyophilized bank, it can take longer. Refrigerated cultures need only a day or so.

Worst case   A set of conditions encompassing upper and lower processing limits and circumstances, including those within standard operating procedures, which pose the greatest chance of process or product failure, when compared to ideal conditions. Such conditions do not necessarily induce product or process failure.

Yeast   A single-celled fungus.

Yeast artificial chromosome (YAC)   The yeast artificial chromosome (YAC) vector is capable of carrying a large DNA fragment (up to 2 Mb), but its transformation efficiency is very low. A vector constructed from the telomeric, centromeric, and replication origin sequences is needed for replication in yeast cells used to clone pieces of DNA.

Yield The amount of target molecules that can be recovered from cross-flow filtration or chromatography. Also called recovery.

Appendix III
Bibliography

CHAPTER 1: THE FRONTIERS OF BIOTECHNOLOGY AND
CHAPTER 2: MARKETING OPPORTUNITIES

Anton PS, Silberglitt R, Schneider J. *The Global Technology Revolution: Bio/Nano/Materials Trends and Their Synergies with Information Technology by 2015.* RAND, National Defense Research Institute, Arlington, VA, 2001.

Biotech 2030: Eight visions of the future, www.biospace.com/articles/, January 6, 2000.

Biotech mania, research and development in the new millennium, *R&D Magazine* June 1999; 41(7):22–27.

Biotech on the move, *MIT Technology Review* November/December 1999; 102(6):67–69.

Biotech trends 100, *MIT Technology Review* November/December 1999; 102(6):91–92.

Biotechnology for the 21st century, New Horizons, Biotechnology Research Subcommittee, Committee on Fundamental Science, National Science and Technology Council, http://www.nal.usda.gov/bic/bio21/, July 1995.

Biotechnology Industry Organization (BIO), *Introductory Guide to Biotechnology*, 2000, http://www.bio.org/aboutbio/guidetoc.html.

Biotechnology: The science and the impact (conference proceedings), Netherlands Congress Centre, the Hague, http://www.usemb.nl/bioproc.htm, January 20–21, 2000.

Biotechnology, Union of Concerned Scientists, http://www.ucsusa.org/agriculture/biotechnology.html.

Caplan A. Silence = disaster: to succeed biotech will have to answer many vexing ethical questions, Forbes ASAP, http://www.forbes.com/asap/99/0531/082.htm, May 31, 1999, pp. 82–84.

Carey J, Freundlich N, Flynn J, Gross N. The biotech century — there's a revolution brewing in the lab, and the payoff will be breathtaking, *Business Week*, March 10, 1999; (3517):78–90.

Carrington D. How the code was cracked, BBC News Online, http://news.bbc.co.uk/hi/english/in_depth/sci_tech/2000/human_genome/newsid_760000/760849.stm, May 30, 2000.

Cho MK, Magnus D, Chaplain AL, McGee D. Ethical considerations in synthesizing a minimal genome, *Science*, December 10, 1999; 286(5447):2087–2090.

Dennis C, Gallagher R, Campbell P (eds.), The human genome, special issue on the human genome, *Nature*, February 15, 2001; 409(6822):791–794.

Eiseman E. Cloning human beings: recent scientific and policy developments, RAND, MR-1099.0-NBAC, http://www.rand.org/publications/MR/MR1099.pdf, August 1999.

Eisen J. Microbial and plant genomics, Biotechnology: The science and the impact (conference proceedings), Netherlands Congress Centre, the Hague, http://www.usemb.nl/bioproc.htm, January 20–21, 2000.

Global issues: biotechnology, U.S. Department of State, International Information Programs, http://usinfo.state.gov/topical/global/biotech/.

Gorman S. Future pharmers of America, *National Journal*, February 2, 1999; 31(6):355–356.

Gunter B, Kinderlerer J, Beyleveld D. The media and public understanding of biotechnology: a survey of scientists and journalists, *Science Communication*, June 1999; 20(4):373–394.

Hapgood F. Garage biotech is here or just around the corner: will genetic modification for fun and profit become a homegrown industry? *Civilization*, April/May 2000; 46–51.

Hutchinson III CA, Peterson SN, Gill SR, Cline RT, White O, Frazer CM, Smith HO, Venter JC. Transponson mutagenesis and a minimal mycoplasma genome, *Science*, December 10, 1999; 286(5447):2165–2169.

Industry in 2010: beyond the millennium, FT.com life sciences: pharmaceuticals, http://www.ft.com/ftsur-veys/q4b1a.htm, November 17, 1999.

International Human Genome Sequencing Consortium (IHGSC), Initial sequencing and analysis of the human genome, *Nature*, February 15, 2001; 409(6822):860–921.

Jasny BR and Kennedy D. (eds.), The human genome, special issue on the human genome, *Science*, February 16, 2001; 291(5507):.

Lederberg J. Science and technology: biology and biotechnology, *Social Research*, Fall 1997; 64(3):1157–1161.

Logan T, Schibsted E, Frankel A, McGrane S, Amer S. Bioworlds: emerging pharma, it's all about drugs, Forbes ASAP, http://www.forbes.com/asap/99/0531/044.htm, May 31, 1999, pp. 44–57.

Long C. Picture biotechnology: promises and problems, The American Enterprise, http://www.theamericanen-terprise.org/taeso98p.htm, September 1, 1998, pp. 55–58.

Matzke MA and Matzke AJM. Cloning problems don't surprise plant biologists, *Science*, June 30, 2000; 288(5475):2318.

Mironesco C. Parliamentary technology assessment of biotechnologies: a review of major TA reports in the European Union and the USA, *Science and Public Policy*, October 1998; 25(5):327–342.

Morton O. First fruits of the new tree of knowledge, Newsweek.com, February 3, 1999. http://www.newsweek.com.

Pennisi E and Vogel G. Animal cloning: clones: a hard act to follow, *Science*, June 9, 2000; 288(5472):1722–1727.

Pfeiffer EW (ed.), Will biotech top the net? Forbes ASAP, special issue on biotechnology, http://www.forbes.com/asap/99/0531/, May 31, 1999.

Poste G. The conversion of genetics and computing: implications for medicine, society, and individual identity, Presentation to the Science and Technology Policy Institute, Summary by Danilo Pelletiere, www.rand.org/centers/stpi/newsci/Poste.html, April 19, 1999.

PricewaterhouseCoopers LLP, Pharma 2005—an industrial revolution in R&D, 1998. http://www.pwcglobal.com.

PricewaterhouseCoopers LLP, Pharma 2005—silicon rally: the race to e-R&D, 1999. http://www.pwcglobal.com.

Rotman D. The next biotech harvest, *MIT Technology Review*, September/October 1998.

Slavkin HC. Insights on human health: announcing the biotechnology century, National Institute of Dental and Craniofacial Research, www.nidr.nih. gov/slavkin/slav0999.htm, November 11, 1999.

Smith HO, Hutchinson III, CA, Pfannkoch C, Venter, JC. Generating a synthetic genome by whole genome assembly: ΩX174 bacteriophage from synthetic oligonucleotides. *PNAS*, 2003; 100(26):15440–15445.

Stone A. This fund makes biotech bets a bit less risky, *Business Week*, July 12, 1999:20–23.

Systems biology in the post-genomics era, *Signals Magazine*, http://recap/coom.signalsmag.nsf/DP91D8DF, February 2, 2000.

The biotech century, *Business Week*, March 10, 1997:79–92.

The third generation of pharmaceutical research and development: introduction, Glaxo Wellcome, October 21, 1999.

Thiel KA. Big picture biology, www.BioSpace.com/articles/, July 14, 1999.

Venter JC et al., The sequence of the human genome, *Science*, February 16, 2001; 291(5507):1304–1351.

We are now starting the century of biology: already, genetic engineering is transforming medicine and agriculture—and that's just scratching the surface, *Business Week*, http://www.business-week.com/1998/35/b3593020.htm, August 24–31, 1998.

Weiss R. Human cloning's "numbers game," *Washington Post*, October 10, 2000, p. A01.

Zorpette G and Ezzell C (eds.), Your bionic future, *Scientific American Presents*, September 1999.

Zucker LG, Darby MR and Brewer MB, Intellectual human capital and the birth of U.S. biotechnology enterprises, *The American Economic Review*, March 1998; 88(1):290–306.

CHAPTER 3: MANUFACTURING OVERVIEW

Asenjo JA and Patrick I. Large-scale protein purification. In: *Protein Purification Applications. A Practical Approach.* Harris ELV, Angal S, editors. IRL Press, Oxford, 1990: 1–28.

Bõdeker BGD, Newcomb R, Yuan P, Braufman A, Kelsey W. Production of recombinant factor VIII from perfusion cultures: I. Large-scale fermentation. In: *Animal Cell Technology. Products of Today, Prospects for Tomorrow*. Spier RE, Griffiths JB, Berthold W, editors. Butterworth Heinemann, Oxford, 1994: 580–583.

Bylund F, Castan A, Mikkola R, Veide A, Larsson G. Influence of scale-up on the quality of recombinant human growth hormone. *Biotechnol Bioeng* 2000; 69(2):119–128.

Davis CJA. Large-scale chromatography: Design and operation. In: *Bioseparation and bioprocessing*. Vol. I. Biochromatography, membrane separations, modeling, validation. Subramanian G, editor. Wiley-VCH 1998: 125–143.

Gerstner JA. Economics of displacement chromatography — a case study: Purification of oligonucleotides. *BioPharm* 1996; 9(1):30–35.

Janson J-C. Scaling up of affinity chromatography, technological and economical aspects. In: *Affinity Chromatography and Related Techniques*. Gribnau TCJ, editor. Elsevier, Amsterdam, 1982: 503–512.

King LA and Possee RD. Scaling up the production of recombinant protein in insect cells; laboratory bench level. In: *The Baculovirus Expression System. A Laboratory Guide*. Chapman and Hall, London, 1992: 171–179.

Munshi CB, Fryxell KB, Lee HC, Branton WD. Large-scale production of human CD38 in yeast by fermentation. *Methods Enzymol* 1997; 280:318–330.

Rathore AS, Latham P, Levine H, Curling J, Kaltenbrunner O. Costing issues in the production of biopharmaceuticals. *BioPharm International* 2004; 17(2):46–55.

Sadana A and Beelaram AM. Efficiency and economics of bioseparation: some case studies. *Bioseparation* 1994; 4(4):221–235.

Sofer G, Hagel L. Economy. In: *Handbook of Process Chromatography: A Guide to Optimization, Scale-Up and Validation*. Academic Press, San Diego, CA, 1997: 227–243.

Sofer G and Hagel L. *Handbook of Process Chromatography: A Guide to Optimization, Scale-Up and Validation*. Academic Press, San Diego, CA, 1997.

Sofer GK and Nystrom LE. Economics. In: *Process Chromatography. A Practical Guide*. Sofer GK, Nystrom LE, editors. Academic Press, London, 1989: 107–116.

Sofer GK and Nystrom LE. *Process Chromatography. A Practical Guide*. Academic Press, London, 1989.

Walter JK. Strategies and considerations for advanced economy in downstream processing of biopharmaceutical proteins. In: *Bioseparation and Bioprocessing* Vol. II. *Processing, Quality and Characterization, Economics, Safety and Hygiene*. Subramanian G, editor. Wiley-VCH 1998: 447–460.

Walter JK, Werz W, Berthold W. Process scale considerations in evaluation studies and scale-up. *Dev Biol Stand* 1996; 88:99–108.

Walter JK, Werz W, Berthold W. Virus removal and inactivation — concept and data for process validation of downstream processing. *Biotech Forum Europe* 1992; 9:560–564.

Warner TN and Nochumsen S. Rethinking the economics of chromatography. New technologies and hidden costs. *BioPharm International* 2003; 16(1):58–60.

Wheelwright SM. *Protein Purification: Design and Scale-Up of Downstream Processing*. John Wiley and Sons, 1993.

Yamamoto S, Nomura M, Sano Y. Resolution of proteins in linear gradient elution ion-exchange and hydrophobic interaction chromatography. *J Chromatogr* 1987; 409:101–110.

CHAPTER 4: GENETICALLY MODIFIED CELLS

Abrahmsen L, Moks T, Nilsson B, Uhlén M. Secretion of heterologous gene products to the culture medium of *Escherichia coli*. *Nucleic Acids Res* 1986; 14:7487–7500.

Adams JM. On the release of the formyl group from nascent protein. *J Mol Biol* 1968; 33:571–589.

Adams TE, MacIntosh B, Brandon MR, Wordsworth P, Puri NK. Production of methionyl-minus ovine growth hormone in *Escherichia coli* and one-step purification. *Gene* 1992; 122:371–375.

Adari H, Andrews B, Ford PJ, Hannig G, Brosius J, Makrides SC. Expression of the human T-cell receptor V5.3 in *Escherichia coli* by thermal induction of the trc promoter: nucleotide sequence of the lacIts gene. *DNA Cell Biol* 1995; 14:945–950.

Adhya S and Gottesman M. Promoter occlusion: transcription through a promoter may inhibit its activity. *Cell* 1982; 29:939–944.

Airenne KJ and Kulomaa MS. Rapid purification of recombinant proteins fused to chicken avidin. *Gene* 1995; 167:63–68.

Amann E, Brosius J, Ptashne M. Vectors bearing a hybrid trp-lac promoter useful for regulated expression of cloned genes in *Escherichia coli*. *Gene* 1983; 25:167–178.

Amrein KE, Takacs B, Stieger M, Molnos J, Flint NA, Burn P. Purification and characterization of recombinant human p50csk protein-tyrosine kinase from an *Escherichia coli* expression system overproducing the bacterial chaperones GroES and GroEL. *Proc Natl Acad Sci USA* 1995; 92:1048–1052.

Anderson KP, Low MA, Lie YS, Keller GA, Dinowitz M. Endogenous origin of defective retroviruslike particles from a recombinant Chinese hamster ovary cell line. *Virology* 1991; 181(1):305–311.

Andrews B, Adari H, Hannig G, Lahue E, Gosselin M, Martin S, Ahmed A, Ford JP, Hayman EG, Makrides SC. A tightly regulated high level expression vector that utilizes a thermosensitive lac repressor: production of the human T cell receptor V5.3 in *Escherichia coli*. *Gene* 1996; (182):101–109.

Aranha H. Viral clearance strategies for biopharmaceutical safety. Part 1: General considerations. *BioPharm* 2001; 14(1):28–35.

Ariga O, Andoh Y, Fujishita Y, Watari T, Sano Y. Production of thermophilic-amylase using immobilized transformed *Escherichia coli* by addition of glycine. J Ferment Bioeng 1991; 71:397–402.

Aristidou AA, San K-Y, Bennett GN. Modification of central metabolic pathway in *Escherichia coli* to reduce acetate accumulation by heterologous expression of the *Bacillus subtilis* acetolactate synthase gene. *Biotechnol Bioeng* 1994; 44:944–951.

Aristidou AA, San K-Y, Bennett GN. Metabolic engineering of *Escherichia coli* to enhance recombinant protein production through acetate reduction. *Biotechnol Prog* 1995; 11:475–478.

Aristidou AA, Yu P, San K-Y. Effects of glycine supplement on protein production and release in recombinant *Escherichia coli*. *Biotechnol Lett* 1995; 15:331–336.

Bachmair A, Finley D, Varshavsky A. *In vivo* half-life of a protein is a function of its amino-terminal residue. *Science* 1986; 234:179–186.

Bachmair A and Varshavsky A. The degradation signal in a short-lived protein. *Cell* 1989; 56:1019–1032.

Backman K, O'Connor MJ, Maruya A, Ere M. Use of synchronous site-specific recombination *in vivo* to regulate gene expression. *BioTechnol* 1984; 2:1045–1049.

Backman K and Ptashne M. Maximizing gene expression on a plasmid using recombination *in vitro*. *Cell* 1978; 13:65–71.

Backman K, Ptashne M, Gilbert W. Construction of plasmids carrying the cI gene of bacteriophage. *Proc Natl Acad Sci USA* 1976; 73:4174–4178.

Baker RT, Smith SA, Marano R, McKee J, Board PG. Protein expression using cotranslational fusion and cleavage of ubiquitin. Mutagenesis of the glutathione-binding site of human Pi class glutathione S-transferase. *J Biol Chem* 1994; 269:25381–25386.

Baker TA, Grossman AD, Gross CA. A gene regulating the heat shock response in *Escherichia coli* also affects proteolysis. *Proc Natl Acad Sci USA* 1984; 81:6779–6783.

Balakrishnan R, Bolten B, Backman KC. A gene cassette for adapting *Escherichia coli* strains as hosts for att-Int-mediated rearrangement and pL expression vectors. *Gene* 1994; 138:101–104.

Balbas P and Bolivar F. Design and construction of expression plasmid vectors in *Escherichia coli*. *Methods Enzymol* 1990; 185:14–37.

Baneyx F and Georgiou G. Construction and characterization of *Escherichia coli* strains deficient in multiple secreted proteases: protease III degrades high-molecular-weight substrates *in vivo*. *J Bacteriol* 1991; 173:2696–2703.

Baneyx F and Georgiou G. Degradation of secreted proteins in *Escherichia coli*. *Ann NY Acad Sci* 1992; 665:301–308.

Baneyx F and Georgiou G. Expression of proteolytically sensitive polypeptides in *Escherichia coli*. In: *Stability of Protein Pharmaceuticals. A. Chemical and Physical Pathways of Protein Degradation*. Ahern TJ and Manning MC, editors. Plenum Press, New York, 1992: 69–108.

Bardwell JCA. Building bridges: disulfide bond formation in the cell. Mol Microbiol 1994; 14:199–205.

Bardwell JCA, McGovern K, Beckwith J. Identification of a protein required for disulfide bond formation *in vivo*. *Cell* 1991; 67:581–589.

Barrick DK, Villanueba K, Childs J, Kalil R, Schneider D Lawrence CE, Gold L, Stormo GD. Quantitative analysis of ribosome binding sites in *E. coli*. *Nucleic Acids Res* 1994; 22:1287–1295.

Battistoni A, Carri MT, Steinkuhler C, Rotilio G. Chaperonins dependent increase of Cu,Zn superoxide dismutase production in *Escherichia coli*. *FEBS Lett* 1993; 322:6–9.

Bauer KA, Ben-Bassat A, Dawson M, de la Puente VT, Neway JO. Improved expression of human interleukin-2 in high-cell-density fermentor cultures of *Escherichia coli* K-12 by a phosphotransacetylase mutant. *Appl Environ Microbiol* 1990; 56:1296–1302.

Bechhofer D. 5 mRNA stabilizers. In: *Control of Messenger RNA Stability*. Belasco JG and Brawerman G, editors. Academic Press, Inc., San Diego, CA, 1993: 31–52.

Bechhofer DH and Dubnau D. Induced mRNA stability in *Bacillus subtilis*. *Proc Natl Acad Sci USA* 1987; 84:498–502.

Becker J and Craig EA. Heat-shock proteins as molecular chaperones. *Eur J Biochem* 1994; 219:11–23.

Bedouelle H and Duplay P. Production in *Escherichia coli* and one-step purification of bifunctional hybrid proteins which bind maltose. Export of the Klenow polymerase into the periplasmic space. *Eur J Biochem* 1988; 171:541–549.

Belasco JG. mRNA degradation in prokaryotic cells: an overview. In: *Control of Messenger RNA Stability*. Belasco JG and Brawerman G, editors. Academic Press, Inc., San Diego, CA 1993: 3–12.

Belasco JG and Brawerman G, editors. *Control of Messenger RNA Stability*. Academic Press, Inc., San Diego, CA, 1993.

Belasco JG and Higgins CF. Mechanisms of mRNA decay in bacteria: a perspective. *Gene* 1988; 72:15–23.

Belasco JG, Nilsson G, von Gabain A, Cohen SN. The stability of *E. coli* gene transcripts is dependent on determinants localized to specific mRNA segments. *Cell* 1986; 46:245–251.

Belt A. Characterization of cultures used for biotechnology and industry. In: *Maintaining Cultures for Biotechnology and Industry*. Hunter-Cevera JC and Belt A, editors. Academic Press, New York, 1996: 251–258.

Ben-Bassat A, Bauer K, Chang S-Y, Myambo K, Boosman A, Chang S. Processing of the initiation methionine from proteins: properties of the *Escherichia coli* methionine aminopeptidase and its gene structure. *J Bacteriol* 1987; 169:751–757.

Bentley WE, Mirjalili N, Andersen DC, Davis RH, Kompala DS. Plasmid-encoded protein: the principal factor in the "metabolic burden" associated with recombinant bacteria. *Biotechnol. Bioeng* 1990; 35:668–681.

Berg KL, Squires C, Squires CL. Ribosomal RNA operon antitermination. Function of leader and spacer region boxB-boxA sequences and their conservation in diverse microorganisms. *J Mol Biol* 1989; 209:345–358.

Berkow R. (ed.). *The Merck Manual of Diagnosis and Therapy*, 16th ed. Merck Research Laboratories, Rahway, NJ 1992: 24–30.

Bernard, H-U, Remaut E, Hersheld MV, Das HK, Helinski DR, Yanofsky C, Franklin N. Construction of plasmid cloning vehicles that promote gene expression from the bacteriophage lambda pL promoter. *Gene* 1979; 5:59–76.

Better M, Chang CP, Robinson RR, Horwitz AH. *Escherichia coli* secretion of an active chimeric antibody fragment. *Science* 1988; 240:1041–1043.

Betton J-M and Hofnung M. Folding of a mutant maltose-binding protein of *Escherichia coli* which forms inclusion bodies. *J Biol Chem* 1996; 271:8046–8052.

Birikh KR, Lebedenko EN, Boni IV, Berlin YA. A high-level prokaryotic expression system: synthesis of human interleukin 1 and its receptor antagonist. *Gene* 1995; 164:341–345.

Bishai WR, Rappuoli R, Murphy JR. High-level expression of a proteolytically sensitive diphtheria toxin fragment in *Escherichia coli*. *J Bacteriol* 1987; 169:5140–5151.

Björnsson A, Mottagui-Tabar S, Isaksson LA. Structure of the C-terminal end of the nascent peptide influences translation termination. *EMBO J* 1996; 15:1696–1704.

Blackwell JR and Horgan R. A novel strategy for production of a highly expressed recombinant protein in an active form. *FEBS Lett* 1991; 295:10–12.

Blight MA, Chervaux C, Holland IB. Protein secretion pathways in *Escherichia coli*. *Curr Opin Biotechnol* 1994; 5:468–474.

Blondel A, Nageotte R, Bedouelle H. Destabilizing interactions between the partners of a bifunctional fusion protein. *Protein Eng* 1996; 9:231–238.

Blum P, Ory J, Bauernfeind J, Krska J. Physiological consequences of DnaK and DnaJ overproduction in *Escherichia coli*. *J Bacteriol* 1992; 174:7436–7444.

Blum P, Velligan M, Lin N, Matin A. DnaK-mediated alterations in human growth hormone protein inclusion bodies. *BioTechnol* 1992; 10:301–304.

Boni IV, Isaeva DM, Musychenko ML, Tzareva NV. Ribosome-messenger recognition: mRNA target sites for ribosomal protein S1. *Nucleic Acids Res* 1991; 19:155–162.

Bowden GA and Georgiou G. The effect of sugars on β-lactamase aggregation in *Escherichia coli*. *Biotechnol Prog* 1988; 4:97–101.

Bowden GA and Georgiou G. Folding and aggregation of β-lactamase in the periplasmic space of *Escherichia coli*. *J Biol Chem* 1990; 265:16760–16766.

Bowden GA, Baneyx F, Georgiou G. Abnormal fractionation of β-lactamase in *Escherichia coli*: evidence for an interaction of β-lactamase with the inner membrane in the absence of a leader peptide. *J Bacteriol* 1992; 174:3407–3410.

Bowden GA, Paredes AM, Georgiou G. Structure and morphology of protein inclusion bodies in *Escherichia coli*. *BioTechnol* 1991; 9:725–730.

Bowie JU. and Sauer RT. Identification of C-terminal extensions that protect proteins from intracellular proteolysis. *J Biol Chem* 1989; 264:7596–7602.

Brenner S, Jacob F, Meselson M. An unstable intermediate carrying information from genes to ribosomes for protein synthesis. *Nature* (London) 1961; 190:576–581.

Brewer SJ and Sassenfeld HM. The purification of recombinant proteins using C-terminal polyarginine fusions. *Trends Biotechnol* 1985; 3:119–122.

Brinkmann U, Mattes RE, Buckel P. High-level expression of recombinant genes in *Escherichia coli* is dependent on the availability of the dnaY gene product. *Gene* 1989; 85:109–114.

Brizzard BL, Chubet RG, Vizard DL. Immunoaffinity purification of FLAG epitope-tagged bacterial alkaline phosphatase using a novel monoclonal antibody and peptide elution. *BioTech* 1994; 16:730–734.

Brosius J. Compilation of superlinker vectors. *Methods Enzymol* 1992; 216:469–483.

Brosius J and Holy A. Regulation of ribosomal RNA promoters with a synthetic lac operator. *Proc Natl Acad Sci USA* 1984; 81:6929–6933.

Brosius J, Ere M, Storella J. Spacing of the 10 and 35 regions in the tac promoter. Effect on its *in vivo* activity. *J Biol Chem* 1985; 260:3539–3541.

Brosius J, Ullrich A, Raker MA, Gray A, Dull TJ, Gutell RG, Noller F. Construction and fine mapping of recombinant plasmids containing the rrnB ribosomal RNA operon of *E. coli*. Plasmid 1981; 6:112–118.

Brown WC and Campbell JL. A new cloning vector and expression strategy for genes encoding proteins toxic to *Escherichia coli*. *Gene* 1993; 127:99–103.

Buchner J. Supervising the fold: functional principles of molecular chaperones. *FASEB J* 1996; 10:10–19.

Buell G, Schulz M-F, Selzer G, Chollet A, Movva NR, Semon D, Escanez S, Kawashima E. Optimizing the expression in *E. coli* of a synthetic gene encoding somatomedin-C (IGF-I). *Nucleic Acids Res* 1985; 13:1923–1938.

Bujard H, Gentz R, Lanzer M, Stueber D, Mueller M, Ibrahimi I, Haeuptle M-T, Dobberstein B. A T5 promoter-based transcription-translation system for the analysis of proteins *in vitro* and *in vivo*. *Methods Enzymol* 1987; 155:416–433.

Bukrinsky MI, Barsov EV, Shilov AA. Multicopy expression vector based on temperature-regulated lac repressor: expression of human immunodeficiency virus env gene in *Escherichia coli*. *Gene* 1988; 70:415–417.

Bula C and Wilcox KW. Negative effect of sequential serine codons on expression of foreign genes in *Escherichia coli*. *Protein Expression Purif* 1996; 7:92–103.

Bulmer M. Codon usage and intragenic position. *J Theor Biol* 1988; 133:67–71.

Butler JS, Springer M, Grunberg-Manago M. AUU-to-AUG mutation in the initiator codon of the translation initiator factor IF3 abolishes translational autocontrol of its own gene (infC) *in vivo*. *Proc Natl Acad Sci USA* 1987; 84:4022–4025.

Cabilly S. Growth at sub-optimal temperatures allows the production of functional, antigen-binding Fab fragments in *Escherichia coli*. *Gene* 1989; 85:553–557.

Carter P. Site-specific proteolysis of fusion proteins. In: *Protein Purification: From Molecular Mechanisms to Large-Scale Processes*. Ladisch MR, Willson RC, Painton C-C, Builder SE, editors. American Chemical Society Symposium Series no. 427. American Chemical Society, Washington, DC 1990: 181–193.

Caspers P, Stieger M, Burn P. Overproduction of bacterial chaperones improves the solubility of recombinant protein tyrosine kinases in *Escherichia coli. Cell Mol Biol* 1994, 40:635–644.

Caulcott CA and Rhodes M. Temperature-induced synthesis of recombinant proteins. *Trends Biotechnol* 1986; 4:142–146.

Chale M, Tu Y, Euskirchen G, Ward, WW, Prasher DC. Green fluorescent protein as a marker for gene expression. *Science* 1994; 263:802–805.

Chalmers JJ, Kim E, Telford JN, Wong EY, Tacon WC, Shuler LM, Wilson DB. Effects of temperature on *Escherichia coli* overproducing β-lactamase or human epidermal growth factor. *Appl Environ Microbiol* 1990; 56:104–111.

Chamberlin MJ. New models for the mechanism of transcription elongation and its regulation. *Harvey Lect* 1994; 88:1–21.

Chang CN, Kuang W-J, Chen EY. Nucleotide sequence of the alkaline phosphatase gene of *Escherichia coli. Gene* 1986; 44:121–125.

Charbit A, Molla A, Saurin W, Hofnung M. Versatility of a vector for expressing foreign polypeptides at the surface of gram-negative bacteria. *Gene* 1988; 70:181–189.

Chau V, Tobias JW, Bachmair A, Marriott D, Ecker D, Gonda DK, Varshavsky A. A multiubiquitin chain is confined to a specific lysine in a targeted short-lived protein. *Science* 1989, 243:1576–1583.

Cheah KC, Harrison S, King R, Crocker L, Wells JRE, Robins A. Secretion of eukaryotic growth hormones in *Escherichia coli* is influenced by the sequence of the mature proteins. *Gene* 1994; 138:9–15.

Chen BPC and Hai TW. Expression vectors for affinity purification and radiolabeling of proteins using *Escherichia coli* as host. *Gene* 1994; 139:73–75.

Chen C-YA, Beatty JT, Cohen SN, Belasco JG. An intercistronic stem-loop structure functions as an mRNA decay terminator necessary but insufficient for puf mRNA stability. *Cell* 1988; 52:609–619.

Chen C-YA and Belasco JG. Degradation of puf LMX mRNA in Rhodobacter capsulatus is initiated by nonrandom endonucleolytic cleavage. *J Bacteriol* 1990; 172:4578–4586.

Chen G-FT and Inouye M. Suppression of the negative effect of minor arginine codons on gene expression: preferential usage of minor codons within the rst 25 codons of the *Escherichia coli* genes. *Nucleic Acids Res* 1990; 18:1465–1473.

Chen G-FT and Inouye M. Role of the AGA/AGG codons, the rarest codons in global gene expression in *Escherichia coli. Genes Dev* 1994; 8:2641–2652.

Chen HY, Bjerknes M, Kumar R, Jay E. Determination of the optimal aligned spacing between the Shine-Dalgarno sequence and the translation initiation codon of *Escherichia coli* mRNAs. *Nucleic Acids Res* 1994; 22:4953–4957.

Chen HY, Pomeroy-Cloney L, Bjerknes M, Tam J, Jay E. The influence of adenine-rich motifs in the 3 portion of the ribosome binding site on human IFN- gene expression in *Escherichia coli. J Mol Biol* 1994; 240:20–27.

Chen K-S, Peters TC, Walker JR. A minor arginine tRNA mutant limits translation preferentially of a protein dependent on the cognate codon. *J Bacteriol* 1990; 172:2504–2510.

Chen L-H, Emory SA, Bricker AL, Bouvet P, Belasco JG. Structure and function of a bacterial mRNA stabilizer: Analysis of the 5 untranslated region of ompA mRNA. *J Bacteriol* 1991; 173:4578–4586.

Chen W, Kallio PT, Bailey JE. Construction and characterization of a novel cross-regulation system for regulating cloned gene expression in *Escherichia coli. Gene* 1993; 130:15–22.

Chen W, Kallio PT, Bailey JE. Process characterization of a novel cross-regulation system for cloned protein production in *Escherichia coli. Biotechnol Prog* 1995; 11:397–402.

Cheng Y-SE, Kwoh DY, Kwoh TJ, Soltvedt BC, Zipser D. Stabilization of a degradable protein by its overexpression in *Escherichia coli. Gene* 1981; 14:121–130.

Chesshyre JA and Hipkiss AR. Low temperatures stabilize interferon-2 against proteolysis in *Methylophilus methylotrophus* and *Escherichia coli. Appl Microbiol Biotechnol* 1989; 31:158–162.

Chopra AK, Brasier AR, Das M, Xu X-J, Peterson JW. Improved synthesis of *Salmonella typhimurium* enterotoxin using gene fusion expression systems. *Gene* 1994; 144:81–85.

Chou C-H, Aristidou AA, Meng S-Y, Bennett GN, San K-Y. Characterization of a pH-inducible promoter system for high-level expression of recombinant proteins in *Escherichia coli. Biotechnol Bioeng* 1995; 47:186–192.

Chou C-H, Bennett GN, San K-Y. Effect of modified glucose uptake using genetic engineering techniques on high-level recombinant protein production in *Escherichia coli* dense cultures. *Biotechnol Bioeng* 1994; 44:952–960.

Clarke AR. Molecular chaperones in protein folding and translocation. *Curr Opin Struct Biol* 1996; 6:43–50.

Cloney LP, Bekkaoui DR, Hemmingsen SM. Coexpression of plastid chaperonin genes and a synthetic plant Rubisco operon in *Escherichia coli*. *Plant Mol Biol* 1993; 23:1285–1290.

Cole PA. Chaperone-assisted protein expression. *Structure* 1996; 4:239–242.

Coleman J, Inouye M, Nakamura K. Mutations upstream of the ribosome-binding site affect translational efficiency. *J Mol Biol* 1985; 181:139–143.

Collier DN, Strobel SM, Bassford Jr. JP. SecB-independent export of *Escherichia coli* ribose-binding protein (RBP): some comparisons with export of maltose-binding protein (MBP) and studies with RBP-MBP hybrid proteins. J Bacteriol 1990; 172:6875–6884.

Collins-Racie M, Follettie T, Williams MJ, McCoy JM. Histidine patch thioredoxins. Mutant forms of thioredoxin with metal chelating affinity that provide for convenient purifications of thioredoxin fusion proteins. *J Biol Chem* 1996; 271:5059–5065.

Collins-Racie LA, McColgan JM, Grant KL, DiBlasio-Smith EA, Coy J, LaVallie ER. Production of recombinant bovine enterokinase catalytic subunit in *Escherichia coli* using the novel secretory fusion partner DsbA. *BioTechnol* 1995; 13:982–987.

Condon C, Squires C, Squires CL. Control of rRNA transcription in *Escherichia coli*. *Microbiol Rev* 1995; 59:623–645.

Cornelis P, Sierra JC, Lim Jr. A, Malur A, Tungpradabkul S, Tazka H, Leitao A, Martins CV, di Perna C, Brys L, De Baetselier P, Hamers, R. Development of new cloning vectors for the production of immunogenic outer membrane fusion proteins in *Escherichia coli*. *BioTechnol* 1996; 14:203–208.

Craigen WJ, Lee CC, Caskey CT. Recent advances in peptide chain termination. *Mol Microbiol* 1990; 4:861–865.

Crameri A, Whitehorn AE, Tate E, Stemmer WPC. Improved green fluorescent protein by molecular evolution using DNA shuffling. *Nat Biotechnol* 1996; 14:315–319.

Cronan JE, Jr. Biotination of proteins *in vivo*. A post-translational modification to label, purify, and study proteins. *J Biol Chem* 1990; 265:10327–10333.

Cull MG, Miller JF, Schatz PJ. Screening for receptor ligands using large libraries of peptides linked to the C terminus of the lac repressor. *Proc Natl Acad Sci USA* 1992; 89:1865–1869.

Cumming DA. Improper glycosylation and the cellular editing of nascent proteins. In: *Stability of Protein Pharmaceuticals. B. In vivo Pathways of Degradation and Strategies for Protein Stabilization.* Ahern TJ and Manning MC, editors. Plenum Press, New York, 1992: 1–42.

d'Aubenton Carafa Y, Brody E, Thermes C. Prediction of rho-independent *Escherichia coli* transcription terminators. A statistical analysis of their RNA stem-loop structures. *J Mol Biol* 1990; 216:835–858.

Dalbøge H, Dahl H-HM, Pedersen J, Hansen JW, Christensen T. A novel enzymatic method for production of authentic hGH from an *Escherichia coli* produced hGH-precursor. *BioTechnol* 1987; 5:161–164.

Dale GE, Broger C, Langen H, D'Arcy A, Stuber D. Improving protein solubility through rationally designed amino acid replacements: solubilization of the trimethoprim-resistant type S1 dihydrofolate reductase. *Protein Eng* 1994; 7:933–939.

Dale GE, Schönfeld HJ, Langen H, Stieger M. Increased solubility of trimethoprim-resistant type S1 DHFR from *Staphylococcus aureus* in *Escherichia coli* cells overproducing the chaperonins GroEL and GroES. *Protein Eng* 1994; 7:925–931.

Das A. Overproduction of proteins in *Escherichia coli*: vectors, hosts, and strategies. *Methods Enzymol* 1990; 182:93–112.

Datar RV, Cartwright T, Rosen C-G. Process economics of animal cell and bacterial fermentations: a case study analysis of tissue plasminogen activator. *BioTechnol* 1993; 11:349–357.

de Boer HA, Comstock LJ, Vasser M. The tac promoter: a functional hybrid derived from the trp and lac promoters. *Proc Natl Acad Sci USA* 1983; 80:21–25.

de Boer HA and Kastelein RA. Biased codon usage: an exploration of its role in optimization of translation. In: *Maximizing Gene Expression*. Reznikoff WS and Gold L, editors. Butterworths, Boston. 1986: 225–285.

de la Torre JC, Ortin J, Domingo E, Delamarter J, Allet B, Davies J, Bertrand KP, Wray Jr., LV, Reznikoff WS. Plasmid vectors based on Tn10 DNA: gene expression regulated by tetracycline. *Plasmid* 1984; 12:103–110.

de Smit MH and van Duin J. Secondary structure of the ribosome binding site determines translational efficiency: a quantitative analysis. *Proc Natl Acad Sci USA* 1990; 87:7668–7672.

de Smit MH and van Duin J. Control of translation by mRNA secondary structure in *Escherichia coli*. A quantitative analysis of literature data. *J Mol Biol* 1994; 244:144–150.

de Smit MH and van Duin J. Translational initiation on structured messengers. Another role for the Shine-Dalgarno interaction. *J Mol Biol* 1994; 235:173–184.

De Sutter K, Hostens K, Vandekerckhove J, Fiers W. Production of enzymatically active rat protein disulfide isomerase in *Escherichia coli*. *Gene* 1994; 141:163–170.

Del Tito Jr., BJ, Ward JM, Hodgson J, Gershater CJL, Edwards H, Wysocki LA, Watson FA, Sathe G, Kane JF. Effects of a minor isoleucyl tRNA on heterologous protein translation in *Escherichia coli*. *J Bacteriol* 1995; 177:7086–7091.

Denèe P, Kovarik S, Ciora T, Gosselet N, Bénichou J-C, Latta M, Guinet F, Ryter A, Mayaux J-F. Heterologous protein export in *Escherichia coli*: influence of bacterial signal peptides on the export of human interleukin 1. *Gene* 1989; 85:499–510.

Derman AI, Prinz WA, Belin D, Beckwith J. Mutations that allow disulfide bond formation in the cytoplasm of *Escherichia coli*. *Science* 1993; 262:1744–1747.

Derom C, Gheysen D, Fiers W. High-level synthesis in *Escherichia coli* of the SV40 small-t antigen under the control of the bacteriophage lambda pL promoter. *Gene* 1982; 17:45–54.

Derynck R, Remaut E, Saman E, Stanssens P, De Clercq E, Content J, Fiers W. Expression of human fibroblast interferon gene in *Escherichia coli*. *Nature* (London) 1980; 287:193–197.

Deuschle U, Kammerer W, Gentz R, Bujard H. Promoters of *Escherichia coli*: a hierarchy of *in vivo* strength indicates alternate structures. *EMBO J* 1986; 5:2987–2994.

Devlin PE, Drummond JR, Toy P, Mark DF, Watt KWK, Devlin JJ. Alteration of amino-terminal codons of human granulocyte-colony-stimulating factor increases expression levels and allows efficient processing by methionine aminopeptidase in *Escherichia coli*. *Gene* 1988; 65:13–22.

di Guan C, Li P, Riggs PD, Inouye H. Vectors that facilitate the expression and purification of foreign peptides in *Escherichia coli* by fusion to maltose-binding protein. *Gene* 1988; 67:21–30.

Doherty AJ, Connolly BA, Worrall AF. Overproduction of the toxic protein, bovine pancreatic DNaseI, in *Escherichia coli* using a tightly controlled T7-promoter-based vector. *Gene* 1993; 136:337–340.

Donovan WP and Kushner SR. Amplification of ribonuclease II (rnb) activity in *Escherichia coli* K-12. *Nucleic Acids Res* 1983; 11:265–275.

Donovan WP and Kushner SR. Polynucleotide phosphorylase and ribonuclease II are required for cell viability and mRNA turnover in *Escherichia coli* K-12. *Proc Natl Acad Sci USA* 1986; 83:120–124.

Dreyfus M. What constitutes the signal for the initiation of protein synthesis on *Escherichia coli* mRNAs? *J Mol Biol* 1988; 204:79–94.

Dubendorff JW and Studier FW. Controlling basal expression in an inducible T7 expression system by blocking the target T7 promoter with lac repressor. *J Mol Biol* 1991; 219:45–59.

Duffaud GD, March PE, Inouye M. Expression and secretion of foreign proteins in *Escherichia coli*. *Methods Enzymol* 1987; 153:492–507.

Duvoisin RM, Belin D, Krisch HM. A plasmid expression vector that permits stabilization of both mRNAs and proteins encoded by the cloned genes. *Gene* 1986; 45:193–201.

Dykes CW, Bookless AB, Coomber BA, Noble SA, Humber DC, Hobden AN. Expression of atrial natriuretic factor as a cleavable fusion protein with chloramphenicol acetyltransferase in *Escherichia coli*. *Eur J Biochem* 1988; 174:411–416.

Easton AM., Gierse JK, Seetharam R, Klein BK, Kotts CE. Production of bovine insulin-like growth factor 2 (bIGF2) in *Escherichia coli*. *Gene* 1991; 101:291–295.

Edalji R, Pilot-Matias TJ, Pratt SD, Egan DA, Severin JM, Gubbins EG, Petros AM, Fesik SW, Burres NS, Holzman TF. High-level expression of recombinant human FK-binding protein from a fusion precursor. *J Protein Chem* 1992; 11:213–223.

Ehretsmann CP, Carpousis AJ, Krisch HM. mRNA degradation in procaryotes. *FASEB J* 1992; 6:3186–3192.

Eliasson M, Olsson A, Palmcrantz E, Wiberg K, Inganas M, Guss B, Lindberg M, Uhlén M. Chimeric IgG-binding receptors engineered from staphylococcal protein A and streptococcal protein G *J Biol Chem* 1988; 263:4323–4327.

Ellis RJ and Hartl FU. Protein folding in the cell: competing models of chaperonin function. *FASEB J* 1996; 10:20–26.

Elvin CM, Thompson PR, Argall ME, Hendry P, Stamford NPJ, Lilley E, Dixon NE. Modified bacteriophage lambda promoter vectors for overproduction of proteins in *Escherichia coli*. *Gene* 1990; 87:123–126.

Emory SA and Belasco JG. The ompA 5 untranslated RNA segment functions in *Escherichia coli* as a growth-rate-regulated mRNA stabilizer whose activity is unrelated to translational efficiency. *J Bacteriol* 1990; 172:4472–4481.

Emory SA, Bouvet P, Belasco JG. A 5-terminal stem-loop structure can stabilize mRNA in *Escherichia coli*. *Genes Dev* 1992; 6:135–148.

Enfors S-O. Control of *in vivo* proteolysis in the production of recombinant proteins. *Trends Biotechnol* 1992; 10:310–315.

Ernst JF and Kawashima E. Variations in codon usage are not correlated with heterologous gene expression in *Saccharomyces cerevisiae* and *Escherichia coli*. *J Biotechnol* 1988; 7:1–9.

Eyre-Walker A and Bulmer M. Reduced synonymous substitution rate at the start of enterobacterial genes. *Nucleic Acids Res* 1993; 21:4599–4603.

Fahey RC, Hunt JS, Windham GC. On the cysteine and cystine content of proteins. Differences between intracellular and extracellular proteins. *J Mol Evol* 1977; 10:155–160.

Falkenberg C, Björck L, Åkerström B. Localization of the binding site for streptococcal protein G on human serum albumin. Identification of a 5.5-kilodalton protein G binding albumin fragment. *Biochemistry* 1992; 31:1451–1457.

Faxen M, Plumbridge J, Isaksson LA. Codon choice and potential complementarity between mRNA downstream of the initiation codon and bases 1471-1480 in 16S ribosomal RNA affects expression of glnS. *Nucleic Acids Res* 1991; 19:5247–5251.

Figge J, Wright C, Collins CJ, Roberts TM, Livingston DM. Stringent regulation of stably integrated chloramphenicol acetyl transferase genes by *E. coli* lac repressor in monkey cells. *Cell* 1988; 52:713–722.

Firpo MA, Connelly MP, Goss DJ, Dahlberg AE. Mutations at two invariant nucleotides in the 3-minor domain of *Escherichia coli* 16 S rRNA affecting translational initiation and initiation factor 3 function. *J Biol Chem* 1996; 271:4693–4698.

Ford CF, Suominen I, Glatz CE. Fusion tails for the recovery and purification of recombinant proteins. *Protein Expression Purif* 1991; 2:95–107.

Forsberg G. Site specific cleavage of recombinant fusion proteins expressed in *Escherichia coli* and characterization of the products. Ph.D. dissertation. Royal Institute of Technology, Stockholm, Sweden, 1992.

Forsberg G, Baastrup B, Rondahl H, Holmgren E, Pohl G, Hartmanis M, Lake M. An evaluation of different enzymatic cleavage methods for recombinant fusion proteins, applied on des(1-3)insulin-like growth factor I. *J Protein Chem* 1992; 11:201–211.

Freundlich M, Ramani N, Mathew E, Sirko A, Tsui P. The role of integration host factor in gene expression in *Escherichia coli*. *Mol Microbiol* 1992; 6:2557–2563.

Friedman DI. Integration host factor: a protein for all reasons. *Cell* 1988; 55:545–554.

Friefeld BR, Korn R, de Jong PJ, Sninsky JJ, Horwitz MS. The 140-kDa adenovirus DNA polymerase is recognized by antibodies to *Escherichia coli*-synthesized determinants predicted from an open reading frame on the adenovirus genome. *Proc Natl Acad Sci USA* 1985; 82:2652–2656.

Frorath B, Abney CC, Berthold H, Scanarini M, Northemann W. Production of recombinant rat interleukin-6 in *Escherichia coli* using a novel highly efficient expression vector pGEX-3T. *BioTech* 1992; 12:558–563.

Fuchs J. Isolation of an *Escherichia coli* mutant deficient in thioredoxin reductase. *J Bacteriol* 1977; 129:967–972.

Fuchs P, Breitling F, Dubel S, Seehaus T, Little M. Targeting recombinant antibodies to the surface of *Escherichia coli*: fusion to a peptidoglycan associated lipoprotein. *BioTechnol* 1991; 9:1369–1372.

Fuh G, Mulkerrin MG, Bass S, McFarland N, Brochier M, Bourell JH, Light DR, Wells JA. The human growth hormone receptor. Secretion from *Escherichia coli* and disulfide bonding pattern of the extracellular binding domain. *J Biol Chem* 1990; 265:3111–3115.

Fujimoto K, Fukuda T, Marumoto R. Expression and secretion of human epidermal growth factor by *Escherichia coli* using enterotoxin signal sequences. *J Biotechnol* 1988; 8:77–86.

Gaal T, Barkei J, Dickson RR, de Boer HA, de Haseth PL, Alavi H, Gourse RL. Saturation mutagenesis of an *Escherichia coli* rRNA promoter and initial characterization of promoter variants. *J Bacteriol* 1989; 171:4852–4861.

Gafny R, Cohen S, Nachaliel N, Glaser G. Isolated P2 rRNA promoters of *Escherichia coli* are strong promoters that are subject to stringent control. *J Mol Biol* 1994; 243:152–156.

Galas DJ, Eggert M, Waterman MS. Rigorous pattern-recognition methods for DNA sequences. Analysis of promoter sequences from *Escherichia coli*. *J Mol Biol* 1985; 186:117–128.

Garcia GM, Mar PK, Mullin DA, Walker JR, Prather NE. The *E. coli* dnaY gene encodes an arginine transfer RNA. *Cell* 1986; 45:453–459.

Gardella TJ, Rubin D, Abou-Samra A-B, Keutmann HT, Potts Jr. JT, Kronenberg HM, Nussbaum SR. Expression of human parathyroid hormone-(1-84) in *Escherichia coli* as a factor X-cleavable fusion protein. *J Biol Chem* 1990; 265:15854–15859.

Gates CM, Stemmer WPC, Kaptein R, Schatz PJ. Affinity selective isolation of ligands from peptide libraries through display on a lac repressor "headpiece dimer." *J Mol Biol* 1996; 255:373–386.

Georgiou G. Expression of proteins in bacteria. In: *Protein Engineering: Principles and Practice*. Cleland JL and Craik CS, editors. Wiley Liss, New York, 1996: 101–127.

Georgiou G, Poetschke HL, Stathopoulos C, Francisco JA. Practical applications of engineering Gram-negative bacterial cell surfaces. *Trends Biotechnol* 1993; 11:6–10.

Georgiou G, Stephens DL, Stathopoulos C, Poetschke HL, Mendenhall J, Earhart CF. Display of β-lactamase on the *Escherichia coli* surface: outer membrane phenotypes conferred by Lpp-OmpA β-lactamase fusions. *Protein Eng* 1996, 9:239–247.

Georgiou G and Valax P. Expression of correctly folded proteins in *Escherichia coli*. *Curr Opin Biotechnol* 1996; 7:190–197.

Germino J and Bastia D. Rapid purification of a cloned gene product by genetic fusion and site specific proteolysis. *Proc Natl Acad Sci USA* 1984; 81:4692–4696.

Germino J, Gray JG, Charbonneau H, Vanaman T, Bastia D. Use of gene fusions and protein-protein interaction in the isolation of a biologically active regulatory protein: The replication initiator protein of plasmid R6K. *Proc Natl Acad Sci USA* 1983; 80:6848–6852.

Gething M-J and Sambrook J. Protein folding in the cell. *Nature* (London) 1992; 355:33–45.

Gheysen D, Iserentant D, Derom C, Fiers W. Systematic alteration of the nucleotide sequence preceding the translation initiation codon and the effects on bacterial expression of the cloned SV40 small-t antigen gene. *Gene* 1982; 17:55–63.

Ghrayeb J, Kimura H, Takahara M, Hsiung H, Masui Y, Inouye M. Secretion cloning vectors in *Escherichia coli*. *EMBO J* 1984; 3:2437–2442.

Giacomini A, Ollero FJ, Squartini A, Nuti MP. Construction of multipurpose gene cartridges based on a novel synthetic promoter for high-level gene expression in gram-negative bacteria. *Gene* 1994; 144:17–24.

Giladi H, Goldenberg D, Koby S, Oppenheim AB. Enhanced activity of the bacteriophage PL promoter at low temperature. *Proc Natl Acad Sci USA* 1995; 92:2184–2188.

Giladi H, Koby S, Gottesman ME, Oppenheim AB. Supercoiling, integration host factor, and a dual promoter system, participate in the control of the bacteriophage pL promoter. *J Mol Biol* 1992; 224:937–948.

Gilbert HF. Protein chaperones and protein folding. *Curr Opin Biotechnol* 1994; 5:534–539.

Giordano TJ, Deuschle U, Bujard H, McAllister WT. Regulation of coliphage T3 and T7 RNA polymerases by the lac repressor-operator system. *Gene* 1989; 84:209–219.

Goeddel DV. Systems for heterologous gene expression. *Methods Enzymol* 1990; 185:3–7.

Goeddel DV, Kleid DG, Bolivar F, Heyneker HL, Yansura DG, Crea R, Hirose T, Kraszewski A, Itakura K, Riggs AD. Expression in *Escherichia coli* of chemically synthesized genes for human insulin. *Proc Natl Acad Sci USA* 1979; 76:106–110.

Goff SA, Casson LP, Goldberg AL. Heat shock regulatory gene htpR influences rates of protein degradation and expression of the lon gene in *Escherichia coli*. *Proc Natl Acad Sci USA* 1984; 81:6647–6651.

Goff SA and Goldberg AL. Production of abnormal proteins in *E. coli* stimulates transcription of lon and other heat shock genes. *Cell* 1985; 41:587–595.

Goff SA and Goldberg AL. An increased content of protease La, the lon gene product, increases protein degradation and blocks growth in *E. coli*. *J Biol Chem* 1987; 262:4508–4515.

Gold L. Posttranscriptional regulatory mechanisms in *Escherichia coli*. *Annu Rev Biochem* 1988; 57:199–233.

Gold L. Expression of heterologous proteins in *Escherichia coli*. *Methods Enzymol* 1990; 185:11–14.

Gold L and Stormo GD. High-level translation initiation. *Methods Enzymol* 1990; 185:89–93.

Goldberg AL. The mechanism and functions of ATP-dependent proteases in bacterial and animal cells. *Eur J Biochem* 1992; 203:9–23.

Goldberg AL and Dice JF. Intracellular protein degradation in mammalian and bacterial cells. *Annu Rev Biochem* 1974, 43:835–869.

Goldberg AL and Goff SA. The selective degradation of abnormal proteins in bacteria. In: *Maximizing Gene Expression*. Reznikoff W and Gold L, editors. Butterworths, Boston, 1986: 287–314.

Goldberg AL, Goff SA, Casson LP. Hosts and methods for producing recombinant products in high yields. U.S. patent 4,758,512. July 1988.

Goldberg AL and St. John AC. Intracellular protein degradation in mammalian and bacterial cells. Part 2. *Annu Rev Biochem* 1976; 45:747–803.

Goldman E, Rosenberg AH, Zubay G, Studier FW. Consecutive low-usage leucine codons block translation only when near the 5 end of a message in *Escherichia coli*. *J Mol Biol* 1995; 245:467–473.

Goldstein MA and Doi RH. Prokaryotic promoters in biotechnology. *Biotechnol Annu Rev* 1995; 1:105–128.

Goldstein J, Lehnhardt S, Inouye M. Enhancement of protein translocation across the membrane by specific mutations in the hydrophobic region of the signal peptide. *J Bacteriol* 1990; 172:1225–1231.

Goldstein J, Pollitt NS, Inouye M. Major cold shock protein of *Escherichia coli*. *Proc Natl Acad Sci USA* 1990; 87:283–287.

Goloubinoff P, Gatenby AA, Lorimer GH. GroE heat-shock proteins promote assembly of foreign prokaryotic ribulose bisphosphate carboxylase oligomers in *Escherichia coli*. *Nature* (London) 1989; 337:44–47.

Gonda DK, Bachmair A, Wünning I, Tobias JW, Lane WS, Varshavsky A. Universality and structure of the N-end rule. *J Biol Chem* 1989; 264:16700–16712.

Gorski K, Roch J-M, Prentki P, Krisch HM. The stability of bacteriophage T4 gene 32 mRNA: a 5 leader sequence that can stabilize mRNA transcripts. *Cell* 1985; 43:461–469.

Gottesman S. Minimizing proteolysis in *Escherichia coli*: genetic solutions. *Methods Enzymol* 1990; 185:119–129.

Gottesman S and Maurizi MR. Regulation by proteolysis: energy-dependent proteases and their targets. *Microbiol Rev* 1992; 56:592–621.

Gourse RL, de Boer HA, Nomura M. DNA determinations of rRNA synthesis in *E. coli*: growth rate dependent regulation, feedback inhibition, upstream activation, antitermination. *Cell* 1986; 44:197–205.

Gouy M and Gautier C. Codon usage in bacteria: correlation with gene expressivity. *Nucleic Acids Res* 1982; 10:7055–7074.

Gram H, Ramage P, Memmert K, Gamse R, Kocher HP. A novel approach for high level production of a recombinant human parathyroid hormone fragment in *Escherichia coli*. *BioTechnol* 1994; 12:1017–1023.

Grauschopf U, Winther JR, Korber P, Zander T, Dallinger P, Bardwell JCA. Why is DsbA such an oxidizing disulfide catalyst? *Cell* 1995; 83:947–955.

Gray GL, Baldridge JS, McKeown KS, Heyneker HL, Chang CN. Periplasmic production of correctly processed human growth hormone in *Escherichia coli*: natural and bacterial signal sequences are interchangeable. *Gene* 1985; 39:247–254.

Gren EJ. Recognition of messenger RNA during translational initiation in *Escherichia coli*. *Biochimie* 1984; 66:1–29.

Grentzmann G, Brechemier-Baey D, Heurgué V, Mora L, Buckingham RH. Localization and characterization of the gene encoding release factor RF3 in *Escherichia coli*. *Proc Natl Acad Sci USA* 1994; 91:5848–5852.

Grisshammer R, Duckworth R, Henderson R. Expression of a rat neurotensin receptor in *Escherichia coli*. *Biochem J* 1993; 295:571–576.

Gronenborn B. Overproduction of phage lambda repressor under control of the lac promoter of *Escherichia coli*. *Mol Gen Genet* 1976; 148:243–250.

Gros F, Hiatt H, Gilbert W, Kurland CG, Risebrough RW, Watson JD. Unstable ribonucleic acid revealed by pulse labelling of *Escherichia coli*. *Nature* (London) 1961; 190:581–585.

Gross G, Mielke C, Hollatz I, Blöcker H, Frank R. RNA primary sequence or secondary structure in the translational initiation region controls expression of two variant interferon-α genes in *Escherichia coli*. *J Biol Chem* 1990; 265:17627–17636.

Gualerzi CO and Pon CL. Initiation of mRNA translation in prokaryotes. *Biochemistry* 1990; 29:5881–5889.

Guan K and Dixon JE. Eukaryotic proteins expressed in *Escherichia coli*: an improved thrombin cleavage and purification procedure of fusion proteins with glutathione S-transferase. *Anal Biochem* 1991; 192:262–267.

Guan X and Wurtele ES. Reduction of growth and acetyl-CoA carboxylase activity by expression of a chimeric streptavidin gene in *Escherichia coli*. *Appl Microbiol Biotechnol* 1996; 44:753–758.

Guarneros G, Montanez C, Hernandez T, Court D. Posttranscriptional control of bacteriophage int gene expression from a site distal to the gene. *Proc Natl Acad Sci USA* 1982; 79:238–242.

Guilhot C, Jander G, Martin NL, Beckwith J. Evidence that the pathway of disulfide bond formation in *Escherichia coli* involves interactions between the cysteines of DsbB and DsbA. *Proc Natl Acad Sci USA* 1995; 92:9895–9899.

Gutman GA and Hateld GW. Nonrandom utilization of codon pairs in *Escherichia coli*. *Proc Natl Acad Sci USA* 1989; 86:3699–3703.

Hall MN, Gabay J, Débarbouillé M, Schwartz M. A role for mRNA secondary structure in the control of translation initiation. *Nature* (London) 1982; 295:616–618.

Hammarberg B, Nygren P-A, Holmgren E, Elmblad A, Tally M, Hellman U, Moks T, Uhlén M. Dual affinity fusion approach and its use to express recombinant human insulin-like growth factor II. *Proc Natl Acad Sci USA* 1989; 86:4367–4371.

Hansson M, Ståhl S, Hjorth R, Uhlén M, Moks T. Single-step recovery of a secreted recombinant protein by expanded bed adsorption. *BioTechnol* 1994; 12:285–288.

Harley CB and Reynolds RP. Analysis of *E. coli* promoter sequences. *Nucleic Acids Res* 1987; 15:2343–2361.

Hartz D, McPheeters DS, Gold L. Influence of mRNA determinants on translation initiation in *Escherichia coli*. *J Mol Biol* 1991; 218:83–97.

Hasan N and Szybalski W. Control of cloned gene expression by promoter inversion *in vivo*: construction of improved vectors with a multiple cloning site and the ptac promoter. *Gene* 1987; 56:145–151.

Hasan N and Szybalski W. Construction of lacIts and lacIqts expression plasmids and evaluation of the thermosensitive lac repressor. *Gene* 1995. 163:35–40.

Hawley DK and McClure WR. Compilation and analysis of *Escherichia coli* promoter DNA sequences. *Nucleic Acids Res* 1983; 11:2237–2255.

Hay RJ. Animal cells in culture. In: Maintaining Cultures for Biotechnology and Industry. Hunter-Cevera JC and Belt A, editors. Academic Press, New York, 1996: 161–178.

Hayashi MN and Hayashi M. Cloned DNA sequences that determine mRNA stability of bacteriophage X174 *in vivo* are functional. *Nucleic Acids Res* 1985, 13:5937–5948.

Hayes SA and Dice JF. Roles of molecular chaperones in protein degradation. *J Cell Biol* 1996; 132:255–258.

He BA, McAllister WT, Durbin RK. Phage RNA polymerase vectors that allow efficient gene expression in both prokaryotic and eukaryotic cells. *Gene* 1995; 164:75–79.

Hedgpeth J, Ballivet M, Eisen H. Lambda phage promoter used to enhance expression of a plasmid-cloned gene. *Mol Gen Genet* 1978; 163:197–203.

Hein R and Tsien RY. Engineering green fluorescent protein for improved brightness, longer wavelengths and fluorescence resonance energy transfer. *Curr Biol* 1996; 6:178–182.

Helke A, Geisen RM, Vollmer M, Sprengart ML, Fuchs E. An unstructured messenger RNA region and a 5 hairpin represent important elements of the *E. coli* translation initiation signal determined by using the bacteriophage T7 gene 1 translation start site. *Nucleic Acids Res* 1993; 21:5705–5711.

Hellebust H, Murby M, Abrahmsén L, Uhlén M, Enfors S-O. Different approaches to stabilize a recombinant fusion protein. *BioTechnol* 1989; 7:165–168.

Hellman J and Mäntsä P. Construction of an *Escherichia coli* export-affinity vector for expression and purification of foreign proteins by fusion to cyclomaltodextrin glucanotransferase. *J Biotechnol* 1992; 23:19–34.

Hénaut A and Danchin A. Analysis and predictions from *Escherichia coli* sequences, or *E. coli* in silico. In: *Escherichia coli and Salmonella: Cellular and Molecular Biology*, vol. 2. Neidhardtrtiss III FC, Ingraham JL, Lin ECC, Low KB, Magasanik B, Wznikoff, R, Riley M, Schaechter M, Umbarger HE, editors. ASM Press, Washington, DC, 1996: 2047–2066.

Hendrick JP and Hartl F-U. The role of molecular chaperones in protein folding. *FASEB J* 1995; 9:1559–1569.

Herbst B, Kneip S, Bremer E. pOSEX: vectors for osmotically controlled and finely tuned gene expression in *Escherichia coli*. *Gene* 1994; 151:137–142.

Hernan RA, Hui HL, Andracki ME, Noble RW, Sligar SG, Walder JA, Walder RY. Human hemoglobin expression in *Escherichia coli*: importance of optimal codon usage. *Biochemistry* 1992; 31:8619–8628.

Higgins CF, Causton HC, Dance GSC, Mudd EA. The role of the 3 end in mRNA stability and decay. In: *Control of Messenger RNA Stability*. Belasco JG and Brawerman G, editors. Academic Press, San Diego, 1993: 13–30.

Hirel P-H, Schmitter J-M, Dessen P, Fayat G, Blanquet S. Extent of N-terminal methionine excision from *Escherichia coli* proteins is governed by the side-chain length of the penultimate amino acid. *Proc Natl Acad Sci USA* 1989; 86:8247–8251.

Hochuli E, Döbeli H, Schacher A. New metal chelate adsorbent selective for proteins and peptides containing neighbouring histidine residues. *J Chromatogr* 1987; 411:177–184.

Hockney RC. Recent developments in heterologous protein production in *Escherichia coli*. *Trends Biotechnol* 1994; 12:456–463.

Hodgson J. Expression systems: a user's guide. *BioTechnol* 1993; 11:887–893.

Hoffman CS and Wright A. Fusions of secreted proteins to alkaline phosphatase: an approach for studying protein secretion. *Proc Natl Acad Sci USA* 1985; 82:5107–5111.

Høgset A, Blingsmo OR, Saether O, Gautvik VT, Holmgren E, Josephson S, Gabrielsen OS, Gordeladze OJ, Alestrøm P, Gautvik KM. Expression and characterization of a recombinant human parathyroid hormone secreted by *Escherichia coli* employing the staphylococcal protein A promoter and signal sequence. *J Biol Chem* 1990; 265:7338–7344.

Holland IB, Kenny B, Steipe B, Plückthun A. Secretion of heterologous proteins in *Escherichia coli*. *Methods Enzymol* 1990; 182:132–143.

Holmgren A. Thioredoxin and glutaredoxin systems. *J Biol Chem* 1989; 264:13963–13966.

Hopp TP, Prickett KS, Price VL, Libby RT, March CJ, Cerretti DP, Urdal DL, Conlon PJ. A short polypeptide marker sequence useful for recombinant protein identification and purification. *BioTechnol* 1988; 6:1204–1210.

Horii T, Ogawa T, Ogawa H. Organization of the recA gene of *Escherichia coli*. *Proc Natl Acad Sci USA* 1980; 77:313–317.

Hsiung HM, Cantrell A, Luirink J, Oudega B, Veros AJ, Becker GW. Use of bacteriocin release protein in *E. coli* for excretion of human growth hormone into the culture medium. *BioTechnol* 1989; 7:267–271.

Hsiung HM and MacKellar WC. Expression of bovine growth hormone derivatives in *Escherichia coli* and the use of the derivatives to produce natural sequence growth hormone by cathepsin C cleavage. *Methods Enzymol* 1987; 153:390.

Hsiung H. M., N. G. Mayne, and G. W. Becker. High-level expression, efficient secretion and folding of human growth hormone in *Escherichia coli*. Bio/Technology 1986; 4:991–995.

Hsu LM, Giannini JK, Leung T-WC, Crosthwaite JC. Upstream sequence activation of *Escherichia coli* argT promoter *in vivo* and *in vitro*. *Biochemistry* 1991; 30:813–822.

Huh KR, Cho EH, Lee SO, Na DS. High level expression of human lipocortin (annexin) 1 in *Escherichia coli*. *Biotechnol Lett* 1996; 18:163–168.

Hui A, Hayick J, Dinkelspiel K, de Boer HA. Mutagenesis of the three bases preceding the start codon of the β-galactosidase mRNA and its effect on translation in *Escherichia coli*. *EMBO J* 1984; 3:623–629.

Hummel M, Herbst H, Stein H. Gene synthesis, expression in *Escherichia coli* and purification of immunoreactive human insulin-like growth factors I and II. Application of a modified HPLC separation technique for hydrophobic proteins. *Eur J Biochem* 1989; 180:555–561.

Humphreys DP, Weir N, Mountain A, Lund PA. Human protein disulfide isomerase functionally complements a dsbA mutation and enhances the yield of pectate lyase C in *Escherichia coli*. *J Biol Chem* 1995; 270:28210–28215.

Hüttenhofer A and Noller HF. Footprinting mRNA-ribosome complexes with chemical probes. *EMBO J* 1994; 13:3892–3901.

Hwang C, Sinskey AJ, Lodish HF. Oxidized redox state of glutathione in the endoplasmic reticulum. *Science* 1992; 257:1496–1502.

ICH. Quality of biotechnological products: viral safety evaluation of biotechnology products derived from cell lines of human or animal origin. ICH Harmonised Tripartite Guideline. *Dev Biol Stand* 1998; 93:177–201.

Ikehara M, Ohtsuka E, Tokunaga T, Nishikawa S, Uesugi S, Tanaka T, Aoyama Y, Kikyodani S, Fujimoto K, Yanase K, Fuchimura K, and Morioka H. Inquiries into the structure-function relationship of ribonuclease T1 using chemically synthesized coding sequences. *Proc Natl Acad Sci USA* 1986; 83:4695–4699.

Ikemura T. Codon usage and tRNA content in unicellular and multicellular organisms. *Mol Biol Evol* 1985; 2:13–34.

Ingram LO, Conway T, Clark DP, Sewell GW, Preston JF. Genetic engineering of ethanol production in *Escherichia coli*. *Appl Environ Microbiol* 1987; 53:2420–2425.

Inouye S and Inouye M. Up-promoter mutations in the lpp gene of *Escherichia coli*. *Nucleic Acids Res* 1985; 13:3101–3110.

Inouye H, Michaelis S, Wright A, Beckwith J. Cloning and restriction mapping of the alkaline phosphatase structural gene (phoA) of *Escherichia coli* and generation of deletion mutants *in vitro*. *J Bacteriol* 1981; 146:668–675.

Irwin B, Heck JD, Hateld GW. Codon pair utilization biases influence translational elongation step times. *J Biol Chem* 1995; 270:22801–22806.

Iserentant D and W. Fiers. Secondary structure of mRNA and efficiency of translation initiation. *Gene* 1980; 9:1–12.

Itakura K, Hirose T, Crea R, Riggs AD, Heyneker HL, Bolivar F, Boyer HW. Expression in *Escherichia coli* of a chemically synthesized gene for the hormone somatostatin. *Science* 1977; 198:1056–1063.

Ito K, Kawakami K, Nakamura Y. Multiple control of *Escherichia coli* lysyl-tRNA synthetase expression involves a transcriptional repressor and a translational enhancer element. *Proc Natl Acad Sci USA* 1993; 90:302–306.

Ivanov I, Alexandrova R, Dragulev B, Saraffova A, AbouHaidar MG. Effect of tandemly repeated AGG triplets on the translation of CAT-mRNA in *E. coli*. *FEBS Lett* 1992; 307:173–176.

Iwakura M, Obara K, Kokubu T, Ohashi S, Izutsu H. Expression and purification of growth hormone-releasing factor with the aid of dihydrofolate reductase handle. *J Biochem* 1992; 112:57–62.

Izard J, Parker MW, Chartier M, Duché D, Baty D. A single amino acid substitution can restore the solubility of aggregated colicin A mutants in *Escherichia coli*. *Protein Eng* 1994; 7:1495–1500.

Jacob F and Monod J. Genetic regulatory mechanisms in the synthesis of proteins. *J Mol Biol* 1961; 3:318–356.

Jacques N, Guillerez J, Dreyfus M. Culture conditions differentially affect the translation of individual *Escherichia coli* mRNAs. *J Mol Biol* 1992; 226:597–608.

Jensen EB and Carlsen S. Production of recombinant human growth hormone in *Escherichia coli*: expression of different precursors and physiological effects of glucose, acetate, and salts. *Biotechnol Bioeng* 1990; 36:1–11.

Johnson DL, Middleton SA, McMahon F, Barbone FP, Kroon D, Tsao E, Lee WH, Mulcahy LS, and Jolliffe LK. Refolding, purification, and characterization of human erythropoietin binding protein produced in *Escherichia coli*. *Protein Expression Purif* 1996; 7:104–113.

Johnson ES, Gonda DK, Varshavsky A. cis-trans recognition and subunit-specific degradation of short-lived proteins. *Nature* (London) 1990; 346:287–291.

Jones PG, Krah R, Tafuri SR, Wolffe AP. DNA gyrase, CS7.4, and the cold shock response in *Escherichia coli*. *J Bacteriol* 1992; 174:5798–5802.

Josaitis CA, Gaal T, Gourse RL. Stringent control and growth-rate-dependent control have nonidentical promoter sequence requirements. *Proc Natl Acad Sci USA* 1995; 92:1117–1121.

Josaitis CA, Gaal T, Ross W, Gourse RL. Sequences upstream of the 35 hexamer of rrnB P1 affect promoter strength and upstream activation. *Biochim Biophys Acta* 1990; 1050:307–311.

Kadokura H, Yoda K, Watanabe S, Kikuchi Y, Tamura G, Yamasaki M. Enhancement of protein secretion by optimizing protein synthesis: isolation and characterization of *Escherichia coli* mutants with increased secretion ability of alkaline phosphatase. *Appl Microbiol BioTechnol* 1994; 41:163–169.

Kane JF. Effects of rare codon clusters on high-level expression of heterologous proteins in *Escherichia coli*. *Curr Opin Biotechnol* 1995; 6:494–500.

Kane JF and Hartley DL. Formation of recombinant protein inclusion bodies in *Escherichia coli*. *Trends Biotechnol* 1988; 6:95–101.

Kastelein RA, Berkhout B, van Duin J. Opening the closed ribosome-binding site of the lysis cistron of bacteriophage MS2. *Nature* (London) 1983; 305:741–743.

Kato C, Kobayashi T, Kudo T, Furusato T, Murakami Y, Tanaka T, Baba H, Oishi T, Ohtsuka E, Ikehara M, Yanagida T, Kato H, Moriyama S, Horikoshi K. Construction of an excretion vector and extracellular production of human growth hormone from *Escherichia coli*. *Gene* 1987; 54:197–202.

Kaufmann A, Stierhof Y-D, Henning U. New outer membrane-associated protease of *Escherichia coli* K–12. *J Bacteriol* 1994; 176:359–367.

Kavanaugh JS, Rogers PH, Arnone A. High-resolution X-ray study of deoxy recombinant human hemoglobins synthesized from globins having mutated amino termini. *Biochemistry* 1992; 31:8640–8647.

Keiler KC, Waller PRH, Sauer RT. Role of a peptide tagging system in degradation of proteins synthesized from damaged messenger RNA. *Science* 1996; 271:990–993.

Kelman Z, Yao N, O'Donnell M. *Escherichia coli* expression vectors containing a protein kinase recognition motif, His6-tag and hemagglutinin epitope. *Gene* 1995; 166:177–178.

Kendall RL, Yamada R, Bradshaw RA. Cotranslational amino-terminal processing. *Methods Enzymol* 1990; 185:398–407.

Kenealy WR, Gray JE, Ivanoff LA, Tribe DE, Reed DL, Korant BD, Petteway Jr. SR. Solubility of proteins overexpressed in *Escherichia coli*. *Dev Ind Microbiol* 1987; 28:45–52.

Kern I and Ceglowski P. Secretion of streptokinase fusion proteins from *Escherichia coli* cells through the hemolysin transporter. *Gene* 1995; 163:53–57.

Khosla C and Bailey JE. Characterization of the oxygen-dependent promoter of the Vitreoscilla hemoglobin gene in *Escherichia coli*. *J Bacteriol* 1989; 171:5995–6004.

Khosla C, Curtis JE, Bydalek P, Swartz JR, Bailey JE. Expression of recombinant proteins in *Escherichia coli* using an oxygen-responsive promoter. *BioTechnol* 1990; 8:554–558.

Kikuchi Y, Yoda K, Yamasaki M, Tamura G. The nucleotide sequence of the promoter and the amino-terminal region of alkaline phosphatase structural gene (phoA) of *Escherichia coli*. *Nucleic Acids Res* 1981; 9:5671–5678.

Kim, J-S and Raines RT. Ribonuclease S-peptide as a carrier in fusion proteins. *Protein Sci* 1993; 2:348–356.

Kim J-S and Raines RT. Peptide tags for a dual affinity fusion system. *Anal Biochem* 1994; 219:165–166.

Kitai K, Kudo T, Nakamura S, Masegi T, Ichikawa Y, Horikoshi K. Extracellular production of human immunoglobulin G Fc region (hIgG-Fc) by *Escherichia coli*. *Appl Microbiol Biotechnol* 1988; 28:52–56.

Kitano K, Fujimoto S, Nakao M, Watanabe T, Nakao Y. Intracellular degradation of recombinant proteins in relation to their location in *Escherichia coli* cells. *J Biotechnol* 1987; 5:77–86.

Kleerebezem M and Tommassen J. Expression of the pspA gene stimulates efficient protein export in *Escherichia coli*. *Mol Microbiol* 1993; 7:947–956.

Knappik A, Krebber C, Plückthun A. The effect of folding catalysts on the *in vivo* folding process of different antibody fragments expressed in *Escherichia coli*. *BioTechnol* 1993; 11:77–83.

Knappik A and Plückthun A. An improved affinity tag based on the FLAG peptide for the detection and purification of recombinant antibody fragments. *BioTechniques* 1994; 17:754–761.

Knappik A and Plückthun A. Engineered turns of a recombinant antibody improve its *in vivo* folding. *Protein Eng* 1995; 8:81–89.

Knott JA, Sullivan CA, Weston A. The isolation and characterization of human atrial natriuretic factor produced as a fusion protein in *Escherichia coli*. *Eur J Biochem* 1988; 174:405–410.

Knowles P. The role of the β-lactamase signal sequence in the secretion of proteins by *Escherichia coli*. *J Biol Chem* 1984; 259:2149–2154.

Ko JH, Park DK, Kim IC, Lee SH, Byun SM. High-level expression and secretion of streptokinase in *Escherichia coli*. *Biotechnol Lett* 1995; 17:1019–1024.

Kobayashi M, Nagata K, Ishihama A. Promoter selectivity of *Escherichia coli* RNA polymerase: effect of base substitutions in the promoter 35 region on promoter strength. *Nucleic Acids Res* 1990; 18:7367–7372.

Koken MHM, Odijk HHM, van Duin M, Fornerod M, Hoeijmakers JHJ. Augmentation of protein production by a combination of the T7 RNA polymerase system and ubiquitin fusion: overproduction of the human DNA repair protein, ERCC1, as a ubiquitin fusion protein in *Escherichia coli*. *Biochem Biophys Res Commun* 1993; 195:643–653.

Köhler K, Ljungquist C, Kondo A, Veide A, Nilsson B. Engineering proteins to enhance their partition coefficients in aqueous two-phase systems. *BioTechnol* 1991; 9:642–646.

Krueger JK, Kulke MN, Schutt C, Stock J. Protein inclusion body formation and purification. *BioPharm* 1989; 2:40–45.

Kozak M. Comparison of initiation of protein synthesis in prokaryotes, eukaryotes, and organelles. *Microbiol Rev* 1983; 47:1–45.

Kushner SR. mRNA decay. In: Escherichia coli *and Salmonella: Cellular and Molecular Biology*, Vol. 1. Neidhardt FC, Curtiss III R, Ingraham JL, Lin ECC, Low KB, Magasanik B, Reznikoff WS, Riley M, Schaechter M, Umbarger HE, editors. ASM Press, Washington, DC, 1996: 849–860.

Kwon S, Kim S, Kim E. Effects of glycerol on β-lactamase production during high cell density cultivation of recombinant *Escherichia coli*. *Biotechnol Prog* 1996; 12:205–208.

Landick R, Turnbough Jr. CL, Yanofsky C. Transcription attenuation. In: Escherichia coli *and Salmonella: Cellular and Molecular Biology*, Vol. 1. Neidhardt FC, Curtiss III R, Ingraham JL, Lin ECC, Low KB, Magasanik B, Reznikoff WS, Riley M, Schaechter M, Umbarger HE, editors. ASM Press, Washington, DC, 1996: 1263–1286.

Lange R and Hengge-Aronis R. The cellular concentration of the s subunit of RNA polymerase in *Escherichia coli* is controlled at the levels of transcription, translation, and protein stability. *Genes Dev* 1994; 8:1600–1612.

Langer T, Lu C, Echols H, Flanagan J, Hayer MK, Hartl FU. Successive action of DnaK, DnaJ and GroEL along the pathway of chaperone-mediated protein folding. *Nature* (London) 1992; 356:683–689.

Lanzer M and Bujard H. Promoters largely determine the efficiency of repressor action. *Proc Natl Acad Sci USA* 1988; 85:8973–8977.

LaVallie ER, DiBlasio EA, Kovacic S, Grant KL, Schendel PF, McCoy JM. A thioredoxin gene fusion expression system that circumvents inclusion body formation in the *E. coli* cytoplasm. *BioTechnol* 1993; 11:187–193.

LaVallie ER and McCoy JM. Gene fusion expression systems in *Escherichia coli*. *Curr Opin Biotechnol* 1995; 6:501–506.

Le Calvez H, Green JM, Baty D. Increased efficiency of alkaline phosphatase production levels in *Escherichia coli* using a degenerate PelB signal sequence. *Gene* 1996; 170:51–55.

Lee C, Li P, Inouye H, Brickman ER, Beckwith J. Genetic studies on the instability of β-galactosidase to be translocated across the *Escherichia coli* cytoplasmic membrane. *J Bacteriol* 1989; 171:4609–4616.

Lee H-W, Joo J-H, Kang S, Song I-S, Kwon J-B, Han MH, Na DS. Expression of human interleukin-2 from native and synthetic genes in *E. coli*: no correlation between major codon bias and high level expression. *Biotechnol Lett* 1992; 14:653–658.

Lee J, Cho MW, Hong E-K, Kim K-S, Lee J. Characterization of the nar promoter to use as an inducible promoter. *Biotechnol Lett* 1996; 18:129–134.

Lee N, Zhang S-Q, Cozzitorto J, Yang J-S, Testa D. Modification of mRNA secondary structure and alteration of the expression of human interferon-1 in *Escherichia coli*. *Gene* 1987; 58:77–86.

Lee SC and Olins PO. Effect of overproduction of heat shock chaperones GroESL and DnaK on human procollagenase production in *Escherichia coli*. *J Biol Chem* 1992; 267:2849–2852.

Lee SY. High cell-density culture of *Escherichia coli*. *Trends Biotechnol* 1996; 14:98–105.

Lehnhardt S, Pollitt S, Inouye M. The differential effect on two hybrid proteins of deletion mutations within the hydrophobic region of the *Escherichia coli* ompA signal peptide. *J Biol Chem* 1987; 262:1716–1719.

Lei S-P, Lin H-C, Wang S-S, Callaway J, Wilcox G. Characterization of the *Erwinia carotovora* pelB gene and its product pectate lyase. *J Bacteriol* 1987; 169:4379–4383.

Li SC, Squires CL, Squires C. Antitermination of *E. coli* rRNA transcription is caused by a control region segment containing lambda nut-like sequences. *Cell* 1984; 38:851–860.

Liang S-M, Allet B, Rose K, Hirschi M, Liang C-M, Thatcher DR. Characterization of human interleukin 2 derived from *Escherichia coli*. *Biochem J* 1985; 229:429–439.

Lindsey DF, Mullin, DA, Walker JR. Characterization of the cryptic lambdoid prophage DLP12 of *Escherichia coli* and overlap of the DLP12 integrase gene with the tRNA gene argU. *J Bacteriol* 1989; 171:6197–6205.

Lisser S and Margalit H. Compilation of *E. coli* mRNA promoter sequences. *Nucleic Acids Res* 1993; 21:1507–1516.

Little M, Fuchs P, Breitling F, Dübel S. Bacterial surface presentation of proteins and peptides: an alternative to phage technology? *Trends Biotechnol* 1993; 11:3–5.

Little S, Campbell CJ, Evans IJ, Hayward EC, Lilley RJ. A short N-proximal region of prochymosin inhibits the secretion of hybrid proteins from *Escherichia coli*. *Gene* 1989; 83:321–329.

Ljungquist C, Lundeberg J, Rasmussen A-M, Hornes E, Uhlén M. Immobilization and recovery of fusion proteins and B-lymphocyte cells using magnetic separation. *DNA Cell Biol* 1993; 12:191–197.

Lo AC, MacKay RM, Seligy VL, Willick GE. Bacillus subtilis -1,4-endoglucanase products from intact and truncated genes are secreted into the extracellular medium by *Escherichia coli*. *Appl Environ Microbiol* 1988; 54:2287–2292.

Lofdahl S, Guss B, Uhlén M, Philipson L, Lindberg M. Gene for staphylococcal protein A. *Proc Natl Acad Sci USA* 1983; 80:697–701.

Lorimer GH. A quantitative assessment of the role of chaperonin proteins in protein folding *in vivo*. *FASEB J* 1996; 10:5–9.

Lovatt A, McMutrie D, Black J, Doherty I. Validation of quantitative PCR assays. Addressing virus contamination concerns. *BioPharm* 2002; 15(3):22–32.

Lu ZJ, DiBlasio-Smith EA, Grant KL, Warne NW, LaVallie ER. Histidine patch thioredoxins. *J Biol Chem* 1996; (271):5059–5065.

Lu ZJ, Murray KS, Van Cleave V, LaVallie ER, Stahl ML, J. Expression of thioredoxin random peptide libraries of *E. coli* cell surface as functional fusions to flagellin: a system designed for exploring protein–protein interaction. *BioTechnol* 1995; (13):366–372.

Luli GW and Strohl WR. Comparison of growth, acetate production and acetate inhibition of *Escherichia coli* strains in batch and fed-batch fermentations. *Appl Environ Microbiol* 1990; 56:1004–1011.

Lundeberg J, Wahlberg J, Uhlén M. Affinity purification of specific DNA fragments using a lac repressor fusion protein. *Genet Anal Tech Appl* 1990; 7:47–52.

MacFerrin KD, Chen L, Terranova MP, Schreiber SL, Verdine GL. Overproduction of proteins using expression-cassette polymerase chain reaction. *Methods Enzymol* 1993; 217:79–102.

MacIntyre S and Henning U. The role of the mature part of secretory proteins in translocation across the plasma membrane and in regulation of their synthesis in *Escherichia coli*. *Biochimie* 1990; 72:157–167.

Mackman N, Baker K, Gray L, Haigh R, Nicaud J-M, Holland IB. Release of a chimeric protein into the medium from *Escherichia coli* using therminal secretion signal of haemolysin. *EMBO J* 1987; 6:2835–2841.

Makoff AJ and Smallwood AE. The use of two-cistron constructions in improving the expression of a heterologous gene in *E. coli*. *Nucleic Acids Res* 1990; 18:1711–1718.

Makrides S. Strategies for achieving high level expression of genes in *E. coli.*, Microbiol Rev 1996; 60(3):512–538.

Makrides SC, Nygren P-Å, Andrews B, Ford PJ, Evans KS, Hayman EG, Adari H, Levin J, Uhlén M, Toth CA. Extended *in vivo* half-life of human soluble complement receptor type 1 fused to albumin-binding receptor. *J Pharmacol Exp Ther* 1996, 277:534–542.

Malke H and Ferretti JJ. Streptokinase: cloning, expression and secretion by *Escherichia coli*. *Proc Natl Acad Sci USA* 1984; 81:3557–3561.

Manning M (ed.). *Stability of Protein Pharmaceuticals. A. Chemical and Physical Pathways of Protein Degradation*. Plenum Press, New York,.

Marino MH. Expression systems for heterologous protein production. *BioPharm* 1989; 2:18–33.

Marston FAO. The purification of eukaryotic polypeptides synthesized in *Escherichia coli*. *Biochem J* 1986; 240:1–12.

Martin J and Hartl FU. Molecular chaperones in cellular protein folding. *Bioessays* 1994; 16:689–692.

Masuda K, Kamimura T, Kanesaki M, Ishii K, Imaizumi A, Sugiyama T, Suzuki Y, Ohtsuka E. Efficient production of the C-terminal domain of secretory leukoprotease inhibitor as a thrombin-cleavable fusion protein in *Escherichia coli*. *Protein Eng* 1996; 9:101–106.

Matin A. Starvation promoters of *Escherichia coli*. Their function, regulation, and use in bioprocessing and bioremediation. *Ann NY Acad Sci* 1994; 721:277–291.

Maurizi MR. Proteases and protein degradation in *Escherichia coli*. *Experientia* 1992; 48:178–201.

McCarthy JEG and Brimacombe R. Prokaryotic translation: the interactive pathway leading to initiation. *Trends Genet* 1994; 10:402–407.

McCarthy JEG and Gualerzi C. Translational control of prokaryotic gene expression. *Trends Genet* 1990; 6:78–85.

McCarthy JEG, Schairer HU, Sebald W. Translational initiation frequency of atp genes from *Escherichia coli*: identification of an intercistronic sequence that enhances translation. *EMBO J* 1985; 4:519–526.

McCarthy JEG, Sebald W, Gross G, Lammers R. Enhancement of translational efficiency by the *Escherichia coli* atpE translational initiation region: its fusion with two human genes. *Gene* 1986, 41:201–206.

Meerman HJ and Georgiou G. Construction and characterization of a set of *E. coli* strains deficient in all known loci affecting the proteolytic stability of secreted recombinant proteins. *BioTechnol* 1994; 12:1107–1110.

Meerman HJ and Georgiou G. High-level production of proteolytically sensitive secreted proteins in *Escherichia coli* strains impaired in the heat-shock response. *Ann NY Acad Sci* 1994; 721:292–302.

Mertens N, Remaut E, Fiers W. Tight transcriptional control mechanism ensures stable high-level expression from T7 promoter-based expression plasmids. *BioTechnol* 1995, 13:175–179.

Mertens N, Remaut E, Fiers W. Versatile, multi-featured plasmids for high-level expression of heterologous genes in *Escherichia coli*: overproduction of human and murine cytokines. *Gene* 1995; 164:9–15.

Michaelis S and Beckwith J. Mechanism of incorporation of cell envelope proteins in *Escherichia coli*. *Annu Rev Microbiol* 1982; 36:435–465.

Mikuni O, Ito K, Moffat J, Matsumura K, McCaughan K, Nobukuni T, Tate W, Nakamura Y. Identification of the prfC gene, which encodes peptide-chain-release factor 3 of *Escherichia coli*. *Proc Natl Acad Sci USA* 1994; 91:5798–5802.

Miller CG. Protein degradation and proteolytic modification. In: *Escherichia coli and Salmonella: Cellular and Molecular Biology*, Vol. 1. Neidhardt FC, Curtiss III R, Ingraham JL, Lin ECC, Low KB, Magasanik B, Reznikoff WS, Riley M, Schaechter M, Umbarger HE, editors. ASM Press, Washington, DC, 1996: 938–954.

Minas W and Bailey JE. Co-overexpression of prlF increases cell viability and enzyme yields in recombinant *Escherichia coli* expressing *Bacillus stearothermophilus* β-amylase. *Biotechnol Prog* 1995; 11:403–411.

Minor PD. Ensuring safety and consistency in cell culture production processes: viral screening and inactivation. *Trends Biotechnol* 1994; 12(7):257–261.

Minor PD. Significance of contamination with viruses of cell lines used in the production of biological medicinal products. In: *Animal Cell Technology. Products of Today, Prospects for Tomorrow*. Spier RE, Griffiths JB, Berthold W, editors. Butterworth Heinemann, Oxford, 1994: 741–748.

Misoka F, Fuwa T, Yoda K, Yamasaki M, Tamura G. Secretion of human interferon-α induced by using secretion vectors containing a promoter and signal sequence of alkaline phosphatase gene of *Escherichia coli*. *J Biochem* 1985; 97:1429–1436.

Misoka F, Miyake T, Miyoshi K-I, Sugiyama M, Sakamoto S, Fuwa T. Overproduction of human insulin-like growth factor-II in *Escherichia coli*. *Biotechnol Lett* 1989; 11:839–844.

Mitraki A and King J. Protein folding intermediates and inclusion body formation. *BioTech* 1989; 7:690–697.

Mohsen A-WA and Vockley J. High-level expression of an altered cDNA encoding human isovaleryl-CoA dehydrogenase in *Escherichia coli*. *Gene* 1995; 160:263–267.

Moks T, Abrahmsén L, Holmgren E, Bilich M, Olsson A, Uhlén M, Pohl G, Sterky C, Hultberg H, Josephson S, Holmgren A, Jörnvall H, Nilsson B. Expression of human insulin-like growth factor I in bacteria: use of optimized gene fusion vectors to facilitate protein purification. *Biochemistry* 1987; 26:5239–5244.

Moks T, Abrahmsén L, Osterlöf B, Josephson S, Ostling M, Enfors S-O, Persson I, Nilsson B, Uhlén M. Large-scale affinity purification of human insulin-like growth factor I from culture medium of *Escherichia coli*. *BioTechnol* 1987; 5:379–382.

Moore JT, Uppal A, Maley F, Maley GF. Overcoming inclusion body formation in a high-level expression system. *Protein Expression Purif* 1993; 4:160–163.

Morino T, Morita M, Seya K, Sukenaga Y, Kato K, Nakamura T. Construction of a runaway vector and its use for a high-level expression of a cloned human superoxide dismutase gene. *Appl Microbiol Biotechnol* 1988, 28:170–175.

Morioka-Fujimoto K, Marumoto R, Fukuda T. Modified enterotoxin signal sequences increase secretion level of the recombinant human epidermal growth factor in *Escherichia coli*. *J Biol Chem* 1991; 266:1728–1732.

Mottagui-Tabar, S, Björnsson A, Isaksson LA. The second to last amino acid in the nascent peptide as a codon context determinant. *EMBO J* 1994; 13:249–257.

Müller-Hill, B, Crapo L, Gilbert W. Mutants that make more lac repressor. *Proc Natl Acad Sci USA* 1968; 59:1259–1264.

Mukhija R, Rupa P, Pillai D, Garg LC. High-level production and one-step purification of biologically active human growth hormone in *Escherichia coli*. *Gene* 1995; 165:303–306.

Munro S and Pelham HRB. An Hsp70-like protein in the ER: identity with the 78 kd glucose-regulated protein and immunoglobulin heavy chain binding protein. *Cell* 1986; 46:291–300.

Murby M, Cedergren L, Nilsson J, Nygren P-Å, Hammarberg B, Nilsson B, Enfors S-O, Uhlén M. Stabilization of recombinant proteins from proteolytic degradation in *Escherichia coli* using a dual affinity fusion strategy. *Biotechnol Appl Biochem* 1991; 14:336–346.

Murby M, Samuelsson E, Nguyen TN, Mignard L, Power U, Binz H, Uhlén M, Ståhl S. Hydrophobicity engineering to increase solubility and stability of a recombinant protein from respiratory syncytial virus. *Eur J Biochem* 1995; 230:38–44.

Murby M, Uhlén M, Ståhl S. Upstream strategies to minimize proteolytic degradation upon recombinant production in *Escherichia coli*. *Protein Expression Purif* 1996; 7:129–136.

Nagahari K, Kanaya S, Munakata K, Aoyagi Y, Mizushima S. Secretion into the culture medium of a foreign gene product from *Escherichia coli*: use of the ompF gene for secretion of human β-endorphin. *EMBO J* 1985; 4:3589–3592.

Nagai K, Perutz MF, Poyart C. Oxygen binding properties of human mutant hemoglobins synthesized in *Escherichia coli*. *Proc Natl Acad Sci USA* 1985; 82:7252–7255.

Nagai K and Thøgersen HC. Generation of globin by sequence-specific proteolysis of a hybrid protein produced in *Escherichia coli*. *Nature* (London) 1984; 309:810–812.

Nagai K and Thøgersen HC. Synthesis and sequence-specific proteolysis of hybrid proteins produced in *Escherichia coli*. *Methods Enzymol* 1987; 153:461–481.

Nagai H, Yuzawa H, Yura T. Interplay of two cis-acting mRNA regions in translational control of 32 synthesis during the heat shock response of *Escherichia coli*. *Proc Natl Acad Sci USA* 1991; 88:10515–10519.

Nakamura K and Inouye M. Construction of versatile expression cloning vehicles using the lipoprotein gene of *Escherichia coli*. *EMBO J* 1982; 1:771–775.

Nakashima K, Kanamaru K, Mizuno T, Horikoshi K. A novel member of the cspA family of genes that is induced by cold shock in *Escherichia coli*. *J Bacteriol* 1996; 178:2994–2997.

Neri D, De Lalla C, Petrul H, Neri P, Winter G. Calmodulin as a versatile tag for antibody fragments. *BioTechnol* 1995; 13:373–377.

Newbury SF, Smith NH, Robinson EC, Hiles ID, Higgins CF. Stabilization of translationally active mRNA by prokaryotic REP sequences. *Cell* 1987; 48:297–310.

Nguyen TN, Hansson M, Ståhl S, Bächi T, Robert A, Domzig W, Binz H, Uhlén M. Cell-surface display of heterologous epitopes on Staphylococcus xylosus as a potential delivery system for oral vaccination. *Gene* 1993; 128:89–94.

Nicaud J-M, Mackman N, Holland IB. Current status of secretion of foreign proteins by microorganisms. *J Biotechnol* 1986; 3:255–270.

Nierlich DP and Murakawa GJ. The decay of bacterial messenger RNA. *Prog Nucleic Acid Res Mol Biol* 1996; 52:153–216.

Nilsson B and Abrahmsén L. Fusions to staphylococcal protein A. *Methods Enzymol* 1990; 185:144–161.

Nilsson B, Forsberg G, Moks T, Hartmanis M, Uhlén M. Fusion proteins in biotechnology and structural biology. *Curr Opin Struct Biol* 1992; 2:569–575.

Nilsson J, Nilsson P, Williams Y, Pettersson L, Uhlén M, Nygren P-Å. Competitive elution of protein A fusion proteins allows specific recovery under mild conditions. *Eur J Biochem* 1994; 224:103–108.

Nishi T and Itoh S. Enhancement of transcriptional activity of the *Escherichia coli* trp promoter by upstream AT-rich regions. *Gene* 1986; 44:29–36.

Nishihara T, Iwabuchi T, Nohno T. A T7 promoter vector with a transcriptional terminator for stringent expression of foreign genes. *Gene* 1994; 145:145–146.

Nomura M, Gourse R, Baughman G. Regulation of the synthesis of ribosomes and ribosomal components. *Annu Rev Biochem* 1984; 53:75–118.

Nordström K and Uhlin BE. Runaway-replication plasmids as tools to produce large quantities of proteins from cloned genes in bacteria. *BioTechnol* 1992; 10:661–666.

Nossal NG and Heppel LA. The release of enzymes by osmotic shock from *Escherichia coli* in exponential phase. *J Biol Chem* 1966; 241:3055–3062.

Novotny J, Ganju RK, Smiley ST, Hussey RE, Luther MA, Recny MA, Siliciano RF, Reinherz EL. A soluble, single-chain T-cell receptor fragment endowed with antigen-combining properties. *Proc Natl Acad Sci USA* 1991; 88:8646–8650.

Nygren P-Å, Ljungquist C, Tromborg H, Nustad K, Uhlén M. Species-dependent binding of serum albumins to the streptococcal receptor protein G. *Eur J Biochem* 1990; 193:143–148.

Nygren P-Å, Ståhl S, Uhlén M. Engineering proteins to facilitate bioprocessing. *Trends Biotechnol* 1994; 12:184–188.

Nygren P-Å, Uhlén M, Flodby P, Andersson R, Wigzell H. *In vivo* stabilization of a human recombinant CD4 derivative by fusion to a serum-albumin-binding receptor. *Vaccines* 1991; 91:363–368.

O'Connor CD and Timmis KN. Highly repressible expression system for cloning genes that specify potentially toxic proteins. *J Bacteriol* 1987; 169:4457–4462.

Obukowicz MG, Staten NR, Krivi GG. Enhanced heterologous gene expression in novel rpoH mutants of *Escherichia coli*. *Appl Environ Microbiol* 1992; 58:1511–1523.

Obukowicz MG, Turner MA, Wong EY, Tacon WC. Secretion and export of IGF-1 in *Escherichia coli* strain JM101. *Mol Gen Genet* 1988; 215:19–25.

Oka T, Sakamoto S, Miyoshi K-I, Fuwa T, Yoda K, Yamasaki M, Tamura G, Miyake T. Synthesis and secretion of human epidermal growth factor by *Escherichia coli*. *Proc Natl Acad Sci USA* 1985; 82:7212–7216.

Olins D, Chaplin D, Gordon JI. Compartmentalization of mammalian proteins produced in *Escherichia coli*. *J Biol Chem* 1990; 265:13066–13073.

Olins PO, Devine CS, Rangwala SH, Kavka KS. The T7 phage gene 10 leader RNA, a ribosome-binding site that dramatically enhances the expression of foreign genes in *Escherichia coli*. *Gene* 1988; 73:227–235.

Olins PO and Lee SC. Recent advances in heterologous gene expression in *Escherichia coli*. *Curr Opin Biotechnol* 1993; 4:520–525.

Olins PO and Rangwala SH. A novel sequence element derived from bacteriophage T7 mRNA acts as an enhancer of translation of the lacZ gene in *Escherichia coli*. *J Biol Chem* 1989; 264:16973–16976.

Olins PO and Rangwala SH. Vector for enhanced translation of foreign genes in *Escherichia coli*. *Methods Enzymol* 1990; 185:115–119.

Olsen MK, Rockenbach SK, Curry KA, Tomich C-SC. Enhancement of heterologous polypeptide expression by alterations in the ribosome-binding-site sequence. *J Biotechnol* 1989; 9:179–190.

Omer CA, Diehl RE, Kral AK. Bacterial expression and purification of human protein prenyltransferases using epitope-tagged, translationally coupled systems. *Methods Enzymol* 1995; 250:3–12.

Ong E, Gilkes NR, Warren RAJ, Miller Jr. RC, Kilburn DG. Enzyme immobilization using the cellulose-binding domain of a Cellulomonas mi exoglucanase. *BioTechnol* 1989; 7:604–607.

Ong E, Greenwood JM, Gilkes NR, Kilburn DG, Miller Jr. RC, Warren RAJ. The cellulose-binding domains of cellulases: tools for biotechnology. *Trends Biotechnol* 1989; 7:239–243.

Oppenheim AB, Giladi H, Goldenberg D, Kobi S, Azar I. Vectors and transformed host cells for recombinant protein production at reduced temperatures. International patent application WO 96/ 03521. February 1996.

Pace CN, Shirley BA, McNutt M, Gajiwala K. Forces contributing to the conformational stability of proteins. *FASEB J* 1996; 10:75–83.

Persson M, Bergstrand MG, Bulow L, Mosbach K. Enzyme purification by genetically attached polycysteine and polyphenylalanine affinity tails. *Anal Biochem* 1988; 172:330–337.

Petersen C. Control of functional mRNA stability in bacteria: Multiple mechanisms of nucleolytic and non-nucleolytic inactivation. *Mol Microbiol* 1992; 6:277–282.

Pilot-Matias TJ, Pratt SD, Lane BC. High-level synthesis of the 12-kDa human FK506-binding protein in *Escherichia coli* using translational coupling. *Gene* 1993; 128:219–225.

Platt T. Transcriptional termination and the regulation of gene expression. *Annu Rev Biochem* 1986; 55:339–372.

Pluckthun A. Mono- and bivalent antibody fragments produced in *Escherichia coli*: engineering, folding and antigen binding. *Immunol Rev* 1992; 130:151–188.

Podhajska AJ, Hasan N, Szybalski W. Control of cloned gene expression by promoter inversion *in vivo*: construction of the heat-pulse-activated att-nutL-p-att-N module. *Gene* 1985; 40:163–168.

Pohlner J, Krämer J, Meyer TF. A plasmid system for high-level expression and *in vitro* processing of recombinant proteins. *Gene* 1993; 130:121–126.

Pollitt S and Zalkin H. Role of primary structure and disulfide bond formation in β-lactamase secretion. *J Bacteriol* 1983; 153:27–32.

Pollock MR and Richmond MH. Low cyst(e)ine content of bacterial extracellular proteins: its possible physiological signicance. *Nature* (London) 1962; 194:446–449.

Poole ES, Brown CM, Tate WP. The identity of the base following the stop codon determines the efficiency of *in vivo* translational termination in *Escherichia coli*. *EMBO J* 1995; 14:151–158.

Prickett KS, Amberg DC, Hopp TP. A calcium-dependent antibody for identification and purification of recombinant proteins. *Bio-Techniques* 1989; 7:580–589.

Proba K, Ge LM, Plückthun A. Functional antibody single-chain fragments from the cytoplasm of *Escherichia coli*: influence of thioredoxin reductase (TrxB). *Gene* 1995; 159:203–207.

Proudfoot AEI, Power CA, Hoogewerf AJ, Montjovent M-O, Borlat F, Offord RE, Wells TNC. Extension of recombinant human RANTES by the retention of the initiating methionine produces a potent antagonist. *J Biol Chem* 1996; 271:2599–2603.

Pugsley AP. The complete general secretory pathway in gram-negative bacteria. Microbiol Rev 1993; 57:50–108.

Pugsley AP and Schwartz M. Export and secretion of proteins by bacteria. *FEMS Microbiol Rev* 1985; 32:3–38.

Ramesh V, De A, Nagaraja V. Engineering hyperexpression of bacteriophage Mu C protein by removal of secondary structure at the translation initiation region. *Protein Eng* 1994; 7:1053–1057.

Rao L, Ross W, Appleman JA, Gaal T, Leirmo S, Schlax PJ, Record MT, Gourse RL. Factor independent activation of rrnB P1 — an "extended" promoter with an upstream element that dramatically increases promoter strength. *J Mol Biol* 1994; 235:1421–1435.

Remaut E, Stanssens P, Fiers W. Plasmid vectors for high-efficiency expression controlled by the pL promoter of coliphage lambda. *Gene* 1981; 15:81–93.

Richardson JP. Transcription termination. *Crit Rev Biochem Mol Biol* 1993; 28:1–30.

Richardson JP and Greenblatt J. Control of RNA chain elongation and termination. In: Escherichia coli *and* Salmonella: Cellular and Molecular Biology. Vol. 1. Neidhardt FC, Curtiss III R., Ingraham JL, Lin ECC, Low KB, Magasanik B, Reznikoff WS, Riley M, Schaechter M, Umbarger HE, editors. ASM Press, Washington, DC, 1996: 822–848.

Rinas U, Tsai LB, Lyons D, Fox GM, Stearns G, Fieschko J, Fenton D, Bailey JE. Cysteine to serine substitutions in basic broblast growth factor: effect on inclusion body formation and proteolytic susceptibility during *in vitro* refolding. *BioTechnol* 1992; 10:435–440.

Ringquist S, Shinedling S, Barrick D, Green L, Binkley J, Stormo GD, Gold L. Translation initiation in *Escherichia coli*: sequences within the ribosome-binding site. *Mol Microbiol* 1992; 6:1219–1229.

Robben J, Massie G, Bosmans E, Wellens B, Volckaert G. An *Escherichia coli* plasmid vector system for high-level production and purification of heterologous peptides fused to active chloramphenicol acetyltransferase. *Gene* 1993; 126:109–113.

Roberts TM, Kacich R, Ptashne M. A general method for maximizing the expression of a cloned gene. *Proc Natl Acad Sci USA* 1979; 76:760–764.

Robertson JS. Strategy for adventitious agent assays. *Dev Biol Stand* 1996; 88:37-40.

Rogers S, Wells R, Rechsteiner M. Amino acid sequences common to rapidly degraded proteins: the PEST hypothesis. *Science* 1986; 234:364–368.

Ron D and Dressler H. pGSTag — a versatile bacterial expression plasmid for enzymatic labeling of recombinant proteins. *BioTechniques* 1992; 13:866–869.

Rosenberg AH, Goldman E, Dunn JJ, Studier FW, Zubay G. Effects of consecutive AGG codons on translation in *Escherichia coli*, demonstrated with a versatile codon test system. *J Bacteriol* 1993; 175:716–722.

Rosenberg AH and Studier FW. T7 RNA polymerase can direct expression of influenza virus cap-binding protein (PB2) in *Escherichia coli*. *Gene* 1987; 59:191–200.

Rosenberg M and Court D. Regulatory sequences involved in the promotion and termination of RNA transcription. *Annu Rev Genet* 1979; 13:319–353.

Ross J. mRNA stability in mammalian cells. Microbiol Rev 1995; 59:423–450.

Ross W, Gosink KK, Salomon J, Igarashi K, Zou C, Ishihama A, Severinov K, Gourse RL. A third recognition element in bacterial promoters: DNA binding by the subunit of RNA polymerase. *Science* 1993; 262:1407–1413.

Rudolph R and Lilie H. *In vitro* folding of inclusion body proteins. *FASEB J* 1996; 10:49–56.

Russell DR and Bennett GN. Cloning of small DNA fragments containing the *Escherichia coli* tryptophan operon promoter and operator. *Gene* 1982; 17:9–18.

Russell DR and Bennett GN. Construction and analysis of *in vivo* activity of *E. coli* promoter hybrids and promoter mutants that alter the 35 to 10 spacing. *Gene* 1982; 20:231–243.

Sagawa H, Ohshima A, Kato I. A tightly regulated expression system in *Escherichia coli* with SP6 RNA polymerase. *Gene* 1996; 168:37–41.

Saier Jr. MH. Differential codon usage: a safeguard against inappropriate expression of specialized genes? *FEBS Lett* 1995; 362:1–4.

Saier Jr. MH, Werner PK, Muller M. Insertion of proteins into bacterial membranes: mechanism, characteristics, and comparisons with the eucaryotic process. *Microbiol Rev* 1989; 53:333–366.

Sali A, Shakhnovich E, Karplus M. How does a protein fold? Nature (London) 1994; 369:248–251.

Samuelsson E, Moks T, Nilsson B, Uhlén M. Enhanced *in vitro* refolding of insulin-like growth factor I using a solubilizing fusion partner. *Biochemistry* 1994; 33:4207–4211.

Samuelsson E, Wadensten H, Hartmanis M, Moks T, Uhlén M. Facilitated *in vitro* refolding of human recombinant insulin-like growth factor I using a solubilizing fusion partner. *BioTechnol* 1991; 9:363–366.

San K-Y, Bennett GN, Aristidou AA, Chou CH. Strategies in high-level expression of recombinant protein in *Escherichia coli. Ann N Acad Sci* 1994; 721:257–267.

San K-Y, Bennett GN, Chou C-H, Aristidou AA. An optimization study of a pH-inducible promoter system for high-level recombinant protein production in *Escherichia coli. Ann NY Acad Sci* 1994; 721:268–276.

Sandler P and Weisblum B. Erythromycin-induced stabilization of ermA messenger RNA in Staphylococcus aureus and Bacillus subtilis. *J Mol Biol* 1988; 203:905–915.

Sandler P and Weisblum B. Erythromycin-induced ribosome stall in the ermA leader: a barricade to 5-to-3 nucleolytic cleavage of the ermA transcript. *J Bacteriol* 1989; 171:6680–6688.

Sandman K, Grayling RA, Reeve JN. Improved N-terminal processing of recombinant proteins synthesized in *Escherichia coli. BioTechnol* 1995; 13:504–506.

Sano T and Cantor CR. Expression vectors for streptavidin-containing chimeric proteins. *Biochem Biophys Res Commun* 1991; 176:571–577.

Sano, T, Glazer AN, Cantor CR. A streptavidin-metallothio-nein chimera that allows specific labeling of biological materials with many different heavy metal ions. *Proc Natl Acad Sci USA* 1992; 89:1534–1538.

Sarmientos P, Duchesne M, P. Denèe P, Boiziau J, Fromage N, Del-porte N, Parker F, Lelievre Y, Mayaux J-F, Cartwright T. Synthesis and purification of active human tissue plasminogen activator from *Escherichia coli. BioTechnol* 1989; 7:495–501.

Sassenfeld HM. Engineering proteins for purification. *Trends Biotechnol* 1990; 8:88–93.

Sassenfeld, HM and Brewer SJ. A polypeptide fusion designed for the purification of recombinant proteins. *BioTechnol* 1984; 2:76–81.

Sato K, Sato MH, Yamaguchi A, Yoshida M. Tetracycline/H antiporter was degraded rapidly in *Escherichia coli* cells when truncated at last transmembrane helix and this degradation was protected by overproduced GroEL/ES. *Biochem Biophys Res Commun* 1994; 202:258–264.

Schatz G and Dobberstein B. Common principles of protein translocation across membranes. *Science* 1996; 271:1519–1526.

Schatz PJ. Use of peptide libraries to map the substrate specificity of a peptide-modifying enzyme: a 13 residue consensus peptide species biotinylation in *Escherichia coli. BioTechnol* 1993; 11:1138–1143.

Schatz PJ and Beckwith J. Genetic analysis of protein export in *Escherichia coli. Annu Rev Genet* 1990; 24:215–248.

Schauder B, Blöcker H, Frank R, McCarthy JEG. Inducible expression vectors incorporating the *Escherichia coli* atpE translational initiation region. *Gene* 1987; 52:279–283.

Schauder B and McCarthy JEG. The role of bases upstream of the Shine-Dalgarno region and in the coding sequence in the control of gene expression in *Escherichia coli*: translation and stability of mRNAs *in vivo. Gene* 1989; 78:59–72.

Schein CH. Optimizing protein folding to the native state in bacteria. *Curr Opin Biotechnol* 1991; 2:746–750.

Schein CH. Production of soluble recombinant proteins in bacteria. *BioTechnol* 1989; 7:1141–1149.

Schein CH. Solubility and secretability. *Curr Opin Biotechnol* 1993; 4:456–461.

Schein CH, Boix E, Haugg M, Holliger KP, Hemmi S, Frank G. Secretion of mammalian ribonucleases from *Escherichia coli* using the signal sequence of murine spleen ribonuclease. *Biochem J* 1992; 283:137–144.

Scherer GFE, Walkinshaw MD, Arnott S, Morré DJ. The ribosome binding sites recognized by *E. coli* ribosomes have regions with signal character in both the leader and protein coding segments. *Nucleic Acids Res* 1980; 8:3895–3907.

Schertler GFX. Overproduction of membrane proteins. Curr Opin Struct Biol 1992; 2:534–544.

Schmidt TGM and Skerra A. The random peptide library-assisted engineering of a C-terminal affinity peptide, useful for the detection and purification of a functional Ig Fv fragment. *Protein Eng* 1993; 6:109–122.

Schneider TD, Stormo GD, Gold L, Ehrenfeucht A. Information content of binding sites on nucleotide sequences. *J Mol Biol* 1986; 188:415–431.

Schoner BE, Belagaje RM, Schoner RG. Translation of a synthetic two-cistron mRNA in *Escherichia coli*. *Proc Natl Acad Sci USA* 1986; 83:8506–8510.

Schoner BE, Belagaje RM, Schoner RG. Enhanced translational efficiency with two-cistron expression system. Methods Enzymol 1990; 185:94–103.

Schoner BE, Hsiung HM, Belagaje RM, Mayne NG, Schoner RG. Role of mRNA translational efficiency in bovine growth hormone expression in *Escherichia coli*. *Proc Natl Acad Sci USA* 1984; 81:5403–5407.

Schumperli D, McKenney K, Sobieski DA, Rosenberg M. Translational coupling at an intercistronic boundary of the *Escherichia coli* galactose operon. *Cell* 1982; 30:865–871.

Scolnik E, Tompkins R, Caskey T, Nirenberg M. Release factors differing in specificity for terminator codons. *Proc Natl Acad Sci USA* 1968; 61:768–774.

Sharp PM and Bulmer M. Selective differences among translation termination codons. *Gene* 1988; 63:141–145.

Sharp PM, Cowe E, Higgins DG, Shields DC, Wolfe KH, Wright F. Codon usage patterns in *Escherichia coli*, Bacillus subtilis, Saccharomyces cerevisiae, Schizosaccharomyces pombe, Drosophila melanogaster and *Homo sapiens*: a review of the considerable within-species diversity. *Nucleic Acids Res* 1988; 16:8207–8211.

Shatzman AR. Expression systems. Curr Opin Biotechnol 1995; 6:491–493.

Shean CS and Gottesman ME. Translation of the prophage cI transcript. *Cell* 1992; 70:513–522.

Shen SH. Multiple joined genes prevent product degradation in *Escherichia coli*. *Proc Natl Acad Sci USA* 1984; 81:4627–4631.

Shen T-J, Ho NT, Simplaceanu V, Zou M, Green BN, Tam MF, Ho C. Production of unmodified human adult hemoglobin in *Escherichia coli*. *Proc Natl Acad Sci USA* 1993; 90:8108–8112.

Shine J and Dalgarno L. The 3-terminal sequence of *Escherichia coli* 16S ribosomal RNA: complementarity to nonsense triplets and ribosome binding sites. *Proc Natl Acad Sci USA* 1974; 71:1342–1346.

Shine J and Dalgarno L. Determinant of cistron specificity in bacterial ribosomes. *Nature* (London) 1975; 254:34–38.

Shirakawa M, Tsurimoto T, Matsubara K. Plasmid vectors designed for high-efficiency expression controlled by the portable recA promoter-operator of *Escherichia coli*. Gene 1984; 28:127–132.

Shirano Y and Shibata D. Low temperature cultivation of *Escherichia coli* carrying a rice lipoxygenase L-2 cDNA produces a soluble and active enzyme at a high level. *FEBS Lett* 1990; 271:128–130.

Shuman HA, Silhavy TJ, Beckwith JR. Labeling of proteins with β-galactosidase by gene fusion. Identification of a cytoplasmic membrane component of the *Escherichia coli* maltose transport system. *J Biol Chem* 1980; 255:168–174.

Simon LD, Randolph B, Irwin N, Binkowski G. Stabilization of proteins by a bacteriophage T4 gene cloned in *Escherichia coli*. *Proc Natl Acad Sci USA* 1983; 80:2059–2062.

Simon LD, Tomczak K, St. John AC. Bacteriophages inhibit degradation of abnormal proteins in *E. coli*. *Nature* (London) 1978; 275:424–428.

Singer BS and Gold L. Phage T4 expression vector: protection from proteolysis. *Gene* 1991; 106:1–6.

Skerra A. Bacterial expression of immunoglobulin fragments. *Curr Opin Immunol* 1993; 5:256–262.

Skerra A. Use of the tetracycline promoter for the tightly regulated production of a murine antibody fragment in *Escherichia coli*. Gene 1994; 151: 131–135.

Smith DB and Johnson KS. Single-step purification of polypeptides expressed in *Escherichia coli* as fusions with glutathione S-transferase. *Gene* 1988; 67:31–40.

Snyder WB and Silhavy TJ. Enhanced export of β-galactosidase fusion proteins in prlF mutants is Lon dependent. *J Bacteriol* 1992; 174:5661–5668.

Sprengart ML, Fatscher HP, Fuchs E. The initiation of translation in *E. coli*: apparent base pairing between the 16S rRNA and downstream sequences of the mRNA. *Nucleic Acids Res* 1990; 18:1719–1723.

Sprengart ML, Fuchs E, Porter AG. The downstream box: an efficient and independent translation initiation signal in *Escherichia coli*. *EMBO J* 1996; 15:665–674.

Stadel D, Ecker J, Crooke ST. Ubiquitin fusion augments the yield of cloned gene products in *Escherichia coli*. *Proc Natl Acad Sci USA* 1989; 86:2540–2544.

Stader JA and Silhavy TJ. Engineering *Escherichia coli* to secrete heterologous gene products. *Methods Enzymol* 1990; 185:166–187.

Ståhl S, Nygren P-Å, Sjolander A, Uhlén M. Engineered bacterial receptors in immunology. *Curr Opin Immunol* 1993; 5:272–277.

Stallings G, Glover I, Olins PO. High-level production of active HIV-1 protease in *Escherichia coli. Gene* 1992; 122:263–269.

Stanssens P, Remaut E, Fiers W. Alterations upstream from the Shine-Dalgarno region and their effect on bacterial gene expression. *Gene* 1985; 36:211–223.

Stark MJR. Multicopy expression vectors carrying the lac repressor gene for regulated high-level expression of genes in *Escherichia coli. Gene* 1987; 51:255–267.

Steitz JA and Jakes K. How ribosomes select initiator regions in mRNA: base pair formation between the 3 terminus of 16S rRNA and the mRNA during initiation of protein synthesis in *Escherichia coli. Proc Natl Acad Sci USA* 1975; 72:4734–4738.

Stempfer G, Höll-Neugebauer B, Kopetzki E, Rudolph R. A fusion protein designed for noncovalent immobilization: stability, enzymatic activity, and use in an enzyme reactor. *Nat Biotechnol* 1996; 14:481–484.

Stempfer G, Höll-Neugebauer B, Rudolph R. Improved refolding of an immobilized fusion protein. *Nat Biotechnol* 1996; 14:329–334.

Stermeier M, De Sutter K, Georgiou G. Eukaryotic protein disulfide isomerase complements *Escherichia coli* dsbA mutants and increases the yield of a heterologous secreted protein with disulfide bonds. *J Biol Chem* 1996; 271:10616–10622.

Stormo GD, Schneider TD, Gold LM. Characterization of translational initiation sites in *E. coli. Nucleic Acids Res* 1982; 10:2971–2996.

Strandberg L and Enfors S-O. Factors inuencing inclusion body formation in the production of a fused protein in *Escherichia coli. Appl Environ Microbiol* 1991; 57:1669–1674.

Studier FW and Moffatt BA. Use of bacteriophage T7 RNA polymerase to direct selective high-level expression of cloned genes. *J Mol Biol* 1986; 189:113–130.

Studier FW, Rosenberg AH, Dunn JJ, Dubendorf JW. Use of T7 RNA polymerase to direct expression of cloned genes. *Methods Enzymol* 1990; 185:60–89.

Stueber D and Bujard H. Transcription from efficient promoters can interfere with plasmid replication and diminish expression of plasmid specified genes. EMBO J 1982; 1:1399–1404.

Su X, Prestwood AK, McGraw RA. Production of recombinant porcine tumor necrosis factor alpha in a novel *E. coli* expression system. *BioTechniques* 1992; 13:756–762.

Sugimoto S, Yokoo Y, Hatakeyama N, Yotsuji A, Teshiba S, Hagino H. Higher culture pH is preferable for inclusion body formation of recombinant salmon growth hormone in *Escherichia coli. Biotechnol Lett* 1991; 13:385–388.

Summers RG and Knowles JR. Illicit secretion of a cytoplasmic protein into the periplasm of *Escherichia coli* requires a signal peptide plus a portion of the cognate secreted protein. Demarcation of the critical region of the mature protein. *J Biol Chem* 1989; 264:20074–20081.

Suominen I, Karp M, Lähde M, Kopio A, Glumoff T, Meyer P, aMäntsä P. Extracellular production of cloned β-amylase by *Escherichia coli. Gene* 1987; 61:165–176.

Suter-Crazzolara C, Unsicker K. Improved expression of toxic proteins in *E. coli.* BioTechniques 1995; 19:202–204.

Swamy KHS and Goldberg AL. *E. coli* contains eight soluble proteolytic activities, one being ATP dependent. *Nature* (London) 1981; 292:652–654.

Swamy KHS and Goldberg AL. Subcellular distribution of various proteases in *Escherichia coli. J Bacteriol* 1982; 149:1027–1033.

Szekely M. From DNA to protein: the transfer of genetic information. John Wiley & Sons, Inc., New York, 1980; 13–17.

Tabor S and Richardson CC. A bacteriophage T7 RNA polymer-ase/promoter system for controlled exclusive expression of specific genes. *Proc Natl Acad Sci USA* 1985; 82:1074–1078.

Tacon W, Carey N, and Emtage S. The construction and characterization of plasmid vectors suitable for the expression of all DNA phases under the control of the *E. coli* tryptophan promoter. *Mol Gen Genet* 1980; 177:427–438.

Talmadge K and Gilbert W. Cellular location affects protein stability in *Escherichia coli. Proc Natl Acad Sci USA* 1982; 79:1830–1833.

Tanabe H, Goldstein J, Yang M, Inouye M. Identification of the promoter region of the *Escherichia coli* major cold shock gene, cspA. *J Bacteriol* 1992; 174:3867–3873.

Tarragona-Fiol A, Taylorson CJ, Ward JM, Rabin BR. Production of mature bovine pancreatic ribonuclease in *Escherichia coli*. *Gene* 1992; 118:239–245.

Tate WP and Brown CM. Translational termination: "stop" for protein synthesis or "pause" for regulation of gene expression. *Biochemistry* 1992; 31:2443–2450.

Taylor A, Brown DP, Kadam S, Maus M, Kohlbrenner WE, Weigl D, Turon MC, Katz L. High-level expression and purification of mature HIV-1 protease in *Escherichia coli* under control of the araBAD promoter. *Appl Microbiol Biotechnol* 1992; 37:205–210.

Taylor ME and Drickamer K. Carbohydrate-recognition domains as tools for rapid purification of recombinant eukaryotic proteins. *Biochem* 1991; 4:575–580.

Tessier L-H, Sondermeyer P, Faure T, Dreyer D, Benavente A, Villeval D, Courtney M, Lecocq J-P. The influence of mRNA primary and secondary structure on human IFN-gene expression in *E. coli*. *Nucleic Acids Res* 1984; 12:7663–7675.

Thomann H-U, Ibba M, Hong K-W, Söll D. Homologous expression and purification of mutants of an essential protein by reverse epitope-tagging. *BioTechnol* 1996; 14:50–55.

Thomas CD, Modha J, Razzaq TM, Cullis PM, Rivett AJ. Controlled high-level expression of the lon gene of *Escherichia coli* allows overproduction of Lon protease. *Gene* 1993; 136:237–242.

Thornton JM. Disulfide bridges in globular proteins. *J Mol Biol* 1981; 151:261–287.

Tobias JW, Shrader TE, Rocap G, Varshavsky A. The N-end rule in bacteria. *Science* 1991; 254:1374–1377.

Tolentino GJ, Meng S-Y, Bennett GN, San K-Y. A pH-regulated promoter for the expression of recombinant proteins in *Escherichia coli*. *Biotechnol Lett* 1992; 14:157–162.

Torriani A. Influence of inorganic phosphate in the formation of phosphatases by *Escherichia coli*. *Biochim Biophys Acta* 1960; 38:460–479.

Trudel P, Provost S, Massie B, Chartrand P, Wall L. pGATA: a positive selection vector based on the toxicity of the transcription factor GATA-1 to bacteria. *BioTechniques* 1996; 20:684–693.

Tunner JR, Robertson CR, Schippa S, Matin A. Use of glucose starvation to limit growth and induce protein production in *Escherichia coli*. *Biotechnol Bioeng* 1992; 40:271–279.

Tzareva NV, Makhno VI, Boni IV. Ribosome-messenger recognition in the absence of the Shine-Dalgarno interactions. *FEBS Lett* 1994; 337:189–194.

Uhlén M, Forsberg G, Moks T, Hartmanis M, Nilsson B. Fusion proteins in biotechnology. *Curr Opin Biotechnol* 1992; 3:363–369.

Uhlén M and Moks T. Gene fusions for purpose of expression: an introduction. *Methods Enzymol* 1990; 185:129–143.

Uhlén M, Nilsson B, Guss B, Lindberg M, Gatenbeck S, Philipson L. Gene fusion vectors based on the gene for staphylococcal protein A. *Gene* 1983; 23:369–378.

Ullmann A. One-step purification of hybrid proteins which have β-galactosidase activity. *Gene* 1984; 29:27–31.

van Dijl JM, de Jong A, Smith H, Bron S, Venema G. Signal peptidase I overproduction results in increased efficiencies of export and maturation of hybrid secretory proteins in *Escherichia coli*. *Mol Gen Genet* 1991; 227:40–48.

Varshavsky A. The N-end rule. *Cell* 1992; 69:725–735.

Vasquez JR, Evnin LB, Higaki JN, Craik CS. An expression system for trypsin. *J Cell Biochem* 1989; 39:265–276.

Vellanoweth RL and Rabinowitz JC. The influence of ribosome-binding-site elements on translational efficiency in Bacillus subtilis and *Escherichia coli in vivo*. *Mol Microbiol* 1992; 6:1105–1114.

Villa-Komaroff L, Efstratiadis A, Broome S, Lomedico P, Tizard R, Chick SWL, Gilbert W. A bacterial clone synthesizing proinsulin. *Proc Natl Acad Sci USA* 1978; 75:3727–3731.

von Heijne G. Transcending the impenetrable: how proteins come to with membranes. *Biochim Biophys Acta* 1988; 947:307–333.

von Heijne G. The signal peptide. *J Membr Biol* 1990; 115:195–201.

von Heijne G and Abrahmsén L. Species-specific variation in signal peptide design. Implications for protein secretion in foreign hosts. *FEBS Lett* 1989; 244:439–446.

von Strandmann EP, Zoidl C, Nakhei H, Holewa B, von Strand-mann RP, Lorenz P, Klein-Hitpass L, Ryffel GU. A highly specific and sensitive monoclonal antibody detecting histidine-tagged recombinant proteins. *Protein Eng* 1995; 8:733–735.

Voorma HO. Control of translation initiation in prokaryotes. In: *Translational Control*. Hershey JWB, Mathews MB, and Sonenberg N, editors. Cold Spring Harbor Laboratory Press, Cold Spring Harbor, NY, 1996: 759–777.

Wada K-N, Wada Y, Ishibashi F, Gojobori T, Ikemura T. Codon usage tabulated from the GenBank genetic sequence data. *Nucleic Acids Res* 1992; 20(Suppl.):2111–2118.

Wang L-F, Yu M, White JR, Eaton BT. BTag: a novel six-residue epitope tag for surveillance and purification of recombinant proteins. *Gene* 1996; 169:53–58.

Warburton N, Boseley PG, Porter AG. Increased expression of a cloned gene by local mutagenesis of its promoter and ribosome binding site. *Nucleic Acids Res* 1983; 11:5837–5854.

Ward ES. Expression and secretion of T-cell receptor V and V domains using *Escherichia coli* as a host. *Scand J Immunol* 1991; 34:215–220.

Ward ES, Gupta D, Grifths AD, Jones PT, Winter G. Binding activities of a repertoire of single immunoglobulin variable domains secreted from *Escherichia coli*. *Nature* (London) 1989; 341:544–546.

Ward GA, Stover CK, Moss B, Fuerst TR. Stringent chemical and thermal regulation of recombinant gene expression by vaccinia virus vectors in mammalian cells. *Proc Natl Acad Sci USA* 1995; 92:6773–6777.

Warne SR, Thomas CM, Nugent ME, Tacon WCA. Use of a modified *Escherichia coli* trpR gene to obtain tight regulation of high-copy-number expression vectors. *Gene* 1986; 46:103–112.

Wetzel R. Protein aggregation *in vivo*. Bacterial inclusion bodies and mammalian amyloid. In: *Stability of Protein Pharmaceuticals. B.* In vivo *Pathways of Degradation and Strategies for Protein Stabilization.* Ahern TJ and Manning MC, editors. Plenum Press, New York, 1992: 43–48.

WHO Expert Committee on Biological Standardization. Requirements for the collection, processing and quality control of blood, blood components and plasma derivatives (Requirements for biological substances No 27, revised 1992). 43rd Report, Annex 2. 1994. World Health Organization, Geneva. WHO Technical Report Series, No 840.

WHO. Report of a WHO consultation on medicinal and other products in relation to human and animal transmissible spongiform encephalopathies. WHO/BLG/97.2. 1997. World Health Organization, Geneva.

WHO. WHO requirements for the use of animal cells as *in vitro* substrates for the production of biologicals (Requirements for biological substances No 50). *Dev Biol Stand* 1998; 93:141–171.

Wickner W. Assembly of proteins into membranes. *Science* 1980; 210:861–868.

Wikstrom PM, Lind LK, Berg DE, Björk GR. Importance of mRNA folding and start codon accessibility in the expression of genes in a ribosomal protein operon of *Escherichia coli*. *J Mol Biol* 1992; 224:949–966.

Wilkinson DL and Harrison RG. Predicting the solubility of recombinant proteins in *Escherichia coli*. *Bio-Technol* 1991; 9:443–448.

Wilkinson DL, Ma NT, Haught C, Harrison RG. Purification by immobilized metal affinity chromatography of human atrial natriuretic peptide expressed in a novel thioredoxin fusion protein. *Biotechnol Prog* 1995; 11:265–269.

Williams KL, Emslie KR, Slade MB. Recombinant glycoprotein production in the slime mould Dictyostelium discoideum. *Curr Opin Biotechnol* 1995; 6:538–542.

Wilson BS, Kautzer CR, Antelman DE. Increased protein expression through improved ribosome-binding sites obtained by library mutagenesis. *BioTechniques* 1994; 17:944.

Wilson KS and von Hippel PH. Transcription termination at intrinsic terminators: the role of the RNA hairpin. *Proc Natl Acad Sci USA* 1995; 92:8793–8797.

Wittliff JL, Wenz LL, Dong J, Nawaz Z, Butt TR. Expression and characterization of an active human estrogen receptor as a ubiquitin fusion protein from *Escherichia coli*. *J Biol Chem* 1990; 265:22016–22022.

Wolber V, Maeda K, Schumann R, Brandmeier B, Wiesmüller L, Wittinghofer A. A universal expression-purification system based on the coiled-coil interaction of myosin heavy chain. *BioTechnol* 1992; 10:900–904.

Wong HC and Chang S. Identification of a positive retroregulator that stabilizes mRNAs in bacteria. *Proc Natl Acad Sci USA* 1986; 83:3233–3237.

Wong HC and Chang S. 3-Expression enhancing fragments and method. U.S. patent 4,910,141. March 1990.

Wückthun. Protein folding in the periplasm of *Escherichia coli*. *Mol Microbiol* 1994; 12:685–692.

Xue G-P. ¨Ing, C., and A. Plu Cultivation process and constructs for use therein. International patent application WO 95/11981. May 1995.

Xue G-P, Johnson JS, Smyth DJ, Dierens LM, Wang X, Simpson GD, Gobius KS, Aylward JH. Temperature regulated expression of the tac/lacI system for overproduction of a fungal xylanase in *Escherichia coli*. *Appl Microbiol Biotechnol* 1996; 45:120–126.

Yabuta M, Onai-Miura S, Ohsuye K. Thermo-inducible expression of a recombinant fusion protein by *Escherichia coli* lac repressor mutants. *J Biotechnol* 1995; 39:67–73.

Yamada M, Kubo M, Miyake T, Sakaguchi R, Higo Y, Imanaka T. Promoter sequence analysis in Bacillus and Escherichia: construction of strong promoters in *E. coli. Gene* 1991; 99:109–114.

Yamamoto T and Imamoto F. Differential stability of trp messenger RNA synthesized originating at the trp promoter and pL promoter of lambda trp phage. *J Mol Biol* 1975; 92:289–309.

Yamane,T and Shimizu S. Fed-batch techniques in microbial processes. Adv Biochem Eng 1984; 30:147–194.

Yamano,N, Kawata Y, Kojima H, Yoda K, Yamasaki M. *In vivo* biotinylation of fusion proteins expressed in *Escherichia coli* with a sequence of Propionibacterium freudenreichii transcarboxylase 1.3S biotin subunit. *Biosci Biotechnol Biochem* 1992; 56:1017–1026.

Yang M-T, Scott II HB, Gardner JF. Transcription termination at the thr attenuator. Evidence that the adenine residues upstream of the stem and loop structure are not required for termination. *J Biol Chem* 1995; 270:23330–23336.

Yanisch-Perron C, Vieira J, Messing J. Improved M13 phage cloning vectors and host strains: nucleotide sequences of the M13mp18 and pUC19 vectors. *Gene* 1985; 33:103–119.

Yansura DG. Expression as trpE fusion. *Methods Enzymol* 1990; 185:161–166.

Yansura DG and Henner DJ. Use of *Escherichia coli* trp promoter for direct expression of proteins. *Methods Enzymol* 1990; 185:54–60.

Yasukawa T, Kaneiishii C, Maekawa T, Fujimoto J, Yamamoto T. Increase of solubility of foreign proteins in *Escherichia coli* by coproduction of the bacterial thioredoxin. J Biol Chem 1995; 270:25328–25331.

Yee L and Blanch HW. Recombinant protein expression in high cell density fed-batch cultures of *Escherichia coli. BioTechnol* 1992; 10:1550–1556.

Yike I, Zhang Y, Ye J, Dearborn DG. Expression in *Escherichia coli* of cytoplasmic portions of the cystic fibrosis transmembrane conductance regulator: apparent bacterial toxicity of peptides containing R-domain sequences. *Protein Expression Purif* 1996; 7:45–50.

Young JF, Dusselberger U, Palese P, Ferguson B, Shatzman AR. Efficient expression of influenza virus NS1 nonstructural proteins in *Escherichia coli. Proc Natl Acad Sci USA* 1983; 80:6105–6109.

Yu P, Aristidou AA, San K-Y. Synergistic effects of glycine and bacteriocin release protein in the release of periplasmic protein in recombinant *E. coli. Biotechnol. Lett* 1991; 13:311–316.

Zacharias M, Goringer HU, Wagner R. Analysis of the Fis-dependent and Fis-independent transcription activation mechanisms of the *Escherichia coli* ribosomal RNA P1 promoter. *Biochemistry* 1992; 31:2621–2628.

Zentgraf H, Frey M, Schwinn S, Tessmer C, Willemann B, Samstag Y, Velhagen I. Detection of histidine-tagged fusion proteins by using a high-specific mouse monoclonal anti-histidine tag antibody. *Nucleic Acids Res* 1995; 23:3347–3348.

Zhang J and Deutscher MP. *Escherichia coli* RNase D: sequencing of the rnd structural gene and purification of the overexpressed protein. *Nucleic Acids Res* 1988; 16:6265–6278.

Zhang J and Deutscher MP. Analysis of the upstream region of the *Escherichia coli* rnd gene encoding RNase D. Evidence for translational regulation of a putative tRNA processing enzyme. *J Biol Chem* 1989; 264:18228–18233.

Zhang J and Deutscher MP. A uridine-rich sequence required for isolation of prokaryotic mRNA. *Proc Natl Acad Sci USA* 1992; 89:2605.

Zhang S, Zubay G, Goldman E. Low usage codons in *Escherichia coli*, yeast, fruit fly and primates. *Gene* 1991; 105:61–72.

CHAPTER 5: UPSTREAM PROCESSING

Berry DR. Growth of yeast. In: *Fermentation Process Development of Industrial Organisms*. Neway JO, editor. Marcel Dekker Inc., New York, 1989: 277–311.

Bylund F, Collet E, Enfors SO, Larsson G. Substrate gradient formation in the large-scale bioreactor lowers cell yield and increases by-product formation. *Bioprocess Eng* 1998; 18(3):171–180.

Dale C, Allen A, Fogerty S. Pichia pastoris: A eukaryotic system for the large-scale production of biopharmaceuticals. *BioPharm* 1999; 12(11):36–42.

Handa-Corrigan A. Bioreactors for mammalian cells. In: Mammalian cell biotechnology. A practical approach. Butler M, editor. IRL Press, Oxford, 1991: 139–158.

Hensing MC, Rouwenhorst RJ, Heijnen JJ, van Dijken JP, Pronk JT. Physiological and technological aspects of large-scale heterologous-protein production with yeasts. *Antonie Van Leeuwenhoek* 1995; 67(3):261–279.

Larsson G, Törnquist M, Ståhl Wernesson E, Trägårdh C, Noorman H, Enfors SO. Substrate gradients in bioreactors: origin and consequences. *Bioprocess Eng* 1996; 14(6):281–289.

Lee SY. High cell-density culture of *Escherichia coli. Trends Biotechnol* 1996; 14(3):98–105.

Mizutani S, Mori H, Shimizu S, Sakaguchi S, Kobayashi T. Effect of amino acid supplement on cell yield and gene product in *Escherichia coli* harboring plasmid. *Biotechnol Bioeng* 1986; 28:204–209.

Mori H, Yano T, Kobayashi T, Shimizu S. High density cultivation of biomass in fed-batch system with DO-Stat. *J Chem Eng* Japan 1979; 12:313–319.

Rosenfeld SA, Brandis JW, Ditullio DF, Lee JF, Armiger WB. High-cell-density fermentations based on culture fluorescence. In: *Expression Systems and Processes for rDNA Products*. Hatch RT, Goochee C, Moreira A, Alroy Y, editors. ACS, Washington, DC, 1991: 23–33.

CHAPTER 6: MANUFACTURING SYSTEMS

BACTERIAL SYSTEMS

Andrews B, Adari H, Hannig G, Lahue E, Gosselin M, Martin S, Ahmed A, Ford PJ, Hayman EG, Makrides SC. A tightly regulated high level expression vector that utilizes a thermosensitive lac repressor: production of the human T cell receptor V beta 5.3 in *Escherichia coli. Gene* 1996; 182(1–2): 101–109.

Arthur PM, Duckworth B, Seidman M. High level expression of interleukin-1 beta in a recombinant *Escherichia coli* strain for use in a controlled bioreactor. *J Biotechnol* 1990; 13(1):29–46.

Baneyx F. Recombinant protein expression in *Escherichia coli. Curr Opin Biotechnol* 1999; 10(5):411–421.

Batas B, Chaudhuri JB. Protein refolding at high concentration using size-exclusion chromatography. *Biotechnol Bioeng* 1996; 50(1):16–23.

Bech Jensen E and Carlsen S. Production of recombinant human growth hormone in *Escherichia coli*: expression of different precursors and physiological effects of glucose, acetate and salts. *Biotechnol Bioeng* 1990; 36(1):1–11.

Bermudez-Humaran LG, Langella P, Miyoshi A, Gruss A, Guerra RT, Montes dO-L, Le Loir Y. Production of human papillomavirus type 16 E7 protein in Lactococcus lactis. *Appl Environ Microbiol* 2002; 68(2):917–922.

Berry DR. Growth of yeast. In: *Fermentation Process Development of Industrial Organisms*. Neway JO, editor. Marcel Dekker Inc., New York, 1989: 277–311.

Billman-Jacobe H. Expression in bacteria other than *Escherichia coli. Curr Opin Biotechnol* 1996; 7(5):500–504.

Birnboim HC and Doly J. A rapid alkaline extraction procedure for screening recombinant plasmid DNA. *Nucleic Acids Res* 1979; 7(6):1513–1523.

Breuer S, Marzban G, Cserjan-Puschmann M, Durrschmid E, Bayer K. Off-line quantitative monitoring of plasmid copy number in bacterial fermentation by capillary electrophoresis. *Electrophoresis* 1998; 19(14):2474–2478.

Buchner J and Rudolph R. Renaturation, purification and characterization of recombinant Fab-fragments produced in *Escherichia coli. Biotechnology* (NY) 1991; 9(2):157–162.

Bylund F, Castan A, Mikkola R, Veide A, Larsson G. Influence of scale-up on the quality of recombinant human growth hormone. *Biotechnol Bioeng* 2000; 69(2):119–128.

Bylund F, Collet E, Enfors SO, Larsson G. Substrate gradient formation in the large-scale bioreactor lowers cell yield and increases by-product formation. *Bioprocess Eng* 1998; 18(3):171–180.

Caldwell SR, Varghese J, Puri NK. Large scale purification process for recombinant NS1-OspA as a candidate vaccine for Lyme disease. *Bioseparation* 1996; 6(2):115–123.

Cleland JL, Builder SE, Swartz JR, Winkler M, Chang JY, Wang DI. Polyethylene glycol enhanced protein refolding. *Biotechnology* (NY) 1992; 10(9):1013–1019.

Clemmitt RH and Chase HA. Facilitated downstream processing of a histidine-tagged protein from unclarified *E. coli* homogenates using immobilized metal affinity expanded-bed adsorption. *Biotechnol Bioeng* 2000; 67(2):206–216.

Dahlgren ME, Powell AL, Greasham RL, George HA. Development of scale-down techniques for investigation of recombinant *Escherichia coli* fermentations: acid metabolites in shake flasks and stirred bioreactors. *Biotechnol Prog* 1993; 9(6):580–586.

Dale C, Allen A, Fogerty S. Pichia pastoris: A eukaryotic system for the large-scale production of biopharmaceuticals. *BioPharm* 1999; 12(11):36–42.

de Oliveira JE, Soares CR, Peroni CN, Gimbo E, Camargo IM, Morganti L, Bellini MH, Affonso R, Arkaten RR, Bartolini P, Ribela MT. High-yield purification of biosynthetic human growth hormone secreted in *Escherichia coli* periplasmic space. *J Chromatogr A* 1999; 852(2):441–450.

de Vos WM. Gene expression systems for lactic acid bacteria. *Curr Opin Microbiol* 1999; 2(3):289–295.

Dieye Y, Usai S, Clier F, Gruss A, Piard JC. Design of a protein-targeting system for lactic acid bacteria. *J Bacteriol* 2001; 183(14):4157–4166.

Dobeli H, Andres H, Breyer N, Draeger N, Sizmann D, Zuber MT, Weinert B, Wipf B. Recombinant fusion proteins for the industrial production of disulfide bridge containing peptides: purification, oxidation without concatamer formation, and selective cleavage. *Protein Expr Purif* 1998; 12(3):404–414.

Ejima D, Watanabe M, Sato Y, Date M, Yamada N, Takahara Y. High yield refolding and purification process for recombinant human interleukin-6 expressed in *Escherichia coli*. *Biotechnol Bioeng* 1999; 62(3):301–310.

Fahey EM, Chaudhuri JB, Binding P. Refolding and purification of a urokinase plasminogen activator fragment by chromatography. *J Chromatogr B Biomed Sci Appl* 2000; 737(1–2):225–235.

Fahey EM, Chaudhuri JB, Binding P. Refolding of low molecular weight urokinase plasminogen activator by dilution and size exclusion chromatography — a comparative study. *Sep Sci Technol* 2000; 35:1743–1760.

Feliu JX, Cubarsi R, Villaverde A. Optimized release of recombinant proteins by ultrasonication of *E. coli* cells. *Biotechnol Bioeng* 1998; 58(5):536–540.

Feng M and Glassey J. Physiological state-specific models in estimation of recombinant *Escherichia coli* fermentation performance. *Biotechnol Bioeng* 2000; 69(5):495–503.

Franchi E, Maisano F, Testori SA, Galli G, Toma S, Parente L, de Ferra F, Grandi G. A new human growth hormone production process using a recombinant Bacillus subtilis strain. *J Biotechnol* 1991; 18(1–2):41–54.

Friehs K and Reardon KF. Parameters influencing the productivity of recombinant *E. coli* cultivations. *Adv Biochem Eng Biotechnol* 1993; 48:53–77.

Funaba M and Mathews LS. Recombinant expression and purification of smad proteins. *Protein Expr Purif* 2000; 20(3):507–513.

Gaeng S, Scherer S, Neve H, Loessner MJ. Gene cloning and expression and secretion of Listeria monocytogenes bacteriophage-lytic enzymes in Lactococcus lactis. *Appl Environ Microbiol* 2000; 66(7):2951–2958.

Georgiou G and Valax P. Isolating inclusion bodies from bacteria. *Methods Enzymol* 1999; 309:48–58.

Gibert S, Bakalara N, Santarelli X. Three-step chromatographic purification procedure for the production of a his-tag recombinant kinesin overexpressed in *E. coli*. *J Chromatogr B Biomed Sci Appl* 2000; 737(1–2):143–150.

Goldberg ME, Expert-Bezancon N, Vuillard L, Rabilloud T. Non-detergent sulphobetaines: a new class of molecules that facilitate *in vitro* protein renaturation. *Folding and Design* 1996; 1(1):21–27.

Hannig G and Makrides SC. Strategies for optimizing heterologous protein expression in *Escherichia coli*. *Trends Biotechnol* 1998; 16(2):54–60.

Harder MP, Sanders EA, Wingender E, Deckwer WD. Studies on the production of human parathyroid hormone by recombinant *Escherichia coli*. *Appl Microbiol Biotechnol* 1993; 39(3):329–334.

Hartleib J and Ruterjans H. High-yield expression, purification, and characterization of the recombinant diisopropylfluorophosphatase from Loligo vulgaris. *Protein Expr Purif* 2001; 21(1):210–219.

Hensing MC, Rouwenhorst RJ, Heijnen JJ, van Dijken JP, Pronk JT. Physiological and technological aspects of large-scale heterologous-protein production with yeasts. *Antonie Van Leeuwenhoek* 1995; 67(3):261–279.

Hodgson J. Expression systems: a user's guide. Emphasis has shifted from the vector construct to the host organism. *Biotechnology* (NY) 1993; 11(8):887–893.

Hoffman BJ, Broadwater JA, Johnson P, Harper J, Fox BG, Kenealy WR. Lactose fed-batch overexpression of recombinant metalloproteins in *Escherichia coli* BL21 (DE3): process control yielding high levels of metal-incorporated, soluble protein. *Protein Expr Purif* 1995; 6(5):646–654.

Holms WH. The central metabolic pathways of *Escherichia coli*: relationship between flux and control at a branch point, efficiency of conversion to biomass, and excretion of acetate. *Curr Top Cell Regul* 1986; 28:69–105.

Jung G, Denefle P, Becquart J, Mayaux JF. High-cell density fermentation studies of recombinant *Escherichia coli* strains expressing human interleukin-1 beta. *Ann Inst Pasteur Microbiol* 1988; 139(1):129–146.

Karuppiah N and Sharma A. Cyclodextrins as protein folding aids. *Biochem Biophys Res Commun* 1995; 211(1):60–66.

Kramer W, Elmecker G, Weik R, Mattanovich D, Bayer K. Kinetics studies for the optimization of recombinant protein formation. *Ann NY Acad Sci* 1996; 782:323–333.

Langella P and Le Loir Y. Heterologous protein secretion in Lactococcus lactis: a novel antigen delivery system. *Braz J Med Biol Res* 1999; 32(2):191–198.

Le Loir Y, Gruss A, Ehrlich SD, Langella P. A nine-residue synthetic propeptide enhances secretion efficiency of heterologous proteins in Lactococcus lactis. *J Bacteriol* 1998; 180(7):1895–1903.

Le Loir Y, Nouaille S, Commissaire J, Bretigny L, Gruss A, Langella P. Signal peptide and propeptide optimization for heterologous protein secretion in Lactococcus lactis. *Appl Environ Microbiol* 2001; 67(9):4119–4127.

Lee JY, Yoon CS, Chung IY, Lee YS, Lee EK. Scale-up process for expression and renaturation of recombinant human epidermal growth factor from *Escherichia coli* inclusion bodies. *Biotechnol Appl Biochem* 2000; 31(Pt 3):245–248.

Lee SY. High cell-density culture of *Escherichia coli*. *Trends Biotechnol* 1996; 14(3):98–105.

Lin HY and Neubauer P. Influence of controlled glucose oscillations on a fed-batch process of recombinant *Escherichia coli*. *J Biotechnol* 2000; 79(1):27–37.

Lin LS, Yamamoto R, Drummond RJ. Purification of recombinant human interferon E expressed in *Escherichia coli*. *Methods Enzymol* 1986; 119:183–192.

Listrom CD, Morizono H, Rajagopal BS, McCann MT, Tuchman M, Allewell NM. Expression, purification, and characterization of recombinant human glutamine synthetase. *Biochem J* 1997; 328(Pt 1):159–163.

Liu S, Tobias R, McClure S, Styba G, Shi Q, Jackowski G. Removal of endotoxin from recombinant protein preparations. *Clin Biochem* 1997; 30(6):455–463.

Looker D, Mathews AJ, Neway JO, Stetler GL. Expression of recombinant human hemoglobin in *Escherichia coli*. *Methods Enzymol* 1994; 231:364–374.

Luli GW and Strohl WR. Comparison of growth, acetate production, and acetate inhibition of *Escherichia coli* strains in batch and fed-batch fermentations. *Appl Environ Microbiol* 1990; 56(4):1004–1011.

MacDonald HL and Neway JO. Effects of medium quality on the expression of human interleukin-2 at high cell density in fermentor cultures of *Escherichia coli* K-12. *Appl Environ Microbiol* 1990; 56(3):640–645.

Marczinovits I, Somogyi C, Patthy A, Nemeth P, Molnar J. An alternative purification protocol for producing hepatitis B virus X antigen on a preparative scale in *Escherichia coli*. *J Biotechnol* 1997; 56(2):81-88.

Marston FA. The purification of eukaryotic polypeptides synthesized in *Escherichia coli*. *Biochem J* 1986; 240(1):1–12.

Marston FA and Hartley DL. Solubilization of protein aggregates. *Methods in Enzymology* 1990; 182(20):264–276.

Merten OW. Safety issues of animal products used in serum-free media. *Dev Biol Stand* 1999; 99:167–180.

Miksch G, Neitzel R, Fiedler E, Friehs K, Flaschel E. Extracellular production of a hybrid beta-glucanase from Bacillus by *Escherichia coli* under different cultivation conditions in shaking cultures and bioreactors. *Appl Microbiol Biotechnol* 1997; 47(2):120–126.

Miyoshi A, Poquet I, Azevedo V, Commissaire J, Bermudez-Humaran L, Domakova E, Le Loir Y, Oliveira SC, Gruss A, Langella P. Controlled production of stable heterologous proteins in Lactococcus lactis. *Appl Environ Microbiol* 2002; 68(6):3141–3146.

Muller C and Rinas U. Renaturation of heterodimeric platelet-derived growth factor from inclusion bodies of recombinant *Escherichia coli* using size-exclusion chromatography. *J Chromatogr A* 1999; 855(1):203–213.

Nagai K, Thogersen HC, Luisi BF. Refolding and crystallographic studies of eukaryotic proteins produced in *Escherichia coli*. *Biochem Soc Trans* 1988; 16(2):108–110.

Neubauer P, Hofmann K, Holst O, Mattiasson B, Kruschke P. Maximizing the expression of a recombinant gene in *Escherichia coli* by manipulation of induction time using lactose as inducer. *Appl Microbiol Biotechnol* 1992; 36(6):739–744.

Nilsson J, Stahl S, Lundeberg J, Uhlen M, Nygren PA. Affinity fusion strategies for detection, purification, and immobilization of recombinant proteins. *Protein Expr Purif* 1997; 11(1):1–16.

Novotny J, Ganju RK, Smiley ST, Hussey RE, Luther MA, Recny MA, Siliciano RF, Reinherz EL. A soluble, single-chain T-cell receptor fragment endowed with antigen-combining properties. *Proc Natl Acad Sci USA* 1991; 88(19):8646–8650.

Patra AK, Mukhopadhyay R, Mukhija R, Krishnan A, Garg LC, Panda AK. Optimization of inclusion body solubilization and renaturation of recombinant human growth hormone from *Escherichia coli*. *Protein Expr Purif* 2000; 18(2):182–192.

Pedersen J, Lauritzen C, Madsen MT, Weis DS. Removal of N-terminal polyhistidine tags from recombinant proteins using engineered aminopeptidases. *Protein Expr Purif* 1999; 15(3):389–400.

Petsch D and Anspach FB. Endotoxin removal from protein solutions. *J Biotechnol* 2000; 76(2–3):97–119.

Piard JC, Jimenez-Diaz R, Fischetti VA, Ehrlich SD, Gruss A. The M6 protein of Streptococcus pyogenes and its potential as a tool to anchor biologically active molecules at the surface of lactic acid bacteria. *Adv Exp Med Biol* 1997; 418:545–550.

Pluckthun A, Krebber A, Krebber C, Horn U, Knupfer U, Wenderoth R et al. Producing antibodies in *Escherichia coli*: From PCR to fermentation. In: *Antibody Engineering*. McCafferty J, Hoogenboom H, Chiswell D, editors. JRL Press, Oxford, 1996: 203–252.

Poquet I, Ehrlich SD, Gruss A. An export-specific reporter designed for gram-positive bacteria: application to Lactococcus lactis. *J Bacteriol* 1998; 180(7):1904–1912.

Qureshi GA, Fohlin L, Bergstrom J. Application of high-performance liquid chromatography to the determination of free amino acids in physiological fluids. *J Chromatogr* 1984; 297:91–100.

Riesenberg D. High-cell-density cultivation of *Escherichia coli*. *Curr Opin Biotechnol* 1991; 2(3):380–384.

Riesenberg D, Menzel K, Schulz V, Schumann K, Veith G, Zuber G, Knorre WA. High cell density fermentation of recombinant *Escherichia coli* expressing human interferon alpha 1. *Appl Microbiol Biotechnol* 1990; 34(1):77–82.

Rinas U, Kracke-Helm HA, Schügerl K. Glucose as substrate in recombinant strain fermentation technology. *Appl Microbiol Biotechnol* 1989; 31(2):163–167.

Rosenfeld SA, Nadeau D, Tirado J, Hollis GF, Knabb RM, Jia S. Production and purification of recombinant hirudin expressed in the methylotrophic yeast Pichia pastoris. *Protein Expr Purif* 1996; 8(4):476–482.

Rymaszewski Z, Abplanalp WA, Cohen RM, Chomczynski P. Estimation of cellular DNA content in cell lysates suitable for RNA isolation. *Anal Biochem* 1990; 188(1):91–96.

Sandkvist M and Bagdasarian M. Secretion of recombinant proteins by gram-negative bacteria. *Curr Opin Biotechnol* 1996; 7(5):505–511.

Savijoki K, Kahala M, Palva A. High level heterologous protein production in Lactococcus and Lactobacillus using a new secretion system based on the Lactobacillus brevis S-layer signals. *Gene* 1997; 186(2):255–262.

Schein CH. Production of soluble recombinant proteins in bacteria. *Biotechnology* (NY) 1989; 7(11):1141–1149.

Seeger A and Rinas U. Two-step chromatographic procedure for purification of basic fibroblast growth factor from recombinant *Escherichia coli* and characterization of the equilibrium parameters of adsorption. *J Chromatogr A* 1996; 746(1):17–24.

Skerra A. Bacterial expression of immunoglobulin fragments. *Curr Opin Immunol* 1993; 5(2):256–262.

Steidler L, Robinson K, Chamberlain L, Schofield KM, Remaut E, Le Page RW, Wells JM. Mucosal delivery of murine interleukin-2 (IL-2) and IL-6 by recombinant strains of Lactococcus lactis coexpressing antigen and cytokine. *Infect Immun* 1998; 66(7):3183–3189.

Stratton J, Chiruvolu V, Meagher M. High cell-density fermentation. *Methods Mol Biol* 1998; 103:107–120.

Summers DK and Sherratt DJ. Multimerization of high copy number plasmids causes instability: ColE1 encodes a determinant essential for plasmid monomerization and stability. *Cell* 1984; 36(4):1097–1103.

Swartz JR. Advances in *Escherichia coli* production of therapeutic proteins. *Curr Opin Biotechnol* 2001; 12(2):195–201.

Tandon S and Horowitz P. The effects of lauryl maltoside on the reactivation of several enzymes after treatment with guanidinium chloride. *Biochim Biophys Acta* 1988; 955(1):19–25.

Tarnowski SJ, Roy SK, Liptak RA, Lee DK, Ning RY. Large-scale purification of recombinant human leukocyte interferons. *Methods Enzymol* 2002; 119:153–165.

Thatcher DR. Recovery of therapeutic proteins from inclusion bodies: problems and process strategies. *Biochem Soc Trans* 1990; 18(2):234–235.

Thies MJ and Pirkl F. Chromatographic purification of the C(H)2 domain of the monoclonal antibody MAK33. *J Chromatogr B Biomed Sci Appl* 2000; 737(1–2):63–69.

Thøgersen C, Holtet TL, Etzerodt M. -Denzyme Aps, Assignee. Iterative method of at least five cycles for the refolding of proteins. Patent US 5917018. Issued 29-6-1999. September 18, 1995.

Thompson BG, Kole M, Gerson DF. Control of ammonium concentration in *Escherichia coli* fermentations. *Biotechnol Bioeng* 1985; 27:818–824.

Walsh G. Biopharmaceutical benchmarks. *Nat Biotechnol* 2000; 18(8):831–833.

Warren TC, Miglietta JJ, Shrutkowski A, Rose JM, Rogers SL, Lubbe K, Shih CK, Caviness GO, Ingraham R, Palladino DE. Comparative purification of recombinant HIV-1 and HIV-2 reverse transcriptase: preparation of heterodimeric enzyme devoid of unprocessed gene product. *Protein Expr Purif* 1992; 3(6):479–487.

Weickert MJ, Doherty DH, Best EA, Olins PO. Optimization of heterologous protein production in *Escherichia coli*. *Curr Opin Biotechnol* 1996; 7(5):494–499.

Werner MH, Clore GM, Gronenborn AM, Kondoh A, Fisher RJ. Refolding proteins by gel filtration chromatography. *FEBS Lett* 1994; 345(2–3):125–130.

Wetlaufer DB and Xie Y. Control of aggregation in protein refolding: a variety of surfactants promote renaturation of carbonic anhydrase II. *Protein Sci* 1995; 4(8):1535–1543.

Wlad H, Ballagi A, Bouakaz L, Gu Z, Janson JC. Rapid two-step purification of a recombinant mouse Fab fragment expressed in *Escherichia coli*. *Protein Expr Purif* 2001; 22(2):325–329.

Xu B, Jahic M, Blomsten G, Enfors SO. Glucose overflow metabolism and mixed-acid fermentation in aerobic large-scale fed-batch processes with *Escherichia coli*. *Appl Microbiol Biotechnol* 1999; 51(5):564–571.

Yamane T and Shimizu S. Fed-batch techniques in microbial processes. *Adv Biochem Eng* 1984; 30:147–194.

Yang S. *Influence of Proteolysis on Production of Recombinant Proteins in* Escherichia coli. Royal Institute of Technology (KHT), Stockholm, Sweden, 1995.

Yang ST and Shu CH. Kinetics and stability of GM-CSF production by recombinant yeast cells immobilized in a fibrous-bed bioreactor. *Biotechnol Prog* 1996; 12(4):449–456.

Yang XM. Optimization of a cultivation process for recombinant protein production by *Escherichia coli*. *J Biotechnol* 1992; 23(3):271–289.

Yee L and Blanch HW. Recombinant protein expression in high cell density fed-batch cultures of *Escherichia coli*. *Biotechnology* (NY) 1992; 10(12):1550–1556.

Zardeneta G and Horowitz PM. Micelle-assisted protein folding. Denatured rhodanese binding to cardiolipin-containing lauryl maltoside micelles results in slower refolding kinetics but greater enzyme reactivation. *J Biol Chem* 1992; 267(9):5811–5816.

Zigova J. Effect of RQ and pre-seed conditions on biomass and galactosyl transferase production during fed-batch culture of S. cerevisiae BT150. *J Biotechnol* 2000; 80(1):55–62.

MAMMALIAN SYSTEMS

Ambesi-Impiombato FS, Parks LA, Coon HG. Culture of hormone-dependent functional epithelial cells from rat thyroids. *Proc Natl Acad Sci USA* 1980; 77(6):3455–3459.

Barnes D and Sato G. Methods for growth of cultured cells in serum-free medium. *Anal Biochem* 1980; 102(2):255–270.

Batt BC, Yabannavar VM, Singh V. Expanded bed adsorption process for protein recovery from whole mammalian cell culture broth. *Bioseparation* 1995; 5(1):41–52.

Beck JT, Williamson B, Tipton B. Direct coupling of expanded bed adsorption with a downstream purification step. *Bioseparation* 1999; 8(1-5):201–207.

Berthold W and Kempken R. Interaction of cell culture with downstream purification: a case study. *Cytotechnology* 1994; 15(1–3):229–242.

Bettger WJ and Ham RG. The nutrient requirements of cultured mammalian cells. *Adv Nutr Res* 1982; 4:249–286.

Bödeker BGD, Potere E, Dove G. Production of recombinant factor VIII from perfusion cultures: II. Large-scale purification. In: *Animal Cell Technology. Products of Today, Prospects for Tomorrow.* Spier RE, Griffiths JB, Berthold W, editors. Butterworth Heinemann, Oxford, 1994: 584–587.

Broad D, Boraston R, Rhodes M. Production of recombinant proteins in serum-free media. *Cytotechnology* 1991; 5(1):47–55.

Buntemeyer H, Lutkemeyer D, Lehmann J. Optimization of serum-free fermentation processes for antibody production. *Cytotechnology* 1991; 5(1):57–67.

Cassiman JJ, Brugmans M, Van den BH. Growth and surface properties of dispase dissociated human fibroblasts. *Cell Biol Int Rep* 1981; 5(2):125–132.

CBER/FDA. Points to Consider in the Manufacture and Testing of Monoclonal Antibody Products for Human Use (1997).

CBER/FDA. Points to Consider in the Characterization of Cell Lines Used to Produce Biologicals (1993).

CBER/FDA. Points to Consider in the Production and Testing of New Drugs and Biologicals Produced by Recombinant DNA Technology (1985).

Collodi P, Rawson C, Barnes D. Serum-free culture of carcinoma cell lines. *Cytotechnology* 1991; 5(1):31–46.

Dutton RL. Redox potentiometry: determination of midpoint potentials of oxidation-reduction components of biological electron-transfer systems. *Methods Enzymol* 1978; 54:411–435.

Dutton RL, Scharer JM, Moo-Young M. Descriptive parameter evaluation in mammalian cell culture. *Cytotechnology* 1998; 26(2):139–152.

Fahrner RL, Blank GS, Zapata GA. Expanded bed protein A affinity chromatography of a recombinant humanized monoclonal antibody: process development, operation, and comparison with a packed bed method. *J Biotechnol* 1999; 75(2-3):273–280.

Fahrner RL, Knudsen HL, Basey CD, Galan W, Feuerhelm D, Vanderlaan M, Blank GS. Industrial purification of pharmaceutical antibodies: development, operation, and validation of chromatography processes. *Biotechnol Genet Eng Rev* 2001; 18:301–327.

Gagnon P. *Purification Tools for Monoclonal Antibodies.* Validated Biosystems Inc., Tucson, AZ, 1996.

Gorfien SF, Paul W, Judd D, Tescione L, Jayme DW. Optimized nutrient additives for fed-batch cultures. *BioPharm Int* 2003; 16(4):34–40.

Graf H, Rabaud JN, Egly JM. Ion exchange resins for the purification of monoclonal antibodies from animal cell culture. *Bioseparation* 1994; 4(1):7–20.

Griffiths B. The use of oxidation-reduction potential (ORP) to monitor growth during a cell culture. *Dev Biol Stand* 1983; 55:113–116.

Guilbert LJ and Iscove NN. Partial replacement of serum by selenite, transferrin, albumin and lecithin in haemopoietic cell cultures. *Nature* 1976; 263(5578):594–595.

Hale JE and Beidler DE. Purification of humanized murine and murine monoclonal antibodies using immobilized metal-affinity chromatography. *Anal Biochem* 1994; 222(1):29–33.

Handa-Corrigan A. Bioreactors for mammalian cells. In: *Mammalian Cell Biotechnology. A Practical Approach.* Butler M, editor. IRL Press, Oxford, 1991: 139–158.

Harakas NK, Schaumann JP, Conolly DT, Wittwer AJ, Olander JV, Feder J. Large-scale purification of tissue type plasminogen activator from cultured human cells. *Biotechnol Prog* 2002; 4(3):149–158.

Hewlett G. Strategies for optimising serum-free media. *Cytotechnology* 1991; 5(1):3–14.

Hoshi H, Kan M, Yamane I, Minamoto Y. Hydrocortisone potentiates cell proliferation and promotes cell spreading on tissue culture substrata of human diploid fibroblasts in a serum-free hormone supplemented medium. *Biomed Res* 1982; 3(5):546–552.

Hu WS and Aunins JG. Large-scale mammalian cell culture. *Curr Opin Biotechnol* 1997; 8(2):148–153.

ICH. Quality of biotechnological products: viral safety evaluation of biotechnology products derived from cell lines of human or animal origin. ICH Harmonised Tripartite Guideline. *Dev Biol Stand* 1998; 93:177–201.

ICH Guidance. Derivation and Characterization of Cell Substrates Used for Production of Biotechnological/Biological Products (1997).

Ikonomou L, Bastin G, Schneider YJ, Agathos SN. Design of an efficient medium for insect cell growth and recombinant protein production. *In vitro Cell Dev Biol Anim* 2001; 37(9):549–559.

Invitrogen. *Guide to Baculovirus Expression Vector Systems (BEVS) and Insect Cell Culture Techniques.* Invitrogen life technologies, Carlsbad, CA, 2002.

Jayme DW. Nutrient optimization for high density biological production applications. *Cytotechnology* 1991; 5(1):15–30.

Josic D, Loster K, Kuhl R, Noll F, Reusch J. Purification of monoclonal antibodies by hydroxylapatite HPLC and size exclusion HPLC. *Biol Chem Hoppe Seyler* 1991; 372(3):149–156.

Kaszubska W, Zhang H, Patterson RL, Suhar TS, Uchic ME, Dickinson RW, Schaefer VG, Haasch D, Janis RS, DeVries PJ, Okasinski GF, Meuth JL. Expression, purification, and characterization of human recombinant thrombopoietin in Chinese hamster ovary cells. *Protein Expr Purif* 2000; 18(2):213–220.

Kilburn DG. Monitoring and control of bioreactors. In: *Mammalian Cell Biotechnology.* A practical approach. Butler M, editor. IRL Press, Oxford, 1991: 159–185.

King DJ. *Applications and Engineering of Monoclonal Antibodies.* Taylor & Francis, London, 1998.

Levin W, Daniel RF, Stoner CR, Stoller TJ, Wardwell-Swanson JA, Angelillo YM, Familletti PC, Crowl RM. Purification of recombinant human secretory phospholipase A2 (group II) produced in long-term immobilized cell culture. *Protein Expr Purif* 1992; 3(1):27–35.

Lubiniecki AS and Lupker JH. Purified protein products of rDNA technology expressed in animal cell culture. *Biologicals* 1994; 22(2):161–169.

Luellau E, von Stockar U, Vogt S, Freitag R. Development of a downstream process for the isolation and separation of monoclonal immunoglobulin A monomers, dimers and polymers from cell culture supernatant. *J Chromatogr A* 1998; 796(1):165–175.

Lüllau E, Marison IW, von Stockar U. Ceramic hydroxyapatite: A new tool for separation and analysis of IgA monoclonal antibodies. In: *Animal Cell Technology: From Vaccines to Genetic Medicine.* Carrondo MJT, Griffiths JB, Moreira JLP, editors. Kluwer Academic Publishers, Dordrecht, 1997: 265–269.

Lundgren B and Blüml G. Microcarriers in cell culture production. In: *Bioseparation and Bioprocessing.* Vol. II: *Processing, Quality and Characterization, Economics, Safety and Hygiene.* Subramanian G, editor. Wiley-VCH, 1998: 165–222.

Lutkemeyer D, Ameskamp N, Priesner C, Bartsch EM, Lehmann J. Capture of proteins from mammalian cells in pilot scale using different STREAMLINE adsorbents. *Bioseparation* 2001; 10(1–3):57–63.

Lutkemeyer D, Bretschneider M, Buntemeyer H, Lehmann J. Membrane chromatography for rapid purification of recombinant antithrombin III and monoclonal antibodies from cell culture supernatant. *J Chromatogr* 1993; 639(1):57–66.

Manousos M, Ahmed M, Torchio C, Wolff J, Shibley G, Stephens R, Mayyasi S. Feasibility studies of oncornavirus production in microcarrier cultures. *In Vitro* 1980; 16(6):507–515.

Manzke O, Tesch H, Diehl V, Bohlen H. Single-step purification of bispecific monoclonal antibodies for immunotherapeutic use by hydrophobic interaction chromatography. *J Immunol Methods* 1997; 208(1):65–73.

Matejtschuk P, Baker RM, Chapman GE. Purification and characterization of monoclonal antibodies. In: *Bioseparation and Bioprocessing.* Vol. II. *Processing, Quality and Characterization, Economics, Safety and Hygiene.* Subramanian G, editor. Wiley-VCH, 1998: 223–252.

Mather JP and Sato GH. The growth of mouse melanoma cells in hormone-supplemented, serum-free medium. *Exp Cell Res* 1979; 120(1):191–200.

Maurer HR. Serum-free media and cell cultures. Introductory remarks. *Cytotechnology* 1991; 5(1):1.

Merten OW. Safety issues of animal products used in serum-free media. *Dev Biol Stand* 1999; 99:167–180.

Merten OW and Litwin J. Serum-free medium for fermentor cultures of hybridomas. *Cytotechnology* 1991; 5(1):69–82.

Metcalfe H, Field RP, Froud SJ. The use of 2-hydroxy-2,4,6-cycloheptarin-1-one (tropolone) as a replacement for transferrin. In: *Animal Cell Technology, Products of Today, Prospects for Tomorrow.* Spier RE, Griffiths JB, Berthold W, editors. Butterworth-Heinemann, Oxford, 1994: 88–90.

Morton HC, Atkin JD, Owens RJ, Woof JM. Purification and characterization of chimeric human IgA1 and IgA2 expressed in COS and Chinese hamster ovary cells. *J Immunol* 1993; 151(9):4743–4752.

Murakami H, Yamada K, Shirahata S, Enomoto A, Kaminogawa S. Physiological enhancement of immuno-globulin production of hybridomas in serum-free media. *Cytotechnology* 1991; 5(1):83–94.

Nagata M and Matsumura T. Action of the bacterial neutral protease, dispase, on cultured cells and its application to fluid suspension culture with a review on biomedical application of this protease. *Jpn J Exp Med* 1986; 56(6):297–307.

Nair MP, Kudchodkar BJ, Pritchard PH, Lacko AG. Purification of recombinant lecithin: cholesterol acyltransferase. *Protein Expr Purif* 1997; 10(1):38–41.

Nguyen B, Jarnagin K, Williams S, Chan H, Barnett J. Fed-batch culture of insect cells: a method to increase the yield of recombinant human nerve growth factor (rhNGF) in the baculovirus expression system. *J Biotechnol* 1993; 31(2):205–217.

Ogez JR and Builder SE. Downstream processing of proteins from mammalian cells. *Bioprocess Technol* 1990; 10:393–416.

Page M and Thorpe R. Purification of monoclonal antibodies. *Methods Mol Biol* 1998; 80:113–119.

Price AE, Logvinenko KB, Higgins EA, Cole ES, Richards SM. Studies on the microheterogeneity and *in vitro* activity of glycosylated and nonglycosylated recombinant human prolactin separated using a novel purification process. *Endocrinology* 1995; 136(11):4827–4833.

Prior CP. Large-scale process purification of clinical product from animal cell cultures. *Biotechnology* 1991; 17:445–478.

Propst CL, Von Wedel RJ, Lubiniecki AS. Using mammalian cells to produce products. In: *Fermentation Process Development of Industrial Organisms*. Neway JO, editor. Marcel Dekker Inc., New York, 1989: 221–276.

Ransohoff TC and Levine HL. Purification of monoclonal antibodies. *Bioprocess Technol* 1991; 12:213–235.

Rasmussen L and Toftlund H. Phosphate compounds as iron chelators in animal cell cultures. *In vitro Cell Dev Biol* 1986; 22(4):177–179.

Reichert JM. Monoclonal antibodies in the clinic. *Nat Biotechnol* 2001; 19(9):819–822.

Roddie PH and Ludlam CA. Recombinant coagulation factors. *Blood Rev* 1997; 11(4):169–177.

Schmidt HH, Genschel J, Haas R, Buttner C, Manns MP. Expression and purification of recombinant human apolipoprotein A-I in Chinese hamster ovary cells. *Protein Expr Purif* 1997; 10(2):226–236.

Sellick I. Improve product recovery during cell harvesting. Enhanced TFF may reduce the capacity crunch. *BioProcess Int* 2003; 1(4):62–65.

Summers MD and Smith GE. *A Manual of Methods for Baculovirus Virus Vectors and Insect Cell Culture Procedures*. Texas Agricultural Experimental Station Bulletin No. 1555. Texas A&M University, College Station, TX, 1987.

Tsujimoto M, Adachi H, Kodama S, Tsuruoka N, Yamada Y, Tanaka S, Mita S, Takatsu K. Purification and characterization of recombinant human interleukin 5 expressed in Chinese hamster ovary cells. *J Biochem* (Tokyo) 1989; 106(1):23–28.

Walker ID. Detection, purification, and utilization of murine monoclonal IgM antibodies. *Methods Mol Biol* 1995; 45:183–188.

Wang MY, Kwong S, Bentley WE. Effects of oxygen/glucose/glutamine feeding on insect cell baculovirus protein expression: a study on epoxide hydrolase production. *Biotechnol Prog* 1993; 9(4):355–361.

WHO. WHO requirements for the use of animal cells as *in vitro* substrates for the production of biologicals (Requirements for biological substances No. 50). *Dev Biol Stand* 1998; 93:141–171.

Yabe N, Kato M, Matsuya Y, Yamane I, Iizuka M, Takayoshi H, Suzuki K. Role of iron chelators in growth-promoting effect on mouse hybridoma cells in a chemically defined medium. *In vitro Cell Dev Biol* 1987; 23(12):815–820.

Yamada KM and Olden K. Fibronectins — adhesive glycoproteins of cell surface and blood. *Nature* 1978; 275(5677):179–184.

Yoon SK, Ahn YH, Han K. Enhancement of recombinant erythropoietin production in CHO cells in an incubator without CO_2 addition. *Cytotechnology* 2001; 37(2):119–132.

YEAST SYSTEMS

Bae CS, Yang DS, Lee J, Park YH. Improved process for production of recombinant yeast-derived monomeric human G-CSF. *Appl Microbiol Biotechnol* 1999; 52(3):338–344.

Berry DR. Growth of yeast. In: *Fermentation Process Development of Industrial Organisms*. Neway JO, editor. Marcel Dekker Inc., New York, 1989: 277–311.

Cereghino GP, Cereghino JL, Ilgen C, Cregg JM. Production of recombinant proteins in fermenter cultures of the yeast Pichia pastoris. *Curr Opin Biotechnol* 2002; 13(4):329–332.

Dale C, Allen A, Fogerty S. Pichia pastoris: A eukaryotic system for the large-scale production of biopharmaceuticals. *BioPharm* 1999; 12(11):36–42.

Faber KN, Harder W, Ab G, Veenhuis M. Review: methylotrophic yeasts as factories for the production of foreign proteins. *Yeast* 1995; 11(14):1331–1344.

Feng W, Graumann K, Hahn R, Jungbauer A. Affinity chromatography of human estrogen receptor-alpha expressed in Saccharomyces cerevisiae. Combination of heparin- and 17beta-estradiol-affinity chromatography. *J Chromatogr A* 1999; 852(1):161–173.

Hardy E, Martinez E, Diago D, Diaz R, Gonzalez D, Herrera L. Large-scale production of recombinant hepatitis B surface antigen from Pichia pastoris. *J Biotechnol* 2000; 77(2–3):157–167.

Harrison Jr. RG. Purification of recombinant proteins from yeast. *Bioprocess Technol* 1991; 12:183–191.

Hawthorne TR, Burgi R, Grossenbacher H, Heim J. Isolation and characterization of recombinant annexin V expressed in Saccharomyces cerevisiae. *J Biotechnol* 1994; 36(2):129–143.

Hellwig S, Emde F, Raven NP, Henke M, van Der LP, Fischer R. Analysis of single-chain antibody production in Pichia pastoris using on-line methanol control in fed-batch and mixed-feed fermentations. *Biotechnol Bioeng* 2001; 74(4):344–352.

Hensing MC, Rouwenhorst RJ, Heijnen JJ, van Dijken JP, Pronk JT. Physiological and technological aspects of large-scale heterologous-protein production with yeasts. *Antonie Van Leeuwenhoek* 1995; 67(3):261–279.

Jazwinski SM. Preparation of extracts from yeast. *Methods Enzymol* 1990; 182(13):154–174.

Jones EW. Tackling the protease problem in Saccharomyces cerevisiae. *Methods Enzymol* 1991; 194:428–453.

Juge N, Andersen JS, Tull D, Roepstorff P, Svensson B. Overexpression, purification, and characterization of recombinant barley alpha-amylases 1 and 2 secreted by the methylotrophic yeast *Pichia pastoris*. *Protein Expr Purif* 1996; 8(2):204–214.

Kannan R, Tomasetto C, Staub A, Bossenmeyer-Pourie C, Thim L, Nielsen PF, Rio M. Human pS2/trefoil factor 1: production and characterization in Pichia pastoris. *Protein Expr Purif* 2001; 21(1):92–98.

King DJ, Walton F, Smith BW, Dunn M, Yarranton GT. Recovery of recombinant proteins from yeast. *Biochem Soc Trans* 1988; 16(6):1083–1086.

Merten OW. Safety issues of animal products used in serum-free media. *Dev Biol Stand* 1999; 99:167–180.

Munshi CB, Fryxell KB, Lee HC, Branton WD. Large-scale production of human CD38 in yeast by fermentation. *Methods Enzymol* 1997; 280:318–330.

Niles AL, Maffitt M, Haak-Frendscho M, Wheeless CJ, Johnson DA. Recombinant human mast cell tryptase beta: stable expression in Pichia pastoris and purification of fully active enzyme. *Biotechnol Appl Biochem* 1998; 28(Pt 2):125–131.

Quirk AV, Geisow MJ, Woodrow JR, Burton SJ, Wood PC, Sutton AD, Johnson RA, Dodsworth N. Production of recombinant human serum albumin from Saccharomyces cerevisiae. *Biotechnol Appl Biochem* 1989; 11(3):273–287.

Qureshi GA, Fohlin L, Bergstrom J. Application of high-performance liquid chromatography to the determination of free amino acids in physiological fluids. *J Chromatogr* 1984; 297:91–100.

Reiser J, Glumoff V, Kalin M, Ochsner U. Transfer and expression of heterologous genes in yeasts other than Saccharomyces cerevisiae. *Adv Biochem Eng Biotechnol* 1990; 43:75–102.

Rogelj B, Strukelj B, Bosch D, Jongsma MA. Expression, purification, and characterization of equistatin in Pichia pastoris. *Protein Expr Purif* 2000; 19(3):329–334.

Romanos MA, Scorer CA, Clare JJ. Foreign gene expression in yeast: a review. *Yeast* 1992; 8(6):423–488.

Rosenfeld SA, Nadeau D, Tirado J, Hollis GF, Knabb RM, Jia S. Production and purification of recombinant hirudin expressed in the methylotrophic yeast *Pichia pastoris*. *Protein Expr Purif* 1996; 8(4):476–482.

Sellick I. Improve product recovery during cell harvesting. Enhanced TFF may reduce the capacity crunch. *BioProcess Int* 2003; 1(4):62–65.

Shepard SR, Boucher R, Johnston J, Boerner R, Koch G, Madsen JW, Grella D, Sim BK, Schrimsher JL. Large-scale purification of recombinant human angiostatin. *Protein Expr Purif* 2000; 20(2):216–227.

Steinlein LM, Graf TN, Ikeda RA. Production and purification of N-terminal half-transferrin in Pichia pastoris. *Protein Expr Purif* 1995; 6(5):619–624.

Stratton J, Chiruvolu V, Meagher M. High cell-density fermentation. *Methods Mol Biol* 1998; 103:107–120.

Sudbery PE. The expression of recombinant proteins in yeasts. *Curr Opin Biotechnol* 1996; 7(5):517–524.

van Urk H, Voll WSL, Scheffers WA, van Dijken JP. Transient-state analysis of metabolic fluxes in crabtree-positive and crabtree-negative yeasts. *Appl Environ Microbiol* 1990; 56:281–287.

Werten MW, van den Bosch TJ, Wind RD, Mooibroek H, de Wolf FA. High-yield secretion of recombinant gelatins by *Pichia pastoris*. *Yeast* 1999; 15(11):1087–1096.

Yang ST and Shu CH. Kinetics and stability of GM-CSF production by recombinant yeast cells immobilized in a fibrous-bed bioreactor. *Biotechnol Prog* 1996; 12(4):449–456.

Zhang W, Bevins MA, Plantz BA, Smith LA, Meagher MM. Modeling Pichia pastoris growth on methanol and optimizing the production of a recombinant protein, the heavy-chain fragment C of botulinum neurotoxin, serotype A. *Biotechnol Bioeng* 2000; 70(1):1–8.

Zhou WB, Zhou XS, Zhang YX. [Decolorization and isolation of recombinant hirudin expressed in the methylotrophic yeast *Pichia pastoris*]. *Sheng Wu Gong Cheng Xue Bao* 2001; 17(6):683–687.

Zhu DX, Hua ZC, Liang XF, Zhang XK, Ding Y, Zhu JQ, Han KK. Purification and characterization of the biologically active human truncated macrophage colony-stimulating factor expressed in Saccharomyces cerevisiae. *Biol Chem Hoppe Seyler* 1993; 374(9):903–908.

Zigova J, Mahle M, Paschold H, Malissard M, Berger EG, Weuster-Botz D. Fed-batch production of a soluble -1,4-galactosyltransferase with Saccharomyces cerevisiae. *Enzyme Microbial Tech* 1999; 25(3–5):201–207.

Zigova J. Effect of RQ and pre-seed conditions on biomass and galactosyl transferase production during fed-batch culture of S. cerevisiae BT150. *J Biotechnol* 2000; 80(1):55–62.

INSECT CELL SYSTEMS

Airenne KJ, Laitinen OH, Alenius H, Mikkola J, Kalkkinen N, Arif SA, Yeang HY, Palosuo T, Kulomaa MS. Avidin is a promising tag for fusion proteins produced in baculovirus-infected insect cells. *Protein Expr Purif* 1999; 17(1):139–145.

Airenne KJ, Oker-Blom C, Marjomaki VS, Bayer EA, Wilchek M, Kulomaa MS. Production of biologically active recombinant avidin in baculovirus-infected insect cells. *Protein Expr Purif* 1997; 9(1):100–108.

Altmann F, Staudacher E, Wilson IB, Marz L. Insect cells as hosts for the expression of recombinant glycoproteins. *Glycoconj J* 1999; 16(2):109–123.

Baldock D, Graham B, Akhlaq M, Graff P, Jones CE, Menear K. Purification and characterization of human Syk produced using a baculovirus expression system. *Protein Expr Purif* 2000; 18(1):86–94.

Bezzine S, Ferrato F, Lopez V, de Caro A, Verger R, Carriere F. One-step purification and biochemical characterization of recombinant pancreatic lipases expressed in insect cells. *Methods Mol Biol* 1999; 109:187–202.

Brushia RJ, Forte TM, Oda MN, La Du BN, Bielicki JK. Baculovirus-mediated expression and purification of human serum paraoxonase 1A. *J Lipid Res* 2001; 42(6):951–958.

Budde RJ, Ramdas L, Ke S. Recombinant pp60c-src from baculovirus-infected insect cells: purification and characterization. *Prep Biochem* 1993; 23(4):493–515.

Caron AW, Archambault J, Massie B. High level recombinant protein production in bioreactors using the baculovirus-insect cell expression system. *Biotechnol Bioeng* 1990; 36(11):1133–1140.

Cerione RA, Leonard D, Zheng Y. Purification of baculovirus-expressed Cdc42Hs. *Methods Enzymol* 1995; 256:11–15.

Cha HJ, Dalal NG, Pham MQ, Bentley WE. Purification of human interleukin-2 fusion protein produced in insect larvae is facilitated by fusion with green fluorescent protein and metal affinity ligand. *Biotechnol Prog* 1999; 15(2):283–286.

Cha HJ, Dalal NG, Vakharia VN, Bentley WE. Expression and purification of human interleukin-2 simplified as a fusion with green fluorescent protein in suspended Sf-9 insect cells. *J Biotechnol* 1999; 69(1):9–17.

Chan LC, Greenfield PF, Reid S. Optimising fed-batch production of recombinant proteins using the baculovirus expression vector system. *Biotechnol Bioeng* 1998; 59(2):178–188.

Churgay LM, Kovacevic S, Tinsley FC, Kussow CM, Millican RL, Miller JR, Hale JE. Purification and characterization of secreted human leptin produced in baculovirus-infected insect cells. *Gene* 1997; 190(1):131–137.

Ciaccia AV, Cunningham EL, Church FC. Characterization of recombinant heparin cofactor II expressed in insect cells. *Protein Expr Purif* 1995; 6(6):806–812.

Das T, Johns PW, Goffin V, Kelly P, Kelder B, Kopchick J, Buxton K, Mukerji P. High-level expression of biologically active human prolactin from recombinant baculovirus in insect cells. *Protein Expr Purif* 2000; 20(2):265–273.

Debanne MT, Pacheco-Oliver MC, O'Connor-McCourt MD. Purification of the extracellular domain of the epidermal growth factor receptor produced by recombinant baculovirus-infected insect cells in a 10-L reactor. In: *Baculovirus Expression Protocols*. Richardson CD, editor. Humana Press, Totowa, NJ, 1995: 349–361.

Dobers J, Zimmermann-Kordmann M, Leddermann M, Schewe T, Reutter W, Fan H. Expression, purification, and characterization of human dipeptidyl peptidase IV/CD26 in Sf9 insect cells. *Protein Expr Purif* 2002; 25(3):527–532.

Doerfler W and Bohm P (eds.). *The Molecular Biology of Baculoviruses. Current Topics in Microbiology and Immunology*. Vol. 131. Springer Verlag, Berlin-Heidelberg, 1987.

Dutton RL, Scharer JM, Moo-Young M. Descriptive parameter evaluation in mammalian cell culture. *Cytotechnology* 1998; 26(2):139–152.

Fabbro D, Batt D, Rose P, Schacher B, Roberts TM, Ferrari S. Homogeneous purification of human recombinant GST-Akt/PKB from Sf9 cells. *Protein Expr Purif* 1999; 17(1):83–88.

Farrell PJ, Lu M, Prevost J, Brown C, Behie L, Iatrou K. High-level expression of secreted glycoproteins in transformed lepidopteran insect cells using a novel expression vector. *Biotechnol Bioeng* 1998; 60(6):656–663.

Flamand M, Chevalier M, Henchal E, Girard M, Deubel V. Purification and renaturation of Japanese encephalitis virus nonstructural glycoprotein NS1 overproduced by insect cells. *Protein Expr Purif* 1995; 6(4):519–527.

Frech M, Cussac D, Chardin P, Bar-Sagi D. Purification of baculovirus-expressed human Sos1 protein. *Methods Enzymol* 1995; 255:125–129.

Goosen MF. Large-scale insect cell culture: methods, applications and products. *Curr Opin Biotechnol* 1991; 2(3):365–369.

Graber SG, Figler RA, Garrison JC. Expression and purification of G-protein alpha subunits using baculovirus expression system. *Methods Enzymol* 1994; 237:212–226.

Grossmann M, Wong R, Teh NG, Tropea JE, East-Palmer J, Weintraub BD, Szkudlinski MW. Expression of biologically active human thyrotropin (hTSH) in a baculovirus system: effect of insect cell glycosylation on hTSH activity *in vitro* and *in vivo*. *Endocrinology* 1997; 138(1):92–100.

Hasegawa M, Kawano Y, Matsumoto Y, Hidaka Y, Fujii J, Taniguchi N, Wada A, Hirayama T, Shimonishi Y. Expression and characterization of the extracellular domain of guanylyl cyclase C from a baculovirus and Sf21 insect cells. *Protein Expr Purif* 1999; 15(3):271–281.

Hepler JR, Kozasa T, Gilman AG. Purification of recombinant Gq alpha, G11 alpha, and G16 alpha from Sf9 cells. *Methods Enzymol* 1994; 237:191–212.

Hermanson IL and Turchi JJ. Overexpression and purification of human XPA using a baculovirus expression system. *Protein Expr Purif* 2000; 19(1):1–11.

Hill RM, Brennan SO, Birch NP. Expression, purification, and functional characterization of the serine protease inhibitor neuroserpin expressed in Drosophila S2 cells. *Protein Expr Purif* 2001; 22(3):406–413.

Hoenicka M, Becker EM, Apeler H, Sirichoke T, Schroder H, Gerzer R, Stasch JP. Purified soluble guanylyl cyclase expressed in a baculovirus/Sf9 system: stimulation by YC-1, nitric oxide, and carbon monoxide. *J Mol Med* 1999; 77(1):14–23.

Huang YW, Lu ML, Qi H, Lin SX. Membrane-bound human 3beta-hydroxysteroid dehydrogenase: overexpression with His-tag using a baculovirus system and single-step purification. *Protein Expr Purif* 2000; 18(2):169–174.

Hughes PR and Wood HA. *In vivo* and *in vitro* bioassay methods for baculoviruses. In: *The Biology of Baculoviruses*. Vol II. Granados RR and Federici BA, editors. CRC Press Inc. 1986: 1–30.

Hunninghake D and Grisolia S. A sensitive and convenient micromethod for estimation of urea, citrulline, and carbamyl derivatives. *Anal Biochem* 1966; 16(2):200–205.

Ignoffo CM. Evaluation of *in vivo* specificity of insect viruses. In: *Baculoviruses for Insect Pest Control: Safety Considerations*. Summers M, Engler R, Falcon LA, Vail PV, editors. American Society for Microbiology, Washington, DC, 1975: 52–57.

Iizuka M and Fukuda K. Purification of the bovine nicotinic acetylcholine receptor alpha-subunit expressed in baculovirus-infected insect cells. *J Biochem* (Tokyo) 1993; 114(1):140–147.

Ikonomou L, Bastin G, Schneider YJ, Agathos SN. Design of an efficient medium for insect cell growth and recombinant protein production. *In vitro Cell Dev Biol Anim* 2001; 37(9):549–559.

Invitrogen. *Guide to Baculovirus Expression Vector Systems (BEVS) and Insect Cell Culture Techniques.* Invitrogen Life Technologies, Carlsbad, CA, 2002.

Ishihara K, Satoh I, Nittoh T, Kanaya T, Okazaki H, Suzuki T, Koyama T, Sakamoto T, Ide T, Ohuchi K. Preparation of recombinant rat interleukin-5 by baculovirus expression system and analysis of its biological activities. *Biochim Biophys Acta* 1999; 1451(1):48–58.

Jarvis DL, Kawar ZS, Hollister JR. Engineering N-glycosylation pathways in the baculovirus-insect cell system. *Curr Opin Biotechnol* 1998; 9(5):528–533.

Juntunen K, Rochel N, Moras D, Vihko P. Large-scale expression and purification of the human vitamin D receptor and its ligand-binding domain for structural studies. *Biochem J* 1999; 344(Pt 2):297–303.

Keith MB, Farrell PJ, Iatrou K, Behie LA. Screening of transformed insect cell lines for recombinant protein production. *Biotechnol Prog* 1999; 15(6):1046–1052.

Kilburn DG. Monitoring and control of bioreactors. In: *Mammalian Cell Biotechnology. A Practical Approach.* Butler M, editor. IRL Press, Oxford, 1991: 159–185.

King LA and Possee RD. Insect cell culture media and maintenance of insect cell lines. In: *The Baculovirus Expression System. A Laboratory Guide*. Chapman & Hall, London, 1992: 75–105.

King LA and Possee RD. Production and selection of recombinant virus. In: *The Baculovirus Expression System. A Laboratory Guide*. Chapman & Hall, London, 1992: 127–140.

King LA and Possee RD. Propagation of baculoviruses in insect larvae. In: The Baculovirus Expression System. A Laboratory Guide. Chapman & Hall, London, 1992: 180–194.

King LA and Possee RD. Propagation, titration and purification of AcMNPV in cell culture. In: *The Baculovirus Expression System. A Laboratory Guide*. Chapman & Hall, London, 1992: 106–126.

King LA and Possee RD. Scaling up the production of recombinant protein in insect cells; laboratory bench level. In: *The Baculovirus Expression System. A Laboratory Guide*. Chapman & Hall, London, 1992: 171–179.

King LA and Possee RD. *The Baculovirus Expression System. A Laboratory Guide*. Chapman & Hall, London, 1992.

King LA and Possee RD. The baculoviruses. In: *The Baculovirus Expression System. A Laboratory Guide*. Chapman & Hall, London, 1992: 1–15.

Klaassen CH, Bovee-Geurts PH, Decaluwe GL, DeGrip WJ. Large-scale production and purification of functional recombinant bovine rhodopsin with the use of the baculovirus expression system. *Biochem J* 1999; 342(Pt 2):293–300.

Kost TA and Condreay JP. Recombinant baculoviruses as expression vectors for insect and mammalian cells. *Curr Opin Biotechnol* 1999; 10(5):428–433.

Kozasa T and Gilman AG. Purification of recombinant G proteins from Sf9 cells by hexahistidine tagging of associated subunits. Characterization of alpha 12 and inhibition of adenylyl cyclase by alpha z. *J Biol Chem* 1995; 270(4):1734–1741.

Kunimoto DY, Allison KC, Watson C, Fuerst T, Armstrong GD, Paul W, Strober W. High-level production of murine interleukin-5 (IL-5) utilizing recombinant baculovirus expression. Purification of the rIL-5 and its use in assessing the biologic role of IL-5 glycosylation. *Cytokine* 1991; 3(3):224–230.

Lansmann S, Bartelsen O, Sandhoff K. Purification and characterization of recombinant human acid sphin-gomyelinase expressed in insect Sf21 cells. *Methods Enzymol* 2000; 311:149–156.

Lauritzen C, Pedersen J, Madsen MT, Justesen J, Martensen PM, Dahl SW. Active recombinant rat dipeptidyl aminopeptidase I (cathepsin C) produced using the baculovirus expression system. *Protein Expr Purif* 1998; 14(3):434–442.

Lehr RV, Elefante LC, Kikly KK, O'Brien SP, Kirkpatrick RB. A modified metal-ion affinity chromatography procedure for the purification of histidine-tagged recombinant proteins expressed in Drosophila S2 cells. *Protein Expr Purif* 2000; 19(3):362–368.

Lenhard T and Reilander H. Engineering the folding pathway of insect cells: generation of a stably transformed insect cell line showing improved folding of a recombinant membrane protein. *Biochem Biophys Res Commun* 1997; 238(3):823–830.

Lindsay D and Betenbaugh M. Quantification of cell culture factors affecting recombinant protein yields in baculovirus-infected insect cells. *Biotechnol Bioeng* 1992; 39(6):614–618.

Lorincz Z, Kalabay L, Cseh S, Zavodszky P, Arnaud P, Jakab L. Isolation of human alpha 2HS-glycoprotein synthesized by Sf9 cells. *Acta Microbiol Immunol Hung* 1998; 45(3–4):419–424.

Lowe ME. Human pancreatic procolipase expressed in insect cells: purification and characterization. *Protein Expr Purif* 1994; 5(6):583–586.

Luckow VA and Summers MD. Trends in the development of baculovirus expression vectors. *BioTechnol* 1988; 6(1):47–55.

Maiorella B, Inlow D, Shauger A, Harano D. Large-scale insect cell-culture for recombinant protein production. *BioTechnol* 1988; 6(12):1406–1410.

McCarroll L and King LA. Stable insect cell cultures for recombinant protein production. *Curr Opin Biotechnol* 1997; 8(5):590–594.

Merten OW. Safety issues of animal products used in serum-free media. *Dev Biol Stand* 1999; 99:167–180.

Miller DW, Safer P, Miller LK. An insect baculovirus host-vector system for high-level expression of foreign genes. In: *Genetic Engineering* Vol. 8, *Principles and Methods*. Setlow JK and Hollander A, editors. Plenum Publishing Corp., New York, 1986: 277–298.

Miller LK. Insect viruses. In: *Fields — Virology*. Fields BN, Knipe DM, Howley PM, editors. Lippincott-Raven Publishers, Philadelphia, 1996: 533–556.

Miltenburger HG and David P. Mass production of insect cells in suspension. *Dev Biol Stand* 1980; 46:183–186.

Mitchell DL, Young MA, Entwisle C, Davies AN, Cook RM, Dodd I. Purification and characterisation of recombinant murine interleukin-5 glycoprotein, from a baculovirus expression system. *Biochem Soc Trans* 1993; 21(4):332S.

Moody AJ, Hejnaes KR, Marshall MO, Larsen FS, Boel E, Svendsen I, Mortensen E, Dyrberg T. Isolation by anion-exchange of immunologically and enzymatically active human islet glutamic acid decarboxylase 65 overexpressed in Sf9 insect cells. *Diabetologia* 1995; 38(1):14–23.

Murhammer DW and Goochee CF. Scale-up of insect cultures: protective effects of pluronic F-68. *BioTechnol* 1988; 6(12):1411–1418.

Nguyen B, Jarnagin K, Williams S, Chan H, Barnett J. Fed-batch culture of insect cells: a method to increase the yield of recombinant human nerve growth factor (rhNGF) in the baculovirus expression system. *J Biotechnol* 1993; 31(2):205–217.

Nielsen LK, Smyth GK, Greenfield PF. Accuracy of the endpoint assay for virus titration. *Cytotechnology* 1992; 8(3):231–236.

Niu PD, Lefevre F, Mege D, La Bonnardiere C. Atypical porcine type I interferon. Biochemical and biological characterization of the recombinant protein expressed in insect cells. *Eur J Biochem* 1995; 230(1):200–206.

Ohtaki T, Ogi K, Kitada C, Hinuma S, Onda H. Purification of recombinant human pituitary adenylate cyclase-activating polypeptide receptor expressed in Sf9 insect cells. *Ann NY Acad Sci* 1996; 805:590–594.

Ohtaki T, Ogi K, Masuda Y, Mitsuoka K, Fujiyoshi Y, Kitada C, Sawada H, Onda H, Fujino M. Expression, purification, and reconstitution of receptor for pituitary adenylate cyclase-activating polypeptide. large-scale purification of a functionally active G protein-coupled receptor produced in Sf9 insect cells. *J Biol Chem* 1998; 273(25):15464–15473.

O'Reilly DR, Miller LK, Luckow VA. *Baculovirus Expression Vectors: A Laboratory Manual*. W. H. Freeman and Co., New York, 1992.

O'Riordan CR, Erickson A, Bear C, Li C, Manavalan P, Wang KX, Marshall J, Scheule RK, McPherson JM, Cheng SH. Purification and characterization of recombinant cystic fibrosis transmembrane conductance regulator from Chinese hamster ovary and insect cells. *J Biol Chem* 1995; 270(28):17033–17043.

Overton LK, Patel I, Becherer JD, Chandra G, Kost TA. Expression of tissue inhibitor of metalloproteinases by recombinant baculovirus-infected insect cells cultured in an airlift fermentor. In: *Baculovirus Expression Protocols*. Richardson CD, editor. Humana Press, Totowa, NJ, 1995: 225–242.

Peng S, Sommerfelt M, Logan J, Huang Z, Jilling T, Kirk K, Hunter E, Sorscher E. One-step affinity isolation of recombinant protein using the baculovirus/insect cell expression system. *Protein Expr Purif* 1993; 4(2):95–100.

Pennock GD, Shoemaker C, Miller LK. Strong and regulated expression of *Escherichia coli* beta-galactosidase in insect cells with a baculovirus vector. *Mol Cell Biol* 1984; 4(3):399–406.

Pfeifer TA. Expression of heterologous proteins in stable insect cell culture. *Curr Opin Biotechnol* 1998; 9(5):518–521.

Porfiri E, Evans T, Bollag G, Clark R, Hancock JF. Purification of baculovirus-expressed recombinant Ras and Rap proteins. *Methods Enzymol* 1995; 255:13–21.

Power JF, Reid S, Radford KM, Greenfield PF, Nielsen LK. Modelling and optimization of the baculovirus expression system in batch suspension culture. *Biotechnol Bioeng* 1994; 44(6):710–719.

Ren Y, Busch R, Durban E, Taylor C, Gustafson WC, Valdez B, Li YP, Smetana K, Busch H. Overexpression of human nucleolar proteins in insect cells: characterization of nucleolar protein p120. *Protein Expr Purif* 1996; 7(2):212–219.

Reuveny S, Kim YJ, Kemp CW, Shiloach J. Production of recombinant proteins in high density insect cultures. *Biotechnol Bioeng* 1993; 42(2):235–239.

Rice JW, Rankl NB, Gurganus TM, Marr CM, Barna JB, Walters MM, Burns DJ. A comparison of large-scale Sf9 insect cell growth and protein production: stirred vessel vs. airlift. *Biotechniques* 1993; 15(6):1052–1059.

Rodewald HR, Langhorne J, Eichmann K, Kupsch J. Production of murine interleukin-4 and interleukin-5 by recombinant baculovirus. *J Immunol Methods* 1990; 132(2):221–226.

Rubinfeld B and Polakis P. Purification of baculovirus-produced Rap1 GTPase-activating protein. *Methods Enzymol* 1995; 255:31–38.

Sanghani PC and Moran RG. Purification and characteristics of recombinant human folylpoly-γ-glutamate synthetase expressed at high levels in insect cells. *Protein Expr Purif* 2000; 18(1):36–45.

Sellick I. Improve product recovery during cell harvesting. Enhanced TFF may reduce the capacity crunch. *BioProcess Int* 2003; 1(4):62–65.

Settleman J and Foster R. Purification and GTPase-activating protein activity of baculovirus expressed p190. *Methods Enzymol* 1995; 256:105–113.

Smith GE, Summers MD, Fraser MJ. Production of human beta interferon in insect cells infected with a baculovirus expression vector. *Mol Cell Biol* 1983; 3(12):2156–2165.

Sondergaard L. Drosophila cells can be grown to high cell densities in a bioreactor. *Biotechnol Tech* 1996; 10(3):161–166.

Spivak JL, Avedissian LS, Pierce JH, Williams D, Hankins WD, Jensen RA. Isolation of the full-length murine erythropoietin receptor using a baculovirus expression system. *Blood* 1996; 87(3):926–937.

Sumathy S, Palhan VB, Gopinathan KP. Expression of human growth hormone in silkworm larvae through recombinant Bombyx mori nuclear polyhedrosis virus. *Protein Expr Purif* 1996; 7(3):262–268.

Summers MD and Smith GE. *A Manual of Methods for Baculovirus Virus Vectors and Insect Cell Culture Procedures*. Texas Agricultural Experimental Station Bulletin No. 1555. Texas A&M University, College Station, TX, 1987.

Susa M, Luong-Nguyen NH, Crespo J, Maier R, Missbach M, McMaster G. Active recombinant human tyrosine kinase c-Yes: expression in baculovirus system, purification, comparison to c-Src, and inhibition by a c-Src inhibitor. *Protein Expr Purif* 2000; 19(1):99–106.

Tennagels N, Hube-Magg C, Wirth A, Noelle V, Klein HW. Expression, purification, and characterization of the cytoplasmic domain of the human IGF-1 receptor using a baculovirus expression system. *Biochem Biophys Res Commun* 1999; 260(3):724–728.

Tom RL, Caron AW, Massie B, Kamen AA. Scale-up of recombinant virus and protein production in stirred-tank reactors. In: *Baculovirus Expression Protocols*. Richardson CD, editor. Humana Press, Totowa, NJ, 1995: 203–224.

Tramper J, Williams JB, Joustra D. Shear sensitivity of insect cells in suspension. *Enzyme Microb Technol* 1986; 8:33–36.

Valtanen H, Lehti K, Lohi J, Keski-Oja J. Expression and purification of soluble and inactive mutant forms of membrane type 1 matrix metalloproteinase. *Protein Expr Purif* 2000; 19(1):66–73.

Wang MY, Kwong S, Bentley WE. Effects of oxygen/glucose/glutamine feeding on insect cell baculovirus protein expression: a study on epoxide hydrolase production. *Biotechnol Prog* 1993; 9(4):355–361.

Weinglass AB and Baldwin SA. Characterisation and purification of recombinant GLUT1 expressed in insect cells. *Biochem Soc Trans* 1996; 24(3):478S.

Weiss SA, Godwin GP, Gorfien SF, Whitford WG. Insect cell culture in serum-free media. In: *Baculovirus Expression Protocols*. Richardson CD, editor. Humana Press, Totowa, NJ, 1995: 79–95.

Wells PA, Garlick RL, Lyle SB, Tuls JL, Poorman RA, Brideau RJ, Wathen MW. Purification of a recombinant human respiratory syncytial virus chimeric glycoprotein using reversed-phase chromatography and protein refolding in guanidine hydrochloride. *Protein Expr Purif* 1994; 5(4):391–401.

WHO. WHO requirements for the use of animal cells as *in vitro* substrates for the production of biologicals (Requirements for biological substances No. 50). *Dev Biol Stand* 1998; 93:141–171.

Withers BE, Keller PR, Fry DW. Expression, purification and characterization of focal adhesion kinase using a baculovirus system. *Protein Expr Purif* 1996; 7(1):12–18.

Xu W, Simons FE, Peng Z. Expression and rapid purification of an Aedes aegypti salivary allergen by a baculovirus system. *Int Arch Allergy Immunol* 1998; 115(3):245–251.

Zhang J, Alfonso P, Thotakura NR, Su J, Buergin M, Parmelee D, Collins AW, Oelkuct M, Gaffney S, Gentz S, Radman DP, Wagner GF, Gentz R. Expression, purification, and bioassay of human stanniocalcin from baculovirus-infected insect cells and recombinant CHO cells. *Protein Expr Purif* 1998; 12(3):390–398.

Zhang J, Kalogerakis N, Behie LA, Iatrou K. A two-stage bioreactor system for the production of recombinant proteins using genetically engineered baculovirus/insect cell system. *Biotechnol Bioeng* 1993; 42:357–366.

TRANSGENIC ANIMAL SYSTEMS

Carver A. Recombinant protein production in lactating animals — Transgenic livestock represent an ideal route for the production of recombinant proteins. *Pharm Biotechnol Int* 1996; 3.

Carver A, Wright G, Cottom D, Cooper J, Dalrymple M, Temperley S, Udell M, Reeves D, Percy J, Scott A. Expression of human alpha 1 antitrypsin in transgenic sheep. *Cytotechnology* 1992; 9(1–3): 77–84.

Carver AS, Dalrymple MA, Wright G, Cottom DS, Reeves DB, Gibson YH, Keenan JL, Barrass JD, Scott AR, Colman A, Garner I. Transgenic livestock as bioreactors: Stable expression of human alpha-1-antitrypsin by a flock of sheep. *Biotechnology* 1993; 11(Nov.):1263–1270.

Clark AJ, Bessos H, Bishop JO, Brown P, Harris S, Lathe R, McClenaghan M, Prowse C, Simons JP, Whitelaw CBA, Wilmut I. Expression of human anti-hemophilic factor IX in the milk of transgenic sheep. *Biotechnology* 1989; 7(5):487–492.

Clark AJ. The mammary gland as a bioreactor: Expression, processing, and production of recombinant proteins. *J Mammary Gland Biol Neoplasia* 1998; 3(3):337–350.

Cole KD, Lee TK, Lubon H. Aqueous two-phase partitioning of milk proteins: application to human protein-C secreted in pig milk — recombinant protein-C purification from transgenic pig milk two-phase system extraction. *Appl Biochem Biotechnol* 1997; 67(1–2):97–112.

Dalton JC, Bruley DF, Kang KA, Drohan WN. Separation of recombinant human protein C from transgenic animal milk using immobilized metal affinity chromatography. *Adv Exp Med Biol* 1997; 411:419–428.

Dave AS and Bruley DF. Separation of human protein C from components of transgenic milk using immobilized metal affinity chromatography. *Adv Exp Med Biol* 1999; 471:639–647.

Degener A, Belew M, Velander WH. Expanded bed purification of a recombinant protein from the milk of transgenic livestock. *Abstr Pap Am Chem Soc* 1996; 211(1 (Mar. 24)):P87.

Degener A, Belew M, Velander WH. Zn(2+)-selective purification of recombinant proteins from the milk of transgenic animals. *J Chromatogr A* 1998; 799(1–2):125–137.

Denman J, Hayes M, O'Day C, Edmunds T, Bartlett C, Hirani S, Ebert KM, Gordon K, McPherson JM. Transgenic expression of a variant of human tissue-type plasminogen activator in goat milk: purification and characterization of the recombinant enzyme. *Biotechnology* 1991; 9(9):839–843.

Drohan WN, Wilkins TD, Latimer E, Zhou D, Velander W, Lee TK, Lubon H. A scalable method for the purification of recombinant human protein C from the milk of transgenic swine. *Adv Bioprocess Eng* 1994; 501–507.

Drohan WN, Zhang DW, Paleyanda RK, Chang R, Wroble M, Velander W, Lubon H. Inefficient processing of human protein C in the mouse mammary gland. *Transgenic Res* 1994; 3(6):355–364.

Ebert KM, Selgrath JP, DiTullio P, Denman J, Smith TE, Memon MA, Schindler JE, Monastersky GM, Vitale JA, Gordon K. Transgenic production of a variant of human tissue-type plasminogen activator in goat milk: generation of transgenic goats and analysis of expression. *Biotechnology* (NY) 1991; 9(9):835–838.

Echelard Y. Recombinant protein production in transgenic animals. *Curr Opin Biotechnol* 1996; 7(5):536–540.

Goldman M. Processing challenges for transgenic milk products. *BioProcess Int* 2003; 1(10):60–63.

Harris DP, Andrews AT, Wright G, Pyle DL, Asenjo JA. The application of aqueous two-phase systems to the purification of pharmaceutical proteins from transgenic sheep milk. *Bioseparation* 1997; 7(1):31–37.

Hennighausen L. The mammary gland as a bioreactor: production of foreign proteins in milk. *Protein Expr Purif* 1990; 1(1):3-8.

Houdebine LM. Expression of recombinant proteins in the milk of transgenic animals. *Rev Fr Transfus Hemobiol* 1993; 36(1):49–72.

Houdebine LM. Production of pharmaceutical proteins from transgenic animals. *J Biotechnol* 1994; 34(3):269–287.

Houdebine LM. The production of pharmaceutical proteins from the milk of transgenic animals. *Reprod Nutr Dev* 1995; 35(6):609–617.

Houdebine LM. Transgenic animal bioreactors. *Transgenic Res* 2000; 9(4–5):305–320.

Hoyer LW, Drohan WN, Lubon H. Production of human therapeutic proteins in transgenic animals. *Vox Sang* 1994; 67(Suppl. 3):217–220.

Kutzko JP, Sherman LT, Hayes ML. Genzyme Transgenics Corporation, Assignee. Purification of biological active peptides from milk. Patent US 6268487. Issued 31-7-2001. May 13, 1996.

Ladisch MR, Rudge SR, Ruettimann KW, Lin JK. Bioseparations of milk proteins. In: *Bioproducts and Bioprocesses*. A Fiechter, H Okada, RD Tanner, editors. Springer-Verlag, Berlin-Heidelberg, 1989: 209–221.

Larrick JW and Thomas DW. Producing proteins in transgenic plants and animals. *Curr Opin Biotechnol* 2001; 12(4):411–418.

Lee VW and Antonsen KP. PPL Therapeutics Scotland Ltd, Assignee. Purification of alpha-1 proteinase inhibitor. Patent US 6194553. Issued 27-2-2001.

Logan JS and Martin MJ. Transgenic swine as a recombinant production system for human hemoglobin. *Methods Enzymol* 1994; 231:435–445.

Lubon H. Transgenic animal bioreactors in biotechnology and production of blood proteins. *Biotechnol Annu Rev* 1998; 4:1–54.

Lubon H, Paleyanda RK, Velander WH, Drohan WN. Blood proteins from transgenic animal bioreactors. *Transfus Med Rev* 1996; 10(2):131–143.

Niemann H, Halter R, Carnwath JW, Herrmann D, Lemme E, Paul D. Expression of human blood clotting factor VIII in the mammary gland of transgenic sheep. *Transgenic Res* 1999; 8(3):237–247.

O'Donnell JK, Martin MJ, Logan JS, Kumar R. Production of human hemoglobin in transgenic swine: an approach to a blood substitute. *Cancer Detect Prev* 1993; 17(2):307–312.

Pollock DP, Kutzko JP, Birck-Wilson E, Williams JL, Echelard Y, Meade HM. Transgenic milk as a method for the production of recombinant antibodies. *J Immunol Methods* 1999; 231(1–2):147–157.

Prunkard D, Cottingham I, Garner I, Bruce S, Dalrymple M, Lasser G, Bishop P, Foster D. High-level expression of recombinant human fibrinogen in the milk of transgenic mice. *Nat Biotechnol* 1996; 14(July):867–871.

Rohricht P. Transgenic protein production. The technology and major players. *BioPharm* 1999; 12(3):46–49.

Rohricht P. Transgenic protein production. Part 2: Process economics. *BioPharm* 1999; 12(9):52–54.

Rudolph N. Technologies and economics for protein production in transgenic animal milk. *Gen Eng News* 1997; 17(18):16.

Ruiz Jr. LP, Binion SB, Clark DR, Cady ME. Production of pharmaceutical products from milk — computer model application in assessment of economics of large-scale recombinant protein production in cattle transgenic animal milk. *J Cell Biochem* 1990; (Suppl.14D):17.

Strijker R. Production of proteins in milk of transgenic cows — human recombinant lactoferrin production via mamma tissue-specific gene expression in cattle transgenic animal milk. *Meded Fac Landbouwwet Rijksuniv Gent* 1994; 59(4a):1733–1736.

Stromqvist M, Houdebine M, Andersson JO, Edlund A, Johansson T, Viglietta C, Puissant C, Hansson L. Recombinant human extracellular superoxide dismutase produced in milk of transgenic rabbits. *Transgenic Res* 1997; 6(4):271–278.

Swanson ME, Martin MJ, O'Donnell JK, Hoover K, Lago W, Huntress V, Parsons CT, Pinkert CA, Pilder S, Logan JS. Production of functional human hemoglobin in transgenic swine. *Biotechnology* (NY) 1992; 10(5):557–559.

Udell M and McCreath G. PPL Therapeutics Scotland Ltd, Assignee. Purification of fibrinogen from fluids by precipitation and hydrophobic chromatography. Patent WO0017239; EP1115745. Issued 30-3-2000. September 24, 1998.

van Berkel PH, Welling MM, Geerts M, van Veen HA, Ravensbergen B, Salaheddine M, Pauwels EK, Pieper F, Nuijens JH, Nibbering PH. Large scale production of recombinant human lactoferrin in the milk of transgenic cows. *Nat Biotechnol* 2002; 20(5):484–487.

Van Cott KE. Transgenic animals as drug factories: A new source of recombinant protein therapeutics. *Expert Opinion on Investigational Drugs* 1998; 7(10):1683–1690.

Van Cott KE, Williams B, Velander WH, Gwazdauskas F, Lee T, Lubon H, Drohan WN. Affinity purification of biologically active and inactive forms of recombinant human protein C produced in porcine mammary gland. *J Mol Recognit* 1996; 9(5-6):407–414.

Velander WH. Recovering recombinant proteins from milk of transgenic animals is feasible. *Genet Technol News* 1989; 9(12):4.

Velander WH, Johnson JL, Page RL, Russell CG, Subramanian A, Wilkins TD, Gwazdauskas FC, Pittius C, Drohan WN. High-level expression of a heterologous protein in the milk of transgenic swine using the cDNA encoding human protein C. *Proc Natl Acad Sci USA* 1992; 89(24):12003–12007.

Velander WH, Morcol T, Akers RM, Boyle PL, Johnson JL, Drohan WN. The recovery of therapeutic proteins from milk — protein-C gene cloning and expression in pig or cattle transgenic animal; recombinant protein purification. *J Cell Biochem* 1990; (Suppl.14D):36.

Velander WH, Page RL, Morcol T, Russell CG, Canseco R, Young JM, Drohan WN, Gwazdauskas FC, Wilkins TD, Johnson JL. Production of biologically active human protein C in the milk of transgenic mice. *Ann NY Acad Sci* 1992; 665:391–403.

Wall RJ, Pursel VG, Shamay A, McKnight RA, Pittius CW, Hennighausen L. High-level synthesis of a heterologous milk protein in the mammary glands of transgenic swine. *Proc Natl Acad Sci USA* 1991; 88(5):1696–1700.

Wilkins TD and Velander W. Isolation of recombinant proteins from milk. *J Cell Biochem* 1992; 49(4):333–338.

Wright G. Manufacturing from transgenics: Scale up and production issues. *J Biotechnol Health Care* 1997; 4(3):247–254.

Wright G, Carver A, Cottom D, Reeves D, Scott A, Simons P, Wilmut I, Garner I, Colman A. High level expression of active human alpha-1-antitrypsin in the milk of transgenic sheep — expression as beta-lactoglobulin fusion protein in transgenic animal milk. *Biotechnology* 1991; 9(9):830–834.

Wright G, Colman A, Cottom D, Williams M. Licensing of protein products from the milk of transgenic animals. Validation for pathogen removal — A strategy. *Dev Biol Stand* 1996; 88:269–276.

Wright G and Colman A. Purification of recombinant proteins from sheep's milk. In: *Transgenic Animals. Generation and Use.* Harwood Academic Publishers, Amsterdam, Netherlands, 1997: 469–471.

Wright G and Noble J. Production of transgenic protein. In: *Bioseparation and Bioprocessing.* Vol. II. *Processing, Quality and Characterization, Economics, Safety and Hygiene.* Subramanian G, editor. Wiley-VCH, New York, 1998: 67–79.

Young MW et al. Production of biopharmaceutical proteins in the milk of transgenic dairy animals. *BioPharm* 1997; 10(6):34–38.

Ziomek CA. Minimization of viral contamination in human pharmaceuticals produced in the milk of transgenic goats. *Dev Biol Stand* 1996; 88:265–268.

CHAPTER 7: DOWNSTREAM PROCESSING

PROTEIN REFOLDING

Ahmed AK, Schaffer SW, Wetlaufer DB. Nonenzymic reactivation of reduced bovine pancreatic ribonuclease by air oxidation and by glutathione oxidoreduction buffers. *J Biol Chem* 1975; 250(21):8477–8482.

Ambrosius D and Rudolph R. Boehringer Mannheim GmbH, Assignee. Process for the reactivation of denatured protein. Patent US 5618927. Issued 8-4-1997. Filed July 2, 1992.

Batas B and Chaudhuri JB. Protein refolding at high concentration using size-exclusion chromatography. *Biotechnol Bioeng* 1996; 50(1):16–23.

Berdichevsky Y, Lamed R, Frenkel D, Gophna U, Bayer EA, Yaron S, Shoham Y, Benhar I. Matrix-assisted refolding of single-chain Fv-cellulose binding domain fusion proteins. *Protein Expr Purif* 1999; 17(2):249–259.

Brinkmann U, Buchner J, Pastan I. Independent domain folding of Pseudomonas exotoxin and single-chain immunotoxins: influence of interdomain connections. *Proc Natl Acad Sci USA* 1992; 89(7):3075–3079.

Buchner J and Rudolph R. Renaturation, purification and characterization of recombinant Fab-fragments produced in *Escherichia coli*. *Biotechnology* (NY) 1991; 9(2):157–162.

Cerletti N, McMaster GK, Cox D, Schmitz A, Meyhack B. Ciba-Geigy Corporation, Assignee. Process for refolding recombinantly produced TGF-.beta.-like proteins. Patent US 5650494. Issued 22-7-1997.

Cerletti N, McMaster GK, Cox D, Schmitz A, Meyhack B. Novartis AG, Assignee. Process for the production of biologically active protein (e.g. TGF). Patent EP 0433225. Issued 7-4-1999. Filed November 27, 1990.

Cleland JL, Builder SE, Swartz JR, Winkler M, Chang JY, Wang DI. Polyethylene glycol enhanced protein refolding. *Biotechnology* (NY) 1992; 10(9):1013–1019.

Creighton TE. Process for the production of a protein. Patent US 4977248. Issued 11-12-1990. Filed August 10, 1989.

Daugherty DL, Rozema D, Hanson PE, Gellman SH. Artificial chaperone-assisted refolding of citrate synthase. *J Biol Chem* 1998; 273(51):33961–33971.

De Bernardez Clark E. Protein refolding for industrial processes. *Curr Opin Biotechnol* 2001; 12(2):202–207.

De Bernardez Clark E. Refolding of recombinant proteins. *Curr Opin Biotechnol* 1998; 9(2):157–163.

De Bernardez Clark E, Schwarz E, Rudolph R. Inhibition of aggregation side reactions during *in vitro* protein folding. *Methods Enzymol* 1999; 309:217–236.

Fahey EM, Chaudhuri JB, Binding P. Refolding and purification of a urokinase plasminogen activator fragment by chromatography. *J Chromatogr B Biomed Sci Appl* 2000; 737(1–2):225–235.

Fahey EM, Chaudhuri JB, Binding P. Refolding of low molecular weight urokinase plasminogen activator by dilution and size exclusion chromatography — a comparative study. *Sep Sci Technol* 2000; 35:1743–1760.

Goldberg ME, Expert-Bezancon N, Vuillard L, Rabilloud T. Non-detergent sulphobetaines: a new class of molecules that facilitate *in vitro* protein renaturation. *Folding and Design* 1996; 1(1):21–27.

Hagel P, Gerding JJ, Fieggen W, Bloemendal H. Cyanate formation in solutions of urea. I. Calculation of cyanate concentrations at different temperature and pH. *Biochim Biophys Acta* 1971; 243(3):366–373.

Hejnaes KR, Bayne S, Norskov L, Sorensen HH, Thomsen J, Schaffer L, Wollmer A, Skriver L. Development of an optimized refolding process for recombinant Ala-Glu-IGF-1. *Protein Eng* 1992; 5(8):797–806.

Holtet TL, Etzerodt M, Thøgersen HC. Denzyme Aps, Holtet TL, Etzerodt M, Thøgersen HC, Assignees. Improved method for the refolding of proteins. Patent WO 9418227. Issued 18-8-1994. Filed February 4, 1993.

Huxtable S, Zhou H, Wong S, Li N. Renaturation of 1-aminocyclopropane-1-carboxylate synthase expressed in *Escherichia coli* in the form of inclusion bodies into a dimeric and catalytically active enzyme. *Protein Expr Purif* 1998; 12(3):305–314.

Karuppiah N and Sharma A. Cyclodextrins as protein folding aids. *Biochem Biophys Res Commun* 1995; 211(1):60–66.

Kiefhaber T, Rudolph R, Kohler HH, Buchner J. Protein aggregation *in vitro* and *in vivo*: a quantitative model of the kinetic competition between folding and aggregation. *Biotechnology* (NY) 1991; 9(9):825–829.

Kim CS and Lee EK. Effect of operating parameters in *in vitro* renaturation of a fusion protein of human growth hormone and glutathione S-transferase from inclusion body. *Process Biochem* 2000; 36:111–117.

Lilie H, Schwarz E, Rudolph R. Advances in refolding of proteins produced in *E. coli*. *Curr Opin Biotechnol* 1998; 9(5):497–501.

Machida S, Ogawa S, Xiaohua S, Takaha T, Fujii K, Hayashi K. Cycloamylose as an efficient artificial chaperone for protein refolding. *FEBS Lett* 2000; 486(2):131–135.

Marston FA and Hartley DL. Solubilization of protein aggregates. *Meth Enzymol* 1990; 182(20):264–276.

Michaelis U, Rudolph R, Jarsch M, Kopetzki E, Burtscher H, Schumacher G. Boehringer Mannheim GmbH, Assignee. Process for the production and renaturation of recombinant, biologically active, eukaryotic alkaline phosphatase. Patent US 5434067. Issued 18-7-1995. Filed July 30, 1993.

Misawa S and Kumagai I. Refolding of therapeutic proteins produced in *Escherichia coli* as inclusion bodies. *Biopolymers* 1999; 51(4):297–307.

Muller C and Rinas U. Renaturation of heterodimeric platelet-derived growth factor from inclusion bodies of recombinant *Escherichia coli* using size-exclusion chromatography. *J Chromatogr A* 1999; 855(1):203–213.

Nozaki Y. The preparation of guanidine hydrochloride. *Meth Enzymol* 1972; 26(Pt.C):43–50.

Odorzynski TW and Light A. Refolding of the mixed disulfide of bovine trypsinogen and glutathione. *J Biol Chem* 1979; 254(10):4291–4295.

Qi ZH and Sikorski CT. Controlled delivery using cyclodextrin technology. *Pharm Technol Europe* 2001; 13(11):17–27.

Rogl H, Kosemund K, Kuhlbrandt W, Collinson I. Refolding of *Escherichia coli* produced membrane protein inclusion bodies immobilised by nickel chelating chromatography. *FEBS Lett* 1998; 432(1–2):21–26.

Rozema D and Gellman SH. Artificial chaperone-assisted refolding of denatured-reduced lysozyme: modulation of the competition between renaturation and aggregation. *Biochemistry* 1996; 35(49):15760–15771.

Rozema D and Gellman SH. Artificial chaperone-assisted refolding of carbonic anhydrase B *J Biol Chem* 1996; 271(7):3478–3487.

Rozema D and Gellman SH. Artificial chaperones: Protein refolding via sequential use of detergent and cyclodextrin. *J Am Chem Soc* 1995; 117(8):2373–2374.

Rudolph R, Fischer S, Mattes R. Boehringer Mannheim GmbH, Assignee. Process for the activating of gene-technologically produced, heterologous, disulphide bridge-containing eukaryotic proteins after expression in prokaryotes. Patent US 5593865. Issued 14-1-1997. Filed June 1, 1995.

Rudolph R and Fischer S. Boehringer Mannheim GmbH, Assignee. Process for obtaining renatured proteins. Patent US 4933434. Issued 12-6-1990. Filed January 13, 1989.

Rudolph R and Lilie H. *In vitro* folding of inclusion body proteins. *FASEB J* 1996; 10(1):49–56.

Stark GR, Stein WH, Moore S. Reactions of the cyanate present in aqueous urea with amino acids and proteins. *J Biol Chem* 1960; 235(4):3177–3181.

Stockel J, Doring K, Malotka J, Jahnig F, Dornmair K. Pathway of detergent-mediated and peptide ligand-mediated refolding of heterodimeric class II major histocompatibility complex (MHC) molecules. *Eur J Biochem* 1997; 248(3):684–691.

Sundari CS, Raman B, Balasubramanian D. Artificial chaperoning of insulin, human carbonic anhydrase and hen egg lysozyme using linear dextrin chains — a sweet route to the native state of globular proteins. *FEBS Lett* 1999; 443(2):215–219.

Tandon S and Horowitz P. The effects of lauryl maltoside on the reactivation of several enzymes after treatment with guanidinium chloride. *Biochim Biophys Acta* 1988; 955(1):19–25.

Tandon S and Horowitz PM. Detergent-assisted refolding of guanidinium chloride-denatured rhodanese. The effects of the concentration and type of detergent. *J Biol Chem* 1987; 262(10):4486–4491.

Thøgersen C, Holtet TL, Etzerodt M. Denzyme Aps, Assignee. Iterative method of at least five cycles for the refolding of proteins. Patent US 5917018. Issued 29-6-1999. Filed September 18, 1995.

Tsumoto K, Shinoki K, Kondo H, Uchikawa M, Juji T, Kumagai I. Highly efficient recovery of functional single-chain Fv fragments from inclusion bodies overexpressed in *Escherichia coli* by controlled introduction of oxidizing reagent — application to a human single-chain Fv fragment. *J Immunol Meth* 1998; 219(1–2):119–129.

Werner MH, Clore GM, Gronenborn AM, Kondoh A, Fisher RJ. Refolding proteins by gel filtration chromatography. *FEBS Lett* 1994; 345(2–3):125–130.

West SM, Chaudhuri JB, Howell JA. Improved protein refolding using hollow-fibre membrane dialysis. *Biotechnol Bioeng* 1998; 57(5):590–599.

Wetlaufer DB and Xie Y. Control of aggregation in protein refolding: a variety of surfactants promote renaturation of carbonic anhydrase II. *Protein Sci* 1995; 4(8):1535–1543.

Zardeneta G and Horowitz PM. Micelle-assisted protein folding. Denatured rhodanese binding to cardiolipin-containing lauryl maltoside micelles results in slower refolding kinetics but greater enzyme reactivation. *J Biol Chem* 1992; 267(9):5811–5816.

FILTRATION AND PROTEIN PRECIPITATION

Arakawa T and Timasheff SN. Preferential interactions of proteins with salts in concentrated solutions. *Biochemistry* 1982; 21(25):6545–6552.

Mochizuki S and Zydney AL. Theoretical analysis of pore size distribution effects on membrane transport. *J Membr Sci* 1993; 82(3):211–227.

Nakatsuka S and Michaels AS. Transport and separation of proteins by ultrafiltration through sorptive and non-sorptive membranes. *J Membr Sci* 1992; 69(3):189–211.

Saksena S and Zydney AL. Effect of solution pH and ionic strength on the separation of albumin from immunoglobulins (IgG) by selective filtration. *Biotechnol Bioeng* 1994; 43(10):960–968.

Scopes RK. *Protein Purification: Principles and Practice.* 3rd ed. Springer Verlag, New York, 1994.

Scopes RK. Separation by precipitation. In: *Protein Purification: Principles and Practice.* Springer Verlag, New York, 1987: 41–71.

van Reis R, Gadam S, Frautschy LN, Orlando S, Goodrich EM, Saksena S, Kuriyel R, Simpson CM, Pearl S, Zydney AL. High performance tangential flow filtration. *Biotechnol Bioeng* 1997; 56(1):71–82.

van Reis R and Zydney AL. Protein ultrafiltration. In: *Encyclopedia of Bioprocess Technology: Fermentation, Biocatalysis, and Bioseparation.* Flickinger MC and Drew SW, editors. Wiley, New York, 1999: 2197–2214.

Zeman L.J and Zydney AL. *Microfiltration and Ultrafiltration: Principles and Applications.* Marcel Dekker, New York, 1996.

EXPANDED BED ADSORPTION SYSTEMS

Barnfield Frej A-K, Hjorth R, Hammarström Å. Pilot scale recovery of recombinant annexin v from unclarified *Escherichia coli* homogenate using expanded bed adsorption. *Biotech Bioeng* 1994; 44:922–929.

Barnfield Frej A-K, Johansson HJ, Johansson S., Leijon P. Expanded bed adsorption at production scale: Scale-up verification, process example and sanitization of column and adsorbent. *Bioprocess Eng* 1997; 16:57–63.

Batt BC, Yabannavar VM, Singh V. Expanded bed adsorption process for protein recovery from whole mammalian cell culture broth. *Bioseparations* 1995; 5:41–52.

Buijs A and Wesselingh JA. Batch fluidized ion-exchange column for streams containing suspended particles. *J Chromatogr* 1980; 201:319–327.

Burns MA and Graves DJ. Continuous affinity chromatography using a magnetically stabilized fluidized bed. *Biotechnol Prog* 1985; 1:95–103.

Chang Y-K and Chase HA. Development of operating conditions for protein purification using expanded bed techniques: The effect of the degree of bed expansion on adsorption performance. *Biotech Bioeng* 1996; 49:512–526.

Chang Y-K and Chase HA. Ion exchange purification of G6PDH from unclarified yeast cell homogenates using expanded bed adsorption. *Biotech Bioeng* 1996; 49:204–216.

Chang Y-K, McCreath GE, Chase HA. Development of an expanded bed technique for an affinity purification of G6PDH from unclarified yeast cell homogenates. *Biotech Bioeng* 1995; 48:355–366.

Chase HA. Purification of proteins by adsorption chromatography in expanded beds. *Trends Biotech* 1994; 12:296–303.

Chase HA and Draeger MN. Affinity purification of proteins using expanded beds. *J Chromatogr* 1992; 597:129–145.

Chase HA and Draeger MN. Expanded bed adsorption of proteins using ion-exchangers. *Separation Sci Technol* 1992; 27:2021–2039.

Dasari G, Prince I, Hearn MTW. High-performance liquid chromatography of amino acids, peptides and proteins. CXXIV. Physical characterization of fluidized-bed behaviour of chromatographic packing materials. *J Chromatogr* 1993; 631:115–124.

Degener A, Belew M, Velander WH. Expanded bed purification of a recombinant protein from the milk of transgenic livestock. Presented at 211th American Chemical Society National Meeting, New Orleans, Louisiana, USA, March 24–28, 1996.

Draeger MN and Chase HA. Liquid fluidized bed adsorption of proteins in the presence of cells. *Bioseparations* 1991; 2:67–80.

Drohan WN, Wilkins TD, Latimer E, Zhou D, Velander W, Lee TK, Lubon H. A scalable method for the purification of recombinant human protein C from the milk of transgenic swine. *Adv Bioproc Eng* 1994; (269)501–507.

Erickson JC, Finch JD, Greene DC. Direct capture of recombinant proteins from animal cell culture media using a fluidized bed adsorber. In: *Animal Cell Technology: Products for Today, Prospects for Tomorrow.* Griffiths B, Spier RE, Berthold W, editors. Butterworth Heinemann, Oxford, 1994: 557–560.

Gailliot FP, Gleason C, Wilson JJ, Zwarick J. Fluidized bed adsorption for whole broth extraction. *Biotechnol Prog* 1990; 6:370–375.

Hagel L and Sofer G. *Cleaning, Sanitization and Storage. Handbook of Process Chromatography. A Guide to Optimization, Scale up, and Validation*. Academic Press, London, 1997.

Hansson M, Ståhl S, Hjorth R, Uhlén M, Moks T. Single-step recovery of a secreted recombinant protein by expanded bed adsorption. *BioTechnol* 1994; 12:285–288.

Hjorth R, Kämpe S, Carlsson M. Analysis of some operating parameters of novel adsorbents for recovery of proteins in expanded beds. *Bioseparation* 1995; 5:217–223.

McCormick DK. expanded bed adsorption. The first new unit process operation in decades. *BioTechnol* 1993; 11:1059.

McDonald JR, Ong M, Shen C, Parandoosh Z, Sosnowski B, Bussel S, Houston LL. Large-scale purification and characterization of recombinant fibroblast growth factor-saporin mitotoxin. *Protein Expression Purif* 1996; 8:97–108.

Nixon L, Koval CA, Xu L, Noble RD, Slaff GS. The effects of magnetic stabilization on the structure and performance of fluidized beds. *Bioseparations* 1991; 2:217–230.

Noppe W, Hanssens I, De Cuyper M. Simple two-step procedure for the preparation of highly active pure equine milk lysozyme. *J Chromatogr* 1996; 719:327–331.

Roper DK and Lightfoot EN. Estimating plate-heights in stacked membrane chromatography by flow reversal. *J Chromatogr* A 1995; 702:69–80.

Seidel-Morgenstern A. Analysis of boundary conditions in the axial dispersion model by application of numerical laplace inversion. *Chem Eng Sci* 1991; 46:2567–2571.

Swaine DE and Daugulis AJ. Review of liquid mixing in packed bed biological reactors. *Biotechnol Progr* 1988; 4:134–148.

Thömmes J et al. Purification of monoclonal antibodies from whole hybridoma fermentation broth by fluidized bed adsorption. *Biotech Bioeng* 1995; 45:205–211.

Thömmes J, Bader A, Halfar M, Karau A, Kula M-R. Isolation of monoclonal antibodies from cell containing hybridoma broth using a protein A coated adsorbent in expanded beds. *J Chromatogr* A 1996; 752:111–122.

Wright G, Binieda A, Udell M. Protein separation from transgenic milk. *J Chem Tech Biotechnol* 1994; 54:110.

Zurek C, Kubis E, Keup P, Hörlein D, Beunink J, Thömmes J, Kula M-R, Hollenberg CP, Gellissen G. Production of two aprotinin variants in hansenula polymorpha. *Process Biochem* 1996; 31:679–689.

Virus Removal and Inactivation

Aranha H. Viral clearance strategies for biopharmaceutical safety. Part 2: Filtration for viral clearance. *BioPharm* 2001; 14(2):32–43.

Aranha-Creado H and Brandwein H. Application of bacteriophages as surrogates for mammalian viruses: a case for use in filter validation based on precedents and current practices in medical and environmental virology. *PDA J Pharm Sci Technol* 1999; 53(2):75–82.

Aranha-Creado H and Fennington Jr. GJ. Cumulative viral titer reduction demonstrated by sequential challenge of a tangential flow membrane filtration system and a direct flow pleated filter cartridge. *PDA J Pharm Sci Technol* 1997; 51(5):208–212.

Aranha-Creado H, Oshima K, Jafari S, Howard Jr. G, Brandwein H. Virus retention by a hydrophilic triple-layer PVDF microporous membrane filter. *PDA J Pharm Sci Technol* 1997; 51(3):119–124.

Aranha-Creado H, Peterson J, Huang PY. Clearance of murine leukaemia virus from monoclonal antibody solutions by a hydrophilic PVDF microporous membrane filter. *Biologicals* 1998; 26(2):167–172.

Bachrach HL. Reactivity of viruses *in vitro*. *Prog Med Virol* 1966; 8:214–313.

Bellara SR, Cui Z, MacDonald SL, Pepper DS. Virus removal from bioproducts using ultrafiltration membranes modified with latex particle pretreatment. *Bioseparation* 1998; 7(2):79–88.

Berthold W, Werz W, Walter JK. Relationship between nature and source of risk and process validation. *Dev Biol Stand* 1996; 88:59–71.

Bradley DW, Hess RA, Tao F, Sciaba-Lentz L, Remaley AT, Laugharn Jr. JA, Manak M. Pressure cycling technology: a novel approach to virus inactivation in plasma. *Transfusion* 2000; 40(2):193–200.

Brandwein H and Aranha-Creado H. Membrane filtration for virus removal. In: *Advances in Transfusion Safety*. Brown F and Vyas G, editors. Karger, Basel, 2000: 157–163.

Brantley JD and Martin J. Integrity testing of sterilizing grade filters. *Sci Tech R*, PBB-STR-28. Pall Ultrafine Filtration Company, East Hills, NY, 1997.

Brown F, Meyer RF, Law M, Kramer E, Newman JF. A universal virus inactivant for decontaminating blood and biopharmaceutical products. *Biologicals* 1998; 26(1):39–47.

Cameron R, Davies J, Adcock W, MacGregor A, Barford JP, Cossart Y, Harbour C. The removal of model viruses, poliovirus type 1 and canine parvovirus, during the purification of human albumin using ion-exchange chromatographic procedures. *Biologicals* 1997; 25(4):391–401.

Chapman J. Progress in improving the pathogen safety of red cell concentrates. *Vox Sang* 2000; 78(Suppl. 2):203–204.

Charm SE and Landau SH. Thermalizer. High-temperature short-time sterilization of heat-sensitive biological materials. *Ann NY Acad Sci* 1987; 506:608–612.

Charm SE, Landau S, Williams B, Horowitz B, Prince AM, Pascual D. High-temperature short-time heat inactivation of HIV and other viruses in human blood plasma. *Vox Sang* 1992; 62(1):12–20.

Dichtelmuller H, Rudnick D, Breuer B, Ganshirt KH. Validation of virus inactivation and removal for the manufacturing procedure of two immunoglobulins and a 5% serum protein solution treated with beta-propiolactone. *Biologicals* 1993; 21(3):259–268.

Ebeling F, Baer M, Hormila P, Jarventie G, Koistinen P, Katka K, Oksanen K, Perkkio M, Ruutu T, Soppi E. Tolerability and kinetics of a solvent-detergent-treated intravenous immunoglobulin preparation in hypogammaglobulinaemia patients. *Vox Sang* 1995; 69(2):91–94.

Gerba CP, Staggs CH, Alondie MG. Characterization of sewage solid-associated virus and behavior in natural waters. *Water Res* 1978; 12:805–812.

Graf EG, Jander E, West A, Pora H, Aranha-Creado H. Virus removal by filtration. *Dev Biol Stand* 1999; 99:89–94.

Hamalainen E, Suomela H, Ukkonen P. Virus inactivation during intravenous immunoglobulin production. *Vox Sang* 1992; 63(1):6–11.

Henzler HJ and Kaiser K. Avoiding viral contamination in biotechnological and pharmaceutical processes. *Nature Biotechnol* 1998; 16(11):1077–1079.

Horowitz B. Investigations into the application of tri(n-butyl)phosphate/detergent mixtures to blood derivatives. *Curr Stud Hematol Blood Transfus* 1989; (56):83–96.

Hughes B, Bradburne A, Sheppard A, Young D. Evaluation of anti-viral filters. *Dev Biol Stand* 1996; 88:91–98.

ICH. Quality of biotechnological products: viral safety evaluation of biotechnology products derived from cell lines of human or animal origin. ICH Harmonised Tripartite Guideline. *Dev Biol Stand* 1998; 93:177–201.

Lundblad JL and Seng RL. Inactivation of lipid-enveloped viruses in proteins by caprylate. *Vox Sang* 1991; 60(2):75–81.

Mannucci PM and Colombo M. Virucidal treatment of clotting factor concentrates. *Lancet* 1988; 2(8614):782–785.

Miekka SI, Busby TF, Reid B, Pollock R, Ralston A, Drohan WN. New methods for inactivation of lipid-enveloped and non-enveloped viruses. *Haemophilia* 1998; 4(4):402–408.

Oshima KH, Evans-Strickfaden T, Highsmith A. Comparison of filtration properties of hepatitis B virus (HBV), hepatitis C virus(HCV) and simian virus 40 (SV40) using a polyvinylidene fluoride (PVDF) membrane filter. *Vox Sang* 1998; 75(3):181–188.

Oshima KH, Evans-Strickfaden TT, Highsmith AK, Ades EW. The use of a microporous polyvinylidene fluoride (PVDF) membrane filter to separate contaminating viral particles from biologically important proteins. *Biologicals* 1996; 24(2):137–145.

Oshima KH, Highsmith AK, Ades EW. Removal of influenza A virus, phage T1, and PP7 from fluids with a nylon 0.04-μm membrane filter. *Environ Toxicol Water Quality* 1994; 9:165–170.

Pall. Validation guide for Pall UltiporR VFTM Grade DV50 UltipleatTM AB Style virus removal filter cartridges. Pall Ultrafine Filtration Company, Pall Corporation, New York, 1995.

Perreault P and Brantley JD. Characterization of ultrafiltration membranes using mixed dextrans. Pall Ultrafine Filtration Company, Pall Corporation, New York, 1997.

Phillips MW and DiLeo AJ. A validatible porosimetric technique for verifying the integrity of virus-retentive membranes. *Biologicals* 1996; 24(3):243–253.

Prince AM, Stephan W, Brotman B. Beta-propiolactone/ultraviolet irradiation: a review of its effectiveness for inactivation of viruses in blood derivatives. *Rev Infect Dis* 1983; 5(1):92–107.

Quality of biotechnological products: viral safety evaluation of biotechnology products derived from cell lines of human or animal origin. ICH Harmonised Tripartite Guideline. *Dev Biol Stand* 1998; 93:177–201.

Roberts P. Efficient removal of viruses by a novel polyvinylidene fluoride membrane filter. *J Virol Meth* 1997; 65(1):27–31.

Sato T et al. Integrity test of virus removal membranes through gold particle method and liquid forward flow test method. In: *Animal Cell Technology: Basic and Applied Aspects*. Kobayashi T et al., editors. Kluwer Academic Publishers, Norwell, MA, 1994: 517–522.

Sobsey MD. Methods for detecting enteric viruses in water and wastewater. In: *Viruses in Water*. Berg G, Bodily HL, Lennette EH, editors. American Public Health Association, Washington, DC, 1976: 89–127.

Sobsey MD and Glass JS. Influence of water quality on enteric virus concentration by microporous filter methods. *Appl Environ Microbiol* 1984; 47(5):956–960.

Sobsey MD, Moore RS, Glass JS. Evaluating adsorbent filter performance for enteric virus concentrations in tap water. *J Am Water Works Assoc* 1981; 73:542–548.

Sofer G. Virus inactivation in the 1990s — and into the 21st century. Part 4, Culture media, biotechnology products, and vaccines. *BioPharm* 2003; 16(1):50–57.

Tao CZ, Cameron R, Harbour C, Barford JP. The development of appropriate viral models for the validation of viral inactivation procedures. In: *Animal Cell Technology. Products of Today, Prospects for Tomorrow*. Spier RE, Griffiths JB, Berthold W, editors. Butterworth Heinemann, Oxford, 1994: 754–756.

Tipton B, Boose JA, Larsen W, Beck J, O'Brien T. Retrovirus and parvovirus clearance from an affinity column product using adsorptive depth filtration. *BioPharm* 2002; 15(9):43–50.

Troccoli NM, McIver J, Losikoff A, Poiley J. Removal of viruses from human intravenous immune globulin by 35 nm nanofiltration. *Biologicals* 1999; 26(4):321–329.

Tsao IF and Wang HY. Removal and inactivation of viruses by a surface-bonded quaternary ammonium chloride. In: *Downstream Processing and Bioseparation: Recovery and Purification of Biological Products*. Hamel JFP, Hunter JB, Sikdar SK, editors. American Chemical Society, Washington, DC, 1990: 250–267.

Tsurumi T, Osawa N, Hitaka H, Hirasaki T, Yamaguchi K, Manabe S, Yamashiki T. Mechanism of removing monodisperse gold particles from a suspension using cuprammonium regenerated cellulose hollow fibre (BMM hollow fibre). *Polymer J* 1990; 22:304–311.

Virus inactivation in the 1990s – and into the 21st century. *BioPharm Int* 2003; (January): 50–57.

Vollenbroich D, Ozel M, Vater J, Kamp RM, Pauli G. Mechanism of inactivation of enveloped viruses by the biosurfactant surfactin from bacillus subtilis. *Biologicals* 1997; 25(3):289–297.

Walter JK, Nothelfer F, Werz W. Validation of viral safety for pharmaceutical proteins. In: *Bioseparation and Bioprocessing*. Vol. I. *Biochromatography, Membrane Separations, Modeling, Validation*. Subramanian G, editor. Wiley-VCH, New York, 1998: 465–496.

Walter JK, Nothelfer F, Werz W. Virus removal and inactivation. A decade of validation studies: Critical evaluation of the data set. In: *Validation of Biopharmaceutical Manufacturing Processes*. Oxford, London, 1998.

WHO requirements for the use of animal cells as *in vitro* substrates for the production of biologicals (Requirements for biological substances No. 50). *Dev Biol Stand* 1998; 93:141–171.

CHAPTER 8: PURIFICATION TECHNIQUES

AFFINITY CHROMATOGRAPHY (AC)

Aerts JM, Donker-Koopman WE, Murray GJ, Barranger JA, Tager JM, Schram AW. A procedure for the rapid purification in high yield of human glucocerebrosidase using immunoaffinity chromatography with monoclonal antibodies. *Anal Biochem* 1986; 154(2):655–663.

Amersham Pharmacia Biotech. *Affinity Chromatography: Principles and Methods*. Amersham Pharmacia Biotech AB, Uppsala, Sweden, 2001.

Arvidsson P, Ivanov AE, Galaev IY, Mattiasson B. Polymer versus monomer as displacer in immobilized metal affinity chromatography. *J Chromatogr B Biomed Sci Appl* 2001; 753(2):279–285.

Bollag DM, Rozycki MD, Edelstein SJ. *Protein Methods*. 2nd. ed. Wiley-Liss, New-York, 1996.

Brooks SP, Bennett VD, Suelter CH. Homogeneous chicken heart mitochondrial creatine kinase purified by dye-ligand and transition-state analog-affinity chromatography. *Anal Biochem* 1987; 164(1):190–198.

Burton SJ. Affinity chromatography: production and regulatory considerations. *Am Biotechnol Lab* 1996; 14(5):64–66.

Carlsson J, Janson J-C, Sparrman M. Affinity chromtography. In: *Protein Purification: Principles, High-Resolution Methods, and Applications*. Janson J-C and Ryden L, editors. Wiley-Liss, New York, 1998: 375–442.

Fahrner RL, Blank GS, Zapata GA. Expanded bed protein A affinity chromatography of a recombinant humanized monoclonal antibody: process development, operation, and comparison with a packed bed method. *J Biotechnol* 1999; 75(2–3):273–280.

Fahrner RL, Whitney DH, Vanderlaan M, Blank GS. Performance comparison of protein A affinity-chromatography sorbents for purifying recombinant monoclonal antibodies. *Biotechnol Appl Biochem* 1999; 30(Pt 2):121–128.

Gagnon P. *Purification Tools for Monoclonal Antibodies*. Validated Biosystems Inc., Tucson, AZ, 1996.

Hogan Jr. JC, Legomer Partners LP, Assignees. Aminimide-containing molecules and materials as molecular recognition agents. Patent WO9401102. Issued 20-1-1994.

Jankowski WJ, von Muenchhausen W, Sulkowski E, Carter WA. Binding of human interferons to immobolized Cibacron Blue F3GA: The nature of molecular interaction. *Biochemistry* 1976; 15(23):5182–5187.

Janson J-C and Ryden L. *Protein Purification: Principles, High-Resolution Methods, and Applications*. 2nd ed. Wiley-Liss, New York, 1998.

Kiss L, Tar A, Gal S, Toth-Mortinez BL, Hernadi FJ. Modified general affinity adsorbent for large-scale purification of penicillinases. *J Chromatogr* 1988; 448(1):109–116.

Lowe CR, Burton SJ, Burton NP, Alderton WK, Pitts JM, Thomas JA. Designer dyes: "biomimetic" ligands for the purification of pharmaceutical proteins by affinity chromatography. *Trends Biotechnol* 1992; 10(12):442–448.

Miyata K, Yamamoto Y, Ueda M, Kawade Y, Matsumoto K, Kubota I. Purification of natural human interferon-gamma by antibody affinity chromatography: analysis of constituent protein species in the dimers. *J Biochem* (Tokyo) 1986; 99(6):1681–1688.

Moore WM and Spilburg CA. Purification of human collagenases with a hydroxamic acid affinity column. *Biochemistry* 1986; 25(18):5189–5195.

Nilsson J, Stahl S, Lundeberg J, Uhlen M, Nygren PA. Affinity fusion strategies for detection, purification, and immobilization of recombinant proteins. *Protein Expr Purif* 1997; 11(1):1–16.

Scopes RK. *Protein Purification: Principles and Practice*. 3rd. ed. Springer Verlag, New York, 1994.

Secher DS and Burke DC. A monoclonal antibody for large-scale purification of human leukocyte interferon. *Nature* 1980; 285(5765):446–450.

Seeger A and Rinas U. Two-step chromatographic procedure for purification of basic fibroblast growth factor from recombinant *Escherichia coli* and characterization of the equilibrium parameters of adsorption. *J Chromatogr A* 1996; 746(1):17–24.

Sofer G, Hagel L. *Handbook of Process Chromatography: A Guide to Optimization, Scale-Up and Validation*. Academic Press, San Diego, CA, 1997: 80–85, 289–291.

IMMOBILIZED METAL AFFINITY CHROMATOGRAPHY

Andersson L and Porath J. Isolation of phosphoproteins by immobilized metal (Fe3+) affinity chromatography. *Anal Biochem* 1986; 154(1):250–254.

Borrebaeck CAK, Lonnerdal B, Etzler ME. Metal chelate affinity chromatography of the *Dolichos biflorus* seed lectin and its subunits. *FEBS Lett* 1981; 130(2):194–196.

Carlsson J, Porath J, Lonnerdal B. Isolation of lactoferrin from human milk by metal-chelate affinity chromatography. *FEBS Lett* 1977; 75(1):89–92.

Cawston TE and Tyler JA. Purification of pig synovial collagenase to high specific activity. *Biochem J* 1979; 183(3):647–656.

Cha HJ, Dalal NG, Vakharia VN, Bentley WE. Expression and purification of human interleukin-2 simplified as a fusion with green fluorescent protein in suspended Sf-9 insect cells. *J Biotechnol* 1999; 69(1):9–17.

Chen HM, Luo SL, Chen KT, Lii CK. Affinity purification of Schistosoma japonicum glutathione-S- transferase and its site-directed mutants with glutathione affinity chromatography and immobilized metal affinity chromatography. *J Chromatogr A* 1999; 852(1):151–159.

Clemmitt RH and Chase HA. Facilitated downstream processing of a histidine-tagged protein from unclarified *E. coli* homogenates using immobilized metal affinity expanded-bed adsorption. *Biotechnol Bioeng* 2000; 67(2):206–216.

Coppenhaver DH. Nickel chelate chromatography of human immune interferon. *Methods Enzymol* 1986; 119:199–204.

Dalton JC, Bruley DF, Kang KA, Drohan WN. Separation of recombinant human protein C from transgenic animal milk using immobilized metal affinity chromatography. *Adv Exp Med Biol* 1997; 411:419–428.

Feng W, Graumann K, Hahn R, Jungbauer A. Affinity chromatography of human estrogen receptor-alpha expressed in Saccharomyces cerevisiae. Combination of heparin- and 17beta-estradiol-affinity chromatography. *J Chromatogr A* 1999; 852(1):161–173.

Gagnon P. *Purification Tools for Monoclonal Antibodies*. Validated Biosystems, Tucson AZ, 1996: 127–138.

Gibert S, Bakalara N, Santarelli X. Three-step chromatographic purification procedure for the production of a his-tag recombinant kinesin overexpressed in *E. coli*. *J Chromatogr B Biomed Sci Appl* 2000; 737(1–2):143–150.

Grisshammer R and Tucker J. Quantitative evaluation of neurotensin receptor purification by immobilized metal affinity chromatography. *Protein Expr Purif* 1997; 11(1):53–60.

Grundy JE, Wirtanen LY, Beauregard M. Addition of a poly-(6X) His tag to Milk Bundle-1 and purification using immobilized metal-affinity chromatography. *Protein Expr Purif* 1998; 13(1):61–66.

Hartleib J and Ruterjans H. High-yield expression, purification, and characterization of the recombinant diisopropylfluorophosphatase from Loligo vulgaris. *Protein Expr Purif* 2001; 21(1):210–219.

Hermida L, Rodriguez R, Lazo L, Lopez C, Marquez G, Paez R, Suarez C, Espinosa R, Garcia J, Guzman G, Guillen G. A recombinant envelope protein from Dengue virus purified by IMAC is bioequivalent with its immune-affinity chromatography purified counterpart. *J Biotechnol* 2002; 94(2):213–216.

Hochuli E, Bannwarth W, Döbeli H, Gentz R, Stüber D. Genetic approach to facilitate purification of recombinant proteins with a novel metal chelate adsorbent. *BioTechnol* 1988; 6(11):1321–1325.

Horvath Z and Nagydiosi GY. Imino-diacetic-acid-ethyl-cellulose and its chelate forming behaviour — I. *J Inorg Nucl Chem* 1975; 37(1):767–769.

Janson J-C and Rydén L (eds.). *Protein Purification*. 2nd ed. Wiley-Liss, New York, 1998: 311–342.

Jiang F and Mannervik B. Optimized heterologous expression of glutathione reductase from Cyanobacterium anabaena PCC 7120 and characterization of the recombinant protein. *Protein Expr Purif* 1999; 15(1):92–98.

Kågedal L. Immobilized metal ion affinity chromatography. In: *Protein Purification: Principles, High-Resolution Methods, and Applications*. Janson J-C and Ryden L, editors. Wiley-Liss, New York, 1998: 311–342.

Kikuchi H and Watanabe M. Significance of use of amino acids and histamine for the elution of nonhistone proteins in copper-chelate chromatography. *Anal Biochem* 1981; 115(1):109–112.

Liesiene J, Racaityte K, Morkeviciene M, Valancius P, Bumelis V. Immobilized metal affinity chromatography of human growth hormone. Effect of ligand density. *J Chromatogr A* 1997; 764(1):27–33.

Lilius G, Persson M, Bulow L, Mosbach K. Metal affinity precipitation of proteins carrying genetically attached polyhistidine affinity tails. *Eur J Biochem* 1991; 198(2):499–504.

Narayanan SR. Preparative affinity chromatography of proteins. *J Chromatogr A* 1994; 658(2):237–258.

Nordstrom T, Senkas A, Eriksson S, Pontynen N, Nordstrom E, Lindqvist C. Generation of a new protein purification matrix by loading ceramic hydroxyapatite with metal ions — demonstration with poly-histidine tagged green fluorescent protein. *J Biotechnol* 1999; 69(2-3):125–133.

Ohkubo I, Sahashi W, Namikawa C, Tsukada K, Takeuchi T, Sasaki M. A procedure for large scale purification of human plasma amyloid P component. *Clin Chim Acta* 1986; 157(1):95–101.

Oswald T, Hornbostel G, Rinas U, Anspach FB. Purification of (His)6EcoRV [recombinant restriction endonuclease EcoRV fused to a (His)6 affinity domain] by metal-chelate affinity chromatography. *Biotechnol Appl Biochem* 1997; 25(Pt 2):109–115.

Pedersen J, Lauritzen C, Madsen MT, Weis DS. Removal of N-terminal polyhistidine tags from recombinant proteins using engineered aminopeptidases. *Protein Expr Purif* 1999; 15(3):389–400.

Rahimi N, Etchells S, Elliott B. Hepatocyte growth factor (HGF) is a copper-binding protein: a facile probe for purification of HGF by immobilized Cu(II)-affinity chromatography. *Protein Expr Purif* 1996; 7(3):329–333.

Roberts PL, Walker CP, Feldman PA. Removal and inactivation of enveloped and non-enveloped viruses during the purification of a high-purity factor IX by metal chelate affinity chromatography. *Vox Sang* 1994; 67(Suppl.1):69–71.

Schon U and Schumann W. Construction of His6-tagging vectors allowing single-step purification of GroES and other polypeptides produced in Bacillus subtilis. *Gene* 1994; 147(1):91–94.

Smith MC, Furman TC, Ingolia TD, Pidgeon C. Chelating peptide-immobilized metal ion affinity chromatography. A new concept in affinity chromatography for recombinant proteins. *J Biol Chem* 1988; 263(15):7211–7215.

Tallet B, Astier-Gin T, Castroviejo M, Santarelli X. One-step chromatographic purification procedure of a His-tag recombinant carboxyl half part of the HTLV-I surface envelope glycoprotein overexpressed in *Escherichia coli* as a secreted form. *J Chromatogr B Biomed Sci Appl* 2001; 753(1):17–22.

Torres AR, Peterson EA, Evans WH, Mage MG, Wilson SM. Fractionation of granule proteins of granulocytes by copper chelate chromatography. *Biochim Biophys Acta* 1979; 576(2):385–392.

Ueda EK, Gout PW, Morganti L. Ni(II)-based immobilized metal ion affinity chromatography of recombinant human prolactin from periplasmic *Escherichia coli* extracts. *J Chromatogr A* 2001; 922(1–2):165–175.

Westra DF, Welling GW, Koedijk DG, Scheffer AJ, The TH, Welling-Wester S. Immobilised metal-ion affinity chromatography purification of histidine-tagged recombinant proteins: a wash step with a low concentration of EDTA. *J Chromatogr B Biomed Sci Appl* 2001; 760(1):129–136.

Wilkinson DL, Ma NT, Haught C, Harrison RG. Purification by immobilized metal affinity chromatography of human atrial natriuretic peptide expressed in a novel thioredoxin fusion protein. *Biotechnol Prog* 1995; 11(3):265–269.

Witzgall R, O'Leary E, Bonventre JV. A mammalian expression vector for the expression of GAL4 fusion proteins with an epitope tag and histidine tail. *Anal Biochem* 1994; 223(2):291–298.

Wu CY, Blaszczak LC, Smith MC, Skatrud PL. Construction of a modified penicillin-binding protein 2a from methicillin-resistant Staphylococcus aureus and purification by immobilized metal affinity chromatography. *J Bacteriol* 1994; 176(5):1539–1541.

ANION AND CATION EXCHANGE CHROMATOGRAPHY

Amersham Pharmacia Biotech. *Ion Exchange Chromatography: Principles and Methods*. 3rd ed. Amersham Pharmacia Biotech AB, Uppsala, Sweden, 1991.

Amersham-Pharmacia. *FPLC Ion Exchange and Chromatofocusing: Principles and Methods*. Pharmacia, Uppsala, Sweden, 1985.

Becker GW, Tackitt PM, Bromer WW, Lefeber DS, Riggin RM. Isolation and characterization of a sulfoxide and a desamido derivative of biosynthetic human growth hormone. *Biotechnol Appl Biochem* 1988; 10(4):326–337.

Bhikhabhai R, Johansson G, Pettersson G. Isolation of cellulolytic enzymes from Trichoderma reesei QM 9414. *J Appl Biochem* 1984; 6(5–6):336–345.

Bonnerjea J, Oh S, Hoare M, Dunnill P. Protein purification: The right step at the right time. *BioTechnol* 1986; 4(11):954–958.

Bouillenne F, Matagne A, Joris B, Frere JM. Technique for a rapid and efficient purification of the SHV-1 and PSE-2 beta-lactamases. *J Chromatogr B Biomed Sci Appl* 2000; 737(1–2):261–265.

Caldwell SR, Varghese J, Puri NK. Large scale purification process for recombinant NS1-OspA as a candidate vaccine for Lyme disease. *Bioseparation* 1996; 6(2):115–123.

Cervenansky C, Duran R, Karlsson E. Fasciculin: modification of carboxyl groups and discussion of structure-activity relationship. *Toxicon* 1996; 34(6):718–721.

Creighton TE. *Proteins: Structures and Molecular Properties*. 2nd ed. W. H. Freedman and Co., New York, 1993.

Crestfield A, Stein WH, Moore S. Alkylation and identification of the histidine residues at the active site of ribonuclease. *J Biol Chem* 1963; 238(3):2413–2419.

Crestfield A, Stein WH, Moore S. Properties and conformation of the histidine residues at the active site of ribonuclease. *J Biol Chem* 1963; 238(3):2421–2428.

Eterovic VA, Hebert MS, Hanley MR, Bennett EL. The lethality and spectroscopic properties of toxins from Bungarus multicinctus (Blyth) venom. *Toxicon* 1975; 13(1):37–48.

Fägerstam L, Söderberg L, Wahlström L, Fredriksson UB, Plith K, Wallden E. Basic principles used in the selection of Monobeads™ ion exchangers for the separation of biopolymers. *Protides of the Biological Fluids* 1982; 30:621–628.

Gagnon P. *Purification Tools for Monoclonal Antibodies*. Validated Biosystems, Tucson, AZ, 1996: 57–86.

Garrison TR, Apanovitch DM, Dohlman HG. Purification of RGS protein, Sst2, from Saccharomyces cerevisiae and *Escherichia coli*. *Methods Enzymol* 2002; 344:632–647.

Gokana A, Winchenne JJ, Ben Ghanem A, Ahaded A, Cartron JP, Lambin P. Chromatographic separation of recombinant human erythropoietin isoforms. *J Chromatogr A* 1997; 791(1–2):109–118.

Hardy PM. The protein amino acids. In: *Chemistry and Biochemistry of the Amino Acids*. Barrett GC, editor. Chapman & Hall, London, 1985: 6–24.

Hearn MT, Hodder AN, Aguilar MI. High-performance liquid chromatography of amino acids, peptides and proteins. LXXXVI. The influence of different displacer salts on the retention and bandwidth properties of proteins separated by isocratic anion-exchange chromatography. *J Chromatogr* 1988; 443:97–118.

Hearn MT, Hodder AN, Aguilar MI. High-performance liquid chromatography of amino acids, peptides and proteins. LXXXVII. Comparison of retention and bandwidth properties of proteins eluted by gradient and isocratic anion-exchange chromatography. *J Chromatogr* 1988; 458:27–44.

Hearn MTW, Hodder AN, Stanton PG, Aguilar MI. High-performance liquid chromatography of amino acids, peptides and proteins. LXXXIII. Evaluation of retention and bandwidth relationships for proteins separated by isocratic anion-exchange chromatography. *J Chromatogr* 1987; 24:769–776.

Hodder AN, Aguilar MI, Hearn MT. High-performance liquid chromatography of amino acids, peptides and proteins. LXXXIX. The influence of different displacer salts on the retention properties of proteins separated by gradient anion-exchange chromatography. *J Chromatogr* 1989; 476:391–411.

Hodder AN, Aguilar MI, Hearn MT. High-performance liquid chromatography of amino acids, peptides and proteins. XCVII. The influence of the gradient elution mode and displacer salt type on the retention properties of closely related protein variants separated by high-performance anion-exchange chromatography. *J Chromatogr* 1990; 506:17–34.

Janson J-C and Ryden L. Protein Purification: Principles, High-Resolution Methods, and Applications. 2nd ed. Wiley-Liss, New York, 1998.

Jepson SG and Close TJ. Purification of a maize dehydrin protein expressed in *Echerichia coli*. *Protein Expr Purif* 1995; 6(5):632–636.

Kannan R, Tomasetto C, Staub A, Bossenmeyer-Pourie C, Thim L, Nielsen PF, Rio M. Human pS2/trefoil factor 1: production and characterization in Pichia pastoris. *Protein Expr Purif* 2001; 21(1):92–98.

Karlsson E, Ryden L, Brewer J. Ion-exchange chromatography. In: *Protein Purification: Principles, High-Resolution Methods, and Applications*. Janson J-C and Ryden L, editors. Wiley-Liss, New York, 1998: 145–205.

Koide T and Ikenaka T. Studies on soybean trypsin inhibitors. 3. Amino-acid sequences of the carboxyl-terminal region and the complete amino-acid sequence of soybean trypsin inhibitor (Kunitz). *Eur J Biochem* 1973; 32(3):417–431.

Kopaciewicz W and Regnier FE. Mobile phase selection for the high-performance ion-exchange chromatography of proteins. *Anal Biochem* 1983; 133(1):251–259.

Kopaciewicz W, Rounds MA, Fausnaugh J, Regnier FE. Retention model for high-performance ion-exchange chromatography. *J Chromatogr* 1983; 266(August):3–21.

Malmquist G and Lundell N. Characterization of the influence of displacing salts on retention in gradient elution ion-exchange chromatography of proteins and peptides. *J Chromatogr* 1992; 627(1–2):107–124.

Melander WR, el Rassi Z, Horvath C. Interplay of hydrophobic and electrostatic interactions in biopolymer chromatography. Effect of salts on the retention of proteins. *J Chromatogr* 1989; 469:3–27.

Milby KH, Ho SV, Henis JMS. Ion-exchange chromatography of proteins. The effect of neutral polymers in the mobile phase. *J Chromatogr* 1989; 482(1):133–144.

Murphy JP, Atkinson M, Trowern AR, Stevens GB, Atkinson T, Duggleby CJ, Hinton RJ. Amplified expression and large-scale purification of protein L′. *Bioseparation* 1996; 6(2):107–113.

Price AE, Logvinenko KB, Higgins EA, Cole ES, Richards SM. Studies on the microheterogeneity and *in vitro* activity of glycosylated and nonglycosylated recombinant human prolactin separated using a novel purification process. *Endocrinology* 1995; 136(11):4827–4833.

Regnier FE. High-performance ion-exchange chromatography. *Meth Enzymol* 1984; 104:170–189.

Regnier FE. The role of protein structure in chromatographic behavior. *Science* 1987; 238(4825):319–323.

Ren Q, De Roo G, Kessler B, Witholt B. Recovery of active medium-chain-length-poly-3-hydroxyalkanoate polymerase from inactive inclusion bodies using ion-exchange resin. *Biochem J* 2000; 349(Pt 2):599–604.

Righetti PG and Caravaggio T. Isoelectric points and molecular weights of proteins. *J Chromatogr* 1976; 127(11):1–28.

Righetti PG, Tudor G, Ek K. Isoelectric points and molecular-weights of proteins — A new table. *J Chromatogr* 1981; 220(N2):115–194.

Rounds MA and Regnier FE. Evaluation of a retention model for high-performance ion-exchange chromatography using 2 different displacing salts. *J Chromatogr* 1984; 283(January):37–45.

Schaap FG, Specht B, van der Vusse GJ, Borchers T, Glatz JF. One-step purification of rat heart-type fatty acid-binding protein expressed in *Escherichia coli*. *J Chromatogr B Biomed Appl* 1996; 679(1–2):61–67.

Schwaneberg U, Sprauer A, Schmidt-Dannert C, Schmid RD. P450 monooxygenase in biotechnology. I. Single-step, large-scale purification method for cytochrome P450 BM-3 by anion-exchange chromatography. *J Chromatogr A* 1999; 848(1–2):149–159.

Scopes RK. *Protein Purification: Principles and Practice*. 3rd ed. Springer Verlag, New York, 1994.

Seeger A and Rinas U. Two-step chromatographic procedure for purification of basic fibroblast growth factor from recombinant *Escherichia coli* and characterization of the equilibrium parameters of adsorption. *J Chromatogr A* 1996; 746(1):17–24.

Söderberg L et al. Physicochemical considerations in the use of MONOBEADS™ for the separation of biological molecules. *Protides of the Biological Fluids* 1982; 30:629–634.

Sofer G and Hagel L. *Handbook of Process Chromatography*. Academic Press, San Diego 1997, 65–71, 272–279.

Trinh L, Noronha SB, Fannon M, Shiloach J. Recovery of mouse endostatin produced by Pichia pastoris using expanded bed adsorption. *Bioseparation* 2000; 9(4):223–230.

Yao K and Hjerten S. Gradient and isocratic high-performance liquid chromatography of proteins on a new agarose-based anion exchanger. *J Chromatogr* 1987; 385:87–98.

SIZE EXCLUSION CHROMATOGRAPHY

Amersham Pharmacia Biotech. *Gel Filtration: Principles and Methods*. Amersham Pharmacia Biotech AB, Uppsala, Sweden, 2002.

Beldarrain A, Cruz Y, Cruz O, Navarro M, Gil M. Purification and conformational properties of a human interferon alpha2b produced in *Escherichia coli*. *Biotechnol Appl Biochem* 2001; 33(Pt.3):173–182.

Bouillenne F, Matagne A, Joris B, Frere JM. Technique for a rapid and efficient purification of the SHV-1 and PSE-2 beta-lactamases. *J Chromatogr B Biomed Sci Appl* 2000; 737(1–2):261–265.

D'alessio KJ, McQueney MS, Brun KA, Orsini MJ, Debouck CM. Expression in *Escherichia coli*, refolding, and purification of human procathepsin K, an osteoclast-specific protease. *Protein Expr Purif* 1999; 15(2):213–220.

Fahey EM, Chaudhuri JB, Binding P. Refolding and purification of a urokinase plasminogen activator fragment by chromatography. *J Chromatogr B Biomed Sci Appl* 2000; 737(1–2):225–235.

Gagnon P. *Purification Tools for Monoclonal Antibodies*. Validated Biosystems Inc., Tucson, AZ, 1996: 33–56.

Gibert S, Bakalara N, Santarelli X. Three-step chromatographic purification procedure for the production of a his-tag recombinant kinesin overexpressed in *E. coli*. *J Chromatogr B Biomed Sci Appl* 2000; 737(1–2):143–150.

Gruel N, Chapiro J, Fridman WH, Teillaud JL. Purification of soluble recombinant human FcgammaRII (CD32). *Prep Biochem Biotechnol* 2001; 31(4):341–354.

Hagel L and Janson J-C. Size-exclusion chromatography. In: *Chromatography. Part A: Fundamentals and Techniques*. Heftmann E, editor. Elsevier, Amsterdam, 1992: A267–A307.

Hagel L. Gel filtration. In: *Protein Purification: Principles, High-Resolution Methods, and Applications*. Janson J-C and Ryden L, editors. Wiley-Liss, New York, 1998: 79–143.

Loh KC, Yao ZJ, Yap MG, Chung MC. Role of polyethyleneimine in the purification of recombinant human tumour necrosis factor beta. *J Chromatogr A* 1997; 760(2):165–171.

Rolland D, Gauthier M, Dugua JM, Fournier C, Delpech L, Watelet B, Letourneur O, Arnaud M, Jolivet M. Purification of recombinant HBc antigen expressed in *Escherichia coli* and Pichia pastoris: comparison of size-exclusion chromatography and ultracentrifugation. *J Chromatogr B Biomed Sci Appl* 2001; 753(1):51–65.

Sofer G and Hagel L. *Handbook of Process Chromatography: A Guide to Optimization, Scale-Up and Validation.* Academic Press, San Diego, CA, 1997.

Sofer G and Hagel L. Practical implications of chromatography theory. In: *Handbook of Process Chromatography: A Guide to Optimization, Scale-Up and Validation.* Academic Press, San Diego, CA, 1997: 256–318.

Thies MJ and Pirkl F. Chromatographic purification of the C(H)2 domain of the monoclonal antibody MAK33. *J Chromatogr B Biomed Sci Appl* 2000; 737(1–2):63–69.

Trinh L, Noronha SB, Fannon M, Shiloach J. Recovery of mouse endostatin produced by Pichia pastoris using expanded bed adsorption. *Bioseparation* 2000; 9(4):223–230.

REVERSED PHASE CHROMATOGRAPHY

Amersham Pharmacia Biotech. *Reversed Phase Chromatography: Principles and Methods.* Amersham Pharmacia Biotech AB, Uppsala, Sweden, 1999.

Beldarrain A, Cruz Y, Cruz O, Navarro M, Gil M. Purification and conformational properties of a human interferon alpha2b produced in *Escherichia coli. Biotechnol Appl Biochem* 2001; 33(Pt.3): 173–182.

Dorsey JG and Cooper WT. Retention mechanisms of bonded-phase liquid chromatography. *Anal Chem* 1994; 66(17):857A–867A.

Fahrner RL, Lester PM, Blank GS, Reifsnyder DH. Non-flammable preparative reversed-phase liquid chromatography of recombinant human insulin-like growth factor-I. *J Chromatogr A* 1999; 830(1):127–134.

Hearn MT. High-performance liquid chromatography and its application to protein chemistry. *Adv Chromatogr* 1982; 20:1–82.

Hearn MTW. High-performance liquid chromatography of peptides. In: *High-Performance Liquid Chromatography: Advances and Perspectives.* Vol. 3. Horvath C, editor. Academic Press, New York, 1983: 87–155.

Hearn MTW. High-resolution reversed-phase chromatography. In: *Protein Purification: Principles, High-Resolution Methods, and Applications.* Janson J-C and Ryden L, editors. Wiley-Liss, New York, 1998: 239–282.

Janson J-C and Rydén L (eds). *Protein Purification.* 2nd ed. Ed: Wiley-Liss, New York, 1998, 239–282.

Kamp RM and Wittmann-Liebold B. Purification of *Escherichia coli* 50 S ribosomal proteins by high performance liquid chromatography. *FEBS Lett* 1984; 167(1):59–63.

Kroeff EP, Owens RA, Campbell EL, Johnson RD, Marks HI. Production scale purification of biosynthetic human insulin by reversed-phase high-performance liquid chromatography. *J Chromatogr* 1989; 461:45–61.

Mant CT, Zhou NE, Hodges RS. Amino acids and peptides. In: *Chromatography, Part B: Applications.* Heftmann E, editor. Elsevier Science, New York, 1992: B137.

Olson CV, Reifsnyder DH, Canova-Davis E, Ling VT, Builder SE. Preparative isolation of recombinant human insulin-like growth factor 1 by reversed-phase high-performance liquid chromatography. *J Chromatogr A* 1994; 675(1–2):101–112.

Reversed phase chromatography, principles and methods. Amersham Pharmacia Biotech Handbook, 1999.

Sofer G and Hagel L. *Handbook of Process Chromatography.* Academic Press, San Diego 1997: 71–78, 279–284.

Yamamoto S, Nakanishi K, Matsuno R. *Ion Exchange Chromatography of Proteins.* Marcel Dekker, New York, 1988.

HYDOXYPATITE CHROMATOGRAPHY

Aoyama K and Chiba J. Separation of different molecular forms of mouse IgA and IgM monoclonal antibodies by high-performance liquid chromatography on spherical hydroxyapatite beads. *J Immunol Meth* 1993; 162(2):201–210.

Bernardi G, Giro MG, Gaillard C. Chromatography of polypeptides and proteins on hydroxyapatite columns: some new developments. *Biochim Biophys Acta* 1972; 278(3):409–420.

Eis C, Griessler R, Maier M, Weinhausel A, Bock B, Kulbe KD, Haltrich D, Schinzel R, Nidetzky B. Efficient downstream processing of maltodextrin phosphorylase from *Escherichia coli* and stabilization of the enzyme by immobilization onto hydroxyapatite. *J Biotechnol* 1997; 58(3):157–166.

Gagnon P. *Purification Tools for Monoclonal Antibodies.* Validated Biosystems Inc, Tucson, AZ, 1996: 87–102.

Gagnon P. *Purification Tools for Monoclonal Antibodies.* Validated Biosystems Inc., Tucson, AZ 1996.

Gorbunoff MJ and Timasheff SN. The interaction of proteins with hydroxyapatite. III. Mechanism. *Anal Biochem* 1984; 136(2):440–445.

Gorbunoff MJ. Protein chromatography on hydroxyapatite columns. *Meth Enzymol* 1990; 182(26):329–339.

Gorbunoff MJ. The interaction of proteins with hydroxyapatite. I. Role of protein charge and structure. *Anal Biochem* 1984; 136(2):425–432.

Gorbunoff MJ. The interaction of proteins with hydroxyapatite. II. Role of acidic and basic groups. *Anal Biochem* 1984; 136(2):433–439.

Hoenicka M, Becker EM, Apeler H, Sirichoke T, Schroder H, Gerzer R, Stasch JP. Purified soluble guanylyl cyclase expressed in a baculovirus/Sf9 system: stimulation by YC-1, nitric oxide, and carbon monoxide. *J Mol Med* 1999; 77(1):14–23.

Hofmann AF. Thin-layer adsorption chromatography of proteins on hydroxylapatite. *Biochim Biophys Acta* 1962; 60(2):458–460.

Josic D, Loster K, Kuhl R, Noll F, Reusch J. Purification of monoclonal antibodies by hydroxylapatite HPLC and size exclusion HPLC. *Biol Chem Hoppe Seyler* 1991; 372(3): 149–156.

Kadoya T, Ogawa T, Kuwahara H, Okuyama T. High performance liquid chromatography of proteins on a hydroxyapatite column. *J Liq Chromatogr* 1988; 11(14):2951–2967.

Karlsson E, Ryden L, Brewer J. Ion-exchange chromatography. In: *Protein Purification: Principles, High-Resolution Methods, and Applications.* Janson J-C and Ryden L, editors. Wiley-Liss, New York, 1998: 145–205.

Kawasaki T. Hydroxyapatite as liquid chromatographic packing. *J Chromatogr* 1991; 544:147–184.

Kawasaki T, Takahashi S, Ikeda K. Hydroxyapatite high-performance liquid chromatography: column performance for proteins. *Eur J Biochem* 1985; 152(2):361–371.

Kawasaki T. Hydroxyapatite as liquid chromatographic packing. J Chromatogr 1991; 544:147–184.

Luellau E, von Stockar U, Vogt S, Freitag R. Development of a downstream process for the isolation and separation of monoclonal immunoglobulin A monomers, dimers and polymers from cell culture supernatant. *J Chromatogr A* 1998; 796(1):165–175.

Lüllau E, Marison IW, von Stockar U. Ceramic hydroxyapatite: A new tool for separation and analysis of IgA monoclonal antibodies. In: *Animal Cell Technology: From Vaccines to Genetic Medicine.* Carrondo MJT, Griffiths JB, Moreira JLP, editors. Kluwer Academic Publishers, Dordrecht, 1997: 265–269.

O'Riordan CR, Erickson A, Bear C, Li C, Manavalan P, Wang KX, Marshall J, Scheule RK, McPherson JM, Cheng SH. Purification and characterization of recombinant cystic fibrosis transmembrane conductance regulator from Chinese hamster ovary and insect cells. *J Biol Chem* 1995; 270(28):17033–17043.

Ryden L. Evidence for proteolytic fragments in commercial samples of human ceruloplasmin. *FEBS Lett* 1971; 18(2):321–325.

Tiselius A, Hjerten S, Levin O. Protein chromatography on calcium phosphate columns. *Arch Biochem Biophys* 1956; 65:132–155.

Tsujimoto M, Adachi H, Kodama S, Tsuruoka N, Yamada Y, Tanaka S, Mita S, Takatsu K. Purification and characterization of recombinant human interleukin 5 expressed in Chinese hamster ovary cells. *J Biochem* (Tokyo) 1989; 106(1):23–28.

Watanabe Y, Okuno T, Ishigaki K, Takagi T. Assessment study on the high-performance liquid chromatography-type hydroxyapatite chromatography in the presence of sodium dodecyl sulfate. *Anal Biochem* 1992; 202(2):268–274.

HYDROPHOBIC INTERACTION CHROMATOGRAPHY

Amersham Pharmacia Biotech. *Hydrophobic Interaction Chromatography: Principles and Methods.* Amersham Pharmacia Biotech AB, Uppsala, Sweden, 1993.

Eriksson KO. Hydrophobic interaction chromatography. In: *Protein Purification: Principles, High-Resolution Methods, and Applications*. Janson J-C and Ryden L, editors. Wiley-Liss, New York, 1998: 283–309.

Fisher JR, Sharma Y, Iuliano S, Piccioti RA, Krylov D, Hurley J, Roder J, Jeromin A. Purification of myristoylated and nonmyristoylated neuronal calcium sensor-1 using single-step hydrophobic interaction chromatography. *Protein Expr Purif* 2000; 20(1):66–72.

Gagnon P. *Purification Tools for Monoclonal Antibodies*. Validated Biosystems Inc., Tucson, AZ, 1996: 103–126.

Gagnon P and Grund E. Large-scale process development for hydrophobic interaction chromatography, Part 4: Controlling selectivity. *BioPharm* 1996; 9(5): 54–64.

Gagnon P, Grund E, Lindbäck T. Large-scale process development for hydrophobic interaction chromatography, Part 1: Gel selection and development of binding conditions. *BioPharm* 1995; 8(4): 21–27.

Gagnon P, Grund E, Lindbäck T. Large-scale process development for hydrophobic interaction chromatography, Part 2: Controlling process variation. *BioPharm* 1995; 8(5): 36–41.

Gagnon P and Grund E. Large-scale process development for hydrophobic interaction chromatography, Part 3: Factors affecting capacity determination. *BioPharm* 1996; 9(3): 34–39.

Hereld D, Krakow JL, Bangs JD, Hart GW, Englund PT. A phospholipase C from Trypanosoma brucei which selectively cleaves the glycolipid on the variant surface glycoprotein. *J Biol Chem* 1986; 261(29):13813–13819.

Hjerten S. Some general aspects of hydrophobic interaction chromatography. *J Chromatogr* 1973; 87:325–331.

Hofstee BH and Otillio NF. Non-ionic adsorption chromatography of proteins. *J Chromatogr* 1978; 159(1):57–69.

Jandera P and Churacek J. Peptides and proteins. *J Chromatogr Libr* 1985; 31(21):365–379.

Janson J-C and Ryden L. *Protein Purification: Principles, High-Resolution Methods, and Applications*. 2nd ed. Wiley-Liss, New York, 1998: 283–310.

Jepson SG and Close TJ. Purification of a maize dehydrin protein expressed in *Escherichia coli*. *Protein Expr Purif* 1995; 6(5):632–636.

Lau KH, Freeman TK, Baylink DJ. Purification and characterization of an acid phosphatase that displays phosphotyrosyl-protein phosphatase activity from bovine cortical bone matrix. *J Biol Chem* 1987; 262(3):1389–1397.

Mant CT, Zhou NE, Hodges RS. Amino acids and peptides. In: *Chromatography, Part B: Applications*. Heftmann E, editor. Elsevier Science, New York, 1992: B137.

Melander W and Horvath C. Salt effect on hydrophobic interactions in precipitation and chromatography of proteins: an interpretation of the lyotropic series. *Arch Biochem Biophys* 1977; 183(1):200–215.

Porath J, Sundberg L, Fornstedt N, Olsson I. Salting-out in amphiphilic gels as a new approach to hydrophobic adsorption. *Nature* 1973; 245(5426):465–466.

Roos P, Nyberg F, Wide L. Isolation of human pituitary prolactin. *Biochim Biophys Acta* 1979; 588(3):368–379.

Sharma KK and Ortwerth BJ. Bovine lens acylpeptide hydrolase. Purification and characterization of a tetrameric enzyme resistant to urea denaturation and proteolytic inactivation. *Eur J Biochem* 1993; 216(2):631–637.

Shepard SR, Boucher R, Johnston J, Boerner R, Koch G, Madsen JW, Grella D, Sim BK, Schrimsher JL. Large-scale purification of recombinant human angiostatin. *Protein Expr Purif* 2000; 20(2):216–227.

Shukla AA, Sunasara KM, Rupp RG, Cramer SM. Hydrophobic displacement chromatography of proteins. *Biotechnol Bioeng* 2000; 68(6):672–680.

Sofer G and Hagel L. *Handbook of Process Chromatography: A Guide to Optimization, Scale-Up and Validation*. Academic Press, San Diego, CA, 1997: 76–77, 284–288.

Srinivasan R and Ruckenstein E. Role of physical forces in hydrophobic interaction chromatography. *Sep Purif Meth* 1980; 9(2):267–370.

Thies MJ and Pirkl F. Chromatographic purification of the C(H)2 domain of the monoclonal antibody MAK33. *J Chromatogr B Biomed Sci Appl* 2000; 737(1–2):63–69.

Warren TC, Miglietta JJ, Shrutkowski A, Rose JM, Rogers SL, Lubbe K, Shih CK, Caviness GO, Ingraham R, Palladino DE. Comparative purification of recombinant HIV-1 and HIV-2 reverse transcriptase: preparation of heterodimeric enzyme devoid of unprocessed gene product. *Protein Expr Purif* 1992; 3(6):479–487.

Wilson MJ, Haggart CL, Gallagher SP, Walsh D. Removal of tightly bound endotoxin from biological products. *J Biotechnol* 2001; 88(1):67–75.

Zhou WB, Zhou XS, Zhang YX. [Decolorization and isolation of recombinant hirudin expressed in the methylotrophic yeast Pichia pastoris]. *Sheng Wu Gong Cheng Xue Bao* 2001; 17(6):683–687.

CHAPTER 9: QUALITY ASSURANCE SYSTEMS

Adner N and Sofer G. Chromatography cleaning validation. *BioPharm* 1994; 7(3):44–48.

Akers J, McEntire J, Sofer G. A logical plan. *BioPharm* 1994; 7(2):54–56.

Akers J, McEntire J, Sofer G. Identifying the pitfalls. *BioPharm* 1994; 7(1):40–43.

Anderson KP, Low MA, Lie YS, Keller GA, Dinowitz M. Endogenous origin of defective retroviruslike particles from a recombinant Chinese hamster ovary cell line. *Virology* 1991; 181(1):305–311.

ANSI/ISO 17025-1999: General requirements for the competence of testing and calibration laboratories. American Society for Quality, 1999.

ANSI/ISO/ASQ Q9000-2000: Quality management systems — Fundamentals and vocabulary. American Society for Quality, 2000.

ANSI/ISO/ASQ Q9001-2000: Quality management systems — Requirements. American Society for Quality, 2000.

ANSI/ISO/ASQ Q9004-2000: Quality management systems — Guidelines for performance improvement. American Society for Quality, 2000.

Aygoren-Pursun E and Scharrer I. A multicenter pharmacosurveillance study for the evaluation of the efficacy and safety of recombinant factor VIII in the treatment of patients with hemophilia A. German Kogenate Study Group. *Thromb Haemost* 1997; 78(5):1352–1356.

Bacterial Endotoxins/Pyrogens. Inspection Technical Guide: http://www.fda.gov/ora/inspect_ref/itg/itg40.html.

Balanced Scorecard Institute: http://balancedscorecard.org.

Box GEP, Hunter WG, Hunter JS. *Statistics for Experimenters*. J.Wiley, New York, 1978.

Chew NJ and Wiechert E. Harmonizing the validation of analytical procedures. *BioPharm* 1999; 12(8):18–51.

Chudy M, Budek I, Keller-Stanislawski B, McCaustland KA, Neidhold S, Robertson BH, Nubling CM, Seitz R, Lower J. A new cluster of hepatitis A infection in hemophiliacs traced to a contaminated plasma pool. *J Med Virol* 1999; 57(2):91–99.

CMMI-SE/SW, V1.1: Capability Maturity Model Integration for Systems Engineering and Software Engineering, Staged Representation. Software Engineering Institute, Carnegie Mellon University, 2002: http://www.sei.cmu.edu/pub/documents/02.reports/pdf/02tr002.pdf.

Compliance Policy Guide Sec. 130.300 FDA Access to Results of Quality Assurance Program Audits and Inspections* (CPG 7151.02): http://www.fda.gov/ora/compliance_ref/cpg/cpggenl/cpg130-300.html.

Container and Closure Integrity Testing in Lieu of Sterility Testing as a Component of the Stability Protocol for Sterile Products, (1998): http://www.fda.gov/cber/gdlns/contain.htm.

CPGM 7356.002 Compliance Program — Drug Manufacturing Inspections: http://www.fda.gov/cder/dmpq/compliance_guide.htm.

CPMP/ICH/4106/00 Draft Guidance for Good Manufacturing Practice for Active Pharmaceutical Ingredients (released for consultation July 2000).

Criteria for Performance Excellence, Business. Baldrige National Quality Program, NIST 2003: http://baldrige.nist.gov/PDF_files/2003_Business_Criteria.pdf.

Daniel C. *Applications of Statistics to Industrial Experimentation*. J. Wiley, New York, 1976.

Darby SC, Ewart DW, Giangrande PL, Dolin PJ, Spooner RJ, Rizza CR. Mortality before and after HIV infection in the complete UK population of haemophiliacs. UK Haemophilia Centre Directors' Organisation. *Nature* 1995; 377(6544):79–82.

Darling AJ, Boose JA, Spaltro J. Virus assay methods: accuracy and validation. *Biologicals* 1998; 26(2):105–110.

Del Tito Jr. BJ, Tremblay MA, Shadle PJ. Qualification of raw materials for clinical biopharmaceutical manufacturing. *BioPharm* 1996; 9(10):45–49.

Eis-Hubinger AM, Sasowski U, Brackmann HH. Parvovirus B19 DNA contamination in coagulation factor VIII products. *Thromb Haemost* 1999; 81(3):476–477.

European Commission. Annex 13 Manufacture of investigational medicinal products. Vol 4. Good manufacturing practices. F2/AN D(2001). European Commission, Brussels, 2001.

FDA Center for Biologics Evaluation and Research. *Points to Consider in the Manufacture and Testing of Monoclonal Antibody Products for Human Use*. Food and Drug Administration, Rockville, MD, 1997.

FDA Center for Drug Evaluation and Research. *Guideline on General Principles of Process Validation*. FDA, Rockville, MD, 1987.

FDA Center for Drug Evaluation and Research. Part 210 — Current good manufacturing practice in manufacturing, processing, packing, or holding of drugs; General Part 211 — Current good manufacturing practice for finished pharmaceuticals. FDA, Rockville, MD 1996.

FDA Compliance Policy Guide 7132c.08. Process Validation Requirements for Drug Products and Active Pharmaceutical Ingredients Subject to Pre-Market Approval, updated March 12, 2004: http://www.fda.gov/ora/compliance_ref/cpg/cpgdrg/cpg490-100.html.

FDA Office of Biologics Research and Review. *Points to Consider in the Characterization of Cell Lines Used to Produce Biologicals*. Food and Drug Administration, Rockville, MD, 1993.

Framework for Environmental Health Risk Assessment — Final Report, Vol. 1. Presidential/Congressional Commission on Risk Assessment and Risk Management, 1997: http://www.riskworld.com/Nreports/1997/risk-rpt/pdf/EPAJAN.PDF.

Gerber RG, McAllister PR, Smith CA, Smith TM, Zabriskie DW, Gardner AR. Establishment of proven acceptable process control ranges for production of a monoclonal antibody by cultures of recombinant CHO cells. In: *Validation of Biopharmaceutical Manufacturing Processes*. Kelley BD and Ramelmeier RA, editors. ACS, Washington, DC, 1998: 44–54.

Good Manufacturing Practices for Pharmaceutical Products: Main Principles. World Health Organization Technical Report Series, No. 908, 2003: http://www.who.int/medicines/library/qsm/trs908/trs908-4.pdf.

Green C. Validation compliance issues. *J. Val. Technol.* 2000; 6(3), 643–646.

Guidance for Developing Quality Systems for Environmental Program. EPA QA/G-1, November 2002: http://www.epa.gov/quality/qs-docs/g1-final.pdf.

Guidance for Industry — Sterile Drug Products Produced by Aseptic Processing Current Good Manufacturing Practice — September 2004: http://www.fda.gov/cder/guidance/index.htm.

Guidance for Industry — Q7A Good Manufacturing Practice Guidance for Active Pharmaceutical Ingredients. U.S. Department of Health and Human Services/Food and Drug Administration, August 2001: http://www.fda.gov/cder/guidance/index.htm.

Guidance for Industry for the Submission of Documentation for Sterilization Process Validation in Applications for Human and Veterinary Drug Products: http://www.fda.gov/cder/guidance/cmc2.pdf.

Guide for Determining the Impact of Extractables from non-Metallic Materials on the Safety of Biotechnology Products, Draft Guideline, ASTM.

Guide to Inspections of High Purity Water Systems: http://www.fda.gov/ora/inspect_ref/igs/high.html.

Guide to Inspections of Lyophilization of Parenterals: http://www.fda.gov/ora/inspect_ref/igs/lyophi.html.

Guide to Inspections of Microbiological Pharmaceutical Quality Control Laboratories: http://www.fda.gov/ora/inspect_ref/igs/micro.html.

Guide to Inspections of Sterile Drug Substance Manufacturers: http://www.fda.gov/ora/inspect_ref/igs/subst.html.

Guideline for Validation of Limulus Amebocyte Lysate Test as an End Product Endotoxin Test for Human and Animal Parenteral Drugs, Biological Products, and Medical Devices: http://www.fda.gov/cder/guidance/old005fn.pdf.

Guideline of General Principles of Process Validation, May 1987: http://www.fda.gov/cder/guidance/pv.htm.

Haaland PD. *Experimental Design in Biotechnology*. Marcel Dekker, New York, 1989.

Harris RJ, Dougherty RM, Biggs PM, Payne LN, Goffe AP, Churchill AE, Mortimer R. Contaminant viruses in two live virus vaccines produced in chick cells. *J Hyg* (London) 1966; 64(1):1–7.

Heat Exchangers to Avoid Contamination; Inspection Technical Guide: http://www.fda.gov/ora/inspect_ref/itg/itg34.html.

Hepatitis A among persons with hemophilia who received clotting factor concentrate — United States, September–December 1995. MMWR *Morb Mortal Wkly Rep* 1996; 45(2):29–32.

Huber L. Validation of HPLC methods. *BioPharm* 2003; 12(3):64–66.

ICH Harmonized Tripartite Guideline. Specifications: Test Procedures and Acceptance Criteria for Biotechnological Products (Q6B) on 10 March 1999.

ICH Q7A: Good Manufacturing Practice for Active Pharmaceutical Ingredients Geneva, November 2000.

ICH. Guidance on viral safety evaluation of biotechnology products derived from cell lines of human or animal origin; availability — FDA. Notice. *Fed Regist* 1998; 63(185):51074–51084.

ICH. ICH Topic Q5A. Step 4 Consensus Guideline. Quality of biotechnological products: Viral safety evaluation of biotechnology products derived from cell lines of human or animal origin. CPMP/ICH/295/95. 1997. The European Agency for the Evaluation of Medicinal Products, Human Medicines Evaluation Unit, Canary Wharf, London.

ICH. Quality of biotechnological products: viral safety evaluation of biotechnology products derived from cell lines of human or animal origin. ICH Harmonised Tripartite Guideline. *Dev Biol Stand* 1998; 93:177–201.

Investigating Out-of-Specification (OOS). Test Results for Pharmaceutical Production: http://www.fda.gov/cder/guidance/index.htm.

ISO 9000 (ANSI/ASQC Q 90). Quality management and quality assurance standards — guidelines for selection and use.

ISO 9001 (ANSI/ASQC Q 91). Quality systems — model for quality assurance in design/development, production, installation and servicing.

ISO 9002 (ANSI/ASQC Q 92). Quality systems — model for quality assurance in production and installation.

ISO 9003 (ANSI/ASQC Q 93). Quality systems — model for quality assurance in final inspection and test.

ISO 9004 (ANSI/ASQC Q 94) Quality management and quality system elements — guidelines

Juran JM and Gryna FM (eds.). *Quality Planning and Analysis*. 3rd ed. McGraw-Hill, New York, 1993.

Kelley BD, Jennings P, Wright R, Briasco C. Demonstrating process robustness for chromatographic purification of a recombinant protein. *BioPharm* 1997; 10(October):36–46.

Kelley BD, Shi L, Bonam D, Hubbard B. Robustness testing of a chromatographic purification step used in recombinant factor IX manufacture. In: *Validation of Biopharmaceutical Manufacturing Processes*. Kelley BD and Ramelmeier RA, editors. American Chemical Society, Washington, DC, 1998: 93–113.

Kennedy RM and Gonzales L. Minimizing risk from chromatographic media. *BioPharm* 2001; (May):56–58.

King AM, Underwood BO, McCahon D, Newman JW, Brown F. Biochemical identification of viruses causing the 1981 outbreaks of foot and mouth disease in the UK. *Nature* 1981; 293(5832):479–480.

Kuwahara SS. System suitability testing. *BioPharm* 1998; 11(9):65–66.

Lackritz EM, Satten GA, Aberle-Grasse J, Dodd RY, Raimondi VP, Janssen RS, Lewis WF, Notari EP, Petersen LR. Estimated risk of transmission of the human immunodeficiency virus by screened blood in the United States. *N Engl J Med* 1995; 333(26):1721–1725.

Leonard MW, Sefton L, Costigan R, Shi L, Hubbard B, Bonam D et al. Validation of the recombinant coagulation factor IX purification process for the removal of host cell DNA. In: Validation of biopharmaceutical manufacturing processes. Kelley BD and Ramelmeier RA, editors. American Chemical Society, Washington, DC, 1998: 55–68.

Lovatt A, McMutrie D, Black J, Doherty I. Validation of quantitative PCR assays. Addressing virus contamination concerns. *BioPharm* 2002; 15(3):22–32.

Lubiniecki AS, McAllister PR, Smith TM, Shadle PJ. Process evaluation for biopharmaceuticals: what is appropriate in process evaluation? *Dev Biol Stand* 1996; 88:309–315.

Lundblad RL. Approach to assay validation for the development of biopharmaceuticals. *Biotechnol Appl Biochem* 2001; 34(Pt.3):195–197.

Managing the Risks from Medical Product Use: Creating a Risk Management Framework. U.S. FDA, 1999: http://www.fda.gov/oc/tfrm/1999report.html.

Mannucci PM, Santagostino E, Di Bona E, Gentili G, Ghirardini A, Schiavoni M, Mele A. The outbreak of hepatitis A in Italian patients with hemophilia: facts and fancies. *Vox Sang* 1994; 67(Suppl.1):31–35.

Mason RL, Gunst RF, Hess JL. *Statistical Design and Analysis of Experiments*. J.Wiley, New York 1989.

McAllister PR, Shadle PJ, Smith TM, Scott RG, Lubiniecki AS. Use of a statistical strategy to evaluate sources of variability in viral safety experiments for a recombinant biopharmaceutical. *Dev Biol Stand* 1996; 88:111–121.

Medicinal Products Derived from Human Plasma. CPMP/BWP/268/95 final version 2. The European Agency for the Evaluation of Medicinal Products, Human Medicines Evaluation Unit — CPMP Biotechnology Working Party, Canary Wharf, London, 1996.

Montgomery DC. Design and Analysis of Experiments. J.Wiley, New York, 1991.

Nathanson N and Langmuir AD. The Cutter incident. Poliomyelitis following formaldehyde-inactivated polio-virus vaccination in the United States during the spring of 1955. II. Relationship of poliomyelitis to Cutter vaccine. 1963. *Am J Epidemiol* 1995; 142(2):109–140.

ORA Field Management Directive No. 135: http://www.fda.gov/ora/inspect_ref/fmd/fmd135a.html.

Para M. An outbreak of post-vaccinal rabies (rage de laboratoire) in Fortaleza, Brazil, in 1960. Residual fixed virus as the etiological agent. *Bull World Health Organ* 1965; 33(2):177–182.

Powell-Jackson J, Weller RO, Kennedy P, Preece MA, Whitcombe EM, Newsom-Davis J. Creutzfeldt-Jakob disease after administration of human growth hormone. *Lancet* 1985; 2(8449):244–246.

Preamble to the Good Manufacturing Practice Final Regulations — Federal Register Docket No. 73N-0339. 1978: http://www.fda.gov/cder/dmpq/preamble.txt.

Procedures for the Implementation of the Federal Managers' Financial Integrity Act (FMFIA). FDA Staff Manual Guide 2350.1.

Pyrogens: Still a Danger; Inspection Technical Guide: http://www.fda.gov/ora/inspect_ref/itg/itg32.html.

Quality management in the American pharmaceutical Industry. In: *Pharmaceutical Quality*, Prince R, editor. DHI Publishing, River Grove, IL, 2004: chap. 3.

Rathore AS, Kennedy RM, O'Donnell JK, Bemberis I, Kaltenbrunner O. Qualification of a chromatographic column. Why and how to do it. *BioPharm Int* 2003; 16(3):30–40.

Report on FDA Quality System Framework for Pharmaceutical Product Regulation Activities. Quality System Framework Subcommittee, December 2003.

Robertson BH, Alter MJ, Bell BP, Evatt B, McCaustland KA, Shapiro CN, Sinha SD, Souci JM. Hepatitis A virus sequence detected in clotting factor concentrates associated with disease transmission. *Biologicals* 1998; 26(2):95–99.

Santagostino E, Mannucci PM, Gringeri A, Azzi A, Morfini M, Musso R, Santoro R, Schiavoni M. Transmission of parvovirus B19 by coagulation factor concentrates exposed to 100 degrees C heat after lyophilization. *Transfusion* 1997; 37(5):517–522.

Schreiber GB, Busch MP, Kleinman SH, Korelitz JJ. The risk of transfusion-transmitted viral infections. The retrovirus epidemiology donor study. *N Engl J Med* 1996; 334(26):1685–1690.

Shah K and Nathanson N. Human exposure to SV40: review and comment. *Am J Epidemiol* 1976; 103(1): 1–12.

Smith TM, Wilson E, Scott RG, Misczak JW, Bodek JM, Zabriskie DW. Establishment of operating ranges in a purification process for a monoclonal antibody. In: *Validation of Biopharmaceutical Manufacturing Processes*. Kelley BD and Ramelmeier RA, editors. American Chemical Society, Washington, DC, 1998: 80–92.

Sofer G. Analysis. In: *Handbook of Process Chromatography: A Guide to Optimization, Scale-Up and Validation*. Academic Press, San Diego, CA, 1997: 215–226.

Sofer G. Establishing resin lifetime. Key issues and regulatory positions. *BioProcess Int* 2003; 1(1):64–69.

Sofer G and Hagel L. *Handbook of Process Chromatography: A Guide to Optimization, Scale-Up, and Validation*. Academic Press, New York, 1997: 141–214.

Supplier Certification Task Force. Supplier certification — a model program. *PDA J* 1989; 43(43):151–157.

Thornton AC. *Variation Risk Management — Focusing Quality Improvement in Product Development and Products*. John Wiley and Sons, Inc., Hoboken, NJ, 2004.

Tutorials for Continuous Quality Improvement. Clemson University, 1995: http://deming.eng.clemson.edu/pub/tutorials/.

Walter JK, Werz W, Berthold W. Process scale considerations in evaluation studies and scale-up. *Dev Biol Stand* 1996; 88:99–108.

Wang YJ, Lee SD, Hwang SJ, Chan CY, Chow MP, Lai ST, Lo KJ. Incidence of post-transfusion hepatitis before and after screening for hepatitis C virus antibody. *Vox Sang* 1994; 67(2):187–190.

WHO Expert Committee on Biological Standardization. Requirements for the collection, processing and quality control of blood, blood components and plasma derivatives (Requirements for biological substances No. 27, revised 1992). 43rd Report, Annex 2, WHO Technical Report Series, No. 840. World Health Organization, Geneva, 1994.

WHO. Report of a WHO consultation on medicinal and other products in relation to human and animal transmissible spongiform encephalopathies. WHO/BLG/97.2. World Health Organization, Geneva, 1997.

WHO. WHO requirements for the use of animal cells as *in vitro* substrates for the production of biologicals (Requirements for biological substances No. 50*). Dev Biol Stand* 1998; 93:141–171.

Will RG. An overview of Creutzfeldt-Jakob disease associated with the use of human pituitary growth hormone. *Dev Biol Stand* 1991; 75:85–86.

Williams MD, Cohen BJ, Beddall AC, Pasi KJ, Mortimer PP, Hill FG. Transmission of human parvovirus B19 by coagulation factor concentrates. *Vox Sang* 1990; 58(3):177–181.

Willkommen H, Schmidt I, Lower J. Safety issues for plasma derivatives and benefit from NAT testing. *Biologicals* 1999; 27(4):325–331.

Yee TT, Cohen BJ, Pasi KJ, Lee CA. Transmission of symptomatic parvovirus B19 infection by clotting factor concentrate. *Br J Haematol* 1996; 93(2):457–459.

Zhang J, Reddy J, Salmon P, Buckland B, Greasham R. Process characterization studies to facilitate validation of a recombinant protein fermentation. In: *Validation of Biopharmaceutical Manufacturing Processes.* Kelley BD and Ramelmeier RA, editors. American Chemical Society, Washington, DC, 1998:12–27.

CHAPTER 10: QUALITY CONTROL SYSTEMS

Amersham Pharmacia Biotech. *Ion Exchange Chromatography: Principles and Methods.* 3rd ed. Amersham Pharmacia Biotech AB, Uppsala, Sweden, 1991.

Amersham Pharmacia Biotech. *Reversed Phase chromatography: Principles and Methods.* Amersham Pharmacia Biotech AB, Uppsala, Sweden, 1999.

Anders JC. Advances in amino acid analysis. *BioPharm* 2002; 15(4):32–67.

Anderson KP, Low MA, Lie YS, Keller GA, Dinowitz M. Endogenous origin of defective retroviruslike particles from a recombinant Chinese hamster ovary cell line. *Virology* 1991; 181(1):305–311.

Andrews AT. *Electrophoresis: Theory, Techniques and Biochemical and Clinical Applications.* 2nd ed. Oxford University Press, New York, 1986.

Anicetti VR, Keyt BA, Hancock WS. Purity analysis of protein pharmaceuticals produced by recombinant DNA technology. *Trends Biotechnol* (TIBTECH) 1989; 7:342–349.

Aranha H. Viral clearance strategies for biopharmaceutical safety. Part 1: General considerations. *BioPharm* 2001; 14(1):28–35.

Aranha H, Larson R. Prions: Mayhem and management. 1. General considerations. *BioPharm* Supplement 2002; (May):11–43.

Aranha H, Larson R. Prions: Mayhem and management. 3. Detection and decontamination. *BioPharm* Supplement 2002; (May):30–40.

Aranha H. Viral clearance strategies for biopharmaceutical safety. Part 2: Filtration for viral clearance. *BioPharm* 2001; 14(2):32–43.

Aranha-Creado H, Fennington Jr. GJ. Cumulative viral titer reduction demonstrated by sequential challenge of a tangential flow membrane filtration system and a direct flow pleated filter cartridge. *PDA J Pharm Sci Technol* 1997; 51(5):208–212.

Aranha-Creado H, Peterson J, Huang PY. Clearance of murine leukaemia virus from monoclonal antibody solutions by a hydrophilic PVDF microporous membrane filter. *Biologicals* 1998; 26(2):167–172.

Arcelloni C, Fermo I, Banfi G, Pontiroli AE, Paroni R. Capillary electrophoresis for protein analysis: separation of human growth hormone and human insulin molecular forms. *Anal Biochem* 1993; 212(1):160–167.

Atherton D. Successful PTC amino acid analysis at the picomole level. In: *Techniques in Protein Chemistry.* Hugli TE, editor. Academic Press, San Diego, New York, 1989: 273–283.

Atherton D, Fernandez J, DeMott M, Andrews L, Mische SM. Routine protein sequence analysis below 10 picomoles. In: *Techniques in Protein Chemistry IV.* Angeletti RH, editor. Academic Press, San Diego, 1993: 409–418.

Baekkeskov S, Warnock G, Christie M, Rajotte RV, Larsen PM, Fey S. Revelation of specificity of 64K autoantibodies in IDDM serums by high-resolution 2-D gel electrophoresis. Unambiguous identification of 64K target antigen. *Diabetes* 1989; 38(9):1133–1141.

Baker DR. *Capillary Electrophoresis.* Wiley-Interscience, New York, 1995.

Bang FB. A bacterial disease of Limulus polyphemus. *Bull Johns Hopkins Hosp* 1956; 98(5):325–351.

Bank RA, Jansen EJ, Beekman B, te Koppele JM. Amino acid analysis by reverse-phase high-performance liquid chromatography: improved derivatization and detection conditions with 9-fluorenylmethyl chloroformate. *Anal Biochem* 1996; 240(2):167–176.

Barile MF and Razin S. (eds.). *The Mycoplasmas. 1. Cell Biology.* Academic Press, New York, 1979.

Benaroch P, Yilla M, Raposo G, Ito K, Miwa K, Geuze HJ, Ploegh HL. How MHC class II molecules reach the endocytic pathway. *EMBO J* 1995; 14(1):37–49.

BIOTOL. *Analysis of Amino Acids, Proteins and Nucleic Acids.* Butterworth-Heinemann, Oxford, 1992.

Bishop MJ and Rawlings CJ. *Nucleic acid and Protein Sequence Analysis: A Practical Approach.* IRL Press, 1997.

Bollag DM, Rozycki MD, Edelstein SJ. Electrophoresis under denaturing conditions. In: *Protein Methods.* Wiley-Liss, New-York, 1991: 95–142.

Bollag DM, Rozycki MD, Edelstein SJ. Isoelectric focusing and two dimensional gel electrophoresis. In: *Protein Methods.* Wiley-Liss, New York, 1991: 161–180.

Bollag DM, Rozycki MD, Edelstein SJ. Protein concentration determination. In: *Protein Methods.* Wiley-Liss, New York, 1996: chap. 3.

Bollag DM, Rozycki MD, Edelstein SJ. *Protein Methods.* 2nd. ed. Wiley-Liss, New York: 1996.

Bork P. *Advances in Protein Chemistry.* Vol. 54. Academic Press, New York, 2000.

Bradford MM. A rapid and sensitive method for the quantitation of microgram quantities of protein utilizing the principle of protein-dye binding. *Anal Biochem* 1976; 72(1–2):248–254.

Brendel-Thimmel U. [Experiences with the LAL-test from the viewpoint of a filter manufacturer]. *ALTEX* 1995; 12(2):85–88.

Brennan TV and Clarke S. Deamidation and isoaspartate formation in model synthetic peptides: The effects of sequence and solution environment. In: Deamidation and Isoaspartate Formation in Peptides and Proteins. Aswad DW, editor. CRC Press, London, 1995: 65–90.

Bristow AF. Purification of proteins for therapeutic use. In: *Protein Purification Applications. A Practical Approach.* Harris ELV and Angal S, editors. IRL Press, Oxford, 1990: 29–44.

Brown F, Meyer RF, Law M, Kramer E, Newman JF. A universal virus inactivant for decontaminating blood and biopharmaceutical products. *Biologicals* 1998; 26(1):39–47.

Bueler H, Aguzzi A, Sailer A, Greiner RA, Autenried P, Aguet M, Weissmann C. Mice devoid of PrP are resistant to scrapie. *Cell* 1993; 73(7):1339–1347.

Bussian BM and Sander C. How to determine protein secondary structure in solution by Raman spectroscopy: Practical guide and test case DNase I. *Biochemistry* 1989; 28:4271–4277.

Byrjalsen I, Mose LP, Fey SJ, Nilas L, Larsen MR, Christiansen C. Two-dimensional gel analysis of human endometrial proteins: characterization of proteins with increased expression in hyperplasia and adenocarcinoma. *Mol Hum Reprod* 1999; 5(8):748–756.

Carlton JE and Morgan WT. Simple, economical, amino acid analysis based on pre-column derivatization with 9-fluorenylmethyl chloroformate (FMOC). In: *Techniques in Protein Chemistry.* Hugli TE, editor. Academic Press, San Diego, 1989: 266–272.

Celis JE and Bravo R. *Two-Dimensional Gel Electrophoresis of Proteins: Methods and Applications.* Academic Press, New York, 1984.

Chaiken I, Rose S, Karlsson R. Analysis of macromolecular interactions using immobilized ligands. *Anal Biochem* 1992; 201(2):197–210.

Chamberlain P and Mire-Sluis AR. An overview of scientific and regulatory issues for the immunogenicity of biological products. *Dev Biol* (Basel) 2003; 112:3–11.

Chang JY, Knecht R, Jenoe P, Vekemans S. Amino acid analysis at the femtomole level using the dimethylaminoazobenzene sulfonyl chloride precolumn derivatization method: Potential and limitation. In: *Techniques in Protein Chemistry.* Hugli TE, editor. Academic Press, San Diego, New York, 1989: 305–314.

Chapman J. Progress in improving the pathogen safety of red cell concentrates. *Vox Sang* 2000; 78(Suppl.2):203–204.

Chapman KG, Amer G, Boyce C, Brower G, Green C, Hall WE, Harpaz D, Mullendore B. Proposed validation standard VS-1 Non aseptic pharmaceutical processes. *J Validation Technol* 2000; 6(2):502–521.

Charm SE, Landau SH. Thermalizer. High-temperature short-time sterilization of heat-sensitive biological materials. *Ann NY Acad Sci* 1987; 506:608–612.

Charm SE, Landau S, Williams B, Horowitz B, Prince AM, Pascual D. High-temperature short-time heat inactivation of HIV and other viruses in human blood plasma. *Vox Sang* 1992; 62(1):12–20.

Chen RF, Edelhoch H, Steiner RF. Fluorescence of proteins. In: *Physical Principles and Techniques of Protein Chemistry. Part A*. Leach SJ, editor. Academic Press, New York, 1969: 171–244.

Christensen T, Hansen JJ, Sørensen HH, Thomsen J. RP-HPLC of biosynthetic and hypohyseal human growth hormone. In: *High Performance Liquid Chromatography in Biotechnology*. Hancock WS, editor. John Wiley and Sons, New York, 1990: 191–204.

Clore GM and Gronenborn AM. Multidimensional heteronuclear nuclear magnetic resonance of proteins. *Meth Enzymol* 1994; 239:349–363.

Cohen SA and Strydom DJ. Amino acid analysis utilizing phenylisothiocyanate derivatives. *Anal Biochem* 1988; 174(1):1–16.

Coligan JE, Dunn BM, Ploegh HL, Speicher DW, Wingfield PT. Assays for total protein. In: *Current Protocols in Protein Science*. Vol. 1. Coligan JE, Dunn BM, Ploegh HL, Speicher DW, Wingfield PT, editors. Wiley, New York, 1995: 3.4.1–3.4.24.

Coligan JE, Dunn BM, Ploegh HL, Speicher DW, Wingfield PT. Capillary electrophoresis of proteins and peptides. In: *Current Protocols in Protein Science*. Vol. 1. Coligan JE, Dunn BM, Ploegh HL, Speicher DW, Wingfield PT, editors. Wiley, New York, 1995: 10.9.1–10.9.13.

Coligan JE, Dunn BM, Ploegh HL, Speicher DW, Wingfield PT. C-terminal sequence analysis. In: *Current Protocols in Protein Science*. Vol. 1. Coligan JE, Dunn BM, Ploegh HL, Speicher DW, Wingfield PT, editors. Wiley, New York, 1996: 11.8.1–11.8.14.

Coligan JE, Dunn BM, Ploegh HL, Speicher DW, Wingfield PT. Determining the identity and structure of recombinant proteins. In: Current Protocols in Protein Science. Vol. 1. Coligan JE, Dunn BM, Ploegh HL, Speicher DW, Wingfield PT, editors. Wiley, New York, 1996: 7.3.1–7.3.26.

Coligan JE, Dunn BM, Ploegh HL, Speicher DW, Wingfield PT. One-dimensional isoelectric focusing of proteins in slab gels. In: *Current Protocols in Protein Science*. Vol. 1. Coligan JE, Dunn BM, Ploegh HL, Speicher DW, Wingfield PT, editors. Wiley, New York, 1995: 10.2.1–10.2.8.

Coligan JE, Dunn BM, Ploegh HL, Speicher DW, Wingfield PT. One-dimensional electrophoresis using non-denaturing conditions. In: *Current Protocols in Protein Science*. Vol. 1. Coligan JE, Dunn BM, Ploegh HL, Speicher DW, Wingfield PT, editors. Wiley, New York, 1995: 10.3.1–10.3.11.

Coligan JE, Dunn BM, Ploegh HL, Speicher DW, Wingfield PT. One-dimensional SDS gel electrophoresis of proteins. In: *Current Protocols in Protein Science*. Vol. 1. Coligan JE, Dunn BM, Ploegh HL, Speicher DW, Wingfield PT, editors. Wiley, New York, 1995: 10.1.1–10.1.34.

Coligan JE, Dunn BM, Ploegh HL, Speicher DW, Wingfield PT. Protein detection in gels using fixation. In: *Current Protocols in Protein Science*. Vol. 1. Coligan JE, Dunn BM, Ploegh HL, Speicher DW, Wingfield PT, editors. Wiley, New York, 1995: 10.5.1–10.5.12.

Coligan JE, Dunn BM, Ploegh HL, Speicher DW, Wingfield PT. Quantitative amino acid analysis. In: Current Protocols in Protein Science. Vol. 1. Coligan JE, Dunn BM, Ploegh HL, Speicher DW, Wingfield PT, editors. Wiley, New York, 1995: 3.2.1–3.2.3.

Cooper C, Packer N, Williams K. *Amino Acid Analysis Protocols*. Humana Press, Totowa, NJ, 2001.

Cooper JF. Resolving LAL Test interferences. *J Parenter Sci Technol* 1990; 44(1):13–20.

Crabb JW, West KA, Scott Dodson W, Hulmes JD. Amino acid analysis. In: *Current Protocols in Protein Science*. Vol. 1. Coligan JE, Dunn BM, Ploegh HL, Speicher DW, Wingfield PT, editors. Wiley, New York, 1997: 11.9.1–11.9.42.

Cunningham BC and Wells JA. Comparison of a structural and a functional epitope. *J Mol Biol* 1993; 234(3):554–563.

Davis BJ. Disc electrophoresis. II. Method and application to human serum proteins. *Ann NY Acad Sci* 1964; 121:404–427.

Davis GC and Riggin RM. Characterization and establishment of specifications for biopharmaceuticals. *Dev Biol Stand* 1997; 91:49–54.

Depyrogenation. Technical report No. 7. 1985. Parenteral Drug Association Inc, Bethesda, MD.

Dichtelmuller H, Rudnick D, Breuer B, Ganshirt KH. Validation of virus inactivation and removal for the manufacturing procedure of two immunoglobulins and a 5% serum protein solution treated with beta-propiolactone. *Biologicals* 1993; 21(3):259–268.

Dickinson AG and Outram GW. The scrapie replication-site hypothesis and its implication for pathogenesis. In: *Slow Transmissible Diseases of the Nervous System*. Vol. 2. Prusiner SB, Hadlow JW, editors. Academic Press, London, 1979: 13–21.

DiLeo AJ, Vacante DA, Deane EF. Size exclusion removal of model mammalian viruses using a unique membrane system, Part I: Membrane qualification. *Biologicals* 1993; 21(3):275–286.

DiMarchi RD, Long HB, Kroeff EP, Chance RE. Utilization of analytical reversed-phase HPLC in biosynthetic insulin production. In: *High Performance Liquid Chromatography in Biotechnology*. Hancock WS, editor. John Wiley and Sons, New York, 1990: 181–189.

Dinarello CA, O'Connor JV, LoPreste G, Swift RL. Human leukocytic pyrogen test for detection of pyrogenic material in growth hormone produced by recombinant *Escherichia coli*. *J Clin Microbiol* 1984; 20(3):323–329.

Dizdaroglu M. The purification of polypeptide samples by ion-exchange chromatography on silica-based supports. In: *High Performance Liquid Chromatography in Biotechnology*. Hancock WS, editor. John Wiley and Sons, New York, 1990: 263–278.

Doolittle RF. *Of Urfs and Orfs: A Primer on How to Analyze Derived Amino Acid Sequences*. University Science Books, New York, 1986.

Dudkiewicz-Wilczynska J, Snycerski A, Tautt J. Application of high-performance size exclusion chromatography to the determination of erythropoietin in pharmaceutical preparations. *Acta Pol Pharm* 2002; 59(2):83–86.

Dunbar BS. Troubleshooting and artifacts in two-dimensional polyacrylamide gel electrophoresis. In: *Two-Dimensional Electrophoresis and Immunological Techniques*. Dunbar BS, editor. Kluwer Academic/Plenum Publishers, New York, 1987: 173–195.

Dunbar BS, Kimura H, Timmonds TM. Protein analysis using high-resolution two-dimensional polyacrylamide gel electrophoresis. *Meth Enzymology* 1990; 182(34):441–459.

Dunn MJ. *Gel Electrophoresis: Proteins*. Bios Scientific Publishers Ltd, Oxford, U.K., 1993.

Dupont DR, Keim PS, Chui AH, Bello R, Bozzini M, Wilson KJ. A comprehensive approach to amino acid analysis. In: *Techniques in Protein Chemistry*. Hugli TE, editor. Academic Press, San Diego, New York, 1989: 284–294.

Eaton LC. Host cell contaminant protein assay development for recombinant biopharmaceuticals. *J Chromatogr A* 1995; 705(1):105–114.

Ebeling F, Baer M, Hormila P, Jarventie G, Koistinen P, Katka K, Oksanen K, Perkkio M, Ruutu T, Soppi E. Tolerability and kinetics of a solvent-detergent-treated intravenous immunoglobulin preparation in hypogammaglobulinaemia patients. *Vox Sang* 1995; 69(2):91–94.

Edman P. A method for the determination of the amino acid sequence in peptides. *Arch Biochem Biophys* 1949; 22:476–480.

Edman P and Begg G. A protein sequenator. *Eur J Biochem* 1967; 1(1):80–91.

FDA Center for Drug Evaluation and Research (CDER). Guidance for industry — PAT — A framework for innovative pharmaceutical manufacturing and quality assurance. CDS029\CDERGUID\5815dft.doc, 1-21. 25-8-2003 and September 2004: http://www.fda.gov/cder/guidance/6419fnl.htm.

FDA Office of Biologics Research and Review. Points to consider in the production and testing of new drugs and biologics produced by recombinant DNA technology (Draft). October 4, 1985. Food and Drug Administration.

FDA Office of Biologics Research and Review. *Points to Consider in the Characterization of Cell Lines Used to Produce Biologicals*. Food and Drug Administration, Rockville, MD, 1993.

Findlay JBC and Geisow MJ. *Protein Sequencing, a Practical Approach*. IRL Press, Oxford: 1989.

Fischer L. *Gel Filtration Chromatography*. Elsevier/North-Holland Biomedical Press, Amsterdam, 1980.

Fogh J (ed.). *Contamination in Tissue Cultures*. Academic Press, New York, 1973.

Gallagher S and Smith JA. One-dimensional SDS gel electrophoresis of proteins. In: *Current Protocols in Molecular Biology*. Ausubel FM, Brent R, Kingston RE, Moore DD, Seidman JG, Smith JA et al., editors. John Wiley and Sons, New York, 1995: Unit 10.2A

Ganesa C, Granda BW, Mattaliano RJ. Sialylation levels influence oligosaccharide quantitation. Analyzing response variability using high-pH anion-exchange chromatography and pulsed amperometric detection. *BioPharm International* 2003; 16(6):44–52.

Garfin DE. Isoelectric focusing. *Meth Enzymol* 1990; 182(35):459–477.

Garfin DE. One-dimensional gel electrophoresis. *Meth Enzymol* 1990; 182(33):425–441.

Garnick RL. Specifications from a biotechnology industry perspective. *Dev Biol Stand* 1997; 91:31–36.

Garvey JS. *Methods in Immunology: A Laboratory Text for Instruction and Research.* 3rd ed. W. A. Benjamin Inc., London, 1977.

Gerwig GJ and Damm JBL. General strategies for the characterization of carbohydrates from recombinant glycoprotein therapeutics. In: *Bioseparation and Bioprocessing.* Vol. II. *Processing, Quality and Characterization, Economics, Safety and Hygiene.* Subramanian G, editor. Wiley-VCH, New York, 1998: 325–375.

Gianazza E. Isoelectric focusing as a tool for the investigation of post-translational processing and chemical modifications of proteins. *J Chromatogr A* 1995; 705(1):67–87.

Goldschmidt RC and Kimelberg HK. Protein analysis of mammalian cells in monolayer culture using the bicinchoninic assay. *Anal Biochem* 1989; 177(1):41–45.

Goshev I and Nedkov P. Exending the range of application of the biuret reaction: quantitative determination of insoluble proteins. *Anal Biochem* 1979; 95(2):340–343.

Goverman J. 2-D diagonal gel electrophoresis. *Meth Mol Biol* 1999; 112:265–270.

Grabner RW. Merck & Co., Assignee. Process for removing pyrogenic material from aqueous solutions. Patent US3897309. Issued 29-7-1975. Filed February 15, 1974.

Hagel L. Gel filtration. In: *Protein Purification: Principles, High-Resolution Methods, and Applications.* Janson J-C, Ryden L, editors. Wiley-Liss, New York, 1998: 79–143.

Hamalainen E, Suomela H, Ukkonen P. Virus inactivation during intravenous immunoglobulin production. *Vox Sang* 1992; 63(1):6–11.

Hames BD. One-dimensional polyacrylamide gel electrophoresis. In: *Gel Electrophoresis of Proteins: A Practical Approach.* Hames BD, Rickwood D, editors. Oxford University Press, New York, 1990: 1–148.

Hames BD and Rickwood D. *Gel Electrophoresis of Proteins: A Practical Approach.* 3rd ed. Oxford University Press, New York, 2002.

Hamilton WA. Membrane active antibacterial compounds. In: *Inhibition and Destruction of the Microbial Cell.* Hugo WB, editor. Academic Press, New York, 1971: 77–93.

Hancock WS. *High Performance Liquid Chromatography in Biotechnology.* John Wiley and Sons, New York, 1990.

Harding SE. Determination of absolute molecular weights using sedimentation equilibrium analytical ultra-centrifugation. *Meth Mol Biol* 1994; 22:75–84.

Harding SE. Determination of macromolecular homogeneity, shape, and interactions using sedimentation velocity analytical ultracentrifugation. *Meth Mol Biol* 1994; 22:61–73.

Haris PI and Chapman D. Analysis of polypeptide and protein structures using Fourier transform infrared spectroscopy. *Meth Mol Biol* 1994; 22:183–202.

Harper S, Mozdzanowski J, Speicher D. Two-dimensional gel electrophoresis. In: *Current Protocols in Protein Science.* Vol. 1. Coligan JE, Dunn BM, Ploegh HL, Speicher DW, Wingfield PT, editors. Wiley, New York, 1998: 10.4.1–10.4.36.

Hartmann WK, Saptharishi N, Yang XY, Mitra G, Soman G. Characterization and analysis of thermal dena-turation of antibodies by size exclusion high-performance liquid chromatography with quadruple detection. *Anal Biochem* 2004; 325(2):227–239.

Hartree EF. Determination of protein: a modification of the Lowry method that gives a linear photometric response. *Anal Biochem* 1972; 48(2):422–427.

Henzler HJ and Kaiser K. Avoiding viral contamination in biotechnological and pharmaceutical processes. *Nature Biotechnol* 1998; 16(11):1077–1079.

Hochstrasser DF, Harrington MG, Hochstrasser AC, Miller MJ, Merril CR. Methods for increasing the resolution of two-dimensional protein electrophoresis. *Anal Biochem* 1988; 173(2):424–435.

Hoffman K. Strategies for host cell protein analysis. *BioPharm* 2000; 13(5):38–45.

Hojrup P and Magnusson S. Disulfide bridges of bovine factor X. *Biochem J* 1987; 245(3):887–891.

Horowitz B. Investigations into the application of tri(n-butyl)phosphate/detergent mixtures to blood derivatives. *Curr Stud Hematol Blood Transfus* 1989; (56):83–96.

ICH. Quality of biotechnological products: viral safety evaluation of biotechnology products derived from cell lines of human or animal origin. ICH Harmonised Tripartite Guideline. *Dev Biol Stand* 1998; 93:177–201.

Jackson PJ and Bayne SJ. Quality control of protein primary structure by automated sequencing and mass spectrometry. In: *Bioseparation and Bioprocessing*. Vol. II. *Processing, Quality and Characterization, Economics, Safety and Hygiene*. Subramanian G, editor. Wiley-VCH, New York, 1998: 291–323.

Janson J-C and Ryden L. *Protein Purification: Principles, High-Resolution Methods, and Applications*. 2nd ed. Wiley-Liss, New York, 1998.

Jernejc K, Cimerman A, Perdih A. Comparison of different methods for protein determination in Aspergillus niger mycelium. *Appl Microbiol Biotechnol* 1986; 23:445–448.

Johnson Jr. WC. Protein secondary structure and circular dichroism: a practical guide. *Proteins* 1990; 7(3):205–214.

Johnston D. The decline of six sigma. *Pharma Technol Europe* 2003; 15(12):57–61.

Jungbauer A and Lettner HP. Chemical disinfection of chromatographic resins, part 1: Preliminary studies and microbial kinetics. *BioPharm* 1994; 7(5):46–56.

Kiefhaber T, Rudolph R, Kohler HH, Buchner J. Protein aggregation *in vitro* and *in vivo*: a quantitative model of the kinetic competition between folding and aggregation. *Biotechnology* (NY) 1991; 9(9):825–829.

Kilar F. Recent applications of capillary isoelectric focusing. *Electrophoresis* 2003; 24(22–23):3908–3916.

Kinter M and Sherman NE. *Protein Sequencing and Identification Using Tandem Mass Spectrometry*. Wiley-Interscience, New York, 2000.

Kirk PL. Kjeldahl method for total nitrogen. *Anal Chem* 1950; 22(2):354–365.

Kopaciewicz W, Rounds MA, Fausnaugh J, Regnier FE. Retention model for high-performance ion-exchange chromatography. *J Chromatogr* 1983; 266(August):3–21.

Laemmli UK. Cleavage of structural proteins during the assembly of the head of bacteriophage T4. *Nature* 1970; 227(259):680–685.

Lanni F, Dillon ML, Beard JW. Determination of small quantities of nitrogen in serological precipitates and other biological materials. *Proc Soc Exp Biol Med* 1950; 74:4–7.

Laue TM and Rhodes DG. Determination of size, molecular weight, and presence of subunits. Meth Enzymol 1990; 182(43):566–587.

Lee DC et al. PrP(Sc) partitioning during plasma fractionation: development and application of a sensitive Western blot assay. *Thromb Haemost* 1999; 82(Suppl.):757.

Lee DC, Stenland CJ, Hartwell RC, Ford EK, Cai K, Miller JL, Gilligan KJ, Rubenstein R, Fournel M, Petteway Jr. SR. Monitoring plasma processing steps with a sensitive Western blot assay for the detection of the prion protein. *J Virol Meth* 2000; 84(1):77–89.

Liebsch M. [History of the LAL-test: validation and regulatory acceptance]. ALTEX 1995; 12(2):76–80.

Liu S, Tobias R, McClure S, Styba G, Shi Q, Jackowski G. Removal of endotoxin from recombinant protein preparations. *Clin Biochem* 1997; 30(6):455–463.

Lof AL, Gustafsson G, Novak V, Engman L, Mikaelsson M. Determination of total protein in highly purified factor IX concentrates. *Vox Sang* 1992; 63(3):172–177.

Lovatt A, McMutrie D, Black J, Doherty I. Validation of quantitative PCR assays. Addressing virus contamination concerns. BioPharm 2002; 15(3):22-32.

Lowry OH, Rosebrough NJ, Farr AL, Randall RJ. Protein measurement with the Folin phenol reagent. *J Biol Chem* 1951; 193(1):265–275.

Lynch JM and Barbano DM. Kjeldahl nitrogen analysis as a reference method for protein determination in dairy products. *J AOAC Int* 1999; 82(6):1389–1398.

MacGregor I, Hope J, Barnard G, Kirby L, Drummond O, Pepper D, Hornsey V, Barclay R, Bessos H, Turner M, Prowse C. Application of a time-resolved fluoroimmunoassay for the analysis of normal prion protein in human blood and its components. *Vox Sang* 1999; 77(2):88–96.

Malmquist G and Lundell N. Characterization of the influence of displacing salts on retention in gradient elution ion-exchange chromatography of proteins and peptides. *J Chromatogr* 1992; 627(1-2):107–124.

Mannucci PM and Colombo M. Virucidal treatment of clotting factor concentrates. *Lancet* 1988; 2(8614):782–785.

Matsudaira P. Limited N-terminal sequence analysis. *Meth Enzymol* 1990; 182(45):602–613.

Matsudaira PT and Burgess DR. SDS microslab linear gradient polyacrylamide gel electrophoresis. *Anal Biochem* 1978; 87(2):386–396.

McCormic RM. Capillary zone electrophoresis of peptides. In: *Handbook of Capillary Electrophoresis*. Landers JP, editor. CRC Press, Boca Raton, FL, 1994: 287–324.

McCormic RM. Protein capillary electrophoresis: Theoretical and experimental considerations for method development. In: *Handbook of Capillary Electrophoresis*. Landers JP, editor. CRC Press, Boca Raton, FL, 1994: 325–368.

McCullough KZ. Variability in the LAL test. *J Parenter Sci Technol* 1990; 44(1):19–21.

McKinley MP, Bolton DC, Prusiner SB. A protease-resistant protein is a structural component of the scrapie prion. *Cell* 1983; 35(1):57–62.

McRee D. *Practical Protein Crystallography*. 2nd ed. Academic Press, San Diego, 1999.

Meisel J. [Determination of Pyrogens: Comparison of Different Methods]. *ALTEX* 1995; 12(2):89–92.

Meyer VR. *Practical High-Performance Liquid Chromatography*. 3rd. ed. John Wiley & Sons, 1999.

Miekka S, I, Busby TF, Reid B, Pollock R, Ralston A, Drohan WN. New methods for inactivation of lipid-enveloped and non-enveloped viruses. *Haemophilia* 1998; 4(4):402–408.

Moesby L, Hansen EW, Christensen JD. Endotoxin testing of proteins for parenteral administration using the Mono Mac 6 assay. *J Clin Pharm Ther* 2000; 25(4):283–289.

Montgomery DC. Introduction to factorial designs. In: *Design and Analysis of Experiments*. Wiley & Sons, New York, 1991: 197–256.

Moody AJ, Hejnaes KR, Marshall MO, Larsen FS, Boel E, Svendsen I, Mortensen E, Dyrberg T. Isolation by anion-exchange of immunologically and enzymatically active human islet glutamic acid decarboxylase 65 overexpressed in Sf9 insect cells. *Diabetologia* 1995; 38(1):14–23.

Moore S, Spackman DH, Stein WH. Chromatography of amino acids on sulfonated polystyrene resins. An improved system. *Anal Chem* 1958; 30:1185–1190.

Moore S and Stein WH. Chromatography of amino acids on sulfonated polystyrene resins. *J Biol Chem* 1951; 192(2):663–681.

Moore S and Stein WHJ. Photometric ninhydrin method for use in the chromatography of amino acids. *J Biol Chem* 1948; 176:367–388.

Murano G. FDA perspective on specifications for biotechnology products — from IND to PLA. *Dev Biol Stand* 1997; 91:3–13.

Murano G. International Conference on Harmonization — critical discussion of the biotech "specifications" document. *Curr Opin Biotechnol* 2000; 11(3):303–308.

Na DH, Park EJ, Youn YS, Moon BW, Jo YW, Lee SH, Kim WB, Sohn Y, Lee KC. Sodium dodecyl sulfate-capillary gel electrophoresis of polyethylene glycolylated interferon alpha. *Electrophoresis* 2004; 25(3):476–479.

Niwa M, Milner KC, Ribi E, Rudbach JA. Alteration of physical, chemical, and biological properties of endotoxin by treatment with mild alkali. *J Bacteriol* 1969; 97(3):1069–1077.

North MJ. Prevention of unwanted proteolysis. In: *Proteolytical Enzymes*. Beynan RJ and Bond JS, editors. IRL Press, Oxford 1989: 105–124.

Ochia M, Tamura H, Yamamoto A, Aizawa M, Kataoka M, Toyoizumi H, Horiuchi Y. A limulus amoebocyte lysate activating activity (LAL activity) that lacks biological activities of endotoxin found in biological products. *Microbiol Immunol* 2002; 46(8):527–533.

O'Farrell PH. High resolution two-dimensional electrophoresis of proteins. *J Biol Chem* 1975; 250(10):4007–4021.

O'Farrell PZ, Goodman HM, O'Farrell PH. High resolution two-dimensional electrophoresis of basic as well as acidic proteins. *Cell* 1977; 12(4):1133–1141.

Okajima T, Tanabe T, Yasuda T. Nonurea sodium dodecyl sulfate-polyacrylamide gel electrophoresis with high-molarity buffers for the separation of proteins and peptides. *Anal Biochem* 1993; 211(2):293–300.

Ornstein L. Disc electrophoresis. I. Background and theory. *Ann NY Acad Sci* 1964; 121:321–349.

Ouyang J, Wang J, Deng R, Long Q, Wang X. High-level expression, purification, and characterization of porcine somatotropin in Pichia pastoris. *Protein Expr Purif* 2003; 32(1):28–34.

Ozols J. Amino acid analysis. *Meth Enzymol* 1990; 182(44):587–601.

Ozturk SS, Blackie J, Wu P, Taticek R, Konstantinov K, Matanguihan C et al. On-line monitoring for consistent and optimal production of biologicals from mammalian cell cultures. In: *Animal Cell Technology: From Vaccines to Genetic Medicine*. Carrondo MJT, Griffiths JB, Moreira JLP, editors. Kluwer Academic Publishers, Dordrecht, 1997: 205–214.

Patel D. Gel electrophoresis: Essential data. Wiley & Sons, New York, 1994.

Peterson GL. Determination of total protein. *Meth Enzymol* 1983; 91:95–119.

Pierce J and Suelter CH. An evaluation of the Coomassie brillant blue G-250 dye-binding method for quantitative protein determination. *Anal Biochem* 1977; 81(2):478–480.

Prenata AZ. Separation on the basis of size: gel permeation chromatography. In: *Protein Purification Methods. A Practical Approach*. Harris ELV and Angal S, editors. IRL Press, Oxford, 1989: 293–306.

Prince AM, Stephan W, Brotman B. Beta-propiolactone/ultraviolet irradiation: a review of its effectiveness for inactivation of viruses in blood derivatives. *Rev Infect Dis* 1983; 5(1):92–107.

Prusiner SB. Novel proteinaceous infectious particles cause scrapie. *Science* 1982; 216(4542):136–144.

Ptitsyn OB and Pain RH, Semisotnov GV, Zerovnik E, Razgulyaev OI. Evidence for a molten globule state as a general intermediate in protein folding. *FEBS Lett* 1990; 262(1):20–24.

Rawadi G and Dussurget O. Advances in PCR-based detection of mycoplasmas contaminating cell cultures. *PCR Meth Appl* 1995; 4(4):199–208.

Reim DF and Speicher DW. N-terminal sequence analysis of proteins and peptides. In: *Current Protocols in Protein Science*. Vol. 1. Coligan JE, Dunn BM, Ploegh HL, Speicher DW, Wingfield PT, editors. Wiley, New York, 1997: 11.10.01–11.10.38.

Rhodes DG and Laue TM. Determination of purity. *Meth Enzymol* 1990; 182(42):555–565.

Rickwood D, Alec J, Chambers A, Spragg SP. Two-dimensional gel electrophoresis. In: *Gel Electrophoresis of Proteins: A Practical Approach*. Hames BD, Rickwood D, editors. Oxford University Press, New York, 1990: 217–272.

Rihetti PG. *Isoelectric Focusing: Theory, Methodology and Application*. Elsevier Science, Amsterdam, 1983.

Righetti PG, Bossi A, Gelfi C. Conventional isoelectric focusing in gel slabs, in capillaries, and immobilized pH gradients. In: *Gel Electrophoresis of Proteins: A Practical Approach*. Hames BD, Rickwood D, editors. Oxford University Press, New York, 2002: 127–188.

Righetti PG and Hancock W. *Capillary Electrophoresis in Analytical Biotechnology: A Balance of Theory and Practice*. CRC Press, Boca Raton, FL, 1995.

Ritter N and McEntire J. Determining protein concentration. Part 1: Methodology. *BioPharm* 2002; 15(4):12–58.

Robinson AB and Rudd CJ. Deamidation of glutaminyl and asparaginyl residues in peptides and proteins. *Curr Top Cell Regul* 1974; 8:247–295.

Robson RM, Goll DE, Temple MJ. Determination of proteins in "Tris" buffer by the biuret reaction. *Anal Biochem* 1968; 24(2):339–341.

Roe S. *Protein Purification Applications. A Practical Approach*. 2nd ed. Oxford University Press, New York: 2001.

Roe S. Separation based on structure. In: *Protein Purification Methods. A Practical Approach*. Harris ELV and Angal S, editors. IRL Press, Oxford, 1989: 175–244.

Safar J, Wille H, Itri V, Groth D, Serban H, Torchia M, Cohen FE, Prusiner SB. Eight prion strains have PrP(Sc) molecules with different conformations. *Nat Med* 1998; 4(10):1157–1165.

Salinas M, Fando JL, Grisolia S. A sensitive and specific method for quantitative estimation of carbamylation in proteins. *Anal Biochem* 1974; 62(1):166–172.

Sanger F. Chemistry of insulin; determination of the structure of insulin opens the way to greater understanding of life processes. *Science* 1959; 129(3359):1340–1344.

Sapan CV, Lundblad RL, Price NC. Colorimetric protein assay techniques. *Biotechnol Appl Biochem* 1999; 29(Pt.2):99–108.

Schagger H and Von Jagow G. Tricine-sodium dodecyl sulfate-polyacrylamide gel electrophoresis for the separation of proteins in the range from 1 to 100 kDa. *Anal Biochem* 1987; 166(2):368–379.

Schmerr MJ, Jenny AL, Bulgin MS, Miller JM, Hamir AN, Cutlip RC, Goodwin KR. Use of capillary electrophoresis and fluorescent labeled peptides to detect the abnormal prion protein in the blood of animals that are infected with a transmissible spongiform encephalopathy. *J Chromatogr A* 1999; 853(1–2):207–214.

Seamon KB. Specifications for biotechnology-derived protein drugs. *Curr Opin Biotechnol* 1998; 9(3):319–325.

Sedmak JJ, Grossberg SE. A rapid, sensitive, and versatile assay for protein using Coomassie brilliant blue G250. *Anal Biochem* 1977; 79(1–2):544–552.

Seifter S and England S. Analysis for protein modifications and nonprotein cofactors. *Meth Enzymol* 1990; 182(47):626–646.

Shintani H and Polonsky J. *Handbook of Capillary Electrophoresis Applications.* Chapman and Hall, New York, 1997.

Shrivastaw KP, Singh S, Sharma SB, Sokhey J. Quantitation of protein content by biuret method during production of yellow fever vaccine. *Biologicals* 1995; 23(4):299–300.

Sittampalam GS, Ellis RM, Miner DJ, Rickard EC, Clodfelter DK. Evaluation of amino acid analysis as reference method to quantitate highly purified proteins. *J Assoc Off Anal Chem* 1988; 71(4):833–838.

Sjoholm I. In-process testing and limits. *Dev Biol Stand* 1997; 91:73–78.

Smith BJ. *Protein Sequencing Protocols.* 2nd ed. Humana Press, Totowa, NJ, 2002.

Smith PK, Krohn RI, Hermanson GT, Mallia AK, Gartner FH, Provenzano MD, Fujimoto EK, Goeke NM, Olson BJ, Klenk DC. Measurement of protein using bicinchoninic acid. *Anal Biochem* 1985; 150(1):76–85.

Sofer G and Hagel L. Basic properties of peptides, proteins and nucleic acids. In: *Handbook of Process Chromatography: A Guide to Optimization, Scale-Up and Validation.* Academic Press, San Diego, 1997: 244–255.

Sofer G and Hagel L. Purification design, optimization and scale-up. In: *Handbook of Process Chromatography: A Guide to Optimization, Scale-Up and Validation.* Academic Press, San Diego, 1997: 27–113.

Sofer G and Hagel L. Validation. In: *Handbook of Process Chromatography: A Guide to Optimization, Scale-Up and Validation.* Academic Press, San Diego, CA, 1997: 119–187.

Sorensen HH, Thomsen J, Bayne S, Hojrup P, Roepstorff P. Strategies for determination of disulphide bridges in proteins using plasma desorption mass spectrometry. *Biomed Environ Mass Spectrom* 1990; 19(11):713–720.

Spector T. Refinement of the coomassie blue method of protein quantitation. A simple and linear spectrophotometric assay for less than or equal to 0.5 to 50 microgram of protein. *Anal Biochem* 1978; 86(1):142–146.

Stark GR. Modification of proteins with cyanate. *Meth Enzymol* 1972; 25:579–584.

Stein WH and Moore S. The free amino acids of human blood plasma. *J Biol Chem* 1954; 211(2):915–926.

Stoscheck CM. Quantitation of protein. *Meth Enzymol* 1990; 182(6):50–68.

Strickland EH. Aromatic contributions to circular dichroism spectra of proteins. *CRC Crit Rev Biochem* 1974; 2(1):113–175.

Suck R, Petersen A, Weber B, Becker WM, Fiebig H, Cromwell O. Analytical and preparative native polyacrylamide gel electrophoresis: Investigation of the recombinant and natural major grass pollen allergen Phl p 2. *Electrophoresis* 2004; 25(1):14–19.

Teller JD and Kelly KM. A turbidimetric Limulus amebocyte assay for the quantitative determination of Gram negative bacterial endotoxin. *Prog Clin Biol Res* 1979; 29:423–433.

Thomas D, Schultz P, Steven AC, Wall JS. Mass analysis of biological macromolecular complexes by STEM. *Biol Cell* 1994; 80(2–3):181–192.

Thompson M, Owen L, Wilkinson K, Wood R, Damant A. A comparison of the Kjeldahl and Dumas methods for the determination of protein in foods, using data from a proficiency testing scheme. *Analyst* 2002; 127(12):1666–1668.

Troccoli NM, McIver J, Losikoff A, Poiley J. Removal of viruses from human intravenous immune globulin by 35 nm nanofiltration. *Biologicals* 1999; 26(4):321–329.

Tsao IF and Wang HY. Removal and inactivation of viruses by a surface-bonded quaternary ammonium chloride. In: *Downstream Processing and Bioseparation: Recovery and Purification of Biological Products.* Hamel JFP, Hunter JB, Sikdar SK, editors. American Chemical Society, Washington, DC, 1990: 250–267.

Tsuji K, Baczynskyj L, Bronson GE. Capillary electrophoresis-electrospray mass spectrometry for the analysis of recombinant bovine and porcine somatotropins. *Anal Chem* 1992; 64(17):1864–1870.

Van Holde K. Sedimentation analysis of proteins. In: *The Proteins.* Vol. 1. Neurath H, editor. Academic Press, San Diego, 1975: 225–291.

van Leen RW, Bakhuis JG, van Beckhoven RF, Burger H, Dorssers LC, Hommes RW, Lemson PJ, Noordam B, Persoon NL, Wagemaker G. Production of human interleukin-3 using industrial microorganisms. *Biotechnology* (NY) 1991; 9(1):47–52.

van Wezel AL, van der MP, van Beveren CP, Verma I, Salk PL, Salk J. Detection and elimination of cellular nucleic acids in biologicals produced on continuous cell lines. *Dev Biol Stand* 1981; 50:59–69.

Wachtel RE and Tsuji K. Comparison of limulus amebocyte lysates and correlation with the United States Pharmacopeial pyrogen test. *Appl Environ Microbiol* 1977; 33(6):1265–1269.

Walter JK, Nothelfer F, Werz W. Validation of viral safety for pharmaceutical proteins. In: *Bioseparation and Bioprocessing*. Vol. I. *Biochromatography, Membrane Separations, Modeling, Validation*. Subramanian G, editor. Wiley-VCH, New York, 1998: 465–496.

Walter JK, Nothelfer F, Werz W. Virus removal and inactivation. A decade of validation studies: Critical evaluation of the data set. In: *Validation of Biopharmaceutical Manufacturing Processes*. Kelley BD and Ramelmeier RA, editors. American Chemical Society, Washington, DC, 1998: 114–124.

Weber K, Pringle JR, Osborn M. Measurement of molecular weights by electrophoresis on SDS-acrylamide gel. *Meth Enzymol* 1972; 26(Pt.C):3–27.

Wehr T, Rodriguez-Diaz R, Zhu M. *Capillary Electrophoresis of Proteins*. Marcel Dekker, New York, 1998.

Westermeier R. *Electrophoresis in Practice*. 3rd ed. Wiley-VCH, Weinheim, 2001.

Westermeier R. Isoelectric focusing. *Meth Mol Biol* 2004; 244:225–232.

WHO. Acceptability of all substrates for production of biologicals. Report of a WHO study group. Technical Report Series 747. 1987. World Health Organization, Geneva.

Williams KL. Endotoxin as a standard. In: *Endotoxins. Pyrogens, LAL Testing, and Depyrogenation*. Williams KL, editor. Marcel Dekker, New York, 2001: 136–164.

Williams KL. Endotoxins. *Pyrogens, LAL Testing, and Depyrogenation*. 2nd ed. Marcel Dekker, New York, 2001.

Williams KL. LAL assay development, validation, and regulation. In: *Endotoxins. Pyrogens, LAL Testing, and Depyrogenation*. Williams KL, editor. Marcel Dekker, New York, 2001: 214–263.

Williams KL. Pyrogen, endotoxin, and fever: an overview. In: *Endotoxins. Pyrogens, LAL Testing, and Depyrogenation*. Williams KL, editor. Marcel Dekker, New York, 2001: 12–26.

Wu CS. *Column Handbook for Size Exclusion Chromatography*. Academic Press, San Diego, 1999.

Yasuhara T and Nokihara K. High-throughput analysis of total nitrogen content that replaces the classic Kjeldahl method. *J Agric Food Chem* 2001; 49(10):4581–4583.

Zhou H, Watts JD, Aebersold R. A systematic approach to the analysis of protein phosphorylation. *Nat Biotechnol* 2001; 19(4):375–378.

Zishka MK and Nishimura JS. Effect of glycerol on Lowry and biuret methods of protein determination. *Anal Biochem* 1970; 34:291–297.

CHAPTER 11: REGULATORY AFFAIRS

GENERAL/IMMUNOGENICITY

Antonelli G, Simeoni E, Currenti M, De Pisa F, Colizzi V, Pistello M, Dianzani F. Interferon antibodies in patients with infectious diseases. Anti-interferon antibodies. *Biotherapy* 1997; 10(1):7–14.

Balsari A and Caruso A. Natural antibodies to IL-2. *Biotherapy* 1997; 10(1):25–28.

Braun A and Alsenz J. Development and use of enzyme-linked immunosorbent assays (ELISA) for the detection of protein aggregates in interferon-alpha (IFN-alpha) formulations. *Pharm Res* 1997; 14(10):1394–1400.

Braun A, Kwee L, Labow MA, Alsenz J. Protein aggregates seem to play a key role among the parameters influencing the antigenicity of interferon alpha (IFN-alpha) in normal and transgenic mice. *Pharm Res* 1997; 14(10):1472–1478.

Brown F and Mire-Sluis A. *Immunogenicity of Therapeutic Biological Products*. Karger, Basel, 2003.

Bussiere JL. Animal models as indicators of immunogenicity of therapeutic proteins in humans. *Dev Biol* (Basel) 2003; 112:135–139.

Casadevall N, Nataf J, Viron B, Kolta A, Kiladjian JJ, Martin-Dupont P, Michaud P, Papo T, Ugo V, Teyssandier I, Varet B, Mayeux P. Pure red-cell aplasia and antierythropoietin antibodies in patients treated with recombinant erythropoietin. *N Engl J Med* 2002; 346(7):469–475.

Chamberlain P and Mire-Sluis AR. An overview of scientific and regulatory issues for the immunogenicity of biological products. *Dev Biol* (Basel) 2003; 112:3–11.

Christen U, Thuerkauf R, Stevens R, Lesslauer W. Immune response to a recombinant human TNFR55-IgG1 fusion protein: auto-antibodies in rheumatoid arthritis (RA) and multiple sclerosis (MS) patients have neither neutralizing nor agonist activities. *Hum Immunol* 1999; 60(9):774–790.

Claman HN. Tolerance to a protein antigen in adult mice and the effect of nonspecific factors. *J Immunol* 1963; 91:833–839.

Cleland JL, Powell MF, Shire SJ. The development of stable protein formulations: a close look at protein aggregation, deamidation, and oxidation. *Crit Rev Ther Drug Carrier Syst* 1993; 10(4):307–377.

Colby CB, Inoue M, Thompson M, Tan YH. Immunologic differentiation between *E. coli* and CHO cell-derived recombinant and natural human beta-interferons. *J Immunol* 1984; 133(6):3091–3095.

Common Technical Document, ICH Section 3.2.S. (NTA 2B, CTD module 3, July 2001).

Dearman RJ and Kimber I. Determination of protein allergenicity: studies in mice. *Toxicol Lett* 2001; 120(1–3):181–186.

Diamond B. Speculations on the immunogenicity of self proteins. *Dev Biol* (Basel) 2003; 112:29–34.

Dresser DW. Specific inhibition of antibody production. II. Paralysis induced in adult mice by small quantities of protein antigen. *Immunology* 1962; 5:378–388.

Fineberg NS, Fineberg SE, Anderson JH, Birkett MA, Gibson RG, Hufferd S. Immunologic effects of insulin lispro [Lys (B28), Pro (B29) human insulin] in IDDM and NIDDM patients previously treated with insulin. *Diabetes* 1996; 45(12):1750–1754.

Gerrard TL. Possible regulatory changes as a consequence of immunogenicity concerns. *BioProcess Int* 2003; 1(9):64–69.

Huby RD, Dearman RJ, Kimber I. Why are some proteins allergens? *Toxicol Sci* 2000; 55(2):235–246.

Kontsek P, Liptakova H, Kontsekova E. Immunogenicity of interferon-alpha 2 in therapy: structural and physiological aspects. *Acta Virol* 1999; 43(1):63–70.

Koren E, Zuckerman LA, Mire-Sluis AR. Immune responses to therapeutic proteins in humans — clinical significance, assessment and prediction. *Curr Pharm Biotechnol* 2002; 3(4):349–360.

Moore WV and Leppert P. Role of aggregated human growth hormone (hGH) in development of antibodies to hGH. *J Clin Endocrinol Metab* 1980; 51(4):691–697.

Moreland LW, McCabe DP, Caldwell JR, Sack M, Weisman M, Henry G, Seely JE, Martin SW, Yee CL, Bendele AM, Frazier JL, Kohno T, Cosenza ME, Lyons SA, Dayer JM, Cohen AM, Edwards III CK. Phase I/II trial of recombinant methionyl human tumor necrosis factor binding protein PEGylated dimer in patients with active refractory rheumatoid arthritis. *J Rheumatol* 2000; 27(3):601–609.

Nakamura RM and Weigle WO. *In vivo* behavior of homologous and heterologous thyroglobulin and induction of immunologic unresponsiveness to heterologous thyroglobulin. *J Immunol* 1967; 98(4):653–662.

Ottesen JL, Nilsson P, Jami J, Weilguny D, Duhrkop M, Bucchini D, Havelund S, Fogh JM. The potential immunogenicity of human insulin and insulin analogues evaluated in a transgenic mouse model. *Diabetologia* 1994; 37(12):1178–1185.

Palleroni AV, Aglione A, Labow M, Brunda MJ, Pestka S, Sinigaglia F, Garotta G, Alsenz J, Braun A. Interferon immunogenicity: preclinical evaluation of interferon-alpha 2a. *J Interferon Cytokine Res* 1997; 17 (Suppl.1):S23–S27.

Patten PA and Schellekens H. The immunogenicity of biopharmaceuticals. Lessons learned and consequences for protein drug development. *Dev Biol* (Basel) 2003; 112:81–97.

Rice GP, Paszner B, Oger J, Lesaux J, Paty D, Ebers G. The evolution of neutralizing antibodies in multiple sclerosis patients treated with interferon beta-1b. *Neurology* 1999; 52(6):1277–1279.

Rosenberg AS. Immunogenicity of biological therapeutics: a hierarchy of concerns. *Dev Biol* (Basel) 2003; 112:15–21.

Schellekens H. Bioequivalence and the immunogenicity of biopharmaceuticals. *Nat Rev Drug Discov* 2002; 1(6):457–462.

Schellekens H and Casadevall N. Immunogenicity of biopharmaceuticals. The European perspective. *Dev Biol* (Basel) 2003; 112:23–28.

Stickler MM, Estell DA, Harding FA. CD4+ T-cell epitope determination using unexposed human donor peripheral blood mononuclear cells. *J Immunother* 2000; 23(6):654–660.

Swanson SJ. New technologies for the detection of antibodies to therapeutic proteins. *Dev Biol* (Basel) 2003; 112:127–133.

Takacs MA, Jacobs SJ, Bordens RM, Swanson SJ. Detection and characterization of antibodies to PEG-IFN-alpha2b using surface plasmon resonance. *J Interferon Cytokine Res* 1999; 19(7):781–789.

Thorpe R and Wadhwa M. Unwanted immunogenicity of therapeutic biological products. Problems and their consequences. *BioProcess Int* 2003; 1(9):60–63.

Wierda D, Smith HW, Zwickl CM. Immunogenicity of biopharmaceuticals in laboratory animals. *Toxicology* 2001; 158(1–2):71–74.

PROTEIN STABILITY

Hejnaes KR et al. Protein stability in downstream processing. In: *Bioseparation and Bioprocessing*. Subramanian G, editor. Wiley-VCH, Weinheim, 1988: 31–65.
Whitaker JR and Feeney RE. Chemical and physical modifications of proteins by the hydroxyl ion. *CRC Crit Rev Food Sci Nutr* 1983; 19(3):173–212.

PROTEOLYSIS

Kasche V. Mechanism and yields in enzyme catalysed equilibrium and kinetically controlled synthesis of — lactam antibiotics, peptides and other condensation products. *Enzyme Microb Technol* 1986; 8(1):4–16.
North MJ. Prevention of unwanted proteolysis. In: *Proteolytical Enzymes*. Beynan RJ and Bond JS, editors. IRL Press, Oxford 1989: 105–124.

DEAMIDATION

Aswad DW (ed.). Deamidation and Isoaspartate Formation in Peptides and Proteins. CRC Press, London, 1994.
Brange J, Langkjaer L, Havelund S, Volund A. Chemical stability of insulin. 1. Hydrolytic degradation during storage of pharmaceutical preparations. *Pharm Res* 1992; 9(6):715–726.
Brennan TV and Clarke S. Deamidation and isoaspartate formation in model synthetic peptides: The effects of sequence and solution environment. In: *Deamidation and Isoaspartate Formation in Peptides and Proteins*. Aswad DW, editor. CRC Press, London, 1995: 65–90.
Capasso S. Deamidation via cyclic imide of asparaginyl peptides: Dependence on salts, buffers and organic solvents. *Peptide Res* 1991; 4(4):234–238.
Clarke S, Stephenson RC, Lowenson JD. Lability of asparagine and aspartic acid residues in proteins and peptides. Spontaneous deamidation and isomerization reactions. In: *Stability of Protein Pharmaceuticals*. Ahern TJ and Manning MC, editors. Plenum Press, New York, 1992: 1–29.
Flatmark T. On the heterogeneity of beef heart cytochrome c. 3. A kinetic study of the non-enzymic deamidation of the main subfractions (Cy I-Cy 3). *Acta Chem Scand* 1966; 20(6):1487–1496.
Geiger T and Clarke S. Deamidation, isomerization, and racemization at asparaginyl and aspartyl residues in peptides. Succinimide-linked reactions that contribute to protein degradation. *J Biol Chem* 1987; 262(2):785–794.
Johnson BA and Aswad DW. Deamidation and isoaspartate formation during *in vitro* aging of purified proteins. In: *Deamidation and Isoaspartate Formation in Peptides and Proteins*. Aswad DW, editor. CRC Press, London, 1995: 91–113.
Lewis UJ, Cheever EV, Hopkins WC. Kinetic study of the deamidation of growth hormone and prolactin. *Biochim Biophys Acta* 1970; 214(3):498–508.
Manning MC, Patel K, Borchardt RT. Stability of protein pharmaceuticals. *Pharm Res* 1989; 6(11):903–918.
Robinson AB and Rudd CJ. Deamidation of glutaminyl and asparaginyl residues in peptides and proteins. *Curr Top Cell Regul* 1974; 8:247–295.
Wright HT. Sequence and structure determinants of the nonenzymatic deamidation of asparagine and glutamine residues in proteins. *Protein Eng* 1991; 4(3):283–294.

OXIDATION

Cleland JL. Powell MF, Shire SJ. The development of stable protein formulations: A close look at protein aggregation, deamidation, and oxidation. *Crit Rev Ther Drug Carrier Sys* 1993; 10(4):307–377.
Dedman ML, Farmer TH, Morris CJOR. Studies on pituitary adrenocorticotrophin. 3. Identification of the oxidation-reduction centre. *Biochem* J 1961; **78**:348–352.

Harris CM and Hill RL. The carboxymethylation of human metmyoglobin. *J Biol Chem* 1969; 244(8):2195–2203.

Holeysovsky V and Lazdunski M. The structural properties of trypsinogen and trypsin. Alkylation and oxidation of methionines. *Biochim Biophys Acta* 1968; 154(3):457–467.

Morley JS, Tracy HJ, Gregory RA. Structure-function relationships in the active C-terminal tetrapeptide sequence of gastrin. *Nature* 1965; 207(4):1356–1359.

Tashjian AH, Ontjes DA, Munson PL. Alkylation and oxidation of methionine in bovine parathyroid hormone: effects on hormonal activity and antigenicity. *Biochemistry* 1964; 8:1175–1182.

CARBMYLATION

Dirnhuber P and Schütz F. The isomeric transformation of urea into ammonium cyanate in aqueous solutions. *Biochem J* 1948; 42(2):628–632.

Kilmartin JV and Rossi-Bernardi L. Inhibition of CO_2 combination and reduction of the Bohr effect in haemoglobin chemically modified at its alpha-amino groups. *Nature* 1969; 222(200):1243–1246.

Marier JR and Rose D. Determination of cyanate, a study of its accumulation in aqueous solutions of urea. *Anal Biochem* 1964; 7:304–314.

Mun KC and Golper TA. Impaired biological activity of erythropoietin by cyanate carbamylation. *Blood Purif* 2000; 18(1):13–17.

Nowicki C and Santome JA. Modification of lysine 69 reactivity in bovine growth hormone by carbamylation of its N-terminal group. *Int J Pept Protein Res* 1981; 18(1):52–60.

Oimomi M, Hatanaka H, Yoshimura Y, Yokono K, Baba S, Taketomi Y. Carbamylation of insulin and its biological activity. *Nephron* 1987; 46(1):63–66.

Rimon S and Perlmann GE. Carbamylation of pepsinogen and pepsin. *J Biol Chem* 1968; 243(13):3566–3572.

Salinas M, Fando JL, Grisolia S. A sensitive and specific method for quantitative estimation of carbamylation in proteins. *Anal Biochem* 1974; 62(1):166–172.

Shaw DC, Stein WH, Moore S. Inactivation of chymotrypsin by cyanate. *J Biol Chem* 1964; 239(1):PC671–PC673.

Sluyterman LA. Reversible inactivation of papain by cyanate. *Biochim Biophys Acta* 1967; 139(2):439–449.

Stark GR. Modification of proteins with cyanate. *Meth Enzymol* 1972; 25:579–584.

Stark GR. Reactions of cyanate with functional groups of proteins. 3. Reactions with amino and carboxyl groups. *Biochemistry* 1965; 4(6):1030–1036.

Stark GR. Reactions of cyanate with functional groups of proteins. IV. Inertness of aliphatic hydroxyl groups. Formation of carbamyl- and acylhydantoins. *Biochemistry* 1965; 4(11):2363–2367.

Stark GR, Stein WH, Moore S. Reactions of the cyanate present in aqueous urea with amino acids and proteins. *J Biol Chem* 1960; 235(4):3177–3181.

RACEMIZATION

Brennan TV and Clarke S. Deamidation and isoaspartate formation in model synthetic peptides: The effects of sequence and solution environment. In: *Deamidation and Isoaspartate Formation in Peptides and Proteins*. Aswad DW, editor. CRC Press, London, 1995: 65–90.

Hayashi R and Kameda I. Racemization of amino acid residues during alkali-treatment of protein and its adverse effect on pepsin digestibility. *Agric Biol Chem* 1980; 44(4):891–895.

Masters PM and Friedman M. Amino acid racemization in alkali-treated food proteins — chemistry, toxicology, and nutritional consequences. *ACS Symp Ser* 1980; 123(8):165–194.

CYSTEINYL RESIDUES

Benesch RE and Benesch R. The mechanism of disulfide interchange in acid solution; role of sulfenium ions. *J Am Chem Soc* 1958; 80(3):1666–1669.

Gilbert HF. Molecular and cellular aspects of thiol-disulfide exchange. *Adv Enzymol Relat Areas Mol Biol* 1990; 63:69–172.

Misra HP. Generation of superoxide free radical during the autoxidation of thiols. *J Biol Chem* 1974; 249(7):2151–2155.

Torchinsky YM. The role of S-S groups in proteins. In: *Sulfur in Proteins*. Metzler D, editor. Pergamon Press, New York, 1995: 199–217.

HYDROLYSIS

Brennan TV and Clarke S. Deamidation and isoaspartate formation in model synthetic peptides: The effects of sequence and solution environment. In: *Deamidation and Isoaspartate Formation in Peptides and Proteins*. Aswad DW, editor. CRC Press, London, 1995: 65–90.

Piszkiewicz D, Landon M, Smith EL. Anomalous cleavage of aspartyl-proline peptide bonds during amino acid sequence determinations. *Biochem Biophys Res Commun* 1970; 40(5):1173–1178.

Robinson AB and Rudd CJ. Deamidation of glutaminyl and asparaginyl residues in peptides and proteins. *Curr Top Cell Regul* 1974; 8:247–295.

Schultz J. Cleavage at aspartic acid. *Meth Enzymol* 1967; 11(28):255–263.

DENATURATION

Kauzmann W. Some factors in the interpretation of protein denaturation. *Adv Protein Chem* 1959; 14:1–63.

O'Fagain C, Sheehan H, O'Kennedy R, Kilty C. Maintenance of enzyme structure — possible methods for enhancing stability. *Process Biochem* 1988; (December):166–171.

Privalov PL. Stability of proteins: small globular proteins. *Adv Protein Chem* 1979; 33:167–241.

Scopes RK. Separation by precipitation. In: *Protein Purification. Principles and Practice*. Springer-Verlag, New York, 1987: 41–64.

Tanford C. Protein denaturation. Part B. The transition from native to denatured state. *Adv Protein Chem* 1968; 23:218–282.

AGGREGATION

Hartley DL and Kane JF. Properties of inclusion bodies from recombinant *Escherichia coli*. *Biochem Soc Trans* 1988; 16(2):101–102.

Jaenicke R. Folding and association of proteins. *Prog Biophys Molec Biol* 1987; 49:117–237.

Kiefhaber T, Rudolph R, Kohler HH, Buchner J. Protein aggregation *in vitro* and *in vivo*: a quantitative model of the kinetic competition between folding and aggregation. *Biotechnology* (NY) 1991; 9(9):825–829.

Moody AJ, Hejnaes KR, Marshall MO, Larsen FS, Boel E, Svendsen I, Mortensen E, Dyrberg T. Isolation by anion-exchange of immunologically and enzymatically active human islet glutamic acid decarboxylase 65 overexpressed in Sf9 insect cells. *Diabetologia* 1995; 38(1):14–23.

PRECIPITATION

Scopes RK. Separation by precipitation. In: *Protein Purification Principles and Practice*. Springer-Verlag, New York, 1987: 41–64.

CHAPTER 12: INTELLECTUAL PROPERTY ISSUES

American Inventor's Protection Act of 1999: http://www.uspto.gov/web/offices/dcom/olia/aipa/index. htm, USPTO, Washington, D.C.

Amgen Inc. v. Chugai Pharmaceutical Co., 927 F2d 1200 (Fed. Cir. 1991).

Amgen v. United States International Trade Commission 14 USPQ 2d 1016 (Fed. Cir. 1990).

Amgen, Inc. v. Chugai Pharmaceutical Co. Nos. 90-1273, 90-1275 United States Court of Appeals for the Federal Circuit 927 F. 2d 1200.

Aro Mfg. Co. v. Convertible Top Replacement Co. [Patent — Infringement — Replacement Parts]: http://supct.law.cornell.edu/supct/cases/382us252. htm. (377 U.S. 476, 1964).

Aro Mfg. Co. v. Convertible Top Replacement Co. [Patent — Infringement — Replacement Parts]: http://supct.law.cornell.edu/supct/cases/365us336. htm. (365 U.S. 336, 1961).

Aronson v. Quick Point Pencil Co. [Patent — Licensing]: http://supct.law.cornell.edu/supct/cases/440us257. htm. (115 S.Ct. 788, 130 L. Ed. 2d 682, 1995).

Asgrow Seed Co. v. Winterboer [Plant Variety Protection Act of 1970 — Infringement]: http://supct.law.cornell.edu/supct/cases/115s788. htm.

Beecham Group Ltd's Application [1980] RPC 261 (CA).

Bell, 26 USPQ2d 1529 (Fed. Cir. 1993).

Brenner v. Manson [Patent — Process — Utility of Invention]: http://supct.law.cornell.edu/supct/cases/383us519.htm. (383 U.S. 519, 1966).

Budapest Treaty on the International Recognition of the Deposit of Microorganisms for the Purposes of Patent Procedure: http://www.wipo.int/clea/docs/en/wo/wo002en.htm. WIPO, Geneva, Switzerland.

Certain Recombinant Erythropoietin, 10 USPQ2d 1906 (ITC 1989).

Compco Corp. v. Day-Brite Lighting, Inc. [Patent — Unfair Competition — Preemption]: http://supct.law.cornell.edu/supct/cases/376us234.htm. (376 U.S. 234, 1964).

Consolidated Patent Rules. Title 37: Code of Federal Regulations Patents, Trademarks and Copyrights: http://www.uspto.gov/web/offices/pac/mpep/consolidated_rules.pdf. U.S. Printing Office, Washington, DC.

Cornell University Law Library: http://www.law.cornell.edu/topics/patent.html.

Cuno Engineering v. Automatic Devices Corp., 314 United States 84 (1942).

Diamond v. Chakrabarty [Patent — Living Micro-Organism]: http://supct.law.cornell.edu/supct/cases/447us303.htm. (447 U.S. 303, 1980).

du Pont v. Akzo 1950 ICI.

Evans Medical's Patent [1997] SRIS C/100/97 (Pat. Ct.).

GATT Uruguay Round Patent Law Changes, U.S. Patent and Trademark Office: http://www.uspto.gov/web/offices/com/doc/uruguay/SUMMARY.html. USPTO, Washington, DC.

Genentech Inc. v. Wellcome Foundation Ltd., 31 USPQ2d 1161 (Fed. Cir. 1994).

GENENTECH Polypeptide expression.292/85 (OJ 1989, 275).

GENENTECH/Human t-PA (European Patent 93619). T 923/92 (OJ 1996, 564).

Generic Animal Drug and Patent Term Restoration Act of 1988: http://www.fda.gov/opacom/laws/88SUM. Html. FDA, Washington, DC.

Gottschalk v. Benson [Patent — Mathematical Formula]: http://supct.law.cornell.edu/supct/cases/409us63.htm. (409 U.S. 63, 1972).

Graham v. John Deere Co. [Patent — Nonobviousness of Invention]: http://supct.law.cornell.edu/supct/cases/383us1. htm. (447 U.S. 303, 1980).

Graver Tank and Mfg. Co. v. Linde Air Prods. Co. [Patent — Infringement — Equivalents]: http://supct.law.cornell.edu/supct/cases/339us605.htm. (339 U.S. 605, 1950).

Grubb PW. *Patents for Chemicals, Pharmaceuticals and Biotechnology*. Oxford University Press, Oxford, UK, 1999.

Hazeltine Research, Inc. v. Brenner [Patent — Prior Art — Pending Application]: http://supct.law.cornell.edu/supct/cases/382us252.htm. (382 U.S. 252, 1965).

Kohler G and Milstein C. Nature 1975; 256:495–497.

Madey v. Duke Univ., 307 F. 3d 1351 (Fed. Cir. 2002), cert. denied 156 L. Ed. 2d 656 (2003).

Manual of Patent Examining Procedures "Edition 8 (E8)," August 2001. Latest revision February 2003: http://www.uspto.gov/web/offices/pac/mpep/index.html. USPTO, Washington, DC.

Niazi SK. *Filing Patents OnLine: A Professional Guide*. CRC Press, Boca Raton, FL, 2002.

ORTHO/Monoclonal antibody. T 418/89 (OJ 1993, 20).

Parker v. Flook [Patent — Mathematical Formula]: http://supct.law.cornell.edu/supct/cases/437us584. htm: (437 U.S. 584, 1978).

PBG — Final Rule U.S. Patent and Trademark Office: http://www.uspto.gov/web/offices/dcom/olia/pbg/index.html. USPTO, Washington, DC.

S. Cohen et al., Proceedings of the National Academy of Science, 70, 3240 (1973).

Sears, Roebuck & Co. v. Stiffel Co. [Patent — Unfair Competition — Preemption]: http://supct.law.cornell.edu/supct/cases/376us225.htm. (376 U.S. 225, 1964).

TRIPS — Trade-Related Aspects of Intellectual Property Rights. U.S. Patent and Trademark Office: http://www.uspto.gov/web/offices/dcom/olia/globalip/trips.htm. USPTO, Washington, DC.

U.S. Patent and Trademark Office Attorney Database: http://www.uspto.gov/web/offices/dcom/olia/oed/roster/index.html#changing_contact_information. USPTO, Washington, DC.

U.S. Code Title 35: Patent Laws: http://www.uspto.gov/web/offices/pac/mpep/consolidated_laws. pdf. U.S.
    Government Printing Office, Washington, DC.
University of California v. Eli Lilly, 43 USPQ2d 1398 (Fed. Cir. 1997).
Wistar's Application [1983] RPC 255 (Pat. Ct.).

Index

Milton Keynes UK
Ingram Content Group UK Ltd.
UKHW052028071024
449327UK00027B/2468